RADIATION THERAPY PHYSICS

Third Edition

RADIATION THERAPY PHYSICS

Third Edition

William R. Hendee, Ph.D.

Department of Radiology
Medical College of Wisconsin
Milwaukee, Wisconsin

Geoffrey S. Ibbott, Ph.D.

Department of Radiation Physics
University of Texas, M.D. Anderson Cancer Center
Houston, Texas

Eric G. Hendee, M.S.

Department of Radiation Oncology
Waukesha Memorial Hospital
Waukesha, Wisconsin

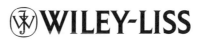

A JOHN WILEY & SONS, INC., PUBLICATION

On the Cover: Helical TomoTherapy research system at the University of Wisconsin, Madison.
Photo courtesy of TomoTherapy, Inc., Middleton Wisconsin

Published by John Wiley & Sons, Inc., Hoboken, New Jersey.
Published simultaneously in Canada.

For general information on our other products and services please contact our Customer Care
Department within the U.S. at 877-762-2974, outside the U.S. at 317-572-3993 or fax 317-572-4002.

Wiley also publishes its books in a variety of electronic formats. Some content that appears in print
however, may not be available in electronic format.

Library of Congress Cataloging-in-Publication Data:

Hendee, William R.
    Radiation therapy physics / William R. Hendee, Geoffrey S. Ibbott, Eric G. Hendee.—3rd ed.
        p.   ;   cm.
    Includes bibliographical references and index.
    ISBN 0-471-39493-9 (cloth : alk. paper)
    1. Radiotherapy.   2. Medical physics.
    [DNLM: 1. Physics.   2. Radiotherapy. WN 250 H495r 2005]   I. Ibbott, Geoffrey S.
II. Hendee, Eric G.   III. Title.
    RM849.H43 2005
    615.8′42—dc22
                                                             2004005205
Printed in the United States of America

10 9 8 7 6 5 4 3

The first and second editions of this text were dedicated to Jack Krohmer. This edition is dedicated to his memory, the many contributions he made to medical physics over a long and productive career, and the inspiration he provided to each of us during the early stages of our own careers.

CONTENTS IN BRIEF

PREFACE   xiii

PREFACE TO THE SECOND EDITION   xv

PREFACE TO THE FIRST EDITION   xvii

1   ATOMIC STRUCTURE AND RADIOACTIVE DECAY   1

2   PRODUCTION OF X RAYS   21

3   INTERACTIONS OF X RAYS AND GAMMA RAYS   35

4   RADIATION UNITS   51

5   MEASUREMENT OF IONIZING RADIATION   79

6   CALIBRATION OF MEGAVOLTAGE BEAMS OF X RAYS AND ELECTRONS   107

7   DOSIMETRY OF RADIATION FIELDS   129

8   TREATMENT PLANNING BY MANUAL METHODS   157

9   DIAGNOSTIC IMAGING AND APPLICATIONS TO RADIATION THERAPY   187

10   COMPUTER SYSTEMS   219

11   COMPUTER-BASED TREATMENT PLANNING   245

12   SOURCES FOR IMPLANT THERAPY   285

13   BRACHYTHERAPY TREATMENT PLANNING   295

14   RADIATION PROTECTION   333

15   QUALITY ASSURANCE   357

16   ADVANCES IN RADIATION THERAPY   413

ANSWERS TO SELECTED PROBLEMS   435

INDEX   439

CONTENTS

PREFACE   xiii

PREFACE TO THE SECOND EDITION   xv

PREFACE TO THE FIRST EDITION   xvii

1 ■ ATOMIC STRUCTURE AND RADIOACTIVE DECAY   1

OBJECTIVES   2

COMPOSITION OF MATTER   2

RADIOACTIVE DECAY   8

TYPES OF RADIOACTIVE DECAY   11

RADIOACTIVE EQUILIBRIUM   15

NATURAL RADIOACTIVITY AND DECAY SERIES   17

ARTIFICIAL PRODUCTION OF RADIONUCLIDES   17

SUMMARY   18

PROBLEMS   19

REFERENCES   20

2 ■ PRODUCTION OF X RAYS   21

OBJECTIVES   22

INTRODUCTION   22

SCATTERING OF ELECTRONS BY ELECTRONS   22

SCATTERING OF ELECTRONS BY NUCLEI   23

HISTORY OF X RAYS   25

CONVENTIONAL X-RAY TUBES   26

X-RAY SPECTRA   30

SUMMARY   34

PROBLEMS   34

REFERENCES   34

3 ■ INTERACTIONS OF X RAYS AND GAMMA RAYS   35

OBJECTIVES   36

INTRODUCTION   36

ATTENUATION OF X RAYS AND GAMMA RAYS   36

X-RAY AND GAMMA-RAY INTERACTIONS   40

SUMMARY   49

PROBLEMS   49

REFERENCES   50

4 ■ RADIATION UNITS   51

OBJECTIVES   52

LOW-ENERGY X-RAY UNITS   52

ISOTOPE TELETHERAPY UNITS   54

LINEAR ACCELERATORS   57

OTHER MEDICAL ACCELERATORS   69

SIMULATORS   73

SUMMARY   76

PROBLEMS   76

REFERENCES   76

5 ■ MEASUREMENT OF IONIZING RADIATION   79

OBJECTIVES   80

INTRODUCTION   80

RADIATION INTENSITY   80

RADIATION EXPOSURE   82

MEASUREMENT OF RADIATION EXPOSURE   84

RADIATION DOSE   92

MEASUREMENT OF RADIATION DOSE   94

ABSORBED DOSE MEASUREMENTS WITH AN IONIZATION CHAMBER   99

DOSE EQUIVALENT   100

RADIATION QUALITY   102

SUMMARY   105

PROBLEMS   105

REFERENCES   106

6 ■ CALIBRATION OF MEGAVOLTAGE BEAMS OF X RAYS AND ELECTRONS 107

OBJECTIVES 108

CALIBRATION STANDARDS AND LABORATORIES 108

CALIBRATION OF LOW-ENERGY X-RAY BEAMS 114

CALIBRATION OF MEGAVOLTAGE BEAMS—THE AAPM PROTOCOL 117

THE IAEA CALIBRATION PROTOCOL 126

SUMMARY 127

PROBLEMS 127

REFERENCES 127

7 ■ DOSIMETRY OF RADIATION FIELDS 129

OBJECTIVES 130

PERCENT DEPTH DOSE 130

TABLES OF PERCENT DEPTH DOSE 135

TISSUE/AIR RATIO 139

DOSE COMPUTATIONS FOR ROTATIONAL THERAPY 142

BACKSCATTER 143

SCATTER/AIR RATIO 144

TISSUE/PHANTOM RATIO 144

ISODOSE CURVES 145

SUMMARY 154

PROBLEMS 154

REFERENCES 155

8 ■ TREATMENT PLANNING BY MANUAL METHODS 157

OBJECTIVES 158

POINT DOSE CALCULATIONS 158

TREATMENT AT STANDARD SSD 160

TREATMENT UNDER ISOCENTRIC CONDITIONS 161

ISODOSE DISTRIBUTIONS FOR MULTIPLE FIELDS 162

DOSE CALCULATIONS FOR IRREGULAR FIELDS 166

OBLIQUE INCIDENCE AND IRREGULAR BEAM SURFACE 168

CORRECTIONS FOR OBLIQUE INCIDENCE AND SURFACE IRREGULARITY 170

EFFECTS OF TISSUE INHOMOGENEITIES 172

CORRECTION FOR THE PRESENCE OF INHOMOGENEITIES 173

SEPARATION OF ADJACENT FIELDS 179

INTEGRAL DOSE 180

DOSE SPECIFICATION FOR EXTERNAL BEAM THERAPY 181

SUMMARY 184

PROBLEMS 185

REFERENCES 185

9 ■ DIAGNOSTIC IMAGING AND APPLICATIONS TO RADIATION THERAPY 187

OBJECTIVES 188

INTRODUCTION 188

RADIOGRAPHY 189

FLUOROSCOPY 196

TREATMENT SIMULATORS 199

COMPUTED TOMOGRAPHY 200

ULTRASONOGRAPHY 203

NUCLEAR MEDICINE 206

EMISSION COMPUTED TOMOGRAPHY 209

MAGNETIC RESONANCE IMAGING 211

FUNCTIONAL MAGNETIC RESONANCE IMAGING 213

SUMMARY 214

PROBLEMS 216

REFERENCES 216

10 ■ COMPUTER SYSTEMS 219

OBJECTIVES 220

HISTORY OF COMPUTERS 220

TERMINOLOGY AND DATA REPRESENTATION 221

CONVERSION FROM ONE SYSTEM TO ANOTHER 223

BITS, BYTES, AND WORDS 223

REPRESENTATION OF DATA 224

COMPUTER ARCHITECTURE 230

COMPUTER SOFTWARE 234

PROGRAMMING LANGUAGES 234

NETWORKING 237

COMPUTER REQUIREMENTS FOR TREATMENT PLANNING 241

SUMMARY 241

PROBLEMS 242

REFERENCES 242

11 ■ COMPUTER-BASED TREATMENT PLANNING   245

OBJECTIVES   246

INTRODUCTION   246

BEAM DATA ENTRY   247

PATIENT DATA ENTRY   248

VIRTUAL SIMULATION TECHNIQUES   252

IMMOBILIZATION AND LOCALIZATION   253

PHOTON BEAM COMPUTATIONAL ALGORITHMS   258

THE ANALYTICAL METHOD   258

MATRIX TECHNIQUES   258

SEMIEMPIRICAL METHODS   259

ELECTRON BEAM COMPUTATIONAL ALGORITHMS   265

SELECTION OF IDEAL TREATMENT PLAN   265

BIOLOGICAL MODELING   267

FORWARD PLANNING   267

INVERSE PLANNING   270

INTENSITY-MODULATED RADIATION THERAPY   270

DYNAMIC DELIVERY TECHNIQUES   277

TOMOTHERAPY   278

TREATMENT PLANNING CHALLENGES   280

SUMMARY   280

PROBLEMS   281

REFERENCES   282

12 ■ SOURCES FOR IMPLANT THERAPY   285

OBJECTIVES   286

RADIUM SOURCES   286

SPECIFICATION OF BRACHYTHERAPY SOURCES   289

RADIUM SUBSTITUTES   290

OPHTHALMIC IRRADIATORS   292

IMPLANTABLE NEUTRON SOURCES   292

RADIATION SAFETY OF BRACHYTHERAPY SOURCES   292

SUMMARY   293

PROBLEMS   293

REFERENCES   294

13 ■ BRACHYTHERAPY TREATMENT PLANNING   295

OBJECTIVES   296

RADIATION DOSE FROM BRACHYTHERAPY SOURCES   296

SIEVERT INTEGRAL   297

ISODOSE DISTRIBUTIONS FROM INDIVIDUAL SEALED SOURCES   300

DESIGN OF IMPLANTS   300

DISTRIBUTION RULES FOR INTERSTITIAL IMPLANTS   302

AIR-KERMA STRENGTH CALCULATION   313

DOSE OVER TREATMENT DURATION   316

PLAQUES   316

REMOTE AFTERLOADING   317

RADIOGRAPHIC LOCALIZATION OF IMPLANTS   318

THREE-DIMENSIONAL IMAGE-BASED IMPLANTS   322

THERAPY WITH RADIOPHARMACEUTICALS   327

INTRAVASCULAR BRACHYTHERAPY   328

SUMMARY   329

PROBLEMS   329

REFERENCES   330

14 ■ RADIATION PROTECTION   333

OBJECTIVES   334

INTRODUCTION   334

EFFECTS OF RADIATION EXPOSURE   336

HISTORY OF RADIATION PROTECTION STANDARDS   337

CURRENT LIMITS ON RADIATION EXPOSURE   338

PROTECTIVE BARRIERS FOR RADIATION SOURCES   341

PROTECTION FOR SEALED RADIOACTIVE SOURCES   352

RADIATION SURVEYS   352

PERSONNEL MONITORING   353

SUMMARY   354

PROBLEMS   354

REFERENCES   355

15 ■ QUALITY ASSURANCE   357

OBJECTIVES   358

INTRODUCTION   358

COMPONENTS OF A QUALITY ASSURANCE PROGRAM   359

PERSONNEL   360

RECOMMENDED QUALITY ASSURANCE PROCEDURES   360

PHYSICS INSTRUMENTATION   361

MEGAVOLTAGE TREATMENT EQUIPMENT   364

QUALITY ASSURANCE PROCEDURES FOR RADIATION THERAPY SIMULATORS 380

CT SIMULATOR QUALITY ASSURANCE 385

IMAGE QUALITY ASSURANCE 387

TREATMENT PLANNING COMPUTER 389

QUALITY ASSURANCE FOR INTENSITY-MODULATED RADIATION THERAPY (IMRT) 394

STEREOTACTIC RADIOSURGERY AND RADIOTHERAPY 397

BRACHYTHERAPY QUALITY ASSURANCE PROCEDURES 399

SUMMARY 409

PROBLEMS 409

REFERENCES 410

16 ■ ADVANCES IN RADIATION THERAPY 413

OBJECTIVES 414

INTRODUCTION 414

HISTORY 414

ALTERED FRACTIONATION 416

BIOLOGICAL MODELING AND PLAN EVALUATION 417

MOLECULAR IMAGING 418

PROTON THERAPY 420

NEUTRON BRACHYTHERAPY 426

NEUTRON CAPTURE THERAPY 427

NEUTRON BEAM THERAPY 428

HEAVY ION AND PION THERAPY 430

CONCLUSIONS 432

REFERENCES 432

ANSWERS TO SELECTED PROBLEMS 435

INDEX 439

PREFACE

When Geoff Ibbott and I published the second edition of *Radiation Therapy Physics* in 1996, we anticipated that the book would be well received. However, the degree of enthusiasm over the book, although rewarding to us, caught our former publisher by surprise. The print run for the book was quickly depleted, and could not be replenished because of a merger under negotiation with a larger publishing house. Consequently, the second edition has been out of print for the past 6 years, and we have been giving permission to teachers and students to photocopy the text for their personal use.

Soon after release of the second edition, Geoff and I realized that a new edition would quickly become necessary, because the techniques of radiation therapy were evolving rapidly and dramatically. Over the past five years, treatment procedures such as conformal and intensity-modulated radiation therapy, high dose-rate and vascular brachytherapy, and image-guided and intraoperative radiation therapy have become standard operating procedures in radiation therapy clinics around the world. In addition, x-ray beams from linear accelerators have replaced ^{60}Co γ rays as the standard teaching model for the parameters of external beam radiation therapy, and several new protocols have been developed for calibrating and applying radiation beams and sources for cancer treatment. These procedures, and others that represent state-of-the-art radiation therapy, are discussed at length in this new edition.

In designing the third edition, Geoff and I had an opportunity to add Eric Hendee as a third member of the writing team. Eric's broad experience in radiation therapy physics, and his ability as a clear writer, make him an excellent member of the team.

In this new edition, we are presenting information in a format that reflects our understanding of the way people learn in today's culture. Throughout the book we make extensive use of self-contained segments, illustrations, highlights, sidebars, examples and problems. We hope that this approach will help students use the book as a primary source of information, rather than simply as a supplement to the classroom. We feel this approach is important because classroom time for learning is becoming a casualty of the increasing emphasis on productivity and accountability in healthcare. It is also important because increasingly each of us is forced to assimilate information in fragments rather than as a continuous process, principally as a product of the Information Age in which we live. Without judging the ultimate societal consequences of this assimilation process, we acknowledge its pervasiveness and have attempted in this text to accommodate it.

The treatment of patients with ionizing radiation is a complex undertaking that requires close collaboration among physicians, physicists, engineers, radiation therapists, dosimetrists and nurses. Together they provide a level of patient care that would be unachievable by any single group working alone. But to achieve maximum success, each member of the team must have a solid foundation in the physics of radiation therapy. It is the intent of this text to provide this foundation. We hope we have done so in a manner that makes learning enriching and enjoyable.

Many people have supported this third edition, including several investigators who have contributed data and illustrations to the text. We are grateful for their help. Luna Han, the book's editor at our new publisher, John Wiley & Sons, Inc., has encouraged and helped us to meet our deadlines without being overbearing. Our editorial assistants, Mary Beth Drapp in Milwaukee and Elizabeth Siller in Houston, have managed to keep the text and the authors organized and focused. We acknowledge that the authors were more of a challenge than the chapters. And, last but certainly not least, Geoff thanks Diane, Eric thanks Lynne, and I thank Jeannie for their forbearance during production of another edition of yet another book.

WILLIAM R. HENDEE

PREFACE TO THE SECOND EDITION

In 1981 the first edition of *Radiation Therapy Physics* was published as a paperback supplement to the second edition of my text *Medical Radiation Physics*. This book addressed the evolving new era of radiation therapy and covered topics such as high-energy x-rays, electron beams, consensus calibration protocols, computerized treatment planning, and the reemergence of sealed-source brachytherapy. It was received by an especially receptive audience, and the publisher's stock of books was soon depleted. The book has been out-of-print for several years, and several physics instructors have told me they have been using photocopies for their classes.

The response to the first edition has been gratifying. However, there was one recurring concern about it. Many readers complained that the book did not cover the fundamentals of radiation physics. They did not like having to buy a text on diagnostic radiologic physics to learn these principles. More recently, several teachers have called to suggest that a new edition be prepared and that it should cover fundamental physics principles as well as their applications to radiation therapy. The publisher, Mosby–Year Book, Inc. also encouraged the preparation of a new edition. This book is my response to this encouragement.

Radiation therapy has changed in many ways since the first edition was released. High-energy x-ray and electron beams have become the preferred approach to the radiation treatment of many cancers, and sealed-source implants have become more common and more complex. Imaging techniques and computers are now used routinely in treatment planning, and sophisticated methods are available for overlaying anatomical images with computer-generated multidimensional treatment plans. Calibration protocols have been extensively revised, and quality assurance in radiation therapy has become almost a subject in itself. A new edition of *Radiation Therapy Physics* is certainly overdue. This second edition is presented in the hope that it will satisfy the needs of radiation physicists, oncologists, and therapists for a text that explains the fundamentals of radiation physics and their applications to the radiation treatment of cancer patients.

In planning the second edition, I had to confront a dilemma. My work schedule simply did not offer enough flexibility to accommodate the efforts that would be required. I needed a co-author. This individual had to be someone who is exceedingly knowledgeable about the physics of radiation therapy. He or she had to be a good writer. Finally, the co-author had to be a person with whom I knew I could work comfortably over the course of a couple of years. One special person came to mind, and I am pleased that Geoff Ibbott agreed to co-write the book with me. Geoff and I have worked as a team on many projects since the late 1960s, including 18 years together at the University of Colorado. If the reader learns half as much from this book as I have learned from Geoff in putting the book together, I will consider the text a success.

Many people have been supportive in the preparation of the second edition. Several investigators have contributed illustrations and data, and I am grateful for their help. Our editor at Mosby, Elizabeth Corra, has been terrific in her persistence and patience. Two individuals, Terri Komar and Claudia Johnson in our respective offices, have been invaluable in their organizational and editorial skills. Finally, Geoff thanks Diane while I remain indebted to Jeannie for their tolerance over the many nights and weekends we have spent in front of the computer. We are not quite sure why they put up with this intrusion into our respective relationships, but we know better than to question it.

WILLIAM R. HENDEE

PREFACE TO THE FIRST EDITION

WHEN THE FIRST edition of *Medical Radiation Physics* was published in 1970, the study of radiology encompassed both diagnostic and therapeutic applications of radiation, and physicians and graduate student trainees in the field were required to understand both applications. Since that time, the field of radiology has bifurcated into two specialties, diagnostic imaging and radiation oncology, and the knowledge required of trainees in either field has expanded greatly. In preparing the second edition of *Medical Radiation Physics*, I confined my text to diagnostic imaging procedures. The present text constitutes a supplement to the second edition of *Medical Radiation Physics* devoted to the physics of radiation therapy. Because it is a supplement, information presented in the second edition on the basic principles of radiologic physics is not duplicated herein. For information on topics such as atomic and nuclear structure, production and interactions of radiation, x-ray generator and tube design, and units and measurement of radiation, the reader is referred to the second edition of *Medical Radiation Physics*. Material in this text is presented with the assumption that the principles of radiologic physics are understood by the reader.

Since publication of the first edition, radiation oncology has progressed from the era of ^{60}Co therapy to a complex clinical specialty employing megavoltage x-ray and electron beams and minicomputers dedicated to the acquisition of dosimetric data and the design of complex treatment plans for radiation therapy patients. This progression is reflected in significant expansion of many sections of the text and the addition of a number of sections related to the current practice of radiation oncology. For example, the chapter on radiation therapy units now includes a lengthy section on linear accelerators, and the chapter on absorbed dose measurements has been expanded to consider problems associated with dose measurements in high-energy x-ray beams. An entire chapter has been added on measurements associated with electron beams, and the chapter on dosimetry of radiation fields now includes sections on tissue-phantom and tissue-maximum ratios, scatter-air ratios, and computational techniques for dose estimates for mantle fields and other fields of irregular shape. Isodose distributions are discussed in part from the perspective of decrement lines, dose gradients, polar coordinates and other methods useful for computer simulation of composite dose distributions. The use of sealed sources such as ^{192}Ir, ^{125}I, and ^{137}Cs is discussed in the chapter on implant therapy, and the chapter on radiation protection has been completely rewritten for greater comprehensibility and relevance to radiation oncology.

In developing this text, I have been greatly helped by Ms. Josephine Ibbott, who prepared new drawings for each chapter, and by Ms. Sarah Bemis, who typed the manuscript and kept the entire project organized. I also wish to thank Geoffrey S. Ibbott, M.S., for his helpful criticism of the entire manuscript and Russell Ritenour, Ph.D., for his assistance in verifying the solutions to problems.

WILLIAM R. HENDEE

CHAPTER

1

ATOMIC STRUCTURE AND RADIOACTIVE DECAY

OBJECTIVES   2

COMPOSITION OF MATTER   2

The Atom   2
Atomic Units   3
Mass Defect and Binding Energy   3
Electron Energy Levels   4
Nuclear Stability   7

RADIOACTIVE DECAY   8

TYPES OF RADIOACTIVE DECAY   11

Alpha Decay   11

Beta Decay   12
Gamma Emission and Internal Conversion   14

RADIOACTIVE EQUILIBRIUM   15

NATURAL RADIOACTIVITY AND DECAY SERIES   17

ARTIFICIAL PRODUCTION OF RADIONUCLIDES   17

SUMMARY   18

PROBLEMS   19

REFERENCES   20

Radiation Therapy Physics, Third Edition, by William R. Hendee, Geoffrey S. Ibbott, and Eric G. Hendee
ISBN 0-471-39493-9 Copyright © 2005 John Wiley & Sons, Inc.

■ OBJECTIVES

By studying this chapter, the reader should be able to:

- Understand the relationship between nuclear instability and radioactive decay.
- Describe the different modes of radioactive decay and the conditions in which they occur.
- Draw and interpret decay schemes.
- Write balanced reactions for radioactive decay.
- State and use the fundamental equations of radioactive decay.
- Perform elementary computations for sample activities.
- Comprehend the principles of transient and secular equilibrium.
- Discuss the principles of the artificial production of radionuclides.

■ COMPOSITION OF MATTER

The composition of matter has puzzled philosophers for centuries and scientists for decades. Even today the mystery continues, as strange new particles are detected in high-energy accelerators used to probe the structure of matter. Various models proposed to explain the composition and mechanics of matter are useful in certain applications but invariably fall short in others. One of the oldest models, the atomic theory of matter devised by early Greek philosophers,[1] remains today as a useful approach to understanding many physical processes, including those important to the study of the physics of radiation therapy. The atomic model is used in this text, but it is important to remember that it is only a model and that the true composition of matter remains an enigma.

The Atom

The atom is the smallest unit of matter that possesses the physical and chemical properties characteristic of one of the 106 elements, of which 92 occur in nature and the others are produced artificially. The atom consists of a central positive core, termed the *nucleus*, surrounded by a cloud of electrons moving in orbits around the nucleus. The nucleus contains most of the mass of the atom and has a diameter of about 10^{-14} m, whereas the electron cloud, and therefore the atom, has a diameter of about 10^{-10} m. The nucleus contains protons and neutrons. In the neutral atom, the number of protons in the nucleus is balanced by an equal number of electrons in the surrounding orbits. An atom with a greater or lesser number of electrons than the number of protons is termed a *negative* or *positive ion*.

An atom can be characterized by the symbolism $_Z^A X$, where A is the number of nucleons (i.e., the number of protons plus the number of neutrons) in the nucleus, Z is the number of protons in the nucleus (or the number of electrons in the neutral atom), and X represents the chemical symbol for the particular element to which the atom belongs. The number of nucleons A is termed the *mass number* of the atom, and Z is called the *atomic number* of the atom. The difference $A - Z$ is the number of neutrons in the nucleus, termed the *neutron number N*. Each element has a characteristic atomic number but can have several mass numbers depending on the number of neutrons N in the nucleus. For example, the element hydrogen has the unique atomic number of 1, signifying the solitary proton that constitutes the hydrogen nucleus, but can have none $\left(_1^1 H\right)$, one $\left(_1^2 H\right)$, or two $\left(_1^3 H\right)$ neutrons. The atomic forms ^{1}H, ^{2}H, and ^{3}H (the subscript 1 can be omitted because it is redundant with the chemical symbol) are said to be isotopes of hydrogen because they contain different numbers of neutrons combined with the single proton characteristic of hydrogen. Isotopes of an element have the same Z but different values of A, reflecting a different neutron number N. Isotones have the same N but different values of Z and A. ^{3}H, ^{4}He, and ^{5}Li are isotones because each nucleus contains two neutrons ($N = 2$). Isobars have the same A but

One philosopher, the Reverend George Berkeley (1685–1753), even suggested that matter cannot be proven to exist.

The atomic theory of matter was supplanted over several centuries by the continuum of matter philosophy of Aristotle and the Stoic philosophers. The atomic theory was revived in 1802 when Dalton developed the Principle of Multiple Proportions.

Protons are particles with a mass of 1.6734×10^{-27} kg and a positive charge of $+1.6 \times 10^{-19}$ coulomb.

Neutrons are particles with a mass of 1.6747×10^{-27} kg and no electrical charge.

Electrons have a mass of 9.108×10^{-31} kg and a negative charge of -1.6×10^{-19} coulomb.

In 1999, physicists at the Lawrence Berkeley Laboratory announced the creation of a new element with 118 protons ($Z = 118$), which then decayed to other new elements ($Z = 116$, $Z = 114$, $Z = 112$, etc.) down to the element with 106 protons ($Z = 106$). In 2001, this announcement was retracted.

different values of Z and N. ^{3}H and ^{3}He are isobars ($A = 3$). Isomers are different energy states of the same atom and therefore have identical values of Z, N, and A. For example ^{99m}Tc and ^{99}Tc are isomers because they are two distinct energy states of the same atom. The m in ^{99m}Tc signifies a metastable energy state that exists for a finite time (6 hours half-life) before changing to ^{99}Tc. The term *nuclide* refers to an atom in any form.

ISOTOPES have the same number of PROTONS.
ISOTONES have the same number of NEUTRONS.
ISOBARS have the same mass number A.
ISOMERS are different ENERGY states of the same atom.

Atomic Units

Units employed to describe dimensions in the macroscopic world are too large to use at the atomic level. Units more appropriate for atomic processes include the atomic mass unit (amu) for mass, electron volt (eV) for energy, nanometer (nm) for distance, and electron charge (e) for electrical charge.

The *amu* is defined as $^1/_{12}$ of the mass of an atom of the most common form of carbon, ^{12}C, which has 6 protons, 6 neutrons, and 6 electrons. By definition, the atomic mass of an atom of ^{12}C is 12.00000 amu. In units of amu, the masses of atomic particles are:

electron = 0.00055 amu
proton = 1.00727 amu
neutron = 1.00866 amu

One amu = 1.66×10^{-27} kg.

Every atom has a characteristic atomic mass A_m. The gram-atomic mass of an isotope is an amount of the isotope in grams that is numerically equivalent to the isotope's atomic mass. For example, one gram-atomic mass of ^{12}C is exactly 12 grams. One gram-atomic mass contains 6.0228×10^{23} atoms, a constant value that is known as Avogadro's number N_A. With these expressions, the following variables can be computed:

Number atoms/g = N_A/A_m
Number electrons/g = $(N_A Z)/A_m$
Number g/atom = A_m/N_A

The electron volt (eV) is a unit of energy equal to the kinetic energy of a single electron accelerated through a potential difference (voltage) of 1 volt. One keV = 10^3 eV, and 1 MeV = 10^6 eV. One nanometer (nm) is 10^{-9} meters. The electron unit of electrical charge = 1.6×10^{-19} coulombs.

Count Amadeo Avogadro (1776–1856) was an Italian physicist and chemist.

Example 1-1

One eV is equal to 1.6×10^{-19} joule of energy.

What is the kinetic energy (E_k) of an electron accelerated through a potential difference of 400,000 volts (400 kilovolts [kV])?

$$E_k = (1 \text{ electron})(400{,}000 \text{ volts})$$

$$= 400{,}000 \text{ eV} = 400 \text{ keV}$$

The angstrom (Å) unit of atomic distance, equal to 10^{-10} m and widely employed in the past, is seldom used today.

Mass Defect and Binding Energy

The neutral ^{12}C atom contains 6 protons, 6 neutrons, and 6 electrons. The mass of the components of this atom can be computed as:

Mass of 6 protons = 6(1.00727 amu) = 6.04362 amu
Mass of 6 neutrons = 6(1.00866 amu) = 6.05196 amu
Mass of 6 electrons = 6(0.00055 amu) = 0.00330 amu
_____
Mass of components of ^{12}C = 12.09888 amu

The equivalence of mass and energy $[E = mc^2]$ is arguably the most notable of Einstein's many contributions to science.

Four forces are thought to exist in nature. In order of increasing strength, they are the (1) gravitational force, (2) electrostatic force, (3) weak force, and (4) nuclear force. An explanation of the common origin of these forces is the objective of the Grand Unified Theory of theoretical physics.

In computing the average binding energy per nucleon as the quotient of the binding energy of the atom divided by the number of nucleons, the small contribution of electrons to the binding energy of the atom is ignored.

The mass of an atom of ^{12}C, however, is 12.00000 amu by definition. That is, the sum of the masses of the components of the ^{12}C atom exceeds the actual mass of the atom, and there is a *mass defect* of 0.09888 amu in the ^{12}C atom. This mass must be supplied to separate the ^{12}C atom into its constituents. The mass defect can be satisfied by supplying energy to the atom according to Einstein's expression $E = mc^2$ for the equivalence of mass and energy. In this expression, E is energy, m is mass, and c is the constant speed of light in a vacuum (3×10^8 m/sec). From the formula for mass-energy equivalence, 1 amu of mass is equivalent to 931 MeV of energy. For example, the energy equivalent to the mass of the electron is (0.00055 amu) (931 MeV/amu) = 0.51 MeV.

The energy associated with the mass defect of ^{12}C is (0.09888 amu)(931 MeV/amu) = 92.0 MeV. The energy equivalent to the mass defect of an atom is known as *the binding energy of the atom* and is the energy required to separate the atom into its constituent parts. Almost all of the binding energy of an atom is associated with the nucleus and reflects the influence of the strong nuclear force that binds particles together in the nucleus. For ^{12}C, the average binding energy per nucleon is 92.0 MeV/12 = 7.67 MeV/nucleon.

Example 1-2

What is the average binding energy per nucleon of ^{16}O with an atomic mass of 15.99492 amu?

$$\text{Mass of 8 protons} = 8(1.00727 \text{ amu}) = 8.05816 \text{ amu}$$
$$\text{Mass of 8 neutrons} = 8(1.00866 \text{ amu}) = 8.06928 \text{ amu}$$
$$\text{Mass of 8 electrons} = 8(0.00055 \text{ amu}) = 0.00440 \text{ amu}$$

$$\text{Mass of components of } ^{16}\text{O} = 16.13184 \text{ amu}$$
$$\text{Mass of } ^{16}\text{O atom} = 15.99492 \text{ amu}$$
$$\text{Mass defect} = 16.13184 \text{ amu} - 15.99492 \text{ amu}$$
$$= 0.13692 \text{ amu}$$
$$\text{Binding energy of } ^{16}\text{O} = (0.13692 \text{ amu})(931 \text{ MeV/amu})$$
$$= 127.5 \text{ MeV}$$
$$\text{Average binding energy per nucleon} = (127.5 \text{ MeV})/16$$
$$= 7.97 \text{ MeV/nucleon}$$

The average binding energy per nucleon is plotted in Figure 1-1 as a function of the mass number of different isotopes. The greatest average binding energies per nucleon occur for isotopes with mass number in the range of 50 to 100. Heavier isotopes gain binding energy by splitting into lighter isotopes. This is equivalent to saying that heavier isotopes release energy when they split into lighter isotopes, a process known as *nuclear fission*. The isotopes ^{233}U, ^{235}U, and ^{239}Pu fission spontaneously when a neutron is added to the nucleus. This process is the origin of the energy released during fission in nuclear reactors and fission weapons. Similarly, energy is released when light isotopes combine to form products with higher average binding energies per nucleon. This latter process is termed *nuclear fusion* and is the source of energy released during a fusion reaction such as that in a "hydrogen" bomb. Controlled nuclear fusion that permits its use for constructive purposes has so far eluded research efforts.

Uncontrolled nuclear fission is the process employed in a uranium or plutonium atomic ("A") bomb. Controlled nuclear fission is the process employed in a nuclear reactor. Uncontrolled nuclear fusion is the process employed in a fusion ("hydrogen") bomb. Efforts to develop controlled fusion have not succeeded so far.

Electron Energy Levels

The model of the atom in which electrons revolve in orbits around the nucleus was developed by Niels Bohr in 1913.[2] This model represented a departure from explanations of the atom that relied on classical physics. In the Bohr model, each orbit or "shell" can hold a maximum number of electrons defined as $2n^2$, where n is the number of the electron shell. The first ($n = 1$ or K) shell can hold up to 2

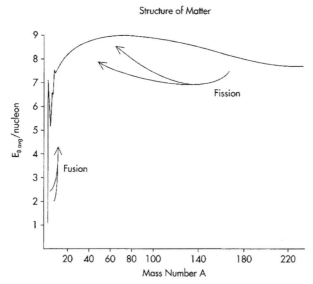

FIGURE 1-1
Average binding energy per nucleon versus mass number.

electrons, the second ($n = 2$ or L) shell can contain up to 8 electrons, the third ($n = 3$ or M) shell can hold up to 18 electrons, and so on. The outermost occupied M, N, or O electron shell, however, can hold no more than 8 electrons, and additional electrons begin to fill the next level to create a new outermost shell before more than 8 electrons are added to an M or higher shell. The number of valence electrons in the outermost shell determines the chemical properties of the atom and the elemental species to which it belongs. Examples of electron orbits in representative atoms are shown in Figure 1-2.

An electron neither gains nor loses energy so long as it remains in a specific electron orbit. Energy is needed, however, to move an electron from one orbit to another farther from the nucleus because work must be done against the attractive electrostatic force of the positive nucleus for the negative electron. Similarly, energy is released when an electron moves from one orbit to another nearer the nucleus. This transition can occur only if a vacancy exists in the nearer orbit, perhaps because an electron has been ejected from that orbit by some physical process. The energy required to remove an electron completely from an atom is defined as the *binding energy of the electron*. The positive charge of the nucleus (i.e., the Z of the atom) and the particular shell from which the electron is removed are the principal influences on the electron's binding energy. Minor influences are the particular energy subshell of the electron within the orbit and the direction of rotation as the electron spins on

"Bohr's work on the atom was the highest form of musicality in the sphere of thought."

A. Einstein as quoted in R. Moore: *Niels Bohr. The Man, His Science and the World They Changed.* Alfred Knopf, New York, 1966.

The maximum number of electrons in a particular electron orbit is defined by the Pauli Exclusion Principle, which states that in any atom (or atomic system), no two electrons can have the same four quantum numbers. The four quantum numbers of an electron are the *principal, azimuthal, magnetic*, and *spin* quantum numbers.

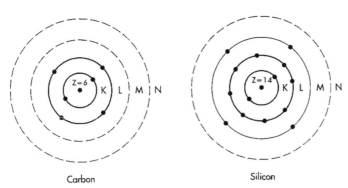

Carbon   Silicon

FIGURE 1-2
Electron "orbits" in the Bohr model of the atom for carbon ($Z = 6$) and silicon ($Z = 14$).

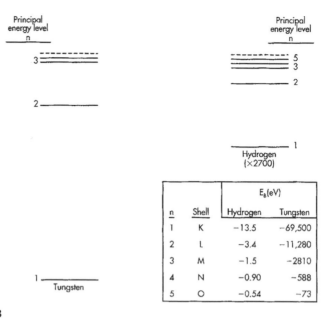

FIGURE 1-3
Binding energies for electrons in hydrogen ($Z = 1$) and tungsten ($Z = 74$). A change in scale is required to show both energy ranges in the same diagram.

its own axis while it revolves in the electron orbit. The electron orbits of a particular atom can be characterized in terms of the binding energies of electrons in the orbits.

Binding energies for electron orbits in hydrogen ($Z = 1$) and tungsten ($Z = 74$) are compared in Figure 1-3. Binding energies are much greater in tungsten than in hydrogen because the higher nuclear charge exerts a stronger attractive force on the electrons. In hydrogen, an electron moving to the K shell from a level farther from the nucleus releases energy usually in the form of ultraviolet radiation. In tungsten, an electron falling into the K shell releases energy usually in the form of an x ray, a form of electromagnetic radiation much more energetic than ultraviolet radiation. The actual energy released equals the difference in binding energy between the electron orbits representing the origin and destination of the electron. For example, an electron moving from the L to the K shell in tungsten releases ($69,500 - 11,280 = 58,220$ eV $= 58.2$ keV) of energy, whereas an electron falling from the M to the K shell in tungsten releases ($69,500 - 2810 = 66,690$ eV $= 66.7$ keV). X rays emitted by electron transitions between orbits are termed characteristic x rays because their energy is defined by the atomic number of the atom and the particular electron shells involved in the transition.

When an electron falls from the L to the K shell in a heavy atom, a vacancy is created in the L shell. This vacancy is usually filled instantly by an electron from a shell farther from the nucleus, usually the M shell. The vacancy created in this shell is then filled by another electron from a more distant orbit. Hence, a vacancy in an inner shell of an atom usually results in a cascade of electrons with the emission of a range of characteristic energies, often as electromagnetic radiation. In tungsten, transitions of electrons into the K and L shell result in the release of x rays, whereas transitions into M and higher shells produce radiations too low in energy to qualify as x rays.

Energy liberated as an electron falls to an orbit closer to the nucleus is not always released as electromagnetic radiation. Instead, it may be transferred to another electron farther from the nucleus, resulting in the ejection of the electron from its orbit. The ejected electron is termed an *Auger electron* and has a kinetic energy equal to the energy transferred to it, decreased by the binding energy required to eject the electron from its orbit. For example, an electron falling from the L to the K shell in tungsten releases 58,220 eV of energy. If this energy is transferred to another electron in the L shell this electron is ejected with a kinetic energy of ($58,220 - 11,280 =$

Characteristic x rays are sometimes called "fluorescence x rays."

X rays from electron transitions from the L to the K shell are termed K_α x rays. X rays resulting from M to K transitions are termed K_β x rays. Similarly, L_α x rays result from M to L transitions, and L_β results from N to L transitions, and so on.

The physicist H. G. J. Moseley studied the x-ray spectra from 38 elements and used his results to refine the Bohr model of the atom. Moseley was killed in 1915 in the ill-fated Dardanelles expedition of World War I.

46,940) eV. Usually an Auger electron is ejected from the same energy level that gave rise to the original transitioning electron. In this case, the kinetic energy of the Auger electron is $E_{bi} - 2E_{bo}$, where E_{bi} is the binding energy of the inner electron orbit that receives the transitioning electron, and E_{bo} is the energy of the orbit that serves as the origin of both the transitioning and the Auger electrons.

Example 1-3

What is the kinetic energy E_k of an Auger electron released from the L shell of gold $[(E_b)_L = 13.335$ keV$]$ as an electron falls from the L to the K shell $[(E_b)_K = 80.713$ keV$]$ in gold?

$$E_k = E_{bi} - 2E_{bo} = [80.713 - 2(13.335)] \text{keV}$$
$$= 54.043 \, \text{keV}$$

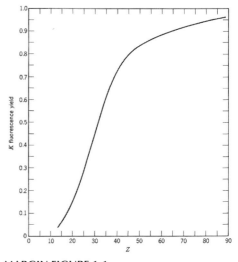

MARGIN FIGURE 1-1
K-shell fluorescence yields as a function of atomic number.[14]

The emission of characteristic electromagnetic radiation and the release of Auger electrons are alternative processes that release energy from an atom during electron transitions. The *fluorescence yield w* defines the probability that an electron vacancy will result in the emission of characteristic radiation as it is filled by an electron from a higher orbit.

$$w = \frac{\text{Number of characteristic radiations emitted}}{\text{Number of electron shell vacancies}}$$

For low-Z nuclides, Auger electrons tend to be emitted more frequently than characteristic radiations, as shown in Margin Figure 1-1. As Z increases, the fluorescence yield also increases, so that characteristic radiations are released more frequently than Auger electrons.[3]

Nuclear Stability

The nuclei of many atoms are stable. In general, it is these atoms that constitute ordinary matter. In stable nuclei of lighter atoms, the number of neutrons is about equal to the number of protons. A high level of symmetry exists in the placement of protons and neutrons into nuclear energy levels similar to the electron shells constituting the extranuclear structure of the atom. The assignment of nucleons to energy levels in the nucleus is referred to as the "shell model" of the nucleus. For heavier stable atoms, the number of neutrons increases faster than the number of protons, suggesting that the higher energy levels are spaced more closely for neutrons than for protons. The number of neutrons (i.e., the neutron number) in nuclei of stable atoms is plotted in Figure 1-4 as a function of the number of protons (i.e., the atomic number). Above $Z = 83$, no stable forms of the elements exist, and the plot depicts the neutron/proton (N/Z) ratio for the least unstable forms of the elements (i.e., isotopes that exist for relatively long periods before changing).

Nuclei that have an imbalance in the N/Z ratio are positioned away from the stability curve depicted in Figure 1-4. These unstable nuclei tend to undergo changes within the nucleus to achieve more stable configurations of neutrons and protons. The changes are accompanied by the emission of particles and electromagnetic radiation (photons) from the nucleus, together with the release of substantial amounts of energy related to an increase in binding energy of the nucleons in their final nuclear configuration. These changes are referred to as *radioactive decay* of the nucleus, and the process is described as *radioactivity*. If the number of protons is different between the initial and final nuclear configurations, Z is changed and the nucleus is transmuted from one elemental form to another. The various processes of radioactive decay are summarized in Table 1-1.

Additional models of the nucleus have been proposed to explain other nuclear properties. For example, the "liquid drop" (also known as the "collective") model was proposed by the Danish physicist Niels Bohr[3] to explain nuclear fission. The model uses the analogy of the nucleus as a drop of liquid.

Radioactivity was discovered in 1896 by Henri Becquerel[4] who observed the emission of radiation (later shown to be beta particles) from uranium salts. A sentence from his 1896 publication reads "We may then conclude from these experiments that the phosphorescent substance in question emits radiations which penetrate paper opaque to light and reduces the salts of silver." Becquerel experienced a skin burn from carrying a radioactive sample in his vest pocket. This is the first known bioeffect of radiation exposure.

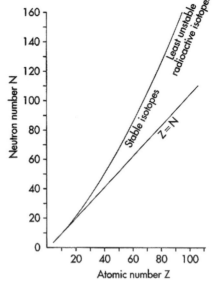

FIGURE 1-4
Number of neutrons (N) in stable (or least unstable) nuclei as a function of the number of protons (atomic number Z).

Equation (1-1) describes the expected decay rate of a radioactive sample. At any moment the actual decay rate may differ somewhat from the expected rate because of statistical fluctuations in the decay rate.

Equation (1-1) depicts a reaction known as a first-order reaction.

The decay constant λ is also called the *disintegration constant*.

The decay constant of a nuclide is truly a constant; it is not affected by external influences such as temperature and pressure, or by magnetic, electrical, or gravitational fields.

The "deltas" in $\Delta N/\Delta t$ signify a very small change in the number of atoms occurring over a very small increment of time Δt. The rate of decay is often written in differential form as dN/dt.

The rutherford (Rf) was once proposed as a unit of activity, where $1\ Rf = 10^6$ dps. The Rf did not gain acceptance in the scientific community and eventually was abandoned. In so doing, science lost an opportunity to honor one of its pioneers.

RADIOACTIVE DECAY

Radioactivity can be described mathematically without reference to the specific mode of decay of a sample of radioactive atoms. The rate of decay (the number of atoms decaying per unit time) is directly proportional to the number of radioactive atoms N present in the sample:

$$\Delta N/\Delta t = -\lambda N \qquad (1\text{-}1)$$

where $\Delta N/\Delta t$ is the rate of decay. The constant λ is the *decay constant* of the particular species of atoms in the sample, and the negative sign reveals that the number of radioactive atoms in the sample is diminishing as the sample decays. The decay constant can be expressed as $-(\Delta N/\Delta t)/N$, revealing that it represents the fractional rate of decay of the atoms. The value of λ is characteristic of the type of atoms in the sample and changes from one nuclide to the next. Units of λ are (time)$^{-1}$. Larger values of λ characterize more unstable nuclides that decay more rapidly.

The rate of decay of a sample of atoms is termed the *activity* A of the sample (i.e., $A = \Delta N/\Delta t$). A rate of decay of 1 atom per second is termed an *activity of 1 becquerel (Bq)*. That is,

$$1\ Bq = 1\ \text{disintegration per second (dps)}$$

TABLE 1-1   Radioactive Decay Processes

Type of Decay	A'	Z'	N'	Comments
Negatron ($\beta-$)	A	$Z+1$	$N-1$	$E_{\beta\text{-mean}} \cong \frac{E_{max}}{3}$
Positron (β^+)	A	$Z-1$	$N+1$	$E_{\beta\text{-mean}} \cong \frac{E_{max}}{3}$
Electron capture	A	$Z-1$	$N+1$	Characteristic + auger electrons
Isomeric transition gamma (γ) emission	A	Z	N	Metastable if $T_{1/2} > 10^{-6}$ sec
Internal conversion (IC)	A	Z	N	IC electrons: characteristic + auger electrons
Alpha (α)	$A-4$	$Z-2$	$N-2$	

A common unit of activity is the megabecquerel (MBq), where 1 MBq = 10^6 dps. An earlier unit of activity, the curie (Ci) is defined as

$$1\,\text{Ci} = 3.7 \times 10^{10}\,\text{dps}$$

Multiples of the curie are the picocurie (10^{-12} Ci), nanocurie (10^{-9} Ci), microcurie (10^{-6} Ci), millicurie (10^{-3} Ci), kilocurie (10^3 Ci), and megacurie (10^6 Ci). The becquerel and the curie are related by 1 Bq = 1 dps = 2.7×10^{-11} Ci. The activity of a radioactive sample per unit mass (e.g., MBq/mg) is known as the *specific activity* of the sample.

The curie was defined in 1910 as the activity of 1 g of radium. Although subsequent measures revealed that 1 g of radium has a decay rate of 3.61×10^{10} dps, the definition of the curie was left as 3.7×10^{10} dps.

Example 1-4

A. $^{60}_{27}$Co has a decay constant of 0.131 y^{-1}. Find the activity in MBq of a sample containing 10^{15} atoms.

$$A = \lambda N = \frac{(0.131\,y^{-1})(10^{15}\,\text{atoms})}{31.54 \times 10^6\,\text{sec/y}}$$

$$= 4.2 \times 10^6\,\text{atoms/s} = 4.2 \times 10^6\,\text{Bq}$$

$$= 4.2\,\text{MBq}$$

B. What is the specific activity of the sample in MBq/g? The gram-atomic mass of ^{60}Co is 59.9338.

$$\text{Sample mass} = \frac{(10^{15}\,\text{atoms})(59.9338\,\text{g/g-atomic mass})}{6.023 \times 10^{23}\,\text{atoms/g-atomic mass}}$$

$$= 9.95 \times 10^{-8}\,\text{g}$$

$$\text{Specific activity} = (4.2\,\text{MBq})/(9.95 \times 10^{-8}\,\text{g})$$

$$= 42 \times 10^6\,\text{MBq/g}$$

Through the process of mathematical integration, an expression for the number N of radioactive atoms remaining in a sample after a time t has elapsed can be shown to equal:

$$N = N_0 e^{-\lambda t} \qquad \text{(1-2)}$$

where N_0 is the number of atoms present at time $t = 0$. This expression can also be written as:

$$A = A_0 e^{-\lambda t} \qquad \text{(1-3)}$$

where A is the activity of the sample at time t, and A_0 is the activity at time $t = 0$.

The number of radioactive atoms N^* that have decayed after time t is $N_0 - N$ or

$$N^* = N_0(1 - e^{-\lambda t}) \qquad \text{(1-4)}$$

The probability that a particular atom will not decay during time t is N/N_0 or $e^{-\lambda t}$, and the probability that the atom will decay during time t is $1 - N/N_0$ or $1 - e^{-\lambda t}$. For small values of λt, the probability of decay ($1 - e^{-\lambda t}$) can be approximated as λt or, expressed as the probability of decay per unit time, p(decay per unit time) $\sim \lambda$.

The *physical half-life* $T_{1/2}$ of a radioactive sample is the time required for half of the atoms in the sample to decay. The half-life is related to the decay constant of the sample through the expression

$$T_{1/2} = (\ln 2)/\lambda = 0.693/\lambda$$

Equation (1-2) reveals that the number N of parent atoms decreases *exponentially* with time.

Radioactive decay must always be described in terms of the probability of decay; whether any particular radioactive nucleus will decay within a specific time period is never certain.

Each radioactive isotope has a unique decay constant and, therefore, a unique half-life.

The average life is often described as the *mean life* for radioactive atoms in a sample.

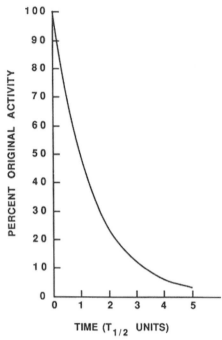

MARGIN FIGURE 1-2A
Percentage of original activity of a radioactive sample as a function of time in units of half-life: Linear plot.

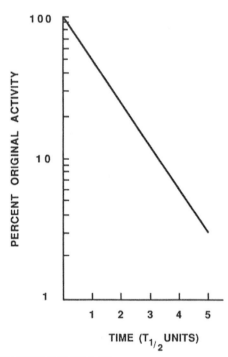

MARGIN FIGURE 1-2B
Percentage of original activity of a radioactive sample as a function of time in units of half-life: Semilogarithmic plot.

where ln 2 is the natural (naperian) logarithm of 2 (logarithm to the base e), and 0.693 is the value of this logarithm. The average life t_{avg} of a radioactive sample, sometimes referred to as the mean life, is the average time for decay of atoms in the sample. The average life is $t_{avg} = 1/\lambda = 1.44(T_{1/2})$.

Example 1-5

What are the half-life and average life of the sample of $^{60}_{27}Co$ described in Example 1-4?

$$T_{1/2} = 0.693/\lambda = 0.693/0.131 \text{ y}^{-1}$$
$$= 5.3 \text{ y}$$
$$T_{avg} = 1.44(T_{1/2}) = 1.44(5.3 \text{ y})$$
$$= 7.63 \text{ y}$$

The percent of original activity remaining in a radioactive sample is depicted in Margin Figure 1-2A as a function of elapsed time. This variable is replotted in Margin Figure 1-2B on a semilogarithmic graph (activity on a vertical logarithmic scale and time on a horizontal linear scale) to yield a straight line. Semilogarithmic plots yield straight lines of variables such as activity that vary according to an exponential relationship and are useful in depicting several quantities in radiation therapy (e.g., radioactive decay, attenuation of radiation, and survival of tumor cells following irradiation).

Example 1-6

The physical half-life of ^{131}I is 8.0 days.
  A. A sample of ^{131}I has a mass of 100 μg. How many ^{131}I atoms are present in the sample?

Number of atoms N
$$= \frac{(\text{Number of grams}) (\text{Number of atoms/g-atomic mass})}{(\text{Number of g/g-atomic mass})}$$
$$= \frac{(100 \times 10^{-6}g)(6.02 \times 10^{23}\text{atoms/g-atomic mass})}{131 \text{ g/g-atomic mass}}$$
$$= 4.6 \times 10^{17}\text{atoms}$$

  B. How many ^{131}I atoms remain after 20 days have elapsed?

$$N = N_0e^{-(0.693\,t/T_{1/2})}$$
$$= (4.6 \times 10^{17} \text{ atoms})e^{-(0.693/8\,d)(20\,d)}$$
$$= 8.1 \times 10^{16} \text{ atoms}$$

  C. What is the activity of the sample after 20 days?

$$A = \lambda N$$
$$= (0.693/8.0\,d)(1/86,400 \text{ s/d})(8.1 \times 10^{16} \text{ atoms})$$
$$= 8.2 \times 10^{10} \text{ atoms/sec}$$
$$= 8.2 \times 10^4 \text{ MBq}$$

  D. What is the specific activity of the ^{131}I sample?

$$SA = 8.2 \times 10^4 \text{ MBq}/0.1\,\text{mg}$$
$$= 8.2 \times 10^5 \text{ MBq/mg}$$

E. What activity should be ordered at 8 AM Monday to provide an activity of 8.2×10^4 MBq at 8 AM on the following Friday?

$$\text{Elapsed time} = 4 \, \text{days}$$

$$N = N_0 e^{-\lambda t}$$

$$8.2 \times 10^4 \, \text{MBq} = N_0 e^{-(0.693/8d)(4d)}$$

$$8.2 \times 10^4 \, \text{MBq} = N_0(0.7072)$$

$$N_0 = 11.6 \times 10^4 \, \text{MBq must be ordered}$$

■ TYPES OF RADIOACTIVE DECAY

The process of radioactive decay often is described by a decay scheme in which energy is depicted on the vertical (y) axis and atomic number is shown on the horizontal (x) axis. A generic decay scheme is illustrated in Figure 1-5. The original nuclide (or "parent") is depicted as $_Z^A X$, and the product nuclide (or "progeny") is denoted as element P, Q, R, or S depending on the decay path. In the path from X to P, the nuclide gains stability by emitting an alpha (α) particle, two neutrons and two protons ejected from the nucleus as a single particle. In this case, the progeny nucleus has an atomic number of $Z - 2$ and a mass number of $A - 4$ and is positioned at reduced elevation in the decay scheme to demonstrate that energy is released as the nucleus gains stability through radioactive decay. The released energy is referred to as the *transition energy*. In the path from X to Q, the nucleus gains stability through the process in which a proton in the nucleus changes to a neutron. This process can be either positron decay or electron capture and yields an atomic number of $Z - 1$ and an unchanged mass number A. The path from X to R represents negatron decay in which a neutron is transformed into a proton, leaving the progeny with an atomic number of $Z + 1$ and an unchanged mass number A. In the path from R to S, the constant Z and constant A signify that no change occurs in nuclear composition. This pathway is termed an isomeric transition between nuclear isomers and results only in the release of energy from the nucleus through the processes of gamma emission and internal conversion.

A decay scheme is a useful way to assimilate and depict the decay characteristics of a radioactive nuclide.

Parent and progeny nuclei were referred to in the past as "mother" and "daughter." The newer and preferred terminology of parent and progeny is used in this text.

The transition energy released during radioactive decay is also referred to as the "disintegration energy" and the "energy of decay."

Neutrons can be transformed to protons, and vice versa, by rearrangement of their constituent quarks.

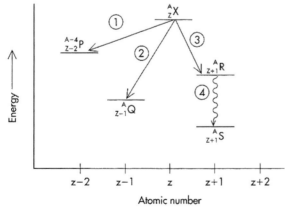

FIGURE 1-5
Symbolic radioactive decay scheme.

Alpha Decay

Alpha decay is a decay process in which greater nuclear stability is achieved by emission of 2 protons and 2 neutrons as a single alpha (α) particle (a nucleus of helium) from the nucleus. Alpha emission is confined to relatively heavy nuclei such

Alpha decay was discovered by Marie and Pierre Curie[5] in 1898 in their efforts to isolate radium, and was first described by Ernest Rutherford[6] in 1899. Alpha particles were identified as helium nuclei by Boltwood and Rutherford in 1911.[7] The Curies shared the 1902 Nobel Prize in Physics with Henri Becquerel.

as ^{226}Ra:

After a lifetime of scientific productivity and two Nobel prizes, Marie Curie died in Paris at the age of 67 from aplastic anemia, probably the result of years of exposure to ionizing radiation.

Rutherford, revered as a teacher and research mentor, was known as "Papa" to his many students.

A radionuclide is a radioactive form of a nuclide.

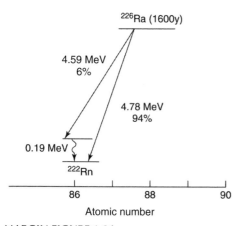

MARGIN FIGURE 1-3A
Radioactive decay scheme: α decay of ^{226}Ra.

Negative and positive electrons emitted during beta decay are created at the moment of decay. They do not exist in the nucleus before decay.

Ernest Rutherford first characterized beta decay in 1899.[6]

The difference in the energy released during decay, and that possessed by the negatron, threatened the concept of energy conservation for several years. In 1933 Wolfgang Pauli[8] suggested that a second particle was emitted during each decay that accounted for the energy not carried out by the negatron. This particle was named the *neutrino* (Italian for "little neutral particle") by Enrico Fermi.

Enrico Fermi was a physicist of astounding insight and clarity who directed the first sustained man-made nuclear chain reaction on December 2, 1942 in the squash court of the University of Chicago stadium. He was awarded the 1938 Nobel Prize in Physics.

$$^{226}_{88}\text{Ra} \rightarrow {}^{222}_{86}\text{Rn} + {}^{4}_{2}\text{He}$$

where $^{4}_{2}$He represents the alpha particle. The sum of mass numbers and the sum of atomic numbers after the transition equal the mass and atomic numbers of the parent before the transition. In α decay, energy is released as kinetic energy of the α particle, and is sometimes followed by energy released during an isomeric transition resulting in emission of a γ ray or conversion electron. Alpha particles are always ejected with energy characteristic of the particular nuclear transition.

An alpha transition is depicted in the margin, in which the parent ^{226}Ra decays directly to the final energy state (ground state) of the progeny ^{222}Rn in 94% of all transitions. In 6% of the transitions, ^{226}Ra decays to an intermediate higher energy state of ^{222}Rn, which then decays to the ground state by isomeric transition. For each of the transition pathways, the transition energy between parent and ground state of the progeny is constant. In the example of ^{226}Ra, the transition energy is 4.78 MeV.

Beta Decay

Nuclei with an N/Z ratio that is above the line of stability tend to decay by a form of beta (β) decay known as negatron emission. In this mode of decay, a neutron is transformed into a proton, and the Z of the nucleus is increased by 1 with no change in A. In this manner, the N/Z ratio is reduced, and the product nucleus is nearer the line of stability. Simultaneously an electron (termed a negative beta particle or negatron) is ejected from the nucleus together with a neutral massless particle, termed a neutrino (actually an "antineutrino" in negatron decay), that carries away the remainder of the released energy that is not accounted for by the negatron. The neutrino (or antineutrino) seldom interacts with matter and is not important to applications of radioactivity in medicine.

The process of negatron emission may be written

$$^{1}_{0}\text{n} \rightarrow {}^{1}_{1}\text{p} + {}^{0}_{-1}\text{e} + \bar{\nu}$$

$$\rightarrow {}^{1}_{1}\text{p} + {}^{0}_{-1}\beta + \bar{\nu}$$

where $^{0}_{-1}e$ depicts the ejected negatron (negative beta particle) and $^{0}_{-1}\beta$ reflects the nuclear origin of the negatron. The symbol $\bar{\nu}$ represents the antineutrino. An example of negatron emission is beta decay of ^{60}Co:

$$^{60}_{27}\text{Co} \rightarrow {}^{60}_{28}\text{Ni} + {}^{0}_{-1}\beta + \bar{\nu} + \text{isomeric transition}$$

with the isomeric transition often accomplished by release of cascading gamma rays of 1.17 and 1.33 MeV. A decay scheme for ^{60}Co is shown in the margin. The transition energy for decay of ^{60}Co is 2.81 MeV.

A discrete amount of energy is released when a negatron is emitted from the nucleus. This energy is depicted as the maximum energy E_{max} of the negatron. Negatrons, however, usually are emitted with some fraction of this energy, and the remainder is carried from the nucleus by the antineutrino. The mean energy of the negatron is $E_{max}/3$. An energy spectrum of 0.31 MeV E_{max} negatrons emitted from ^{60}Co is shown in Figure 1–6. Negatron energy spectra are specific for each negatron transition in every nuclide by this mode of nuclear transformation.

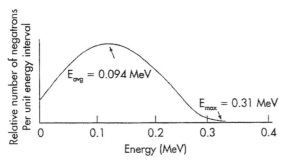

FIGURE 1-6
Energy spectrum of negatrons from $^{60}_{27}$Co.

Example 1-7

Determine the transition energy and the E_{max} of negatrons released during the decay of $^{60}_{27}$Co (atomic mass 59.933814 amu) to $^{60}_{28}$Ni (atomic mass 59.930787 amu).

$$\text{Transition:} \quad {}^{60}_{27}\text{Co}\left[+{}^{0}_{-1}\text{e}\right] \rightarrow {}^{60}_{28}\text{Ni} + {}^{0}_{-1}\beta + \bar{\nu} + \text{isomeric transmission}$$

where the ${}^{0}_{-1}$e on the left side of the transition must be added from outside the atom to balance the additional positive nuclear charge of ^{60}Ni compared with ^{60}Co.

$$\text{Mass difference} = \text{mass}\left({}^{60}_{27}\text{Co} + {}^{0}_{-1}e\right) - \text{mass}\left({}^{60}_{28}\text{Ni} + {}^{0}_{-1}\beta\right)$$

$$= (59.933814 + 0.00055)\,\text{amu} - (59.930787 + 0.00055)\,\text{amu}$$

$$= 0.003027\,\text{amu}$$

$$\text{Transition energy} = (0.003027\,\text{amu})\,(931\,\text{MeV/amu})$$

$$= 2.81\,\text{MeV}$$

The isomeric transition in ^{60}Co accounts for $(1.17 + 1.33) = 2.50$ MeV (Figure 1-3B). Hence the negatron E_{max} is $2.81 - 2.50 = 0.31$ MeV.

    Nuclei below the line of stability are unstable because they have too few neutrons for the number of protons in the nucleus. These nuclei tend to gain stability by a decay process in which a proton is transformed into a neutron, resulting in a unit decrease in Z with no change in A. One possibility for this transformation is positron decay:

$$^{1}_{1}p \rightarrow {}^{1}_{0}n + {}^{0}_{+1}e + \nu$$

$$\rightarrow {}^{1}_{0}n + {}^{0}_{+1}\beta + \nu$$

where ${}^{0}_{+1}\beta$ represents the nuclear origin of the emitted positive electron (positron). A representative positron transition is

$$^{18}_{9}\text{F} \rightarrow {}^{18}_{8}\text{O} + {}^{0}_{+1}\beta + \nu$$

where ν represents the release of a neutrino, a noninteractive particle similar to an antineutrino except with opposite axial spin. In positron decay, the atomic mass of the decay products exceeds the atomic mass of the atom before decay. This difference in mass must be supplied by energy released during decay according to the relationship $E = mc^2$. The energy requirement is 1.02 MeV. Hence, nuclei with a transition energy less than 1.02 MeV cannot undergo positron decay. For nuclei with transition energy greater than 1.02 MeV, the energy in excess of 1.02 MeV is shared among the kinetic energy of the positron, the energy of the neutrino, and the energy released during isomeric transitions. Decay of ^{18}F is depicted in the margin, in which the vertical component of the positron decay pathway represents the 1.02 MeV of energy that is expressed as increased mass of the products of the decay process.

    An alternate pathway to positron decay is electron capture, in which an electron from an extranuclear shell, usually the K shell, is captured by the nucleus and

The antineutrino was detected experimentally by Reines[9] and Cowan in 1953. They used a 10-ton water-filled detector to detect antineutrinos from a nuclear reactor at Savannah River, SC. Reines shared the 1995 Nobel Prize in Physics.

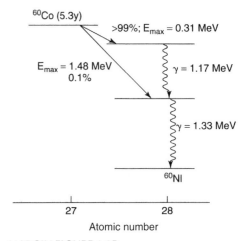

MARGIN FIGURE 1-3B
Radioactive decay scheme: Negatron decay of ^{60}Co.

The emission of positrons from radioactive nuclei was discovered in 1934 by Irene Curie[10] (daughter of Marie Curie) and her husband Frederic Joliet. In bombardments of aluminum by α particles, they documented the following transmutation:

$$^{4}_{2}\text{He} + {}^{27}_{13}\text{Al} \rightarrow {}^{30}_{15}\text{P} + {}^{1}_{0}n$$

$$^{30}_{15}\text{P} \rightarrow {}^{30}_{14}\text{Si} + {}^{0}_{+1}\beta + \upsilon$$

1.02 MeV $= 2m_0c^2$, where m_0 is the mass of the electron.

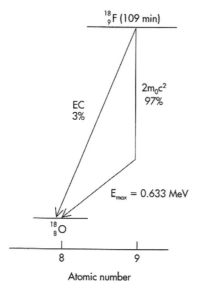

MARGIN FIGURE 1-3C
Radioactive decay scheme: $_{+1}^{0}\beta$: e capture decay of $_9^{18}F$.

Electron capture of K-shell electrons is known as K-capture; electron capture of L-shell electrons is known as L-capture; and so on.

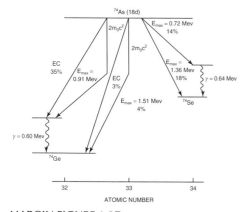

MARGIN FIGURE 1-3D
Complex decay pattern of $_{33}^{74}As$.

Gamma rays were discovered by the French physicist Paul Villard in 1900.[11] Rutherford and Andrade confirmed in 1912 that γ rays and x rays are similar kinds of radiation.

combined with a proton to transform it into a neutron. The process is represented as

$$_1^1p + _{-1}^0e \rightarrow _0^1n + \nu$$

Electron capture does not yield a mass imbalance before and after the transformation. Hence, there is no transition energy prerequisite for electron capture. Low N/Z nuclei with transition energy less than 1.02 MeV can decay only by electron capture. Low N/Z nuclei with transition energy greater than 1.02 MeV can decay by both positron decay and electron capture. For these nuclei, the electron capture branching ratio describes the probability of electron capture, and (1-branching ratio) depicts the probability of positron decay. Usually, positron decay occurs more frequently than electron capture for nuclei that decay by either process. In the figure illustrating electron capture and positron decay in the margin, the branching ratio for electron capture of ^{18}F is 3%.

Example 1-8

Determine the transition energy and E_{max} of positrons released during the transformation of $_9^{18}F$ (atomic mass = 18.000937 amu) to $_8^{18}O$ (atomic mass = 17.999160 amu). There are no isomeric transitions in this decay process.

$$\text{Transition:} \quad _9^{18}F \rightarrow _8^{18}O + _{+1}^0\beta + \nu + _{-1}^0e$$

where the $_{-1}^0e$ on the right side of the transition must be released from the atom to balance the reduced positive nuclear charge of ^{18}O compared with ^{18}F.

$$\text{Mass difference} = \text{mass}\left(_9^{18}F\right) - \text{mass}\left(_8^{18}O + _{+1}^0\beta + _{-1}^0e\right)$$

$$= (18.000937)\,\text{amu} - (17.999160 + 2(0.00055)\,\text{amu}$$

$$= 0.000677\,\text{amu}$$

$$\text{Energy available as } E_{max} = (0.000677\,\text{amu})(931\,\text{MeV/amu})$$

$$= 0.630\,\text{MeV}$$

The energy equivalent to the mass of the $_{+1}^0\beta$ and $_{-1}^0e$ is 2(0.00055 amu) (931 MeV/amu) = 1.02 MeV. Hence the total transition energy is (0.63 + 1.02) MeV = 1.65 MeV.

A few unstable nuclei can decay by negatron decay, positron emission, or electron capture. For example, the decay scheme for ^{74}As in the margin reveals that negatron decay occurs 32% of the time, positron emission occurs with a frequency of 30%, and the nuclide decays by electron capture 38% of the time.

Gamma Emission and Internal Conversion

Frequently during radioactive decay, a product nucleus is formed in an "excited" energy state above the ground energy level. Usually the excited state decays instantly to a lower energy state, often the ground energy level. Occasionally, however, the excited state persists with a finite half-life. An excited energy state that exists for a finite time before decaying is termed a *metastable* energy state and denoted by an m following the mass number (e.g., ^{99m}Tc, which has a half-life of 6 hours). The transition from an excited energy state to one nearer the ground state, or to the ground state itself, is termed an *isomeric transition* because the transition occurs between isomers with no change in Z, N, or A. An isomeric transition can occur by either of two processes: gamma emission or internal conversion.

Gamma rays are high-energy electromagnetic radiation that differ from x rays only in their origin: Gamma rays are emitted during transitions between isomeric energy states of the nucleus, whereas x rays are emitted during electron transitions outside the nucleus. Gamma rays and other electromagnetic radiation are described by their energy E and frequency ν, two properties that are related by the expression $E = h\nu$, where h = Planck's constant ($h = 6.62 \times 10^{-34}$ J-sec). The frequency ν

and wavelength λ of electromagnetic radiation are related by the expression $\nu = c/\lambda$, where c is the speed of light in a vacuum.

No radioactive nuclide decays solely by gamma emission; an isomeric transition is always preceded by a radioactive decay process, such as electron capture or emission of an alpha particle, negatron, or positron. Isomeric transitions for ^{60}Co (as depicted in an earlier marginal figure) yield gamma rays of 1.17 and 1.33 MeV with a frequency of more than 99%. Gamma rays are frequently used in medicine for detection and diagnosis of a variety of ailments, as well as for treatment of cancer.

Internal conversion is a competing process to gamma emission for an isomeric transition between energy states of a nucleus. In a nuclear transition by internal conversion, the released energy is transferred from the nucleus to an inner electron, which is ejected with a kinetic energy equal to the transferred energy reduced by the binding energy of the electron. Internal conversion is accompanied by emission of x rays and Auger electrons as the electron structure of the atom resumes a stable configuration following ejection of the conversion electron. The *internal conversion coefficient* is the fraction of conversion electrons divided by the number of gamma rays emitted during a particular isomeric transition. The conversion coefficient can be expressed in terms of specific electron shells denoting the origin of the conversion electron. The probability of internal conversion increases with Z and the lifetime of the excited state of the nucleus.

RADIOACTIVE EQUILIBRIUM

Some progeny nuclides produced during radioactive decay are themselves unstable and undergo radioactive decay in a continuing quest for stability. For example, ^{226}Ra decays to ^{222}Rn, which, in turn, decays by alpha emission to ^{218}Po. When a radioactive nuclide is produced by radioactive decay of a parent, a condition can be reached in which the rate of production of the progeny equals its rate of decay. In this condition, the number of progeny atoms and therefore the progeny activity reach their highest level and are constant for a moment in time. This constancy reflects an equilibrium condition known as *transient equilibrium* because it exists only momentarily. In cases in which a shorter-lived radioactive progeny is produced by decay of a longer-lived parent, the activity curves for parent and progeny intersect at the moment of transient equilibrium. This intersection reflects the occurrence of equal activities of parent and daughter at that particular moment. After the moment of transient equilibrium has passed, the progeny activity decays with an apparent half-life equal to that of the longer-lived parent. The apparent half-life of the progeny reflects the simultaneous production and decay of the progeny.

If no progeny atoms are present at time $t = 0$, the number N_2 of progeny atoms at any later time t is:

$$N_2 = [\lambda_1/(\lambda_2 - \lambda_1)]N_0(e^{-\lambda_1 t}) \qquad (1\text{-}5)$$

In this expression, N_0 is the number of parent atoms present at time $t = 0$, λ_1 is the decay constant of the parent, and λ_2 is the decay constant of the progeny. If $(N_2)_0$ progeny atoms are present at time $t = 0$, the expression for N_2 is written

$$N_2 = (N_2)_0 e^{-\lambda_2 t} + [\lambda_1/(\lambda_2 - \lambda_1)]N_0(e^{-\lambda_1 t} - e^{-\lambda_2 t})$$

Transient equilibrium for a hypothetical nuclide Y formed by decay of the parent X is illustrated in the margin. The activity of Y is greatest at the moment of transient equilibrium and exceeds the activity of X at all times after transient equilibrium is achieved, provided that no amount of Y is removed from the sample. After transient equilibrium, the activity of progeny Y decays with an apparent half-life equal to that of the parent X. The ratio of activities A_1 and A_2 for X and Y, respectively, is

$$A_1/A_2 = (\lambda_2 - \lambda_1)/\lambda_2$$

In some texts, transient equilibrium is defined as the extended period over which the progeny decays with an apparent half-life equal to the half-life of the parent. This definition is invalid, because no equilibrium exists beyond the moment when the rate of production of the progeny equals its rate of decay.

Equation (1–5) is a Bateman equation. More complex Bateman equations describe progeny activities for sequential phases of multiple radioactive nuclides in transient equilibrium.

The inert gas ^{222}Rn produced by decay of naturally occurring ^{226}Ra is also radioactive, decaying with a half-life of 3.83 days. This radioactive gas, first called "radium-emanation," was characterized initially by Rutherford. Seepage of ^{222}Rn into homes built in areas with significant ^{226}Ra concentrations in the soil is an ongoing concern to homeowners and the Environmental Protection Agency.

In the hypothetical transient equilibrium between parent X and progeny Y, equilibrium occurs

- at only one instant of time
- when Y reaches its maximum activity
- when the activity of Y is neither increasing or decreasing
- when the activities of X and Y are equal

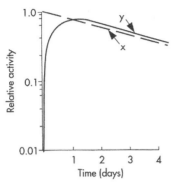

MARGIN FIGURE 1-4A
Transient equilibrium. Hypothetical radionuclide Y formed by decay of parent X.

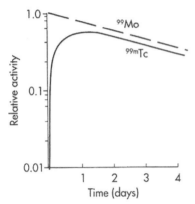

MARGIN FIGURE 1-4B
Transient equilibrium. Formation of ^{99m}Tc by decay of ^{99}Mo.

The ^{99}Mo–^{99m}Tc generator was developed by Powell Richards in 1957.

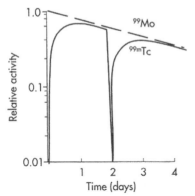

MARGIN FIGURE 1-4C
Transient equilibrium. Reestablishment of equilibrium after "milking" a ^{99m}Tc generator.

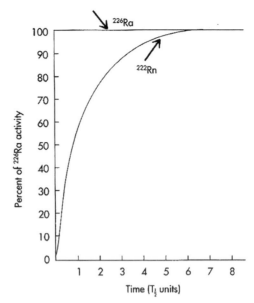

FIGURE 1-7
Growth of activity and secular equilibrium of ^{222}Rn formed by decay of ^{226}Ra.

The principle of transient equilibrium is employed in the production of short-lived nuclides useful in nuclear medicine. The nuclide ^{99m}Tc ($T_{1/2} = 6$ hours), used in more than 85% of all nuclear medicine examinations, is produced in a radionuclide generator in which the progeny ^{99m}Tc is produced by decay of the parent ^{99}Mo ($T_{1/2} = 67$ hours). This process is illustrated in the margin, in which the moment of transient equilibrium is illustrated as the point of greatest activity in the curve for ^{99m}Tc. In this case, the ^{99m}Tc activity never reaches that of the parent ^{99}Mo because not all of the ^{99}Mo atoms decay through the isomeric energy state ^{99m}Tc. In a ^{99m}Tc generator, the progeny atoms are removed periodically by "milking the cow" (i.e., removing activity from the generator) by using saline solution to flush an ion exchange column on which the parent is firmly attached. This process gives rise to abrupt decreases in ^{99m}Tc activity, as depicted in the margin.

When the half-life of the parent greatly exceeds that of the progeny (e.g., by a factor of 10^4 or more), equilibrium of the progeny activity is achieved only after a long period of time has elapsed. The activity of the progeny becomes relatively constant, however, as the progeny activity approaches that of the parent, a condition depicted in Figure 1-7. This condition is known as *secular equilibrium* and is a useful approach for the production of the nuclide ^{222}Rn, which was used at one time in radiation therapy. For radionuclides approaching secular equilibrium, the activities of parent (A_1) and progeny (A_2) are equal, and the number of atoms of parent N_1 (which is essentially N_0 because few atoms have decayed since time $t = 0$) and progeny (N_2) are related by the expression

$$A_1 = A_2$$
$$\lambda_1 N_1 = \lambda_2 N_2$$
$$N_0/(T_{1/2})_1 = N_2/(T_{1/2})_2$$

An intraophthalmic irradiator containing ^{90}Sr sometimes is used to treat various conditions of the eye. The low-energy beta particles from ^{90}Sr are not useful clinically, but the higher-energy beta particles from the progeny ^{90}Y are useful. The relatively short-lived Y ($T_{1/2} = 64$ hours) is contained in the irradiator in secular equilibrium with the longer-lived parent ^{90}Sr ($T_{1/2} = 28$ years) so that the irradiator can be used over many years without replacement. Radium needles and capsules that were formerly used widely in radiation oncology contained many decay products in secular equilibrium with the long-lived ($T_{1/2} = 1600$ years) parent ^{226}Ra.

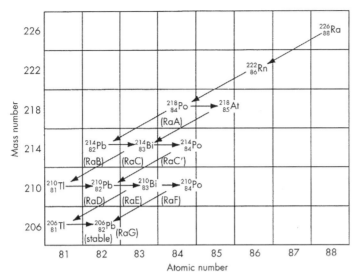

FIGURE 1-8
Uranium ($4n = 2$) decay series.

■ NATURAL RADIOACTIVITY AND DECAY SERIES

Most radionuclides in nature are members of one of three naturally occurring radioactive decay series. Each series consists of a sequence of radioactive transformations that begins with a long-lived radioactive parent and ends with a stable nuclide. In a closed environment such as the earth, intermediate radioactive progeny exist in secular equilibrium with the long-lived parent, and decay with an apparent half-life equal to that of the parent. All naturally occurring radioactive nuclides decay by emitting either alpha or negative beta particles. Hence, each transformation in a radioactive series changes the mass number by either 4 or 0 and changes the atomic number by -2 or $+1$.

The uranium series depicted in Figure 1-8 begins with the isotope ^{238}U and ends with the stable nuclide ^{206}Pb. The parent and each product in this series have a mass number that is divisible by 4 with remainder of 2; the uranium series is also known as the $4n + 2$ series. The naturally occurring isotopes ^{226}Ra and ^{222}Rn are members of the uranium series. The actinium ($4n + 3$) series begins with ^{235}U and ends with ^{207}Pb, and the thorium ($4n$) series begins with ^{232}Th and ends with ^{208}Pb. Members of the hypothetical neptunium ($4n + 1$) series do not occur in nature because no long-lived parent is available. Fourteen naturally occurring radioactive nuclides are not members of a decay series. These nuclides, all with relatively long half-lives, are ^{3}H, ^{14}C, ^{40}K, ^{50}V, ^{87}Rb, ^{115}In, ^{130}Te, ^{138}La, ^{142}Ce, ^{144}Nd, ^{147}Sm, ^{176}Lu, ^{187}Re, and ^{192}Pt.

■ ARTIFICIAL PRODUCTION OF RADIONUCLIDES

Radioactive isotopes with properties useful in biomedical research and clinical medicine may be produced by bombarding selected nuclei with neutrons and high-energy charged particles. Nuclides with excess neutrons that subsequently decay by negatron emission are created by bombarding nuclei with neutrons in a nuclear reactor or from a neutron generator. Typical reactions are

$$^{13}_{6}C + ^{1}_{0}n \rightarrow ^{14}_{6}C + \text{isomeric transition}$$

$$^{31}_{15}P + ^{1}_{0}n \rightarrow ^{32}_{15}P + \text{isomeric transition}$$

Useful isotopes produced by neutron bombardment include ^{3}H, ^{35}S, ^{51}Cr, ^{60}Co,

The first high-energy particle accelerator was the cyclotron developed by Ernest Lawrence in 1931. In 1938, Ernest and his physician brother John used artificially produced ^{32}P to treat their mother who was afflicted with leukemia.

Nuclear transmutation by particle bombardment was first observed by Rutherford[12] in 1919 in his studies of α particles traversing an air-filled chamber. The observed transmutation was

$$^{4}_{2}He + {}^{14}_{7}N \rightarrow {}^{17}_{8}O + {}^{1}_{1}H$$

where $^{4}_{2}He$ represents α particles and $^{1}_{1}H$ depicts protons detected during the experiment. This reaction can be written more concisely as

$$^{14}_{7}N \, (\alpha, p)^{17}_{8}O$$

where $^{14}_{7}N$ represents the bombarded nucleus, $^{17}_{8}O$ the product nucleus, and (α, p) the incident and ejected particles, respectively.

Through their discovery of artificial radioactivity, Irene Curie (the daughter of Marie Curie) and Frederic Joliot paved the way to use of radioactive tracers in biomedical research and clinical medicine.

^{99}Mo, ^{133}Xe, and ^{198}Au. Because the isomeric transition frequently results in prompt emission of a gamma ray, neutron bombardment often is referred to as an (n, γ) reaction. The reaction yields a product nuclide with an increase in A of 1 and no increase in Z. The complete transformation, including radioactive decay that results from neutron bombardment, is demonstrated by the example of ^{60}Co:

$$^{59}_{27}Co + {}^{1}n \rightarrow {}^{60}_{27}Co + \text{isomeric transitions}$$

$$^{60}_{27}Co \rightarrow {}^{60}_{28}Ni + {}^{0}_{-1}\beta + \bar{\nu} + \text{isomeric transitions}$$

The transition can be represented as $^{59}Co(n, \gamma)^{60}Co$. The decay of ^{60}Co occurs with a half-life of 5.3 years. The isomeric transitions accompanying this decay process almost always result in emission of cascading gamma rays of 1.17 and 1.33 MeV.

Radionuclides with excess protons are produced when nuclei are bombarded with high-energy positively charged particles from a particle accelerator. These radionuclides then decay by electron capture and, if the transition energy is adequate, positron decay. A typical reaction is

$$^{11}_{5}B + {}^{1}_{1}P \rightarrow {}^{11}_{6}C + {}^{1}_{0}n$$

where $^{1}_{0}n$ denotes that a neutron is ejected from the nucleus during bombardment so that the parent and progeny nuclei are isobars. This reaction can be represented as $^{11}B(p,n)^{11}C$ and is termed a (p,n) reaction. Other representative charged-particle interactions include

$$^{14}_{7}N + {}^{4}_{2}He \rightarrow {}^{17}_{8}O + {}^{1}_{1}p \quad \text{(an } (\alpha, p) \text{ reaction)}$$

$$^{68}_{30}Zn + {}^{1}_{1}p \rightarrow {}^{67}_{31}Ga + 2{}^{1}_{0}n \quad \text{(a (p, 2n) reaction)}$$

$$^{27}_{13}Al + {}^{4}_{2}He \rightarrow {}^{30}_{15}P + {}^{1}_{0}n \quad \text{(an } (\alpha, n) \text{ reaction)}$$

$$^{12}_{6}C + {}^{1}_{1}p \rightarrow {}^{13}_{7}N + \gamma \quad \text{(a (p, } \gamma) \text{ reaction)}$$

$$^{3}_{1}H + {}^{2}_{1}d \rightarrow {}^{4}_{2}He + {}^{1}_{0}n \quad \text{(a (d, n) reaction)}$$

where d stands for deuteron, a particle composed of a proton and neutron (i.e., a nucleus of deuterium).

Radioactive nuclides are also produced as a result of nuclear fission. These nuclides can be recovered as fission byproducts from the fuel elements used in nuclear reactors. Isotopes such as ^{90}Sr, ^{99}Mo, ^{131}I, and ^{137}Cs can be recovered in this manner.

Fission-produced nuclides (fission byproducts) are often mixed with other stable and radioactive isotopes of the same element, and cannot be separated chemically as a solitary radionuclide.[13] As a consequence, fission byproducts are less useful in research and clinical medicine than are radionuclides that are produced by neutron or charged-particle bombardment.

■ SUMMARY

- Radioactive decay is the consequence of nuclear instability.
  - Negatron decay occurs in nuclei with a high n/p ratio.
  - Positron decay and electron capture occur in nuclei with a low n/p ratio.
  - Alpha decay occurs with heavy unstable nuclei.
  - Isomeric transitions occur between different energy states of nuclei and result in the emission of γ rays and conversion electrons.
- The activity A of a sample is

$$A = A_o e^{-\lambda t}$$

where λ is the decay constant (fractional rate of decay).
- The half-life $T_{1/2}$ is the time required for half of a radioactive sample to decay. The half-life and the decay constant are related by

$$T_{1/2} = 0.693/\lambda$$

- The common unit of activity is the becquerel (Bq), with 1 Bq = 1 disintegration/second.
- Transient equilibrium may exist when the progeny nuclide decays with a $T_{1/2} <$ $T_{1/2}$ parent.
- Secular equilibrium may exist when the progeny nuclide decays with a $T_{1/2} \ll$ $T_{1/2}$ parent.
- Most radioactive nuclides found in nature are members of naturally occurring decay series.

PROBLEMS

1-1. What are the atomic and mass numbers of the oxygen isotope with 17 nucleons? Calculate the mass defect, binding energy, and binding energy per nucleon for this nuclide, with the assumption that the mass defect is associated with the nucleus. The mass of the atom is 16.999133 amu.

1-2. Natural oxygen contains three isotopes with atomic masses in amu of 15.9949, 16.9991, and 17.9992 and relative abundances of 2500:1:5. Determine to three decimal places the average atomic mass of oxygen.

1-3. Determine the energy required to move an electron from the K to the L shell in tungsten and in hydrogen, and explain the difference.

1-4. What is the energy equivalent to the mass of an electron? a proton?

1-5. The energy released during the nuclear explosion at Hiroshima has been estimated as equivalent to that released by 20,000 tons of TNT. Assume that 200 MeV is released when a ^{235}U nucleus absorbs a neutron and fissions and that 3.8×10^9J is released during detonation of 1 ton of TNT. How many nuclear fissions occurred at Hiroshima, and what was the total decrease in mass?

1-6. Group the following nuclides as isotopes, isotones, and isobars:

$$^{14}_{6}C, \ ^{14}_{7}N, \ ^{15}_{7}N, \ ^{15}_{6}C, \ ^{16}_{7}N, \ ^{16}_{8}O, \ ^{17}_{8}O$$

1-7. The half-life of ^{32}P is 14.3 days. What interval of time is required for 100 mCi of ^{32}P to decay to 25 mCi? What time is required for decay of 7/8 of the ^{32}P atoms?

1-8. A radioactive needle contains $^{222}_{86}$Rn ($T_{1/2} = 3.83$ days) in secular equilibrium with $^{226}_{88}$Ra ($T_{1/2} = 1600$ years). How long is required for the $^{222}_{86}$Rn to decay to half of its original activity?

1-9. In nature, $^{226}_{88}$Ra ($T_{1/2} = 1600$ years) exists in secular equilibrium with $^{238}_{92}$U ($T_{1/2} = 4.5 \times 10^9$ years). What fraction of the world's supply of radium will be left after 1600 years?

1-10. What is the mass in grams of 100 MBq of pure ^{32}P? How many ^{32}P atoms constitute 100 MBq? What is the mass in grams of 100 MBq of Na$_3$PO$_4$ if all the phosphorus in the compound is radioactive?

1-11. If a radionuclide decays for an interval of time equal to its average life, what percentage of the original activity remains?

1-12. What are the wavelength and frequency of a 1-MeV photon?

1-13. ^{126}I nuclei decay by negatron emission, positron emission, and electron capture. Write the decay equation for each mode of decay and identify the daughter nuclide.

1-14. How many atoms and grams of ^{90}Y are in secular equilibrium with 50 mCi of ^{90}Sr?

1-15. How many MBq of ^{132}I ($T_{1/2} = 2.3$ hours) should be ordered so that the sample activity will be 500 MBq when it arrives 24 hours later?

1-16. $^{127}_{53}$I is the only stable isotope of iodine. What mode(s) of decay would be expected for ^{131}I? ^{125}I?

1-17. For a nuclide X with the decay scheme

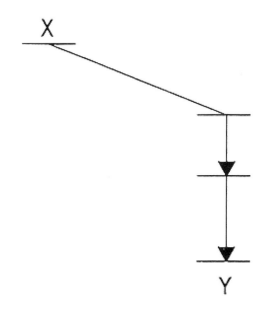

how many gamma rays are emitted per 100 disintegrations of X if the coefficient for interval conversion is 0.25?

1-18. ^{3}H (3.016050 amu) decays to $^3_2$He (3.016030 amu) by negatron emission. What is the transition energy and negatron E_{max} if no isomeric transitions occur?

1-19. $^{11}_6$C (11.011432 amu) decays to $^{11}_5$B (11.009305 amu) by positron emission and electron capture. What is the transition energy and positron E_{max} if no isomeric transitions occur?

REFERENCES

1. Bailey, C. *The Greek Atomists and Epicurus*. New York, Oxford University Press, 1928.

2. Bohr, N. On the constitution of atoms and molecules, *Philos. Mag.* 1913; **26:** 476, 875.

3. Bohr, N. Neutron capture and nuclear constitution. *Nature* 1936; **137:** 344.

4. Becquerel, H. Sur les radiations émises par phosphorescence. *Compt. Rend.* 1896; **122:**420.

5. Curie, P, and Curie, S. Sur une substance nouvelle radio-active, contenue dans la pechblende. *C. R. Hebd. Séances Acad. Sci.* 1898; **127:** 175–178.

6. Rutherford, E. Uranium radiation and the electrical conduction produced by it. *Philos. Mag.* 1899; **27:**109.

7. Boltwood, B., and Rutherford, E. Production of helium by radium. *Philos. Mag.* 1911, **22:**586.

8. Pauli, W. In *Rapports du Septieme Counseil de Physique Solvay, Bruxelles, 1933.* Paris, Gouthier-Villars & Cie, 1934.

9. Reines, F., and Cowan, C. Jr. Detection of the free neutrino. *Physiol. Rev.* 1953, **92:**830.

10. Curie, I., and Joliot, F. Physique nucléaire: Un nouvean type of radioactivité. *Compt. Rend.* 1934; **198:**254.

11. Villard, P. Sur la réfraction des rayons cathodiques et des rayons déviables du radium. *Compt. Rend.* 1900, **130:**1010.

12. Rutherford, E. Collision of α-particles with light atoms. I. Hydrogen, *Philos. Mag.* 1919; **37:**537.

13. Hendee, W. R., and Ritenour, E. R., *Medical Imaging Physics,* 4th edition. New York, John Wiley & Sons, 2001.

14. Broyles, C. D., Thomas, D. A., and Haynes, S. K. K-shell fluorescence yields as a function of atomic number. *Phys. Rev.* 1953; **89:**715.

CHAPTER

2

PRODUCTION OF X RAYS

OBJECTIVES 22

INTRODUCTION 22

SCATTERING OF ELECTRONS BY ELECTRONS 22

SCATTERING OF ELECTRONS BY NUCLEI 23

HISTORY OF X RAYS 25

CONVENTIONAL X-RAY TUBES 26

Electron Source 27
X-Ray Tube Voltage 28

X-RAY SPECTRA 30

SUMMARY 34

PROBLEMS 34

REFERENCES 34

Radiation Therapy Physics, Third Edition, by William R. Hendee, Geoffrey S. Ibbott, and Eric G. Hendee
ISBN 0-471-39493-9 Copyright © 2005 John Wiley & Sons, Inc.

■ OBJECTIVES

After studying this chapter, the reader should be able to:

- Explain the interactions of electrons with electrons, including the concepts of ionization, excitation, work function, specific ionization and linear energy transfer.
- Delineate the interactions of electrons with nuclei, including the concepts of cross section, bremsstrahlung, and the ratio of radiation to collisional energy loss of electrons.
- Describe the components and characteristics of conventional x-ray tubes, including the filament, cathode assembly, tube voltage, modes of rectification, 3ϕ and high frequency generators, x-ray target, target materials, anode, focal spot, and line focus principle.
- Depict x-ray spectra and how spectra are influenced by x-ray tube current and voltage and by beam filtration.

■ INTRODUCTION

X rays are produced during interactions of energetic electrons with atoms in a medium, during which the energy of the electrons is transformed in part to x radiation. An atom is a positively charged nucleus surrounded by a cloud of negative electrons, and an impinging electron can interact with either of theses two constituents: the nucleus or an electron. Interactions of electrons with electrons are considered first, followed by interactions with nuclei.

■ SCATTERING OF ELECTRONS BY ELECTRONS

An energetic electron moving through a medium can interact by transferring part of its energy to an electron in the medium. In this transfer, the impinging electron loses energy and is deflected (scattered) at some angle with respect to its original direction. Electrons are scattered by electrons in a medium with a probability that increases with the Z of the medium and decreases rapidly with increasing energy of the incident electrons.

In an electron–electron interaction, the electron receiving the energy may be raised to a shell farther from the nucleus of the atom to which it belongs, or it may be ejected completely from the atom.

When an electron is raised to a shell farther from the nucleus, the atom is unstable and said to be *excited*. Usually the atom remains in this state only momentarily and quickly regains stability through one or more electron transitions until all vacancies in the lower energy levels are filled.

If an electron is ejected during an electron–electron interaction, its kinetic energy E_k is

$$E_k = E - E_b$$

where E is the energy transferred to the ejected electron, and E_b is its binding energy. If E_b is negligible, the sum of the kinetic energy of the scattered and ejected electrons is equal to the kinetic energy of the original electron before the interaction. When kinetic energy is *conserved* in an interaction, the interaction is said to be *elastic*. If E_b cannot be ignored, kinetic energy is not conserved, and the interaction is said to be *inelastic*.

When an electron is ejected from an atom through a process such as interaction with an incident electron, the atom is said to be *ionized*. The ejected electron and the residual positive ion constitute a *primary ion pair* (IP). In air, an average energy of

The interactions of electrons with electrons and nuclei of a medium are termed "coulombic interactions" because they occur between charged particles in which each particle exerts a coulombic force of attraction or repulsion upon the other.

Elastic scattering interactions of electrons are sometimes referred to as "billiard-ball collisions."

33.97 eV is expended in producing an ion pair. This average value is termed the *work function*, represented by the symbol, $\overline{W}/e$ where

$$\frac{\overline{W}}{e} = 33.97 \text{ eV/IP}$$

The energy needed to overcome the binding energy of the most loosely bound electrons in air is considerably less than the $\overline{W}/e$ quantity. The work function includes not only the electron's binding energy, but also the average kinetic energy of the ejected electron and the average energy lost in the processes of exciting atoms, interacting with nuclei, and increasing the rotational and vibrational energy states of molecules in the medium. On the average, 2.2 atoms are excited for each atom ionized in air by incident electrons.

An electron ejected from an atom may possess enough kinetic energy to ionize nearby atoms. Ion pairs produced by this process are termed *secondary ion pairs*. The number of primary and secondary ion pairs produced per unit path-length of an incident electron is termed the *specific ionization* (SI) of the electron, usually expressed in units of ion pairs per centimeter (IP/cm). In air at standard temperature and pressure (STP), the SI of an electron with a kinetic energy less than 10 MeV can be estimated as

$$SI = 45(v/c)^2 \text{ IP/cm}$$

where v is the velocity of the electron, and c is the speed of light in a vacuum (3×10^8 m/sec).[1] The *linear energy transfer* (LET) is the rate of energy loss along the path of an electron or other ionizing particle. The LET is the product of the specific ionization and the work function [LET $= (SI)(\overline{W}/e)$].

> The work function $\overline{W}/e$ is often referred to as the "W quantity."

> Standard temperature is $0°C$ and standard pressure is one atmosphere or 760 mm Hg.

Example 2-1

Determine the SI and LET of 0.1 MeV electrons in air ($v/c = 0.548$).

$$SI = 45/(v/c)^2 = 45/(0.548)^2$$
$$= 160 \text{ IP/cm}$$
$$LET = (SI)(\overline{W}/e)$$
$$= (160 \text{ IP/cm})(33.97 \text{ eV/IP})(10^{-3} \text{ keV/eV})$$
$$= 5.4 \text{ keV/cm}$$

A positive electron traversing a medium interacts in a manner similar to that of an electron, with one exception. As the positive electron transfers energy to surrounding atoms, it loses kinetic energy and finally combines with a negative electron. The two particles momentarily revolve about each other and then annihilate with release of electromagnetic radiation with a total energy equivalent to the mass of the two particles. Usually the energy is released as two 0.51-MeV photons of electromagnetic energy moving in opposite directions (at 180°). This interaction is termed *pair annihilation*, and the radiation that is produced is referred to as *annihilation radiation*. Annihilation radiation is detected in positron emission tomographic (PET) imaging following administration of a positron-emitting radionuclide to a patient.

> The property of an absorbing medium that influences the rate of energy loss (i.e., the LET) of radiation in the medium is known as the *linear stopping power* of the medium for the radiation. More often the *mass stopping power S_m*, which is the linear stopping power divided by the density of the medium, is used.

> The combination of electron and positron is referred to as positronium.

■ SCATTERING OF ELECTRONS BY NUCLEI

An electron traveling through a medium may be scattered at reduced energy during interaction with a nucleus in the medium. In some interactions, kinetic energy is conserved because the sum of the kinetic energy of the scattered electron and the "recoil" nucleus equals that of the incident electron.

> Backscattering of negatrons and positrons in a radioactive sample is principally a result of elastic scattering by nuclei in the sample.

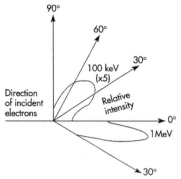

FIGURE 2-1
Relative intensity of bremsstrahlung radiated at different angles for electrons with kinetic energies of 100 keV and 1 MeV. (Data from O. Scherzer[2] and H. Andrews.[3])

The probability of elastic scattering of impinging electrons is about equal for electrons and nuclei in hydrogen. In absorbers of higher Z, elastic scattering by nuclei is more likely because its probability increases with Z^2, whereas the likelihood of elastic scattering by electrons increases with Z. The probability of interaction often is referred to as the *cross section* for the interaction, sometimes expressed in units of *barns*, where 1 barn = 10^{-24} cm^2.

Most scattering interactions of electrons with nuclei are inelastic rather than elastic because the kinetic energy of the interacting particles is not conserved in the interaction. The loss of kinetic energy is expressed as energy released as electromagnetic radiation during the interaction. Energy radiated as an electron (or any charged particle) slows by interacting with a nucleus of an absorbing medium is termed *bremsstrahlung*. A bremsstrahlung photon may possess an energy up to the entire kinetic energy of the incident electron. For low-energy electrons, bremsstrahlung is released predominantly at right angles to the direction of the electrons. The angle narrows for electrons of higher energy (Figure 2-1).

The unit "barn" originated in studies of neutron interactions where a cross section of 10^{-24} cm^2 is so large it is like "hitting the side of a barn."

Bremsstrahlung is German for "braking radiation."

Similarly to elastic scattering of electrons by nuclei, the probability of bremsstrahlung production varies with Z^2 of the medium. Consequently, media of high Z are much more effective in producing bremsstrahlung than are absorbers of low Z. A typical bremsstrahlung spectrum is shown in Figure 2-2. The area under the spectrum (i.e., the amount of bremsstrahlung produced) increases dramatically with the Z of the medium, but the relative shape of the spectrum along the energy axis remains

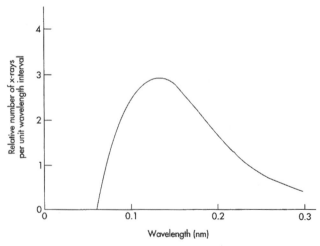

FIGURE 2-2
Bremsstrahlung spectrum for a molybdenum target bombarded by electrons accelerated through 20 kV. (Data from M. Wehr and J. Richard,[5] with permission).

TABLE 2-1 Relative (Percent) Collisional and Radiative Energy Losses of Electrons in Water (Tissue) and Lead[4]

	100 keV	1 MeV	10 MeV	25 MeV
		Water		
Collision	99.9	99	92	80
Radiative	0.1	1	8	20
		Lead		
Collision	97	86	49	25
Radiative	3	14	51	75

constant. The ratio of energy lost by electrons due to inelastic interactions with nuclei (radiative energy loss [bremsstrahlung]), to that lost by excitation and ionization during interactions with electrons (collisional energy loss) is approximately

$$\frac{\text{Radiative energy loss}}{\text{Collisional energy loss}} = \frac{E_k Z}{820}$$

where E_k is the kinetic energy of the incident electrons in MeV, and Z is the atomic number of the medium. For example, bremsstrahlung and ionization-excitation contribute about equal to the energy lost by 10 MeV electrons traversing lead ($Z = 82$). This ratio is important in the design of x-ray tubes used for medical diagnosis and radiation therapy.

The mass stopping power S_m can be separated into a collisional component $(S_m)c$ and a radiative component $(S_m)r$. That is, $S_m = (S_m)_c + (S_m)_r$.

Example 2-2

What is the approximate ratio of radiation to collisional energy loss of 20-MeV electrons in a gold transmission x-ray target ($Z = 79$) used for radiation therapy? Compare this value with the ratio of 0.1-MeV electrons striking a tungsten target ($Z = 74$) in a diagnostic x-ray tube.

$$\frac{\text{Radiation energy loss}}{\text{Collisional energy loss}} = \frac{E_k Z}{820}$$

For 20-MeV electrons in gold:

$$\frac{E_k Z}{820} = \frac{(20)(79)}{820} = 1.9$$

That is, energy released as radiation energy loss (bremsstrahlung) is almost twice that expended in collisional energy losses.

For 0.1-MeV electrons in tungsten:

$$\frac{E_k Z}{820} = \frac{(0.1)(74)}{820} = 0.0090$$

In a diagnostic x-ray tube, almost all (>99%) of the electron energy is expended through collisional energy mechanisms, leading to heat production in the target. Less than 1% of the electron energy is released as radiation energy loss. In radiation therapy, x rays are generated at much higher voltages, and the ratio of x rays to heat is much greater. At a few megavolts, for example, x-ray production may account for 50% or more of the energy delivered by electrons to the x-ray target.

■ HISTORY OF X RAYS

X rays were discovered on November 8, 1895, by Wilhelm Röntgen, a physicist at the University of Würzburg in Germany.[6] Röntgen was studying the properties of "cathode rays" produced by applying a high voltage across a partially evacuated glass

The "x" in x rays was used to denote an "unknown quantity."

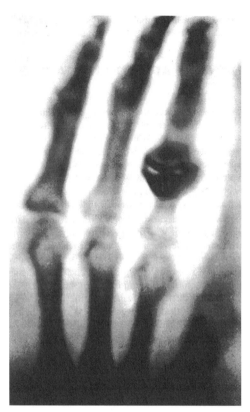

MARGIN FIGURE 2-1
First x-ray image, thought to be a radiograph of the hand of Röntgen's wife.

Röntgen was awarded the first Nobel Prize in Physics in 1901.

Early x-ray tubes were operated with exposed high-voltage cables and terminals, and fatal electrocutions occasionally occurred. The first shock proof x-ray unit was developed by H. F. Waite in 1919.[9]

Röntgen was not the first to acquire an x-ray photograph. In 1890 Alexander Goodspeed of the University of Pennsylvania, with the photographer William Jennings, accidentally exposed some photographic plates to x rays. They were able to explain the images on the developed plates only after Röntgen announced his discovery of x rays.

Coolidge's contributions to x-ray science, in addition to the heated filament, included the focusing cup, embedded x-ray target, and various anode cooling devices.

tube. During his experiments, Röntgen noticed that barium platinocyanide crystals in his laboratory glowed when voltage was applied to the tube. He then determined that the glow diminished but did not disappear when dense objects were placed between the cathode-ray tube and the crystals. The glow could not be caused directly by the cathode rays because it was known that cathode rays could travel no more than a few centimeters in air. Röntgen concluded that the glow was produced by a new type of penetrating radiation released from the cathode-ray tube. He named the new radiation *x rays*.

Over the next few weeks, Röntgen documented several properties of x rays.[7-8] He noted that x rays travel in straight paths, are not affected by magnetic fields, and are attenuated by a material according to its physical density and elemental composition (now characterized as the material's atomic number). He also determined that x rays darken photographic film and used this property to measure the amount of x radiation reaching the film under different experimental conditions. He used photographic film to produce images of objects that are opaque to visible light. His observations are now understood to have resulted from x rays released as residual gas molecules in the cathode-ray tube were ionized by electrons that were emitted as cathode rays interacted with various components of the cathode-ray tube.

Cathode-ray tubes were unreliable sources of x rays and produced radiation at low intensity. In 1913, Coolidge[10] developed the "hot cathode" x-ray tube in which a wire filament was heated with electrical current to release electrons by the process of thermionic emission (sometimes called the Edison effect). The released electrons were repelled by a negative charge on the filament and accelerated toward a positively charged metal target. X rays were released as the high-speed electrons interacted in the target. The Coolidge tube was the prototype for x-ray tubes in use today.

■ CONVENTIONAL X-RAY TUBES

The components of a stationary anode x-ray tube are depicted in Figure 2-3. A filament heated by an electrical current serves as a source of electrons. The electrons are accelerated toward a tungsten target by application of a high potential difference (voltage) between the filament housing (the cathode) and the target (the anode). X rays are produced as the electrons interact with electrons and nuclei of the target atoms. The x rays emerged from the target in all directions and are collimated to produce a useful x-ray beam of defined cross-sectional area. The glass envelope surrounding the components of the x-ray tube is evacuated to prevent the electrons from interacting with gas molecules before they reach the x-ray target. A modern diagnostic x-ray tube with a rotating anode and a dual focus filament is shown in the margin.

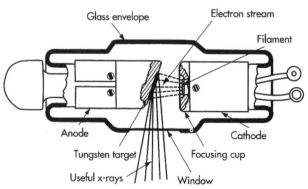

FIGURE 2-3
Simplified x-ray tube with a stationary anode and a heated filament. (From W. Bloom, J. Hollenbach, and J. Morgan.[11])

Electron Source

The filament of the x-ray tube is a metal wire that conducts electricity and has a high melting point. Tungsten (melting point 3370°C) filaments are used in most x-ray tubes. The filament is housed within a negatively charged focusing cup, which, together with the filament, serves as the *cathode assembly* for the x-ray tube. A current of a few amperes (the filament current) is used to heat the filament to a temperature at which thermionic emission occurs. If the released electrons are attracted to the target as soon as they are emitted from the filament, no pile-up of electrons occurs around the filament, and the rate of flow of electrons across the x-ray tube (the tube current) is said to be *filament-emission limited*. In this condition, the tube current can be increased only by heating the filament to a higher temperature through use of a greater filament current. X-ray tubes operating at high voltage or relatively low tube current function in the filament-emission limited condition.

At relatively low voltages across the x-ray tube, electrons released by thermionic emission tend to accumulate around the filament because they are not pulled immediately to the target. This accumulation of electrons is referred to as a space charge. The negative cloud of electrons prevents additional electrons from leaving the filament and thereby limits the tube current. Under this condition, the tube current is said to be *space-charge limited*. Operation of an x-ray tube under space-charge and filament-emission limitations is depicted in Figure 2-4. Space-charge-limited operation is encountered primarily in x-ray tubes operated at relatively low voltages, such as those employed for mammography. At the high voltages usually used for x-ray production in radiation therapy, the x-ray tube functions in the filament-emission-limited condition.

The Coolidge hot-cathode x-ray tube became available commercially in 1917.

Most x-ray tubes employ a target of tungsten or tungsten–rhenium alloy.

The basic necessities for a useful x-ray beam are: (a) electron source; (b) high voltage supply; (c) target for x-ray production; (d) vacuum, (e) collimator.

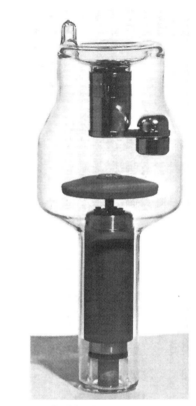

MARGIN FIGURE 2-2
A dual-focus x-ray tube with a rotating anode. (Courtesy of Machlett Laboratories, Inc.)

In a typical diagnostic x-ray tube, the filament is operated at a low voltage (6–12 V) and relatively low current (3–5 A).

X-ray tubes can operate in one of two modes:

- filament-emission limited
- space-charge limited

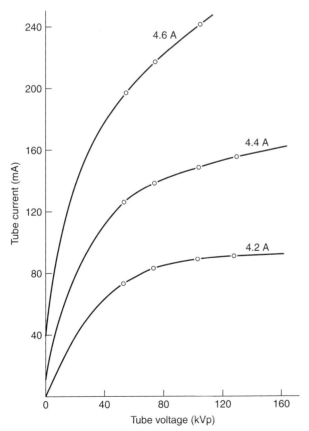

FIGURE 2-4
Influence of tube voltage and filament current on electron flow in a Machlett Dynamax x-ray tube with a rotating anode, 1-mm apparent focal spot, and full-wave rectification.

The focal spot of an x-ray tube is the volume of x-ray target in which electrons are absorbed and x rays are produced. For the most sharply defined x-ray beams, a small focal spot is needed. A small focal spot requires a small or "fine" filament as an electron source. If the filament is too small, however, thermionic emission is limited, and the rate of production of x rays is restricted. In this case, longer exposures are required, and patient motion during an exposure can become troublesome. In any x-ray exposure, a compromise must be reached between (a) use of a small focal spot to provide a sharp x-ray beam and (b) use of a larger focal spot to furnish an x-ray beam of higher intensity.[12–14] This compromise is reflected in the presence of two filaments in most x-ray tubes. The small filament is used when low tube currents can be tolerated and a small focal spot is desired to yield a sharply defined x-ray beam. When patient motion is a problem and higher x-ray intensities are needed to limit exposure times, the large filament is used to provide higher tube currents.

An x-ray tube with two focal spots is called a *dual-focus x-ray tube.*

X-Ray Tube Voltage

The potential difference (voltage) between the filament (cathode) and target (anode) of an x-ray tube influences the intensity and spectral distribution of x rays furnished by the tube. Alternating voltage and current (AC) are used as the source of electrical power for most x-ray tubes because it is the type of electrical power supplied by electrical utilities in most countries. In the United States, alternating current is supplied at a frequency of 60 hertz (Hz), with 1 Hz = 1 cycle per second. With 60 Hz AC, the voltage changes polarity and the current changes direction 120 times each second, with two changes in polarity or direction constituting one cycle. X-ray tubes, however, are designed to operate only when the x-ray target is positive and the filament is negative. Hence, x-ray units must convert the AC furnished by the utility to direct current (DC) for use in the x-ray tube. This conversion is accomplished by the process of *rectification.*

A positive electrode is termed an anode because negative ions (anions) are attracted to it. A negative electrode is referred to as a cathode because positive ions (cations) are attracted to it.

One of the simplest ways to operate an x-ray tube is to use AC and rely on the x-ray tube itself to control the flow of electrons in only one direction, from filament to target. The composition and configuration of the filament is ideal for producing the elevated temperatures necessary to release electrons by thermionic emission. When the filament is negative and the target is positive, these electrons flow to the x-ray target and produce x rays. Under normal circumstances, the x-ray target is not an efficient source of electrons. When the polarity of the alternating voltage is reversed and the target is negative and the filament is positive, electrons are not available from the target, and therefore no electrons flow from target to filament. In this condition, known as *self-rectification*, the x-ray tube itself is rectifying the AC power. Self-rectification is a satisfactory method of controlling electron flow in an x-ray tube, provided that the target does not reach an elevated temperature at which electrons are released from the target by thermionic emission. This provision is satisfied by circumstances in which the tube current is relatively low and the target remains relatively cool. At high tube currents, however, greatly elevated temperatures are achieved by the target. Under these conditions, thermionic emission, and therefore reverse electron flow, can occur. High-energy electrons bombarding the filament can destroy it; hence, self-rectification is employed only in circumstances in which the tube current is intrinsically limited, such as in some low-current generators used for mobile radiography and radiation therapy.[15]

A rectifier is any device that converts alternating current to direct current.

To prevent reverse electron flow across the x-ray tube, devices can be placed in the high-voltage circuit that permit electron flow in only the desired direction (Figure 2-5A). These devices are called rectifiers, and their presence converts AC to DC. With two *rectifiers* in the high-voltage circuit as shown in Figure 2-5A, one pulse of x rays is produced per cycle of the supplied alternating electrical power. This method, termed *half-wave rectification*, is a relatively inefficient use of the supplied power because the reverse half-cycle of the electrical power is discarded. This reverse half-cycle can be captured and used by the process of *full-wave rectification*, which employs the more complex rectification circuit shown in Figure 2-5B.

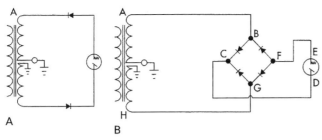

FIGURE 2-5
High-voltage circuit of an x-ray tube. **A**; Half-wave rectification. **B**; Full-wave rectification.

With full-wave rectification, current from both the positive and the negative phases of the voltage waveform emerges from the rectification circuit in a single direction and is always presented to the x-ray tube with the filament at negative potential and the anode at positive potential. In full-wave rectification, the negative pulses in the voltage waveform are essentially "flipped over" so that they also can be used to produce x rays. In this manner, a full-wave rectification circuit converts an AC waveform into a DC waveform with 2 pulses per cycle or 120 pulses per second.

The efficiency of x-ray production can be further increased by maintaining the voltage wave-form at high potential, rather than allowing it to decrease to zero twice during each voltage cycle. Three-phase power permits this goal to be approached. Three-phase (3ϕ) power is supplied through three separate cables connected to the x-ray tube. The voltage waveform in each cable varies slightly out of phase with that in the other two cables. These voltage waveforms are presented to the x-ray tube so that the voltage across the tube is always at or near maximum. The voltage waveforms are full-wave rectified to provide 6 voltage pulses to the x-ray tube during each power cycle. The circuit that supplies the rectified waveforms is known as a 3ϕ, 6-pulse circuit. A refinement of 3ϕ circuitry yields a slight phase delay for the waveform presented to the anode compared with that to the cathode. This refinement, known as a 3ϕ, 12-pulse circuit, provides a smaller ripple (about 3%) in the voltage applied to the x-ray tube compared with a 3ϕ, 6-pulse circuit, for which the ripple may be as great as 12%.

Voltage waveforms across the x-ray tube are depicted in Figure 2-6 for half-wave and full-wave rectification and for 3ϕ and constant potential operation. This latter

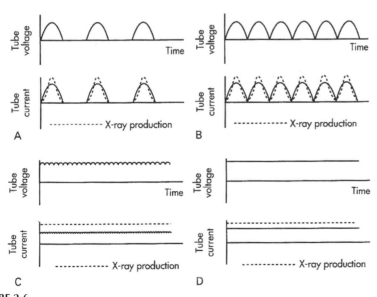

FIGURE 2-6
Voltage and current waveforms across the x-ray tube for (**A**) half-wave rectification, (**B**) full-wave rectification, (**C**) 3-phase, and (**D**) constant potential.

condition is approached in *high-frequency x-ray generators*, in which the voltage pulses are supplied to the x-ray tube at frequencies from 1 to 100 kHz. High-frequency x-ray generators are gaining popularity in diagnostic radiology because they provide the greatest efficiency achievable for x-ray production.

■ X-RAY SPECTRA

Several factors influence the distribution of photon energies in an x-ray beam. The energy of electrons impinging on the target varies with the voltage applied across the x-ray tube. For electrons of a specific energy, bremsstrahlung photons are produced with energies up to a maximum keV equal numerically to the kVp across the x-ray tube. Characteristic x rays are also generated, and these x rays have energies independent of the impinging electrons so long as the threshold energy for characteristic x-ray emission is exceeded.

Every x-ray beam is filtered by materials naturally present in the x-ray beam, including the target, glass envelope of the x-ray tube, insulating oil surrounding the tube, and exit window in the tube housing. These materials are collectively referred to as the inherent filtration of the x-ray beam, usually expressed as millimeters aluminum equivalent (mm Al eq). The inherent filtration in most diagnostic x-ray tubes is about 1 mm Al eq. Additional filtration is always inserted to "harden" the x-ray beam by selectively removing x rays of lower energy. If these x rays were not removed by filtration, they would be absorbed in the patient and increase the patient's radiation dose. In x-ray beams used for diagnosis, the added filtration is usually a few millimeters of aluminum. For the higher-energy *orthovoltage* (a few hundred kVp) x-ray beams employed in radiation therapy, a filter of aluminum, copper, and tin often is used.

Emission spectra for a tungsten-target diagnostic x-ray tube are shown in Figure 2-7 for the three thicknesses of added aluminum filtration. The added filtration decreases the total number of x rays but increases the average energy of the x rays in the beam. These changes are reflected in a decrease in the overall height of the x-ray spectrum and a shift of the spectral peak toward higher energy.

The material used as the target of an x-ray tube affects the x-ray spectrum by influencing the efficiency of x-ray production and determining the energies of the characteristic x rays. The efficiency of x-ray production is the ratio of the energy

kVp depicts the maximum (p = peak) voltage in kilovolts (kV).

Inherent filtration is also referred to as intrinsic filtration.

An x-ray beam of higher average energy is said to be "harder" because it is able to penetrate more dense (i.e., harder) substances such as bone. An x-ray beam of lower average energy is said to be "softer" because it can penetrate only less dense (i.e., softer) substances such as fat and muscle.

A filter of aluminum, copper, and tin is termed a thoreaus filter after its developer, R. Thoreaus, who first described it in 1932.

Although orthovoltage x rays are seldom used today, they once were the mainstay of radiation therapy.

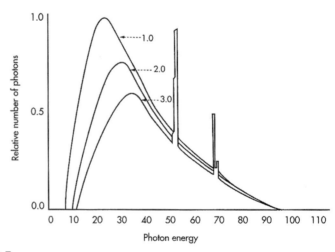

FIGURE 2-7
X-ray spectra for a 100-kVp tungsten target x-ray tube with total filtration values of 1.0, 2.0, and 3.0 mm aluminum. kVp and mAs are the same for the three spectra. (Computer simulation courtesy of Todd Steinberg, St. Louis, MO.)

emitted as x radiation divided by the energy deposited in the target by electrons accelerated from the filament. The rate of energy deposition in the target is the power deposition P_d in watts, where $P_d = VI$, V is the tube voltage in volts, and I is the tube current in amperes. The rate at which energy is released as x-radiation is the emitted power P_r in watts:

$$P_r = 0.9 \times 10^{-9} (Z)(V^2)(I)$$

where Z is the atomic number of the target, and V and I are expressed in units of volts and amperes, respectively. The ratio of these quantities is the x-ray production efficiency:

$$\text{Efficiency} = P_r/P_d = 0.9 \times 10^{-9} (Z)(V)$$

As shown in this equation, the efficiency of x-ray production increases with the atomic number of the target and the voltage across the x-ray tube. At voltages in the range of 100 kVp used in diagnostic radiology, x-ray production is an inefficient process, with less than 1% of the energy that is delivered to the target being released as x radiation. Almost all of the electron energy deposited in the target is degraded to heat, causing an elevated temperature of the target. To prevent the target from overheating, mechanisms are employed to limit the target temperature. These mechanisms include use of large-diameter rotating anodes, beveled targets to spread the deposited energy over a larger target volume, and referral by the operator to tube rating charts to restrict the rate of energy deposition.[16,17]

In the equation $P_d = VI$, the voltage may also be expressed in kilovolts if the current is described in milliamperes.

Example 2-3

In 0.5 sec, 1.25×10^{18} electrons (400 mA) are accelerated across a constant potential difference of 100 kV. At what rate is energy deposited in the x-ray target?

$$P = VI$$
$$= (10^5 \ V)(0.4 \ A)$$
$$= 4 \times 10^4 \text{ watts}$$

Example 2-4

If the x-ray tube in Example 2-3 has a tungsten target ($Z = 74$), determine the power P_r emitted as x radiation and the efficiency of x-ray production.

$$P_r = 0.9 \times 10^{-9} (Z)(V^2)(I)$$
$$= 0.9 \times 10^{-9} (74)(10^5)^2 (0.4)$$
$$= 2.7 \times 10^2 \text{ watts}$$
$$\text{Efficiency} = 0.9 \times 10^{-9} (Z)(V)$$
$$= 0.9 \times 10^{-9} (74)(10^5)$$
$$= 0.67 \times 10^{-2} \cong 0.7\%$$

Approximate efficiency of x-ray production.

KVP	Heat(%)	X rays(%)
50	99.7	0.3
200	99	1
6000	65	35

At tube voltages employed in diagnostic radiology, x rays are emitted approximately at right angles to the incident electrons, and a reflectance target is used to produce an x-ray beam at a 90° angle to the axis of the x-ray tube. At the multi-MV voltages, and therefore greater electron energies employed in radiation therapy, x-ray production is much more efficient, and stationary anodes of reduced mass can be used. At these electron energies, x rays are produced in the forward direction (in the direction of the impinging electrons). In radiation therapy, thin *transmission targets* are used that transmit the x rays with little attenuation on their way from the target to the patient. The efficiency of x-ray production is sufficiently high that anodes of large mass are not required for purposes of heat dissipation. Hence the x rays can be

In radiation therapy the increased efficiency of x-ray production also permits use of stationery rather than rotating x-ray targets.

transmitted in a forward direction through the target without substantial attenuation. Transmission targets frequently employ a cooling mechanism, such as circulating water, to control the target temperature.

The energies of characteristic x rays from an x-ray target reflect the binding energies of electrons in the target, particularly those in the K, L, and M shells. In a typically x-ray spectrum, the principal peak of characteristic x rays reflects electron transitions from the L to the K shell, and a second peak depicts transitions from the M to the K shell. In either case, the x rays have energies slightly below the K binding energies of electrons in the target material. As described in Chapter 3, x rays with energies slightly below the binding energy of K electrons of a material are transmitted through the material with little attenuation. Therefore, a filter of the same material as an x-ray target transmits characteristic x rays from the target with little attenuation. This property is employed in mammographic x-ray tubes, in which a molybdenum target is used to provide characteristic x rays (17–20 keV) of a desirable energy for imaging soft tissue. A molybdenum filter placed in the x-ray beam transmits the characteristic x rays with little attenuation, but absorbs many of the bremsstrahlung photons of lower energies. In all but the heaviest elements, transitions of electrons into the L and higher shells result in the release of electromagnetic radiations that are too low in energy to be classified as x rays, or so low in energy that they are readily absorbed by the inherent and added filtration in the x-ray beam.

As mentioned earlier, interaction of a high-energy electron with a target nucleus can produce a bremsstrahlung photon with any energy up to the total kinetic energy of the electron. Such a photon would possess the maximum energy (and therefore minimum wavelength) of the photons in an x-ray beam generated at a particular tube voltage. Hence the minimum wavelength photons in an x-ray beam are related to the peak kilovoltage applied across the x-ray tube. With λ_{min} expressed in nanometers, the relationship is

$$\text{Maximum photon energy (keV)} = h\nu_{max} = \text{maximum tube voltage (kVp)}$$

But $\nu_{max} = c/\lambda_{min}$, where c is the speed of light in a vacuum:

$$\frac{hc}{\lambda_{min}} = V\,(\text{kVp})$$

$$\lambda_{min} = hc/V\,(\text{kVp})$$

$$\lambda_{min} = 1.24/V\,(\text{kvp})$$

with the minimum wavelength λ_{min} expressed in nm.

In the past, x-ray wavelengths were described in units of angstroms (Å), where $1\,\text{Å} = 10^{-10}m$. The minimum wavelength in angstroms would be $\lambda_{min}\,(\text{Å}) = 12.4/\text{kVp}$. The angstrom is no longer used as a measure of wavelength.

Example 2-5

0.00025 nm ($0.00025 \times 10^{-3}\mu m$) is the λ_{min} of x rays in a therapeutic x-ray beam. What is the maximum energy x ray that corresponds to λ_{min}, and what voltage characterizes the x-ray beam?

$$\lambda_{min} = 1.24/E\,(\text{keV})$$

$$E\,(\text{keV}) = 1.24/\lambda_{min} = 1.24/0.00025\,\text{nm}$$

$$= 4.96\,\text{MeV}$$

Since $E\,(\text{keV}) = V\,(\text{kVp})$, the x-ray beam voltage is "4.96 MV."
Note: At energies above the orthovoltage range, x-ray beams are generated by mechanisms that accelerate electrons uniformly, so the p to designate peak kilovoltage is not used.

The voltage across the x-ray tube determines the maximum x-ray energy and the efficiency of x-ray production. The number of electrons impinging on the target also influences the quantity of x rays during an exposure. The number of electrons is a

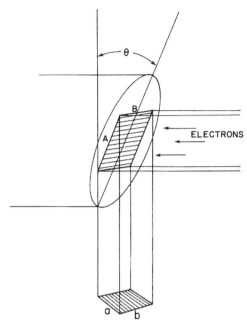

FIGURE 2-8
Line focus principle in which the apparent focal spot is much smaller than the true focal spot.

function of the tube current (milliamperes) and the exposure time (seconds), often expressed as the mAs of the exposure. That is, the kVp influences both the "quality" (energy or penetrating ability) and the quantity of x rays present in the x-ray beam, whereas the mAs influences only the quantity.

Example 2-6

Compute the total number of electrons impinging on the target of an x-ray tube operated at 400 mA for 0.05 sec.

The ampere (A), the unit of electrical current, equals one coulomb per second, and the product of current and time equals the total charge in coulombs. 400 mA = 0.4 A, and one electron = 1.6×10^{-19} coulombs $\{Q \text{ (coulombs)} = [I \text{ (amperes)}] \times [t \text{ (sec)}]\}$:

$$\text{Number of electrons} = \frac{(0.4\text{A})(\text{coulomb/sec-A})(0.05 \text{ sec})}{1.6 \times 10^{-19} \text{ coulombs/electron}} = 1.25 \times 10^{17} \text{ electrons}$$

To produce x-ray images of highest quality, the x rays should emerge from a small volume of reflectance target to provide a sharply defined x-ray beam. This volume of target is referred to as the *focal spot* of the x-ray tube. To reduce the focal spot, the target usually is beveled at a steep angle with respect to the direction of the incident electrons. With the target at a steep angle, the x rays appear to originate from an "apparent focal spot" that appears much smaller than the "true focal spot" (Figure 2-8). This approach to focal spot reduction is termed the *line focus principle* and is widely employed in diagnostic x-ray tubes in which target angles between 6° and 17° are used. The line focus principle is not applicable to most x-ray sources used in radiation therapy because transmission rather than reflectance targets are employed. These sources are discussed in Chapter 4. The line focus principle is important in x-ray tubes employed in x-ray and computed tomography simulators used for treatment planning and patient monitoring in radiation therapy. These simulators are discussed in Chapters 4 and 11.

■ SUMMARY

Features of the production of x rays include:

- The importance of electron interactions with electrons in producing characteristic x rays
- The importance of electron interactions with nuclei in producing bremsstrahlung
- The distinction between elastic and inelastic electron interactions

The work function $\overline{W}/e$ has a value of 33.97 eV/IP in air.

The linear energy transfer is the product of the SI (IP/cm) and the work function.

An x-ray tube may be operated under either space-charge-limited or filament-emission-limited conditions.

X-ray production efficiency may be increased by the use of rectification (self-, half-wave, full-wave) and special x-ray circuits (3-phase and high frequency).

X-ray spectra are influenced by tube current, tube voltage, x-ray circuitry (3∅, high frequency), and beam filtration.

The line-focus principle is employed to reduce the size of the apparent focal spot.

PROBLEMS

2-1. Electrons with a kinetic energy of 1.0 MeV have a SI in air of about 60 IP/cm. What is the LET of these electrons in air?

2-2. 2.0 MeV alpha particles have an LET in air of 0.175 keV/μm. What is the SI of these particles in air if $\overline{W}/e$ is assumed to be 33.97 eV/IP?

2-3. How many electrons flow from the filament to the target each second in an x-ray tube with a tube current of 200 mA? If the tube voltage is a constant 100 kV, what is the power (energy/second) delivered to the target?

2-4. An apparent focal spot of 1 mm is projected from an x-ray target with a "true" focal spot of 5 mm (see diagram below). What is the target angle?

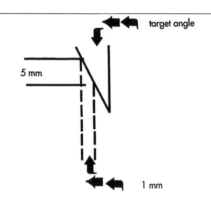

2-5. What is the kinetic energy of electrons accelerated through a potential difference of 250 kV? What fraction of the energy is expended as radiation energy loss as the electrons interact in a tungsten target? What is the λ_{min} of the x rays?

REFERENCES

1. Hendee, W. R., and Ritenour, E. R. *Medical Imaging Physics,* 4th edition. New York, John Wiley & Sons, New York. 2001.
2. Scherzer, O. Radiation emitted on the stopping of protons and fast electrons. *Ann. Physik* 1932; **13**:137.
3. Andrews, H. *Radiation Physics.* Englewood Cliffs, NJ, Prentice-Hall International, 1961.
4. Jayaraman, S., and Lanzl, L. *Clinical Radiotherapy Physics, Vol. 1: Basic Physics and Dosimetry.* Boca Raton, FL, CRC Press, 1996.
5. Wehr, M., Richard, J. *Physics of the Atom.* Reading, MA, Addison-Wesley, 1960, p. 159.
6. Röntgen, W. C. Über eine Art von Strahlen (vorläufige Mitteilung), *Sitzungs-Berichte der Physikalisch-medicinschen Gesellschaft zu Wurzurg* 1895; **9**:132.
7. Donizetti, P. *Shadow and Substance: The Story of Medical Radiography.* Oxford, Pergamon Press, 1967.
8. Glasser, O. *Dr. W.C. Roentgen,* 2nd edition. Springfield, IL, Charles C Thomas, 1958.
9. Feldman, A. Technical history of radiology (1896–1920). *Radiographics* 1989; **9**:1113–1128.
10. Coolidge, W. A powerful roentgen ray tube with a pure electron discharge. *Phys. Rev.* 1913; **2**:409.
11. Bloom, W., Hollenbach, J., and Morgan, J. (eds.) *Medical Radiographic Technic,* 3rd edition. Springfield, IL, Charles C Thomas, 1965.
12. Chaney, E., and Hendee, W. Effects of x-ray tube current and voltage on effective focal-spot size. *Med. Phys.* 1974; **1**:141.
13. Dance, D. R. Diagnostic radiology with x rays. In *The Physics of Medical Imaging,* (S. Webb (ed.). Philadelphia, Institute of Physics, 1988, pp. 20–73.
14. Hendee, W., and Chaney, E. X-ray focal spots: Practical considerations. *Appl. Radiol.* 1974; **3**:25.
15. Curry, T. S., Dowdey, J. E., and Murray, R. C. *Christensen's Physics of Diagnostic Radiology,* 4th edition. Malvern, PA, Lea & Febiger, 1990.
16. Hallock, A. A review of methods used to calculate heat loading of x-ray tubes extending the life of rotating anode x-ray tubes. *Cathode Press* 1958; **15**:1.
17. Johnson, R. Production and interaction of x rays, radiation measurement quantities and units. In *Biomedical Uses of Radiation—Part A: Diagnostic Applications,* W. Hendee (ed.). New York, Wiley-VCH, 1999.

CHAPTER

3

INTERACTIONS OF X RAYS AND GAMMA RAYS

OBJECTIVES 36

INTRODUCTION 36

ATTENUATION OF X RAYS AND GAMMA RAYS 36

X-RAY AND GAMMA-RAY INTERACTIONS 40

Coherent Scattering 41
Photoelectric Interactions 41

Compton Interactions 43
Pair Production 47
Photodisintegration 48
Likelihood of Interactions 48

SUMMARY 49

PROBLEMS 49

REFERENCES 50

Radiation Therapy Physics, Third Edition, by William R. Hendee, Geoffrey S. Ibbott, and Eric G. Hendee
ISBN 0-471-39493-9 Copyright © 2005 John Wiley & Sons, Inc.

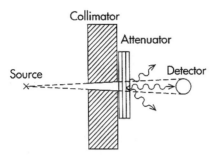

Narrow-beam geometry

MARGIN FIGURE 3-1

Narrow-beam (good) geometry. (From W. R. Hendee and E. R. Ritenour,[1] with permission.)

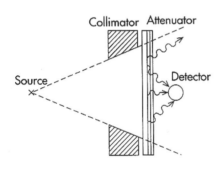

Broad-beam geometry

MARGIN FIGURE 3-2

Broad-beam (poor) geometry for attenuation measurements. (From W. R. Hendee and E. R. Ritenour,[1] with permission.)

X or γ rays impinging on a material may be (1) absorbed, (2) scattered, or (3) transmitted.

Radiation transmitted through a material without interaction is termed *primary radiation*. Radiation scattered in the material is called *secondary radiation* (along with leakage radiation from the radiation source).

Attenuation refers to any process that removes photons from an x- or γ-ray beam.

Narrow-beam and broad-beam geometries are sometimes referred to as "good" and "poor" geometries.

The differential form of the attenuation equation is written $dI/dx = -\mu I$.

■ OBJECTIVES

After studying this chapter, the reader should be able to:

- Perform simple computations related to x- and γ-ray attenuation and transmission.
- Distinguish among various attenuation and absorption coefficients and convert one to another.
- Explain exponential attenuation and broad- and narrow-beam geometry.
- Outline the principles and the variables that influence
  - Photoelectric interactions
  - Compton interactions
  - Pair production
- Compute the energy of Compton-scattered photons.
- Define concepts such as
  - Half- and tenth-value layers
  - Mean free path
  - Linear attenuation coefficient
  - Compton wavelength

■ INTRODUCTION

An x or gamma (γ) ray impinging on a material leads to one of three possible outcomes. The photon may be: (1) absorbed by transfer of its energy to the material through one or more interactions; (2) scattered in a different direction during one or more interactions; or (3) transmitted through the material without interaction. Photons that traverse a material without interaction are referred to as primary photons or *primary radiation*, whereas photons that are scattered are considered *secondary radiation*. If the photon is absorbed or scattered, it is said to have undergone *attenuation*. Attenuation processes can involve single or multiple interactions and can result in transfer of all or only part of the photon's energy to the material. Scattering usually removes photons from an x- or γ-ray beam but does not always do so, especially if the beam is broad or the scattering occurs through small angles. As the distance increases on the far side of a scattering material, the number of scattered photons decreases in an x- or γ-ray beam, because the scatter photons have a greater likelihood of escaping from the beam. A measurement of x- or γ-ray intensity for a narrow beam of photons at a location far from a scatterer is said to be taken under conditions of narrow-beam geometry. A similar measurement obtained near a scatterer or for a broad beam of photons is considered to have been acquired under conditions of broad-beam geometry. These concepts are illustrated in the marginal illustrations.[1]

■ ATTENUATION OF X RAYS AND GAMMA RAYS

The fractional number of photons $\Delta I/I$ attenuated in an infinitesimally thin slab of material of thickness Δx is $\Delta I/I = -\mu \Delta x$, where μ is referred to as the attenuation coefficient.[1] Under conditions of narrow-beam geometry, the number of photons I transmitted through a material of finite thickness x is

$$I = I_0 e^{-\mu x}$$

The fractional transmission is $I/I_0 = e^{-\mu x}$, where I_0 is the number of photons reaching the same point on the far side of the attenuating material in the absence of the material. The expression $e^{-\mu x}$ represents the exponential quantity e raised to the power $-\mu x$, where $e = 2.7183$ as described in Chapter 1. The number I^* of x or γ rays attenuated (absorbed or scattered) in the material is

$$I^* = I_0 - I = I_0 - I_0 e^{-\mu x}$$
$$= I_0(I - e^{-\mu x})$$

The fractional attenuation is $I^*/I_0 = I - e^{-\mu x}$.

The exponent of e must carry no units. Hence, if the thickness x has units of cm, μ must have units of 1/cm (or m and 1/m, mm and 1/mm, and so on). An attenuation coefficient with units of 1/length is called a *linear attenuation coefficient*. The value of the linear attenuation coefficient depends on the energy of the x or γ rays and the composition (atomic number and physical density) of the material.

At times, the dependence of μ on the physical density (g/cm^3) of the attenuating material is troublesome, and a coefficient that is independent of density is desirable. The mass attenuation coefficient has this advantage. The mass attenuation coefficient μ_m is the linear attenuation coefficient divided by the density of the material. Mass attenuation coefficients have units of area/mass, such as cm^2/g or m^2/kg. Thicknesses are expressed in units of mass/area (e.g., g/cm^2 or kg/m^2) when they are used in combination with mass attenuating coefficients. Thicknesses expressed in units of mass per unit area are termed area thicknesses and are computed as the product of the linear thickness (cm or m) times the physical density (g/cm^3 or kg/m^3).

Attenuation coefficients may also have other units. For example, the atomic attenuation coefficient μ_a has units of area/atom (e.g., cm^2/atom or m^2/atom), and corresponding thicknesses have units of atoms/area. Another coefficient encountered occasionally is the electronic attenuation coefficient u_e, with units of area/electron. Corresponding attenuator thicknesses have units of electrons/area. Conversion among attenuation coefficients and computations with different coefficients are illustrated in Example 3-1.

There is no exact analytical expression for transmission of photons under broad-beam conditions. The expression usually encountered is $I = BI_0 e^{-\mu x}$, where B is a *build-up factor* that varies with the area and energy of the photon beam and the nature of the attenuating material.

Use of linear attenuation coefficients may be troublesome in instances where the density of the material (and therefore the value of the coefficient) varies.

The mass attenuation coefficient μ_m may also be written as $\mu_{/\rho}$, where μ is the linear attenuation coefficient and ρ is the density of the absorbing material.

The atomic attenuation coefficient μ_a is related to the linear attenuation coefficient μ by $\mu_a = \mu M/\rho N_a$.

The electronic attenuation coefficient is related to the linear attenuation coefficient μ by $\mu_e = \mu_a/Z = \mu M/\rho N_a Z$.

Relationships among Attenuation Coefficients

Coefficient	Symbol	Unit
Linear	μ	m^{-1}
Mass	μ_m	m^2/kg
Atomic	μ_z	m^2/atom
Electronic	μ_e	m^2/electron

Example 3-1

A. A narrow beam of 5000 monoenergetic photons is reduced to 1000 photons by a copper absorber 2 cm thick. What is the total linear attenuation coefficient of the copper absorber for these photons?

$$I = I_0 e^{-\mu x}$$
$$I/I_0 = e^{-\mu x}$$
$$I_0/I = e^{\mu x}$$
$$\ln I_0/I = \mu x$$
$$\ln\left[\frac{5000}{1000}\right] = \mu[2\text{ cm}]$$
$$\mu = \ln(5)/2\text{ cm} = 1.61/2\text{ cm}$$
$$\mu = 0.81\text{ cm}^{-1}$$

B. What are the total mass (μ_m), atomic (μ_a), and electronic (μ_e) attenuation coefficients? Copper has a density of ρ of 8.9 g/cm^3, a gram-atomic mass M of 63.6, and an atomic number Z of 29.

$$\mu_m = \mu/\rho = 0.81\text{ cm}^{-1}/8.9\text{ g/cm}^3$$
$$= 0.091\text{ cm}^2/\text{g}$$

$$\mu_a = \frac{\mu M}{\rho N_A} = \frac{(0.81\text{ cm}^{-1})(63.6\text{ g/g-atomic mass})}{(8.9\text{ g/cm}^3)(6.02 \times 10^{23}\text{ atoms/g-atomic mass})}$$

$$= 9.6 \times 10^{-24}\text{cm}^2/\text{atom}$$

$$\mu_e = \mu_a/Z = (9.6 \times 10^{-24}\text{cm}^2/\text{atom})/29\text{ electrons/atom}$$

$$= 3.3 \times 10^{-25}\text{cm}^2/\text{electron}$$

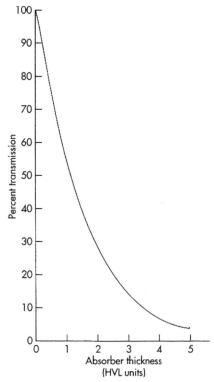

MARGIN FIGURE 3-3

Linear plot of percent transmission of a narrow beam of monoenergetic photons as a function of the thickness of an attenuator in units of HVL.

The mean path length is also called the mean free path or relaxation length.

The half-value layer is sometimes termed the *half-value thickness (HVT)*.

C. An additional 2 cm of copper is added to the copper absorber in part A. How may photons remain in the beam?

$$I = I_0 e^{-\mu x} = 5000 e^{-(0.81\,\text{cm}^{-1})(4\,\text{cm})}$$

$$= 5000 e^{-3.24}$$

$$= 5000(0.0392)$$

$$= 200 \text{ photons}$$

The first 2 cm of copper absorbed 4000 photons (80%), leaving 1000 photons in the beam. An additional 800 photons (80%) is absorbed by the second 2 cm of Cu, leaving 200 photons in the beam.

D. What is the thickness x_e in electrons per square centimeter for the 4-cm absorber?

$$x_e = x_a Z = \frac{x N_a p Z}{M}$$

$$= \frac{(4\,\text{cm})(6.02 \times 10^{23}\,\text{atoms/g-atomic mass})(8.9\,\text{g/cm}^3)\,(29\,\text{electrons/atoms})}{63.6\,\text{g/g-atomic mass}}$$

$$= 9.77 \times 10^{24}\,\text{electrons/cm}^2$$

E. Repeat the calculation in part C using the electronic attenuation coefficient.

$$I = I_0 e^{-\mu x}$$

$$= 5000 e^{-(3.3 \times 10^{-25}\,\text{cm}^2/\text{electron})(9.77 \times 10^{24}\,\text{electrons/cm}^2)}$$

$$= 5000(0.0392)$$

$$= 200 \text{ photons}$$

The mean path length is the average distance traveled by x or γ rays before they interact with a particular material. The mean path length is $1/\mu$, where μ is the linear attenuation coefficient of the material for the particular photons.

The thickness of a material required to reduce the intensity of an x- or γ-ray beam to half under conditions of good geometry is called the *half-value layer (HVL)*. The HVL is related to the attenuation coefficient by the expression HVL = $0.693/\mu$, where 0.693 is the ln 2. In Example 3-1, the HVL is $0.693/0.81\,\text{cm}^{-1} = 0.85\,\text{cm}$ of Cu. Half-value layers can be expressed in other units, such as g/cm^2, atoms/cm^2, or electrons/cm^2.

The expression $I = I_0 e^{-\mu x}$ is termed an exponential equation. A narrow beam of monoenergetic x or gamma rays passed through a material of constant composition is said to be attenuated exponentially. Rewriting the exponential equation in logarithmic form yields

$$\ln(I/I_0) = -\mu x$$

This expression reveals that ln (I/I_0) decreases linearly with increasing thickness of the attenuator. The relationship is depicted in the margin, where I/I_0, expressed as percent transmission, is plotted on both a linear and a logarithmic axis as a function of thickness x of the attenuator on a linear axis. A graph of I/I_0 on a logarithmic axis and x on a linear axis is termed a *semilogarithmic plot*.

For an x- or γ-ray beam to be attenuated exponentially, it must be monoenergetic and measured under conditions of good geometry. A polyenergetic beam such as an x-ray beam from a linear accelerator is not attenuated exponentially because the absorber selectively removes lower-energy x rays from the beam. As a consequence, the beam's average energy, and therefore its attenuation coefficient, changes as the beam proceeds through the material. These changes result in a gradual increase in the penetrating ability of the x-ray beam, as it moves through the attenuator and lower-energy x rays are selectively removed.

From measurements of the HVL of a polyenergetic beam, an effective attenuation coefficient μ_{eff} can be estimated as $\mu_{\text{eff}} = 0.693/\text{HVL}$. The effective energy can then be determined as the energy of monoenergetic photons that have an attenuation coefficient identical to μ_{eff}.

The homogeneity coefficient is the ratio of the first HVL (the thickness of attenuator required to reduce the beam's intensity to half) divided by the second HVL (the thickness required to reduce the intensity from half to one-quarter). For a narrow, monoenergetic beam, the homogeneity coefficient is unity; for polyenergetic beams, it is less than unity.

In general, the attenuation coefficient of a material decreases with increasing energy of incident photons. Consequently, lower-energy photons are attenuated more readily than those of higher energy. A polyenergetic beam becomes more penetrating (it is said to become "harder") after it has traversed an attenuating material because lower-energy photons have been selectively removed from the beam.

Example 3-2

1.2 mm of copper is required to reduce the intensity of an x-ray beam to half, and an additional 1.4 mm is needed to reduce the intensity from half to one-quarter. What are the first HVL, homogeneity coefficient, effective linear and mass attenuation coefficients, and effective energy of the x-ray beam?

$$\text{HVL} = 1.2\,\text{cm Cu}$$

$$\text{Homogeneity coefficient} = \frac{(\text{HVL})_1}{(\text{HVL})_2} = \frac{1.2\,\text{mm Cu}}{1.4\,\text{mm Cu}}$$

$$= 0.86$$

$$\mu_{\text{eff}} = 0.693/\text{HVL} = 0.693/1.2\,\text{mm Cu}$$

$$= 0.58\,\text{mm}^{-1} = 5.8\,\text{cm}^{-1}$$

$$(\mu_{\text{eff}})_m = \mu_{\text{eff}}/\rho = 5.8\,\text{cm}^{-1}/8.9\,\text{g/cm}^3$$

$$= 0.652\,\text{cm}^2/\text{g}$$

Monoenergetic photons of 88 keV have a total mass attenuation coefficient of $0.65\,\text{cm}^2/\text{g}$ in copper. Consequently the effective energy of the x-ray beam is 88 keV.

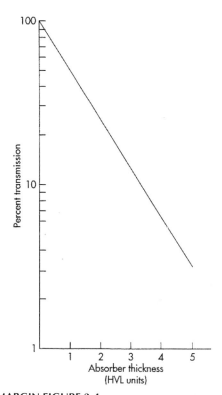

MARGIN FIGURE 3-4
Semilogarithmic plot of percent transmission of a narrow beam of monoenergetic photons as a function of the thickness of an attenuator in units of HVL.

The attenuation coefficient μ describes the removal of photons from an x- or γ-ray beam by either absorption or scattering. To determine the energy removed from the beam by absorptive processes alone (i.e., energy removed by scattering processes is ignored), the energy absorption coefficient μ_{en} must be used, where $\mu_{\text{en}} = \mu[E_a/h\nu]$ and E_a represents the average energy absorbed in the attenuator during interaction of a photon of energy $h\nu^3$. The energy absorption coefficient may also be expressed as the mass energy absorption coefficient $(\mu_{\text{en}})_m$, atomic energy absorption coefficient $(\mu_{\text{en}})_a$, or electronic energy absorption coefficient $(\mu_{\text{en}})_e$, by dividing μ_{en} by the physical density, number of atoms per centimeter, or number of electrons per centimeter.

A closely related concept to the energy absorption coefficient μ_{en} is the energy transfer coefficient μ_{tr}. The energy absorption coefficient equals the energy transfer coefficient corrected for a reduction in energy absorbed in the absorber because of the loss of bremsstrahlung and characteristic x rays. The relationship between μ_{en} and μ_{tr} is $\mu_{\text{en}} = \mu_{\text{tr}}(1-g)$, where g is the fraction of the energy deposited in the absorber by impinging photons that is radiated from the absorber as characteristic x rays and bremsstrahlung. The energy absorption coefficient is used in radiation therapy to estimate the energy absorbed in tissues exposed to a beam of x or gamma rays. Attenuation and energy absorption coefficients for water (a medium that closely simulates muscle) are plotted in Figure 3-1 as a function of photon energy.

A "hard" x-ray beam is able to penetrate dense (i.e., "hard") substances such as bone. A low-energy x-ray beam is said to be "soft" because it is able to penetrate only low-density (i.e., "soft") substances such as "soft tissue"—fat and muscle.

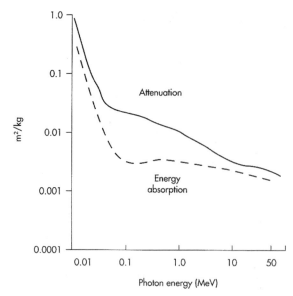

FIGURE 3-1
Total mass attenuation and energy absorption coefficients for water as a function of photon energy.

Example 3-3

The attenuation coefficient is 0.071 cm^{-1} for 1-MeV photons in water. If the energy absorption coefficient for 1-MeV photons in water is 0.031 cm^{-1}, find the average energy absorbed in water per photon interaction.

$$\mu_{en} = \mu \frac{E_a}{h\nu}$$

$$E_a = \frac{\mu_{en}}{\mu}(h\nu)$$

$$= \frac{0.031\,\text{cm}^{-1}}{0.071\,\text{cm}^{-1}}(1\,\text{MeV})$$

$$= 0.44\,\text{MeV}$$

$$= 440\,\text{keV}$$

■ X-RAY AND GAMMA-RAY INTERACTIONS

X rays and γ rays can interact by several different mechanisms, including coherent scattering, photoelectric absorption, Compton scattering, pair production, and photodisintegration. These possibilities can be depicted as

$$e^{-\mu x} = (e^{-\omega x}) \cdot (e^{-\tau x}) \cdot (e^{-\sigma x}) \cdot (e^{-\kappa x}) \cdot (e^{-\pi x}) = e^{-(\omega+\tau+\sigma+\kappa+\pi)x}$$

where $e^{-\mu x}$ is the probability that a photon traverses a medium of thickness x without interacting, and $e^{-\omega x} \ldots e^{-\pi x}$ represent the probabilities that the photon does not interact by specific interaction mechanisms. The total linear attenuation coefficient can be partitioned into separate coefficients for coherent scattering (ω), photoelectric absorption (τ), Compton scattering (σ), pair production (κ), and photodisintegration (π). At times, this expression can be simplified to fewer coefficients because certain mechanisms of interaction are negligible. A diagnostic x-ray beam cannot interact by pair production or photodisintegration because the energy of the x rays is too low. Hence, the expression for μ simplifies to $\mu = \omega + \tau + \sigma$ for a diagnostic x-ray beam. Similarly, a therapeutic x-ray beam may not interact by coherent scattering or photodisintegration, permitting simplification of the expression for μ to $\mu = \tau +$

$\sigma + \kappa$. The individual coefficients for various interactions have equivalent expressions for mass, atomic, and electronic coefficients. For example,

$$\mu_m = \frac{\mu}{\rho}; \quad \omega_m = \frac{\omega}{\rho}; \quad \tau_m = \frac{\tau}{\rho}; \quad \sigma_m = \frac{\sigma}{\rho}; \quad \kappa_m = \frac{\kappa}{\rho}; \quad \pi_m = \frac{\pi}{\rho}$$

Coherent Scattering

Photons are deflected or scattered by the process of *coherent (Rayleigh) scattering*, sometimes referred to as classical scattering.[4] In this interaction, the energy of a photon is transferred completely to an atom, which then radiates the energy of the photon in a slightly different direction (see Margin Figure 3-5). Hence the incoming photon appears to have shifted in direction (i.e., to have been scattered) with no change in energy.

Coherent scattering is negligible for high-energy photons interacting in relatively low-Z tissues, such as those in the body. Hence, it can be ignored in essentially all applications of radiation therapy.

Photoelectric Interactions

A *photoelectric interaction* results in transfer of the total energy of a photon to an inner electron of an atom of the absorbing medium (see Margin Figure 3-6). The electron is ejected from the atom with kinetic energy $E_k = h\nu - E_b$, where $h\nu$ is the energy of the photon and E_b is the binding energy of the ejected electron, termed a *photoelectron*. For low-energy photons, photoelectrons are ejected at close to right angles to the direction of the incident photons. As the energy of incident photons increases, the photoelectrons are ejected increasingly in the direction of the incident photons. Vacancies created by ejected electrons are filled by cascading electrons, resulting in emission of characteristic photons and Auger electrons. When photons interact photoelectrically in tissue, the characteristic photons and Auger electrons have energies less than 0.5 keV and are readily absorbed in tissue in the immediate vicinity of the site of interaction.

Photoelectric interactions occur primarily for x and γ rays of relatively low energy, and the probability of this type of interaction decreases rapidly with increasing photon energy. In general, the mass attenuation coefficient for photoelectric absorption decrease as $(1/h\nu)^3$, where $h\nu$ is the photon energy. Shown in Figure 3-2 are the mass attenuation coefficients for photoelectric interaction in muscle and lead, plotted as a function of photon energy. Discontinuities in the curve for lead, termed *absorption edges*, occur at photon energies equal to the binding energy of electrons in the inner electron shells. Photons with energy less than the binding energy of K-shell electrons cannot eject K electrons from the atom. These photons can interact photoelectrically only with more loosely bound electrons in the L, M, and other shells. Photons with energy greater than the K binding energy selectively interact with K electrons through the photoelectric process. The threshold energy for photoelectric interactions with K-shell electrons causes an abrupt increase in the photoelectric attenuation coefficient at the K-binding energy. In soft tissue, the binding energy of K-shell electrons is too low to be depicted in Figure 3-2. The elements iodine and barium have binding energies of 33 and 36 keV, respectively, and are considered almost ideal absorbers of x rays in the diagnostic energy range. For this reason, they are widely employed as contrast agents in diagnostic radiology.[2]

The probability of photoelectric interaction depends on the atomic number of the absorbing material as well as on the energy of the x or γ rays. In general, the photoelectric mass attenuation coefficient varies directly with Z^3. The likelihood of photoelectric interaction of low-energy photons is almost four times greater in bone ($Z_{eff} = 11.6$) than in an equal mass of soft tissue ($Z_{eff} = 7.4$) because $(11.6/7.4)^3 = 3.8$. The expression Z_{eff} represents the effective atomic number of a multielement absorber, defined as the Z of an imaginary single element that attenuates x and

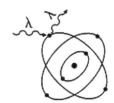

MARGIN FIGURE 3-5
Coherent scattering in which the photon is absorbed and reradiated in a different direction with no significant loss of energy.

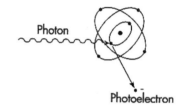

MARGIN FIGURE 3-6
Photoelectric interaction in which the photon disappears and is replaced by an electron ejected from the atom with kinetic energy $E_k = h\nu - E_b$, where E_b is the electron binding energy. Characteristic radiation and Auger electrons are emitted as cascading electrons replace the ejected photoelectron.

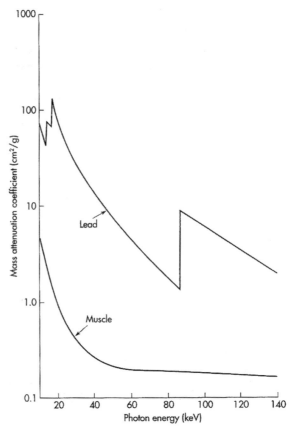

FIGURE 3-2
Mass attenuation coefficient for photons in muscle and lead as a function of photon energy. K- and L-absorption edges are depicted in lead.

Photoelectric interactions

- Involve only bound electrons
- Increase in likelihood with Z^3
- Decrease in likelihood with $(h\nu)^3$
- More than 80% of photoelectric interactions in tissue involve K electrons

gamma rays in the same manner as the absorber. The effective atomic number is discussed further in Chapter 5.

Example 3-4

What is the kinetic energy of a photoelectron ejected from the K shell of lead ($E_b = 88$ keV) by photoelectric absorption of a 200-keV photon?

$$E_k = h\nu = E_b$$
$$= 200\,\text{keV} - 88\,\text{keV}$$
$$= 112\,\text{keV}$$

Selective attenuation of photons by photoelectric interactions in materials with different atomic numbers and different physical densities is one of the principal reasons why low-energy x rays are useful for producing images in diagnostic radiology. Photoelectric interactions rarely occur at the higher photon energies employed in radiation therapy. Hence, differences in atomic number among different media are relatively unimportant in determine the likelihood of photon interactions in radiation therapy. This property is advantageous in therapy because it permits delivery of relatively large doses of soft tissue tumors without excessive doses to higher-Z structures such as bone.

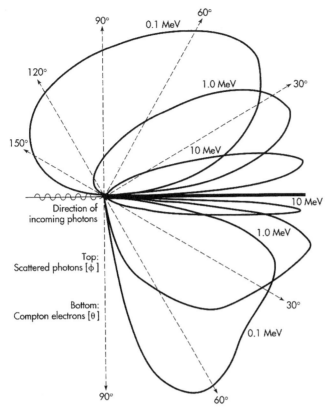

FIGURE 3-3
Electron scattering angle θ as a function of the energy of incident photons. Both θ and ϕ decrease as the energy of incident photons increases.[1]

Compton Interactions

X and γ rays with energies between 30 keV and 30 MeV interact in soft tissue principally by Compton scattering. In this type of photon interaction, part of the energy of the photon is transferred to a loosely bound or "free" electron in the medium (see Margin Figure 3-7). The electron, termed a Compton electron, is set into motion with a kinetic energy equal to the energy transferred by the incident photon, less any binding energy (almost always negligible) that must be overcome in ejecting the electron from its atom. The direction of the Compton electron, defined as the electron scattering angle θ, is confined to the forward hemisphere (i.e., $\pm90°$) with respect to the direction of the incident photon. In the interaction process, the incident photon is scattered with reduced energy at the photon scattering angle ϕ with respect to its original direction. This angle may be any value (i.e., up to $\pm180°$) with respect to the original photon direction. Both θ and ϕ tend to narrow with increasing energy of the incident photon (Figure 3-3).

During a Compton interaction, the change in wavelength ($\Delta\lambda$) in nanometers of the x or γ ray is $\Delta\lambda = 0.00243 (1 - \cos\phi)$, where ϕ is the scattering angle of the photon. The wavelength λ' of the scattered photon is $\lambda' = \lambda + \Delta\lambda$, where λ is the wavelength of the incident photon. The energies $h\nu'$ and E_k of the scattered photon and electron, respectively, are

$$h\nu' = h\nu \left[\frac{1}{1 + \alpha(1 - \cos\phi)} \right]$$

$$E_k = h\nu - h\nu' = h\nu \left[\frac{\alpha(1 - \cos\phi)}{1 + \alpha(1 - \cos\phi)} \right]$$

where $\alpha = h\nu/m_0c^2$ and m_0c^2 is the rest mass energy of the electron (0.511 MeV).

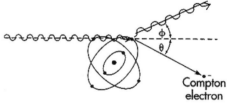

MARGIN FIGURE 3-7
Compton scattering of an incident photon, with the photon scattered at an angle ϕ and the Compton electron ejected at an angle θ with respect to the direction of the incident photon.

Compton scattering is named for Arthur Holly Compton, who in 1927 was awarded the Nobel Prize in Physics for his work on x-ray scattering.

$\Delta\lambda$ is frequently referred to as the *Compton shift* or *Compton wavelength*.[5]

Example 3-5

A 250-keV photon is scattered at an angle of 60° during a Compton interaction. What are the energies of the scattered photon and the Compton electron?

The wavelength λ of the incident photon is

$$\lambda = \frac{1.24}{h\nu} = \frac{1.24}{250\,\text{keV}}$$

$$= 0.005\,\text{nm}$$

The change in wavelength $\Delta\lambda$ during the scattering process is

$$\Delta\lambda = 0.00243(1 - \cos\phi)$$

$$= 0.00243(1 - \cos(60°))$$

$$= 0.00243(1 - 0.5)$$

$$= 0.00122\,\text{nm}$$

The wavelength λ' of the scattered photon is

$$\lambda' = \lambda + \Delta\lambda$$

$$= (0.0050 + 0.0012)\,\text{nm} = 0.0062\,\text{nm}$$

The energy of the scattered photon is

$$h\nu' = \frac{1.24}{\lambda'} = \frac{1.24}{0.0062\,\text{nm}}$$

$$= 200\,\text{keV}$$

The energy of the Compton electron is

$$E_k = h\nu - h\nu' = (250 - 200)\,\text{keV}$$

$$= 50\,\text{keV}$$

The energy of the scattered photon and Compton electron can also be determined with the expressions

$$h\nu' = h\nu \left[\frac{1}{1 + \alpha(1 - \cos\phi)} \right]$$

$$= 250\,\text{keV} \left[\frac{1}{1 + (250/511)(1 - \cos(60°))} \right]$$

$$= 250\,\text{keV} \left[\frac{1}{1 + (0.489)(1 - 0.5)} \right]$$

$$= 250\,\text{keV}\,[0.8]$$

$$= 200\,\text{keV}$$

$$E_k = h\nu' - h\nu = h\nu \left[\frac{\alpha(1 - \cos\phi)}{1 + \alpha(1 - \cos\phi)} \right]$$

$$= 250\,\text{keV} \left[\frac{0.489(0.5)}{1 + 0.489(1 - 0.5)} \right]$$

$$= 250\,\text{keV}\,[0.2]$$

$$= 50\,\text{keV}$$

Example 3-6

A 50-keV photon is scattered by a Compton interaction. What is the maximum energy transferred to the Compton electron?

The energy transferred to the electron is greatest when the change in wavelength is maximum; the change in wavelength is maximum when $\phi = 180°$.

$$\Delta\lambda_{max} = 0.00243[1 - \cos(180°)]\,\text{nm}$$

$$= 0.00243[1 - (-1)]\,\text{nm}$$

$$= 0.00486\,\text{nm}$$

$$\cong 0.005\,\text{nm}$$

The wavelength of a 50-keV photon is

$$\lambda = \frac{1.24}{50\,\text{keV}} = 0.025\,\text{nm}$$

The wavelength λ' of the photon scattered at $180°$ is

$$\lambda' = \lambda + \Delta\lambda$$

$$= (0.025 + 0.005)\,\text{nm} = 0.03\,\text{nm}$$

The energy $h\nu'$ of the scattered photon is

$$h\nu' = \frac{1.24}{\lambda'} = \frac{1.24}{0.03}$$

$$= 41.3\,\text{keV}$$

The energy of the Compton electron is

$$E_k = h\nu - h\nu'$$

$$= (50 - 41.3)\,\text{keV} = 8.7\,\text{keV}$$

When a relatively low-energy photon undergoes a Compton interaction, most of the energy of the incident photon is retained by the scattered photon, and only a small portion of the energy is transferred to the electron.

Example 3-7

A 5-MeV photon is scattered by a Compton interaction. What is the maximum energy transferred to the recoil electron:

The wavelength $\Delta\lambda$ of a 5-MeV photon is

$$\lambda = \frac{1.24}{5000\,\text{keV}} = 0.00025\,\text{nm}$$

The change in wavelength of a photon scattered at $180°$ is 0.005 nm (see Example 3-6). The wavelength λ' of the photon scattered at $180°$ is

$$\lambda' = \lambda + \Delta\lambda$$

$$= (0.00025 + 0.005)\,\text{nm}$$

$$= 0.00525\,\text{nm}$$

The energy of the scattered photon is

$$h\nu' = \frac{1.24}{\lambda'} = \frac{1.24}{0.0052} = 240\,\text{keV}$$

The energy E_k of the Compton electron is

$$E_k = h\nu - h\nu'$$

$$= (5000 - 236)\,\text{keV}$$

$$= 4760\,\text{keV}$$

When a relatively high-energy photon undergoes a Compton interaction, most of the energy of the incident photon is transferred to the electron, and only a small fraction of the energy is retained by the scattered photon.

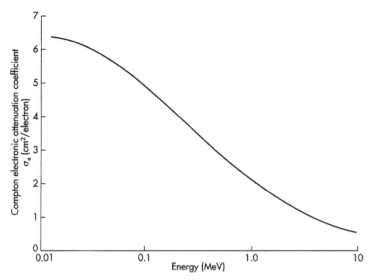

FIGURE 3-4
Compton electronic attenuation coefficient as a function of photon energy.

Example 3-8

Show that, irrespective of the energy of the incident photon, the maximum energy is 255 keV for a photon scattered at 180° and 511 keV for a photon scattered at 90°.

The wavelength λ' of a scattered photon is

$$\lambda' = \lambda + \Delta\lambda$$

For photons at very high energy, λ is very small and may be neglected relative to $\Delta\lambda$.

For a photon scattered at 180°:

$$\lambda' \cong \Delta\lambda = 0.00243(1 - \cos(180°))$$

$$= 0.00243(1 - (-1))$$

$$= 0.00486\,\text{nm}$$

$$h\nu' = \frac{1.24}{\lambda'} = \frac{1.24}{0.00486\,\text{nm}}$$

$$= 255\,\text{keV}$$

For photons scattered at 90°:

$$\lambda \cong \Delta\lambda = 0.00243(1 - \cos(90°))$$

$$= 0.00243(1 - 0)$$

$$= 0.00243\,\text{nm}$$

$$h\nu' = \frac{1.24}{\lambda'} = \frac{1.24}{0.00243\,\text{nm}}$$

$$= 511\,\text{keV}$$

The likelihood of Compton interaction decreases gradually with increasing photon energy, as depicted in Figure 3-4. Because Compton interactions occur principally with loosely bound ("free") electrons, the likelihood of an interaction does not depend on the atomic number of the medium. For the same reason, the Compton mass attenuation coefficient varies directly with the electron density (electrons per gram) of the attenuating material, because a material with a higher electron density provides a higher concentration of electrons with which incident photons can interact. Ordinary hydrogen ($^1_1$H) has an electron density much greater than that of other elements

TABLE 3-1 Variables that Influence Principal Modes of Interaction of X and Gamma Rays

Mode of Interaction	Dependence of Linear Attenuation Coefficient On			
	Photon Energy $h\nu$	Atomic Number Z	Electron Density ρ_e	Physical Density ρ
Photoelectric	$\frac{1}{(h\nu)^3}$	Z^3	—	ρ
Compton	$\frac{1}{h\nu}$	—	ρ_e	ρ
Pair production	$h\nu$ (>1.02 MeV)	Z	—	ρ

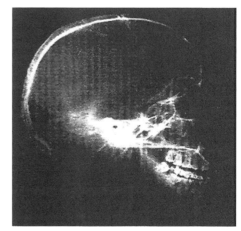

MARGIN FIGURE 3-8
Image obtained at 66 kVp.

In a given mass (1 g, for example), more Compton interactions will occur in fat than in bone. In a given volume (1 cm³, for example), however, more Compton interactions will occur in bone than in fat.

Compton interactions

- Occur with loosely bound electrons
- Have a likelihood of occurrence that is independent of Z
- Have a likelihood of occurrence that decreases slowly with increasing $(h\nu)$
- The fraction of incident photon energy transferred to the Compton electron increases with increasing $(h\nu)$
- The Compton process is the dominant photon interaction in soft tissue between 30 keV and 30 MeV.

Pair production was discovered by C. D. Anderson in 1932.

because hydrogen contains no neutrons. In hydrogen, an electron is present for each nucleon, whereas in other elements one electron is present for every two or more nucleons. Hence, photons interact by Compton interaction more readily in materials with high concentrations of hydrogen. Compared with other tissue constituents, fat has a greater concentration of hydrogen. For this reason, a gram of fat absorbs more energy by Compton interaction than does, for example, a gram of bone. However, the physical density (g/cm³) is greater for bone than for fat. Therefore, a greater number of electrons is present in a given volume of bone than in the same volume of fat, even though the electron density (electrons/g) is greater in fat. Hence a volume of bone attenuates more photons by Compton interaction than does an equal volume of fat or muscle, even though less energy is deposited in each gram of bone compared with the other tissue constituents.

In an image acquired with x rays in the diagnostic energy range (i.e., a radiographic or fluoroscopic image), various tissues can be distinguished because of differences in optical density in the image. These differences are referred to collectively as contrast in the image. Image contrast is a reflection of differences in the transmission of x rays through various regions of the patient. At the higher x-ray energies used in radiation therapy, a localization (*port*) film used to verify alignment of the treatment beam yields an image with greatly subdued contrast compared with a diagnostic image. The difference in the two images is due principally to the difference in the dominant photon interactions contributing to the images. The diagnostic x-ray beam interacts in part by photoelectric interactions that yield a major distinction in x-ray transmission through constituents of different Z within the patient. The higher-energy therapeutic x-ray beam interacts only rarely by photoelectric interaction and almost exclusively by Compton interaction. The transmitted therapy beam used to form the port-film image differs in intensity as a reflection only of variations in the physical and electron densities of various tissues. These properties vary only slightly among muscle, bone, and fat (Table 3-1). Hence the localization port film yields much less contrast compared with the diagnostic x-ray image. This difference is depicted in the margin for a patient examined with a 66-kVp diagnostic x-ray beam and with higher-energy x-ray beams used in radiation therapy.

Pair Production

For an x or γ ray above a threshold energy of 1.02 MeV, pair production is an additional type of interaction available to the photon. This type of interaction occurs near the nucleus of an atom in the absorbing medium and results in complete disappearance of the photon. In its place appear a pair of electrons, one negative and one positive (see Margin Figure 3-11). Pair production exhibits a threshold energy because the photon must possess enough energy to create the mass of the negative and positive electron (2 × 0.51 MeV = 1.02 MeV). Energy in excess of 1.02 MeV is distributed as kinetic energy of the two particles. Although the nucleus recoils slightly when pair production occurs in its vicinity, the energy transferred to the nucleus during the interaction usually can be neglected.

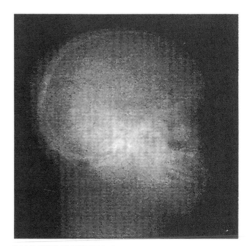

MARGIN FIGURE 3-9
Image obtained at 6 MV.

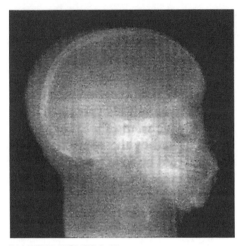

MARGIN FIGURE 3-10
Image obtained at 18 MV, illustrating the loss in image contrast at higher photon energies. (Margin Figures 3-8, 3-9, and 3-10 are provided courtesy of Frances Newman, MS, Medical Physics, University of Colorado.)

Pair and triplet production must occur in the presence of a charged particle (a nucleus or an electron) so that momentum is conserved in the interaction.

The pair-production interaction

- Cannot occur with photons below 1.02 MeV
- Initially increases rapidly for photons above 1.02 MeV
- Increases in likelihood with Z
- Transfers $(h\nu - 1.02 \text{ MeV})$ to the electron–positron pair
- Yields a positron that ultimately interacts with an electron to produce two annihilation photons of 0.51 MeV each.

Most photodisintegration interactions are either (γ, n) or (γ, p) interactions.

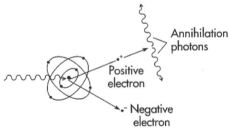

MARGIN FIGURE 3-11
Pair production interaction of a high-energy photon near a nucleus. Annihilation photons are produced when the positron and an electron annihilate each other.

Example 3-9

A 6-MeV photon interacts by pair production. Residual energy is shared equally between the negative and positive electrons. What are the kinetic energies of the particles?

$$h\nu \,(\text{MeV}) = 1.02 + (E_k)_{e-} + (E_k)_{e+}$$
$$(E_k)_{e-} = (E_k)_{e+} = \frac{(h\nu - 1.02)\,\text{MeV}}{2}$$
$$= 2.49\,\text{MeV}$$

Occasionally, pair production occurs near an electron, rather than a nucleus of an atom in the absorbing medium. For 10-MeV photons in soft tissue, for example, about 10% of all pair production interactions occur in the vicinity of an electron. This type of photon interaction is referred to as triplet production because the existing electron receives energy from the photon and is ejected from its atom simultaneously with creation of negative and positive electrons. Hence three ionizing particles, two negative electrons and one positive electron, are set into motion during triplet production. The threshold energy for triplet produce is twice (2.04 MeV) that for pair production. The ratio of triplet to pair production increases with the energy of the incident photons and decreases with increasing atomic number of the medium.

The mass attenuation coefficient κ_m for pair production varies almost linearly with the atomic number of the attenuating material. It also increases slowly with the energy of incident photons above the threshold energy of 1.02 MeV. In diagnostic radiology, pair production is not significant because the x rays do not possess enough energy to undergo this type of interaction. Pair production can be a significant interaction for x rays used in high-energy radiation therapy.

Photodisintegration

Except for pair production, interactions of x and γ rays with nuclei are significant only if the photons have very high energy. *Photodisintegration* interactions occur when photons have enough energy to eject a nuclear particle when they are absorbed by a nucleus. Photodisintegration rarely occurs in tissue but can take place in shielding materials around high-energy accelerators. Photodisintegration interactions also can be used to measure the energy of photons in a high-energy x-ray beam. An example of this procedure is the use of a beryllium foil in combination with elemental silver to calibrate the energy of an x-ray beam. A beryllium foil exposed to high-energy x rays can experience the reaction with a threshold energy of 1.65 MeV. A silver foil adjacent to the beryllium is activated by the ejected neutrons and emits gamma rays (an n, γ reaction). Gamma rays are detected by an external detector only if neutrons are released by the beryllium, signifying that x rays of at least 1.65 MeV are present in the high-energy x-ray beam. By substituting other foils with different threshold energies for the beryllium, the range of energies in the x-ray beam can be determined.

Likelihood of Interactions

The relative importance of photoelectric, Compton, and pair production interactions in different media is depicted in Figure 3-5. In muscle or water ($Z_{\text{eff}} = 7.4$), the probabilities of photoelectric and Compton interactions are equal at a photon energy of 35 keV. However, equal energies are not deposited in tissue at this energy because a photoelectric interaction deposits the total energy of the photon, whereas only part of the photon energy is transferred during a Compton interaction. The energy depositions from photoelectric and Compton interactions are equal at about 60 keV in muscle or water, where more Compton interactions compensate for less energy transferred per interaction.

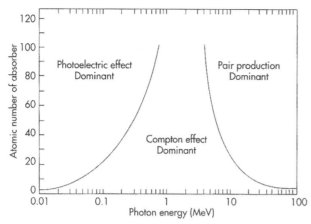

FIGURE 3-5
Relative importance of the three principal interactions of x and γ rays.

A summary of the variables that influence the linear attenuation coefficient for photoelectric, Compton, and pair production interactions is provided in Table 3-1.

■ SUMMARY

- Equations important to photon transmission and attenuation include

$$\mu = \frac{(dI/I)}{x} = \text{fractional rate of attenuation}$$

$$I = I_0 e^{-ux} = \text{number of photons transmitted}$$

$$I^* = I_0(1 - e^{-ux}) = \text{number of photons attenuated}$$

- Useful attenuation and absorption coefficients include μ (linear attenuation), μ_m (mass attenuation), μ_a (atomic attenuation), μ_e (electronic attenuation) and μ_{en} (mass energy absorption).
- Half-value layer measurements should be acquired under conditions of narrow-beam (good) geometry.
- The total attenuation coefficient is the sum of ω (coherent scattering), τ (photoelectric absorption), σ (Compton scattering), κ (pair production), and π photodisintegration.
- The likelihood of pair production varies with Z^3 and $(1/h\nu)^3$.
- The likelihood of Compton scattering varies with $1/h\nu$ and the electron density, but is independent of Z.
- The maximum energy of a photon scattered at 90° is 511 keV, and at 180° it is 255 keV.
- Pair production does not occur for photons below 1.02 MeV in energy.

PROBLEMS

3-1. The tenth-value layer (TVL) is the thickness of a material necessary to reduce the intensity of x or γ rays to 1/10 the intensity with no material present. For conditions of good geometry and monoenergetic photons, show that the TVL equals $2.30/\mu$, where μ is the total linear attenuation coefficient.

3-2. Assume that the exponent μx in the equation $I = I_0 e^{-\mu x}$ is equal to or less than 0.1. Show that, with an error less than

1%, the number of photons transmitted is $I_0(1 - \mu x)$ and the number attenuated is $I_0 \mu x$. (*Hint*: Expand the term $e^{-\mu x}$ into a series.)

3-3. The mass attenuation coefficient of copper is 0.0589 cm²/g for 1.0-MeV photons. The number of 1.0-MeV photons in a narrow beam is reduced to what fraction by a copper absorber 1 cm thick? The density of copper is 8.9 g/cm³.

3-4. Copper has a density of 8.9 g/cm^3 and a gram-atomic mass of 63.56. The total atomic attenuation coefficient of copper is 3.3×10^{-24} cm^2/atom for 5-MeV photons. What thickness of copper in cm is required to attenuate 5-MeV photons to half the original number?

3-5. K- and L-shell binding energies for cesium are 28 keV and 5 keV, respectively. What are the kinetic energies of photoelectrons released from the K and L shells as 30-keV photons interact with cesium?

3-6. Compute the energy of a photon scattered at 45° during a Compton interaction, if the energy of the incident photon is 150 keV. What is the kinetic energy of the Compton electron? Is the energy of the scattered photon increased or decreased if the photon scattering angle is increased to more than 45°?

3-7. A gamma ray of 2.75 MeV from ^{24}Na undergoes pair production in a lead shield. The negative and positive electrons possess equal kinetic energy. What is their kinetic energy?

3-8. Prove that, regardless of the energy of the incident photon, a photon scattered at an angle greater than 60° during a Compton interaction cannot undergo pair production.

3-9. What thickness (cm) of lead is required to reduce the intensity of 2-MeV photons to 0.1% if $\mu_m = 0.046$ cm^2/g and $\rho = 11.3$ g/cm^3 for lead?

3-10. 5 mm of aluminum ($\rho = 2.7$ g/cm^3) transmits 30% of a beam of 30-keV photons. What is the mass attenuation coefficient of aluminum for these photons?

REFERENCES

1. Hendee, W. R., and Ritenour, E. R., *Medical Imaging Physics*, 4th edition. New York, John Wiley & Sons, 2001.
2. Grodstein, G. W. *X-Ray Attenuation Coefficients from 10 keV to 100 MeV*. Washington, DC, U.S. National Bureau of Standards, Pub. No. 583, 1957.
3. Hubbel, J. H. *Photon Cross Section Attenuation Coefficients and Energy Absorption Coefficients from 10 keV to 100 GeV*. Washington, DC, U.S. National Bureau of Standards, Pub. No. 29, 1969.
4. Lord Raleigh. *Philos. Mag.* **41**:274, 1871; **47**:375–284, 1899, reprinted in *Scientific Papers* **1**:87; **4**:397.
5. Niroomand-Rad, A. Production and interaction of high-energy x rays and electrons. In *Biomedical Uses of Radiation. Part B—Therapeutic Applications*, W. Hendee (ed.). New York, Wiley-VCH, 1999, pp. 628–740.

CHAPTER 4

RADIATION UNITS

OBJECTIVES 52

LOW-ENERGY X-RAY UNITS 52

Grenz–Ray Units 52
Contact Therapy Units 52
Superficial Therapy Units 52
Orthovoltage Therapy Units 53
Supervoltage Therapy Units 53
Megavoltage X-Ray Machines 53

ISOTOPE TELETHERAPY UNITS 54

Cobalt Units 54
^{137}Cs Teletherapy Units 57

LINEAR ACCELERATORS 57

Historical Development 58
Major Components of Medical Electron Accelerators 61

OTHER MEDICAL ACCELERATORS 69

Van de Graaff Generators 69
Betatrons 70
Cyclotrons 70
Microtrons 72

SIMULATORS 73

Basic Design 73
Generator 75
X-Ray Tube 75
Image Intensifier 75
Mechanical Subsystems: Collimator 75

SUMMARY 76

PROBLEMS 76

REFERENCES 76

Radiation Therapy Physics, Third Edition, by William R. Hendee, Geoffrey S. Ibbott, and Eric G. Hendee
ISBN 0-471-39493-9 Copyright © 2005 John Wiley & Sons, Inc.

Émil Grubbé of Chicago may have been one of the first practicing radiation therapists. He used an early Crookes x-ray tube and reported treating numerous patients with cancer with this device, beginning in January 1896.

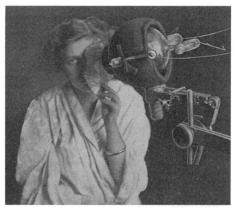

MARGIN FIGURE 4-1

Early photograph of superficial x-ray therapy. Tousey, S., *Medical Electricity and Röntgen Rays.* Philadelphia, W. B. Saunders, 1910.

Radiation therapy was not initially considered a reputable profession. "Roentgenologists who engaged in therapy were looked upon with suspicion. It was difficult to enlist the interest of any qualified roentgenologists in this questionable field." James Ewing, 1934.[1]

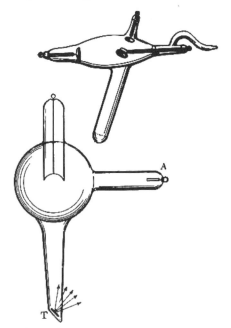

MARGIN FIGURE 4-2

Intracavitary x-ray tubes (1904). *Top*: Cossar's tube for treating carcinoma of the cervix. *Bottom*: Caldwell tube for treating the larynx and other sites such as the cervix or rectum.[2]

■ OBJECTIVES

By studying this chapter, the reader should be able to:

- Discuss the historical developments leading to the design of modern treatment equipment.
- Describe the characteristics of radiation beams produced by treatment equipment found in clinical use.
- Identify the major components of a modern linear accelerator and explain their purpose and function.
- Explain the design and operation of a conventional radiation therapy simulator.
- Compare the operation and clinical utility of linear accelerators with several other megavoltage treatment machines.

■ LOW-ENERGY X-RAY UNITS

The practice of radiation therapy began almost immediately following Roentgen's discovery of x rays. Until the advent of ^{60}Co units in the 1950s, however, most radiation therapy was conducted with x rays generated at potentials below about 300 kV. Since then, many low-energy treatment units have been replaced by megavoltage units. Many radiation oncology departments have retained a low-energy x-ray unit and make frequent use of it, particularly for the treatment of skin lesions.

Grenz–Ray Units

Grenz rays are defined as radiations produced at potentials of less than 20 kV. They are extremely nonpenetrating and consequently have little value in radiation therapy.

Contact Therapy Units

Contact therapy units operate at potentials of 40–50 kV and produce x rays with half-value layers of 1 or 2 mm Al. The x-ray tube is designed so that the surface to be irradiated is placed in contact with the housing, and approximately 2 cm from the target. The combination of low energy and short treatment distance causes an extremely rapid decrease in the depth dose. These x-ray beams are suitable only for treatment of surface lesions.

An advantage of contact therapy units is that their design facilitates use in operating rooms. Contact therapy machines have been used for intraoperative therapy because exposed tissues can be irradiated to high doses, while deeper tissues are spared. Their use is no longer popular because they have largely been replaced by electron-beam units.

Superficial Therapy Units

All x-ray machines operating in the kilovoltage range are primarily suited to treatment of superficial tissues. To distinguish them from *deep* therapy units, machines operating in the range of 50–150 kV are described as *superficial* therapy machines. Aluminum filters of up to 5 or 6 mm are added to increase the penetrating quality of the beam. The resulting half-value layers are generally in the range of 1–8 mm of aluminum.

Glass or stainless-steel cones are used to collimate the beam, and the surface to be treated is placed in contact with the end of the cone. Dose rates as high as several hundred cGy per minute are available. A typical superficial unit is shown in Figure 4-1.

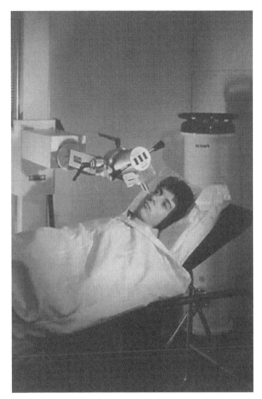

FIGURE 4-1
A representative superficial x-ray unit. (Courtesy of Nucletron Corporation of America.)

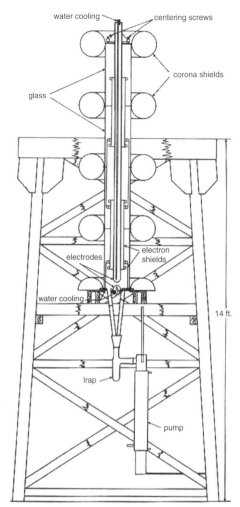

MARGIN FIGURE 4-3
Lauritsen's 750,000-volt unit (1928).[3]

Orthovoltage Therapy Units

As higher-voltage equipment became available, x-ray machines operating in the range of 200–350 kV were developed. For many years, these units provided the most penetrating x-ray beams available to radiation therapists, and consequently they were called *deep therapy* machines. Because their energies are intermediate between those provided by superficial units and so-called supervoltage units, they are also called *orthovoltage* units. A number of orthovoltage units are still in place, particularly outside the United States. They have largely been replaced by linear accelerators with electron beams, which provide more uniform irradiation of tissues than do orthovoltage x rays.

Orthovoltage units are typically equipped with adjustable collimators and a *light localizer*, which aids in placement of the patient for treatment. Relatively short treatment distances, such as 50 cm, are routinely used. At least one modern orthovoltage unit is provided with an internal dose-monitoring system and state-of-the-art digital controls. A representative orthovoltage unit is shown in Figure 4-2.

Supervoltage Therapy Units

A class of treatment units operating in the 500- to 1000-kV range appeared in the late 1940s and 1950s. The use of conventional transformers limited the operation of x-ray machines to about 350 kV. Supervoltage machines relied on devices such as *resonant transformers* to generate higher potentials. Due to the development of alternative high-energy electrical systems and isotope treatment units, supervoltage x-ray generators were promoted for only a few years.

Megavoltage X-Ray Machines

Several types of x-ray machines operating at more than 1000 kV have been developed, including Van de Graaff generators, betatrons, and linear accelerators. Of the

Orthovoltage x-ray units were also known as "deep roentgen therapy" units.

The desire to produce x-rays of up to 1MV for radiation therapy led entrepreneurs such as William Coolidge, R.W. Sorenson, and Charles Lauritsen to design x-ray tubes with cascading sections for electron acceleration. All of these tubes were very long and impractical in the clinical setting. However, one dual-stage Coolidge cascade tube was installed at Memorial Hospital in New York City to study the biological properties of high-energy x rays.

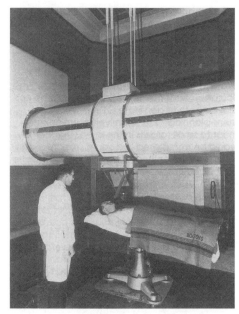

MARGIN FIGURE 4-4
1-MV therapy installation at St. Bartholomew's Hospital, London.

W. F. Mayneord presented a detailed characterization of a new orthovoltage unit at a meeting of the British Institute of Radiology in 1933. During the ensuing discussion, Dr. W. M. Levitt expressed his delight upon hearing about the penetrating ability of 370-kV x-rays: "... depth doses could be obtained at a depth of 10 cm of fifty percent or even more, and more than that was scarcely needed for therapeutic work."[4]

The earliest supervoltage unit was the 30-foot long 1MV x-ray unit installed at St. Bartholomew's Hospital in London in 1931.

Military terms including "cannon," "howitzer," and "bomb" have long been associated with teletherapy sources, although just why this is so isn't entirely clear. Koening reportedly described his teletherapy unit constructed in about 1912 as a "radium cannon." In 1922, Lysholm in Stockholm constructed a device he called a "radium howitzer." By the 1930s, such teletherapy units were referred to by the colloquial but incorrect name "radium bombs," especially in the United Kingdom. However, the term stuck and was used to refer to ^{60}Co units even into the 1960s. (Adapted from Cormack, D., and Munro, P. Cobalt-60: A Canadian Perspective. *Canadian Medical Physics Newsletter* **45**(1), January 1999.)

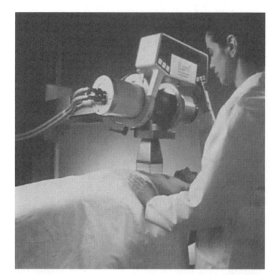

FIGURE 4-2
A representative orthovoltage x-ray unit. (Courtesy of Nucletron Corporation of America.)

three, only linear accelerators are now in widespread use. These units combine the advantages of high dose rates, compact design, and high reliability. Linear accelerators are discussed in detail in later sections of this chapter.

■ ISOTOPE TELETHERAPY UNITS

Cobalt Units

Before 1951, the only teletherapy units were *teleradium units*, which contained a few grams of radium in a sealed capsule. Teleradium units were expensive, furnished a radiation beam of low intensity, and were considered impractical for routine clinical therapy. After World War II, nuclear reactors were constructed to furnish radioactive nuclides for public use. The first high-activity ^{60}Co source for medical use was produced in Canada in 1951. In 1952, Johns and co-workers[5–7] described the first ^{60}Co teletherapy unit. Today, only a few ^{60}Co units are being built, primarily for sale in countries outside the United States and Western Europe. A number of ^{60}Co units, however, are still in use and are valued by radiation oncologists for palliative treatments and for treatment of shallow structures, such as some head-and-neck tumors.

Source Capsule
A standard container for encapsulating ^{60}Co sources has been accepted by manufacturers of teletherapy units (Margin Figure 4-5). The ^{60}Co source is retained within two stainless steel canisters that are welded to prevent escape of the radioactive material. To attenuate gamma rays emitted in undesired directions, shields of tungsten, uranium, or lead surround the source. Gamma rays emitted in the desired direction traverse a thin steel plate and are attenuated only slightly.

Source Exposure Mechanism
Various methods have been devised for exposing and shielding the ^{60}Co source. The two most commonly used techniques are illustrated in Margin Figure 4-6. Some manufacturers mount the source on a metal wheel (Margin Figure 4-6A). The wheel is rotated 180 degrees to expose the source. A motor holds the source in the "on" position. A spring attached to the wheel returns the source to the "off" position when power to the motor is interrupted. An alternative method to expose the source (Margin Figure 4-6B) uses air pressure generated by a small compressor to hold the source in

the "on" position. The source is drawn to the shielded position by a spring when the compressed air is allowed to escape. Both of these designs are considered "fail-safe" in that the source returns to the shielded position if power to the unit is interrupted.

Collimators

With the source in the "on" position, gamma rays from the source capsule enter a diverging channel in the lead or depleted uranium sourcehead. A collimator mounted below the diverging channel is used to vary the size of the radiation beam leaving the sourcehead. Modern ^{60}Co teletherapy units have an interleaved, multivaned collimator with vanes of lead or tungsten (Margin Figure 4-7).

Often a satellite collimator (also referred to as a penumbra trimmer) is attached to the end of the collimator nearest the patient. The satellite collimator sharpens the edge of the radiation beam. To reduce contamination of the gamma ray beam with electrons liberated as photons interact with the collimator, the end of the collimator should be at least 15 cm above the patient's skin.[8] At shorter distances, a significant number of electrons may reach the skin and produce severe skin reactions.

To indicate the location of the gamma-ray beam and assist in the positioning of patients for treatment, a light localizer is provided. A mirror positioned inside the collimator reflects light from a bulb to provide a light field, which is coincident with the radiation beam emerging from the collimator.

Beam Edge Unsharpness

The finite size of a teletherapy source creates an indistinct border for the radiation field. This indistinct border is termed the *geometric penumbra*. The unsharpness at the skin surface and at a depth *d* within the patient is illustrated in Figure 4-3.

The width W of the geometric penumbra at the skin surface is

$$W = c \frac{SSD - SCD}{SCD}$$

where c represents the diameter of the source, SSD is the source-to-skin distance, and SCD is the source-to-collimator distance. The geometric penumbra is independent of the size of the radiation field. The geometric penumbra at the patient's surface could be eliminated by placing the end of the collimator on the skin. Then $SSD = SCD$ and the penumbra $W = 0$. However, this practice must be avoided with high-energy x and gamma beams because electrons from the collimator would contaminate the radiation beam at the skin surface. To minimize the size of the geometric penumbra,

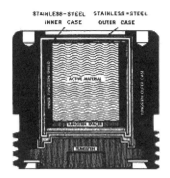

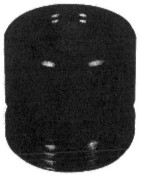

MARGIN FIGURE 4-5

Cross-sectional view (**upper**) and photograph (**lower**) of a standard ^{60}Co source capsule. (Used with permission from Hendee, W. R. *Medical Radiation Physics*, 1st edition, Chicago, Mosby–Year Book, 1970. Courtesy of Picker X-Ray Corporation.)

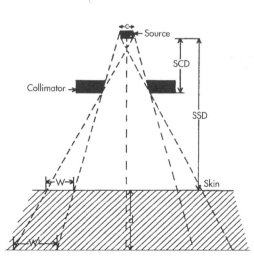

FIGURE 4-3

Diagram of the unsharpness of the beam edge caused by the finite size of a teletherapy source. (Used with permission from Hendee, W. R. *Medical Radiation Physics*, 1st edition, Chicago, Mosby–Year Book, 1970.)

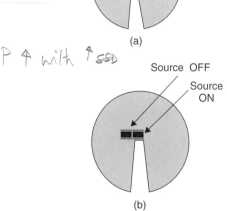

MARGIN FIGURE 4-6

Common methods for exposing and shielding a teletherapy source. (See text.) (Redrawn with permission from Hendee, W. R. *Medical Radiation Physics*, 1st edition, Chicago, Mosby–Year Book, 1970.)

The first teletherapy cobalt source was activated in the AECL NRX reactor at Chalk River, Canada. It was delivered to H. E. Johns and T. A. Watson, M.D., in 1951 following their request in 1949. A second source was requested in 1950 by Eldorado Commercial Products and I. Smith, M.D. at the London (Ontario) Clinic. The source was delivered to London also in 1951. A third source was requested in 1950 by G. Fletcher, M.D. and L.G. Grimmett of the M.D. Anderson Hospital. It was activated in the High Flux Reactor at Oak Ridge, Tennessee. The source was delivered in 1952 and first used clinically in 1954.

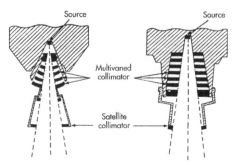

MARGIN FIGURE 4-7
Two type of interleaved, multivaned collimators equipped with satellite collimators. (Used with permission from Hendee, W. R. *Medical Radiation Physics,* 1st edition, Chicago, Mosby–Year, 1970.)

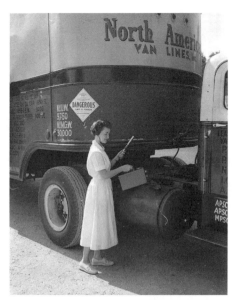

MARGIN FIGURE 4-8
A medical physicist performs a survey of one of the first teletherapy cobalt sources upon its arrival at the M. D. Anderson Hospital in 1952.

sources with high specific activity are constructed with the smallest possible diameter. Such sources can supply a radiation beam of reasonable intensity and relatively small penumbra.

The width W' of the geometric penumbra at the depth d within a patient is

$$W' = c\,\frac{SSD + d - SCD}{SCD} \qquad (4\text{-}1)$$

The geometric penumbra is larger at any depth within the patient than it is on the skin surface.

Example 4-1

Determine the width of the geometric penumbra of a ^{60}Co beam at 10 cm depth in a patient undergoing treatment at 80 cm SSD. The source diameter is 2 cm, and the patient's surface is 35 cm from the distal end of the collimator.

The SCD is $80 - 35 = 45$ cm. From Equation (4-1), the penumbra width at depth is

$$W' = c\,\frac{SSD + d - SCD}{SCD}$$

$$W' = 2\,\frac{80 + 10 - 45}{45}$$

$$W' = 2 \text{ cm}$$

The total penumbra at the surface or at some depth below the surface sometimes is defined as the distance between the 90% and 10% *decrement lines* along the beam edge.[9] Decrement lines are lines through points at which the absorbed dose is a certain percent (e.g., 90%, 80%, 70%, and so forth) of the energy absorbed at the same depth along the central axis of the radiation beam. The total penumbra at the skin surface and at depths below the surface should be considered during treatment planning, particularly when adjacent (abutting) radiation fields are used.

Isocentric Units

Both stand-mounted and isocentrically mounted ^{60}Co teletherapy units have been available and may still be found in radiation therapy departments.

The primary advantage of isocentric treatment units is in setting up patients for treatment. With an isocentric unit, the patient needs only to be positioned once, in preparation for treatment of a single target volume with beams directed from two or more angles. In contrast, a stand-mounted unit often requires that the patient position be changed (i.e., the patient be moved from the supine to the prone position) or that the treatment couch be moved to permit repositioning of the source head. The dosimetric advantages of isocentric treatment are discussed in Chapter 8.

An additional advantage of an isocentric unit is that it permits rotation or *arc therapy*. With arc therapy, the gantry rotates during treatment to move the source head around the isocenter. The patient is positioned so that the center of the target volume is located at the isocenter, and the beam irradiates the target volume during its arc.

Most isocentric teletherapy installations include wall and ceiling lights or lasers that produce narrow light beams that interact at the isocenter. Superposition of the laser beams on marks on the patient's skin permits rapid alignment of the patient for treatment. With most teletherapy units, a counterweight balances the weight of the sourcehead during rotation. Often the counterweight serves as a primary barrier to absorb radiation transmitted by the patient and reduces the shielding required for walls of the treatment room.

^{137}Cs Teletherapy Units

A teletherapy unit with a ^{137}Cs source was described by Brucer in 1956.[10] A few cesium units were used until the early 1990s to treat lesions at relative shallow depths, such as head-and-neck tumors. Collimators and source-exposure mechanisms for most ^{137}Cs units were similar to those for ^{60}Co units, although some ^{137}Cs equipment was supplied with cones rather than collimators. Compared with a ^{60}Co source of equal physical size, the radiation intensity from a source of ^{137}Cs is relatively low because the maximum specific activity is only 3.2×10^{12} Bq/g (87 Ci/g) for ^{137}Cs (Example 4-2) and because gamma rays are emitted during only 83% of all nuclear transitions of ^{137}Cs. Sources of sufficient activity to provide a radiation beam of reasonable intensity at a long treatment distance also furnish a large unsharpness of the beam edge. A smaller source reduces the unsharpness but provides a beam of reasonable intensity only if the treatment distance is short. Consequently, most ^{137}Cs units were used at treatment distances less than 35 cm. The rapid divergence of the beam resulting from the use of short treatment distances caused the distribution of radiation dose within a patient treated with ^{137}Cs photons to resemble that from x rays generated at about 400 kVp.

Example 4-2

What is the maximum specific activity for ^{137}Cs?

Activity is calculated from the number of atoms and the decay constant:

$$A = \lambda N$$

If N is the number of atoms of ^{137}Cs per gram, the activity is the specific activity. For a source of pure ^{137}Cs ($T_{1/2} = 30$ years):

$$\text{Number of atoms/gram } N = \frac{6.02 \times 10^{23} \text{ atoms/g-atomic mass}}{137 \text{ g/g-atomic mass}}$$

$$= 4.4 \times 10^{21} \text{ atom/g}$$

$$\text{Decay constant } \lambda \text{ for } ^{137}Cs = \frac{\ln 2}{(T_{1/2})}$$

$$= \frac{0.693}{30 \text{ y}}$$

$$= 2.3 \times 10^{-2} \text{ y}^{-1}$$

$$= 7.3 \times 10^{-10} \text{ sec}^{-1}$$

$$\text{Specific activity} = \lambda N$$

$$= (7.3 \times 10^{-10} \text{ sec}^{-1}) \cdot (4.4 \times 10^{21} \text{ atoms/g})$$

$$= 3.2 \times 10^{12} \text{ Bq/g}$$

■ LINEAR ACCELERATORS

Modern linear accelerators (*linacs*) are now found in virtually all radiation therapy departments, having replaced most other therapy units. They are used to treat patients with beams of electrons or bremsstrahlung x rays following interactions of electrons in a suitable target. Intense electron beam currents are achievable with an accelerator to provide high dose rates for both x-ray and electron treatments. Hence, treatment times are short even at relatively long target-to-patient distances. Many modern linacs

Only about 50 cobalt units were in clinical use in North America in 2003, of which most were in Canada. However, elsewhere in the world there were approximately 2400 cobalt units in use in 2003. In developing countries, where service capabilities for complex equipment may be limited, a cobalt unit is a relatively trouble-free alternative.

Isocentric units are designed to rotate about an axis located at a fixed distance from the source. ^{60}Co units typically have isocenter distances of 80 cm, although some units with isocenter distances of 95 cm and 100 cm have been made.

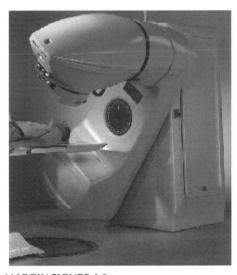

MARGIN FIGURE 4-9
An example of a modern isocentrically mounted ^{60}Co unit. (Courtesy of M. D. S. Nordion, Inc.)

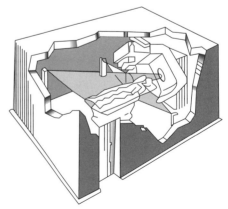

MARGIN FIGURE 4-10
An illustration showing the use of alignment lasers for isocentric positioning of a patient for treatment. (Courtesy of Gammex RMI, Inc.)

In the 1950s and 60s, ^{60}Co units (and to a lesser degree ^{137}Cs units) were by far the most popular units for radiation therapy.

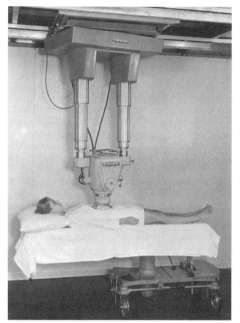

MARGIN FIGURE 4-11
A ^{137}Cs teletherapy unit.

Electron beams were first used for radiation therapy in 1934 by Brasch and Lange in Germany.

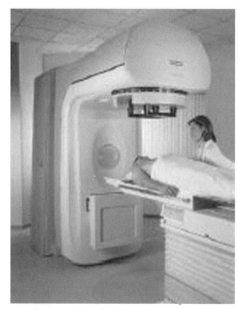

MARGIN FIGURE 4-12
A modern linear accelerator for radiation therapy. (Courtesy of Siemens Medical Systems, Inc.)

provide multiple electron and photon beam energies. These units are stable and compact, and most are mounted within isocentric gantries.

Historical Development

The earliest linear accelerators were so-called direct accelerators, in which charged particles were accelerated by an electric field created by placing a high potential difference over an insulated column. Perhaps the most common example of direct acceleration is a particle accelerator based on the Van de Graaff generator (see section later in this chapter).

In the simplest form of linear accelerator, such as the simple x-ray tube shown in Figure 2-3, electrons are boiled off the cathode surface (which is heated by a filament) and accelerated toward the anode. The accelerating force is provided by a static electric field produced by maintaining the anode at a positive potential V relative to the cathode. The energy acquired by an electron accelerated in this fashion is determined by the voltage V; electrons accelerated through a potential difference of 1 V gain an energy of 1 electron volt (eV). This corresponds to 1.6×10^{-19} joules, although the unit eV (or MeV) is most commonly used.

The velocity of the accelerated electron can be determined from the classical equation for kinetic energy:

$$T = \frac{1}{2}m_e v^2 \tag{4-2}$$

where m_e is the electron's mass and v is its velocity. It is straightforward to calculate the velocity of a 1 eV electron as 1.87×10^7 m/sec, or 6.25% of the speed of light. To accelerate electrons to higher energies requires either that the potential difference be increased (impractical at voltages above a few hundred thousand volts) or that the accelerating force be repeated numerous times. Note that Equation (4-2) cannot be used once the electron becomes *relativistic* (i.e., when its velocity exceeds approximately 20% of the speed of light).

The first linear accelerator was developed by Wideröe in 1928 to accelerate heavy ions.[11] Wideröe's accelerator consisted of a series of metal cylinders, termed *drift tubes*, with alternate cylinders connected to opposite terminals of an oscillating radio frequency voltage (Figure 4-4).

Because adjacent drift tubes are connected to opposite terminals of the power supply, an electric field develops between the ends of the tubes. Ions are accelerated across the gaps between adjacent drift tubes. The accelerating force is described by the equation for force on a charged particle:

$$F = q(E + v \times B) \tag{4-3}$$

where q indicates the charge of the particle, E is the strength of the electric field, v is the velocity of the particle, and B is the strength of the magnetic field. The expression $v \times B$ indicates the *cross product* of velocity and magnetic field strength. When the magnetic field and the velocity are perpendicular, the cross product is

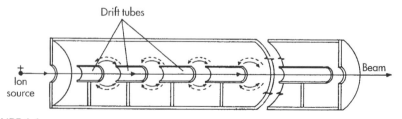

FIGURE 4-4
An early linear accelerator, in which drift tubes were suspended in an evacuated accelerator waveguide and connected to opposite terminals of a power supply.

simply the multiplicative product. When the field and velocity are in the same direction, the cross product is zero. In the case of Wideröe's accelerator the force on the particle is simply the product of charge and electric field strength because B is zero.

While inside the drift tubes, the ions are shielded from the electric fields produced by the radiofrequency voltage. The length of each tube is sufficient to allow ions to drift undisturbed through the tube each time the radiofrequency voltage changes polarity. In this manner, ions are accelerated from one drift tube to the next only after the correct polarity has been established across the gap between tubes. As the energy, and therefore the velocity, of the particles increases, the drift tubes must increase in length. Although useful for accelerating heavy ions, the Wideröe accelerator was not suitable for accelerating electrons because the high speed of the electrons would have required inordinately long drift tubes.

Development of the electron linac was made possible by the invention in the late 1930s and early 1940s of the microwave cavity and by the development of klystron and magnetron tubes as sources of microwave power. In 1944, Cutler showed that a corrugated cylinder could be designed to match the *phase velocity* of a traveling electromagnetic wave to the velocity of an electron beam.[12]

Between 1948 and 1955, the first electron linacs were designed and built by groups working independently in England and in California. Fry and associates[13] at the Telecommunications Research Group, Great Malvern, England (later to become part of the Atomic Energy Research Establishment at Harwell) designed a 0.5-MeV linac in 1946 and accelerated electrons later that same year. Independently, Ginzton and associates[14] in Palo Alto, California, developed a 1.7-MeV accelerator, which became operational in early 1947. By late 1947, both groups had achieved energies of 3.5 to 6 MeV. Also during this period, Chodorow, Ginzton, and Hansen[15] constructed multimegawatt klystrons, having many orders of magnitude greater power than those developed for wartime radar applications. These microwave sources made possible the development of traveling-wave linacs with high beam currents and energies of up to 1000 MeV.

In a microwave accelerator, microwaves are guided into a cylindrical metal tube known as an accelerator waveguide. Simultaneously, electrons or other charged particles are introduced into one end of the accelerator waveguide. The presence of the electromagnetic field induces an electric current within the walls of the accelerator waveguide. The current generates an electric field, which exerts a force on the particles, accelerating them to high velocities.

The microwave power P required to establish the electric field within the accelerator depends on several characteristics of the waveguide:

$$P = \frac{V^2}{ZL}$$

where V is the potential difference developed within the guide through which particles are accelerated, Z is the *shunt impedance* of the accelerator waveguide, and L is the length of the waveguide. The shunt impedance is a measure of the efficiency of the guide. To develop the potential to accelerate particles to an energy of 10 MeV in a structure with a shunt impedance of 100 MΩ/m and a length of 1 m, 1 MW of electromagnetic power is consumed. (*Note*: MΩ represents the quantity "mega ohms," where "ohm" is a unit of impedance). Additional power is consumed by the accelerated particles themselves, as well as by other components of the linac. Consequently, a source of 2 MW or more of microwave power is required. A 2-MW magnetron is often used in low-energy linacs, whereas klystrons with power ratings up to 10 MW are used in higher-energy units.

To regulate the phase velocity of the microwave (the velocity at which a peak of the microwave appears to travel), barriers such as metal discs may be placed in the waveguide at regular intervals (Figure 4-5).

The electric field established by the microwaves develops between the discs. In some accelerator structures, a *forward*-directed field develops between one pair of

The first multi-MV linear accelerator was built by the physicists David Sloan and Ernest Lawrence from a prototype device constructed by Rolf Wideröe.

The term *phase velocity* refers to the velocity of a peak or valley of an electromagnetic wave. A linear accelerator designed by use of this principle allows the crest of the electromagnetic wave to travel at less than the speed of light, permitting the charged particle to keep up. The energy carried by the electromagnetic wave always moves at the speed of light.

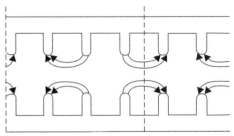

MARGIN FIGURE 4-13
The orientation of the electric field induced by a microwave field in a linear accelerator. The electric field provides an accelerating force on charged particles within the accelerator waveguide. The $\pi/2$ mode is shown in which one wavelength spans four cavities. (From reference 17.)

Microwave frequency bands and frequency range of each band.

Frequency Band	Frequency (GHz)	Wavelength (cm)	Center Frequency (GHz)
L band	0.39–1.55	76.9–19.3	1.30
S band	1.55–5.20	19.4–5.8	3.00
C band	3.90–6.20	7.7–4.8	5.45
X band	6.20–10.90	4.8–2.8	9.38
K band	10.90–36.00	2.8–0.8	24.00
Q band	36.00–46.00	0.8–0.7	34.80
V band	46.00–56.00	0.7–0.5	50.00
W band	56.00–100.00	0.5–0.3	80.00

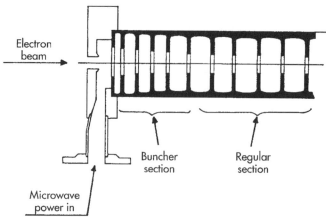

FIGURE 4-5
A disc-loaded waveguide for electron acceleration. The spacing between discs in the "buncher section" is less than that in the "regular section." The buncher section accelerates electrons to relativistic energies and forms them into bunches for efficient acceleration by the regular section.

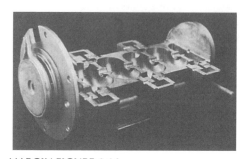

MARGIN FIGURE 4-14
An example of a side-coupled standing-wave linear accelerator waveguide. (Used with permission from Karzmark, C. J., Nunan, C. S., and Tanabe, E. *Medical Electron Accelerators*, New York, McGraw-Hill, 1993.)

The first side-coupled standing wave accelerator was built at Los Alamos National Laboratory in the late 1960s. It accelerated protons and other ions into a target to produce pi mesons (pions). During the 1970s and early 1980s, the *pions* were used for experimental medical treatments.

discs, while a *backward*-directed field develops between the adjacent pair of discs. Consequently a wavelength spans two adjacent cavities (Figure 4-6). Particles in the space between the first pair of discs are accelerated in the forward direction, while particles in the second space (between the second and third discs) are accelerated in the backward direction. Naturally, particles would arrive at the second space only if they were accelerated in the forward direction while in the first space. The distance between the discs is determined by the velocity of the particles:

$$L_n = \frac{v_n}{2\nu}$$

where L_n is the distance between adjacent discs, v_n, is the velocity of the particles, and ν is the frequency of the microwaves. In medical electron linacs, the electrons quickly approach the speed of light as they are accelerated down the waveguide. Consequently the spacing between discs quickly reaches a maximum distance. In the more common $\pi/2$ mode, one wavelength spans four cavities, and particles are accelerated only in alternate cavities. The microwave field has zero intensity in the remaining cavities (see Figure 4-6). The benefits of this design are described later in this chapter.

Early medical linacs were of the *traveling wave* design. Microwaves were injected into one end of the accelerator and traveled to the other end, where they were extracted. As they traveled, they carried the electrons along with them. The extracted microwaves could be conducted back to the proximal end of the accelerator and reinjected. The disc-loaded design limited the shunt impedance to maximum values less than 60 MΩ/m, which restricted the *accelerator gradient*, or attainable electron energy in MeV/m, to fairly low values.

In 1968, Knapp et al.[16] invented the *side-coupled standing wave* accelerator, in which the microwaves were reflected from the ends of the accelerator waveguide. The backward traveling wave interferes with the forward traveling wave, alternately constructively and destructively. The resulting *standing wave* has a magnitude of approximately double that of the traveling wave, and the peak intensity travels along the waveguide at the phase velocity of the traveling wave. In alternate spaces between discs, the magnitude of the wave is always at or near zero (see Figure 4-6).

In standing wave structures, the spaces between discs are optimized by changing the shape of the discs. The resulting *cavities* permit the microwaves to resonate, improving the efficiency with which their energy is transferred to the accelerated electrons. An additional improvement is that the microwave electric field intensity is at or near zero in alternate cavities. Although necessary to conduct the microwave energy, these cavities play no role in accelerating particles. By moving them to the

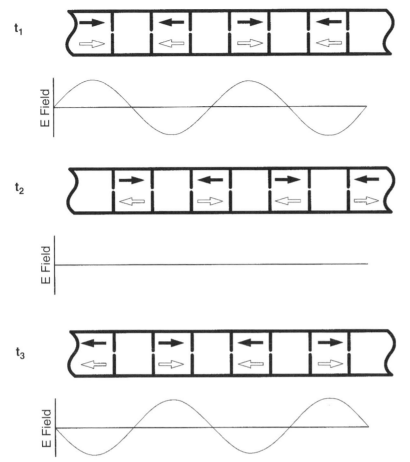

FIGURE 4-6
A schematic of an accelerator waveguide showing separate forward and backward waves and their superposition. In each diagram, the *solid arrows* indicate the positive and negative peaks of a microwave electric field moving from left to right, whereas the *open arrows* indicate a field reflected from the right moving to the left. At t_1 and t_3, the forward and reflected waves superimpose constructively. At t_2, they interfere destructively, and the electric field intensity is zero everywhere. (Redrawn with permission from Karzmark, C. J., Nunan, C. S., and Tanabe, E. *Medical Electron Accelerators*, New York, McGraw-Hill, 1993)

side, off the waveguide axis, the accelerating cavities can be placed closer together. The overall length of the structure becomes shorter, facilitating the placement of the guide in the treatment unit and improving its efficiency.

Major Components of Medical Electron Accelerators

Modern linear accelerators consist of several major subsystems. These components produce the electrical power required to generate microwaves, conduct the microwave power to the accelerator waveguide, and transport the accelerated beam ultimately to the patient.

Modulator and Pulse-Forming Network

Linear accelerators require fairly large amounts of electrical power. The power must be provided in large pulses because linacs accelerate particles in bursts. The *modulator* consists of a power supply that converts the incoming alternating current into direct current, along with a *pulse-forming network* that modulates the current into pulses. A diagram of a modulator appears in Figure 4-7. The direct current charges a bank of capacitors, which store the charge until a pulse is required. The charging cycle

The invention of the side-coupled standing wave electron accelerator allowed the development of a 4-MeV accelerator guide short enough to be mounted colinearly with the x-ray beam. This accelerator guide, introduced in 1970, was installed in a gantry having an 80-cm isocenter. A number of these machines are still in clinical operation today.

The term "linac" is a contraction of "linear accelerator."

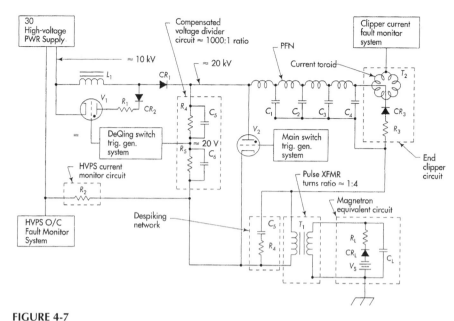

FIGURE 4-7

The modulator and pulse-forming network of a modern medical electron accelerator. (Used with permission from Karzmark, C. J., Nunan, C. S., and Tanabe, E. *Medical Electron Accelerators*, New York, McGraw-Hill, 1993.)

The magnetron was invented by J. T. Randall and H. A. H Boot at the University of Birmingham, England. They achieved power levels of 1 MW in 1940. Their invention enabled the development of radar systems with sufficient spatial resolution to distinguish enemy aircraft from those of the Allies.

In the early 1930s, W. W. Hansen of the Stanford University Physics Department wanted to accelerate electrons by oscillating them with microwaves inside a copper tube. He designed resonant cavities, as an alternative to the conventional resonant circuits of the time, to produce high-power, high-frequency radiowaves.

lasts about a millisecond. On receiving a signal from a timing circuit, a switching tube closes, completing a circuit from the capacitor bank, through a transformer, to ground. The capacitors discharge rapidly, but because of the inductor connecting them, they discharge in sequence. The resulting pulse is nearly square.

The switching tube, or *thyratron*, is a gas-filled triode (Figure 4-7). When the grid is charged positively, electrons flow from the cathode to the anode. The gas within the tube ionizes and conducts larger currents than do other switching devices. At the end of the pulse, the grid voltage is removed, preventing further current flow while the pulse-forming network recharges. This cycle is repeated between 50 and 500 times each second.

The output of the pulse transformer is conducted to the microwave-producing tube, either a magnetron or a klystron. The resulting microwave pulse, similar in shape to the electrical pulse, is about 6 μs long and consists of several megawatts of power.

Magnetrons

The cavity-type magnetron was invented in 1940 by Boot and Randall[17] and made high-definition radar possible in World War II. Magnetrons are commonly used in low-power linear accelerators. A magnetron of this type consists of a cylindrical diode containing a central cathode, which is heated by internal filaments. The coaxial anode is constructed of solid copper with coupled resonant cavities formed in the wall (Figure 4-8).

An axial magnetic field is supplied by a large permanent magnet. When a DC pulse is applied to the diode, electrons from the cathode are accelerated toward the anode and assume a spiral path because of the magnetic field. The individual electrons follow complex cycloidal paths around the cathode. As the electrons swirl along their spiral pathway, they induce intense local variations in the axial magnetic field. The radiofrequency energy induced in the magnetic field by this process is trapped in the resonant cavities. Oscillation of this trapped energy forms varying electrical fields across the lips of each cavity. These varying electrical fields channel electrons to the more positive regions of the anode, and the spiraling electron cloud appears to sweep around the cathode as it tracks the more positive regions. The sweeping electron cloud induces additional intense variations in the magnetic field, which are in resonance and

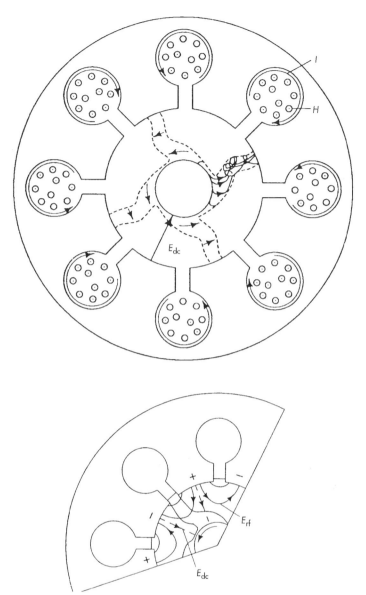

FIGURE 4-8
A cutaway view of a magnetron microwave power tube. (Used with permission from Karzmark, C. J., Nunan, C. S., and Tanabe, E. *Medical Electron Accelerators*, New York, McGraw-Hill, (1993).)

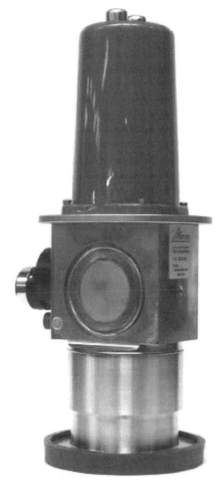

MARGIN FIGURE 4-15
A photograph of a modern magnetron. (Courtesy of E2V Technologies, Ltd.)

coupled with the cavities of the coaxial anode. A loop antenna inserted in one of the cavities taps the radiofrequency energy in the cavities and transfers it to a waveguide for transmission to the accelerator waveguide. Magnetrons transform DC power to radiofrequency power with efficiencies as high as 60%. Typically, such magnetrons provide 2-MW peak power.

The microwave wavelength must be of an appropriate length so that the accelerator components are reasonably easy to design and manufacture. Most modern medical linacs operate with microwaves of about 3000 MHz, in what is known as the *S-band*. (see table in margin note on page 59) The wavelength in a vacuum may be determined from the frequency v and speed of light c as

$$\lambda = \frac{c}{v}$$

For microwaves of 3000 MHz, the wavelength in a vacuum is on the order of 10 cm. In a waveguide, the wavelength is reduced somewhat because the phase velocity of the radiation is reduced.

Hansen's device was named the "rhumbatron" from the Greek word "rhumba" meaning rhythmic oscillations. The electrons moved inside the device in a manner reminiscent (to Hansen) of the sensuous and provocative Latin dance.

It is straightforward to calculate the change in microwave frequency that will reduce the coupling of microwave power to the accelerated beam by 50%. The dependence of power coupling on microwave frequency is characterized by the Q, or quality, of the accelerator. A high Q indicates that a small change in microwave frequency will have a large impact on the efficiency of coupling microwave power to a charged-particle beam.

During operation of a linac, the temperature of various components tends to increase. Changes in temperature may adversely affect the operation of the accelerator and must be avoided. In particular, a temperature rise of the accelerator guide of as little as 1°C may cause sufficient expansion to change the resonant frequency by 60 kHz. A change in resonant frequency of as little as 20 kHz can seriously degrade the performance of the accelerator. This sensitivity means that the frequency of the microwaves must be adjusted to compensate. Consequently the magnetron must be *tunable*, to permit continuous matching of the frequency. Early linacs equipped with fixed-frequency magnetrons required that the operator manually adjust the flow of water around the accelerator waveguide, to regulate the size of the resonant cavities and keep them matched to the microwave frequency. Modern magnetrons are equipped with motor-driven tuners that are controlled by a circuit that senses the microwave frequency.

Klystrons

The principle of the klystron microwave power tube is illustrated in Figure 4-9. The tube requires a low-power radiofrequency oscillator to supply RF power to the first cavity, termed the *buncher*. By application of an accelerating voltage supplied as a DC pulse from the DC power supply (the pulse forming network described earlier),

In 1934, Russell Varian was a graduate student at Stanford, where he met and began working with W. W. Hansen. Russell's brother Sigurd was a pilot for Pan American Airways. Sigurd mentioned to Russell that a way was needed to detect aircraft through cloud cover. Russell proposed to adapt Hansen's rhumbatron to generate high-power microwave fields to power a radar system. The brothers started their own research laboratory but soon realized they had insufficient funds. They applied to Stanford for support and were appointed Research Associates without salary. They were given a budget of $100 for equipment and supplies. This inauspicious start ultimately led to the formation of Varian Associates, which produced the high-power microwave equipment they were seeking. Later, the devices were adapted to linear accelerators.

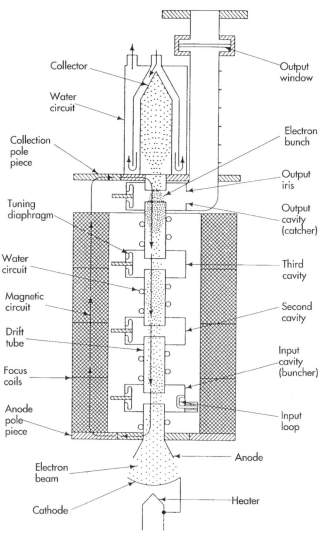

FIGURE 4-9
Schematic cross section of a high-power four cavity klystron power tube.

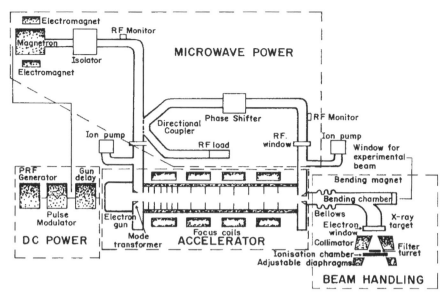

FIGURE 4-10
RF power-handling equipment for a linear accelerator.

electrons with energies of several keV are injected into the cavity. In the buncher cavity, the velocity of the electrons is modulated by the electric field component of the microwave field. This modulation of velocity causes the electrons to group together into closely spaced electron bunches. As the electron bunches arrive at the second cavity, termed the *catcher cavity*, they are decelerated, and their energy is transformed into a pulse of microwave power. High-power klystrons containing additional cavities have achieved direct current-to-microwave conversion efficiencies of up to 55%, with peak powers as high as 24 MW.

Microwave Power-Handling Equipment

Microwaves from the magnetron or klystron are conducted to the accelerator waveguide by rectangular sections of waveguide (Figure 4-10). The microwaves are confined by the metal walls of the waveguide and propagate through a dielectric gas such as freon or sulfur hexafluoride. The dimensions of such waveguides are typically 0.6 λ in width by (0.2–0.5) λ in height. The circular accelerator waveguide is normally energized in the TM_{01} mode, meaning that the magnetic field is transverse to the longitudinal axis of the guide. Consequently, the electric field is axial, and the force exerted by the electric field on the particles accelerates them along the longitudinal axis of the guide.

In single-modality accelerators (those capable of producing only an x-ray beam of selected energy), the waveguide and other microwave power-handling equipment are straightforward. Multimodality accelerators, capable of producing beams of electrons as well as x-ray beams of one or more energies, require alteration of the microwave power delivered to the accelerator structure, so that particles can be accelerated to different energies. Because magnetrons and klystrons are generally adjustable over only small ranges, other means are required to vary the power. One available device is called a *power splitter*. A variable fraction of the power directed to this device is returned to the accelerator waveguide. The remainder is absorbed in a water-filled *load*. Of the power directed to the accelerator waveguide, a portion may be reflected from the guide. A *circulator* or *directional coupler* directs this reflected power away from the magnetron or klystron, to avoid interfering with its operation.

So-called *dual-energy* or *multi-energy* linacs have the capability of producing x-ray beams of two or more energies. They incorporate accelerator waveguides of sufficient length to accelerate electrons to the energy required for the highest-energy photon beam desired, but must be able also to accelerate electrons to lesser energies. This

The low-power RF source used with a klystron is known as the "RF driver" and typically delivers a power level of a few hundred watts.

Waveguides are normally energized in either the transverse magnetic (TM) mode or the transverse electric (TE) mode. Circular waveguides generally support the TM mode, while rectangular waveguides support the TE mode. The variation in magnetic or electric field intensity is described by subscripts. $TM_{m,n}$ indicates that the magnetic field changes by m half-wave lengths around the circumference of the waveguide and by n half-wave lengths along the radius. $TE_{m,n}$ indicates that the electric field varies by m half-wavelengths across the width of the waveguide and by n half-wavelengths across the height. The TE_{10} mode is most commonly used for transporting microwaves from a power-producing device to a circular waveguide, which is used to accelerate particles.

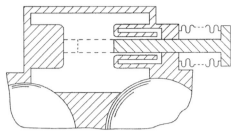

MARGIN FIGURE 4-16

A noncontact-type microwave energy switch for a standing-wave accelerator guide. (Used with permission from Karzmark, C. J., Nunan, C. S., and Tanabe, E. *Medical Electron Accelerators*, New York, McGraw-Hill, 1993.)

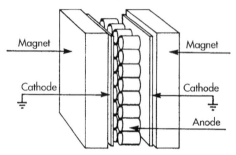

MARGIN FIGURE 4-17

A representative sputter-ion pump.

The term "achromatic" means that the spatial dispersion, or the angular dispersion, of the electron beam is zero at some point along the central trajectory, regardless of the electron momentum. In a *doubly achromatic* magnet, both spatial dispersion and angular dispersion are zero at a point sometimes referred to as the *triple focus*.

The weber is a unit of magnetic flux and describes the integral of the magnetic field strength over a surface. Magnetic field strength is defined by the force exerted by the field on a charged particle,

$$F = qv \times B$$

B therefore is expressed in units of $\frac{newton}{coulomb(m/s)}$, which has been given the special name weber/meter^2:

1 weber/meter^2 = 1 tesla = 10^4 gauss

capability requires radiofrequency power-handling equipment of greater complexity, to ensure that the electron bunches remain focused and that the variation in energy of the electrons remains small. An *energy switch* employed by one manufacturer is shown in Margin Figure 4-16. It provides control over the amount of radiofrequency power passing from the left-hand cavity into the remainder of the guide.

Vacuum Pump

The accelerator guide of a linac requires a high vacuum (on the order of 10^{-8} mm Hg) to prevent power loss and electrical arcing caused by interactions of electrons with gas molecules. Although older models used mechanical fore-pumps and oil diffusion vacuum pumps, all newer models use *sputter-ion (Vac-Ion)* pumps to maintain good vacuum.

A sputter-ion pump typically consists of multiple cylindrical anodes positioned between two cathodes. The cathodes are sandwiched between the poles of a magnet. The cathodes are composed of a reactive sputtering material such as titanium. Electrons ejected spontaneously from the cathode are attracted toward the anode and assume a spiral path in the magnetic field. As a consequence, they oscillate between the cathodes and collide with gas molecules to produce considerable ionization. The resulting positive ions bombard the cathodes, causing ejection (*sputtering*) of neutral atoms of titanium, which are deposited chiefly on the anodes. By this mechanism, gas molecules are continuously removed from the electron accelerator section.

Bending Magnet

Low-energy linacs require short accelerating structures that can be mounted directly in line with the path from the x-ray target to the patient. Higher-energy linacs require longer structures that are often mounted horizontally (or nearly so) within the linac gantry. A *bending magnet* is used to change the direction of the accelerated electron beam from horizontal to vertical. The angle of bend may be 90 degrees, but many accelerators use a 270-degree *achromatic* magnet. As described below, a magnet with multiple 90-degree bends provides greater stability of the resulting photon beam.

The electrons accelerated in a linac do not all reach the bending magnet with exactly the same velocity. The force exerted on an electron in a bending magnet is computed from Newton's law

$$F = ma \qquad (4\text{-}4)$$

and from Equation (4-3) for the force on a particle in an electromagnetic field:

$$F = q(E + v \times B) \qquad (4\text{-}3)$$

A bending magnet is designed so that the magnetic field is perpendicular to the path of the electrons, so the force exerted by the magnetic field is simply

$$F = qvB$$

By substituting the expression for centripetal force, $F = mv^2/r$, and rearranging, the radius of bending of the electron path is shown to be

$$r = \frac{mv}{qB} \qquad (4\text{-}5)$$

Example 4-3

What is the radius of the path of a 10-MeV electron passing through a magnetic field of strength = 7000 gauss (0.7 tesla or 0.7 weber/m^2)?

From Equation (4-5):

$$r = \frac{mv}{qB}$$

where v is the velocity of the 10-MeV electron (99.88% of the speed of light) and m is the mass of the electron. m is related to m_0, the rest mass of the electron (9.11×10^{-31} kg) by

$$m = \frac{m_0}{\sqrt{1 - \dfrac{v^2}{c^2}}}$$

Therefore, $m = 1.86 \times 10^{-29}$ kg. The intensity of the magnetic field $B = 0.7$ weber/m^2 and the charge of an electron $q = 1.6 \times 10^{-19}$ C. Therefore:

$$r = \frac{\left(1.86 \times 10^{-29}\,\text{kg}\right)\left(3 \times 10^8\,\text{m/s}\right)}{\left(1.6 \times 10^{-19}\,\text{C}\right)\left(0.7\,\text{weber/m}^2\right)}$$

$$r = 0.05 \text{ m or } 5 \text{ cm}$$

For a chosen magnetic field strength, electrons with higher energy (higher values of mv) are bent through a larger radius than are lower-energy electrons. As shown in Margin Figure 4-18 of a 90-degree bending magnet, lower-energy electrons strike the target at a different point than the higher-energy component of the beam. However, in a 270° achromatic bending magnet, as shown in Margin Figure 4-19, the low-energy and high-energy components of the beam converge at a point called the *triple focus*. A target positioned at this point intercepts all electrons emerging from the bending magnet. Many bending magnets are equipped with an energy-defining slit consisting of barriers that intercept electrons whose energies vary from the desired energy by more than a selected amount.

X-Ray Target

When an x-ray beam is desired, a *target* of an appropriate material is moved into the path of the electrons. The material usually has a high atomic number (e.g., tungsten) in low-energy linacs, but may be of intermediate atomic number (e.g., copper) in high-energy units. In contrast to conventional x-ray tubes, an accelerator target is generally a *transmission* target, meaning that the generated x rays are transmitted through the target material to reach the patient. The thickness of the target is a compromise between one that ensures every electron interacts and one that absorbs the fewest x rays. The ideal thickness is related to the *radiation length*, the thickness in which $1/e$ of the electron beam is absorbed.

Flattening Filter, Scattering Foil

The x-ray beam from a linac is frequently strongly *forward peaked*. The mean scattering angle subtended by the beam is related to the electron energy by the *Rossi–Griesan* equation:

$$\langle \phi \rangle = \frac{15}{E_0} \sqrt{\frac{X}{X_0}}$$

where $\langle \phi \rangle$ is the mean scattering angle in steradians, E_0 is the energy in MeV of the incident electrons, X is the target thickness, and X_0 is the radiation length. For example, a 15-MeV electron beam incident on a target whose thickness is equal to the radiation length generates a photon beam whose mean scattering angle is only 1 steradian.

A *flattening filter* is used to create a beam of sufficient area and uniformity for clinical use. The effect of a flattening filter on the *raw lobe* of a 10-MV beam is shown in Figure 4-11.

The electron beam exiting from the accelerator waveguide or bending magnet is often no more than 1 or 2 mm in diameter. When the electron beam is to be used for treatment, a *scattering foil* is employed to provide a uniform beam of dimensions suitable for treatment. Modern scattering foils are of complex design, to scatter the

The energy-defining slit of a modern linear accelerator consists of a mechanical barrier placed near the midpoint of the bending magnet. A window in the barrier allows electrons of the selected energy range (correct radius of bend) to pass through. Electrons outside the range are stopped. The choice of barrier material is important to minimize the production of x rays. Nevertheless, the bending magnet is a major source of leakage radiation. If an accelerator is not tuned properly, it can steer a large fraction of the electron beam into the energy slits. The resulting leakage radiation may exceed regulatory limits.

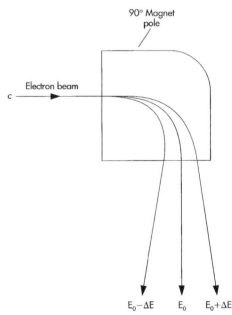

MARGIN FIGURE 4-18
A simple 90° bending magnet, showing the paths of electrons of three energies.

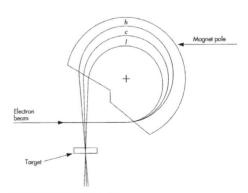

MARGIN FIGURE 4-19
A modern 270° *achromatic* bending magnet, showing the paths of electrons of three energies.

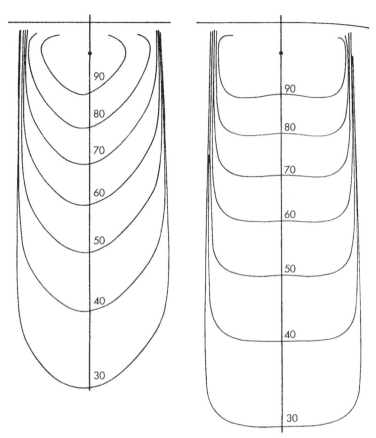

FIGURE 4-11
Isodose distributions for a 10-MV x-ray beam without (**left**) and with (**right**) the beam-flattening filter in place. Lateral horns of the distribution are apparent near the surface for the distribution obtained with the beam-flattening filter.

Bremsstrahlung x rays leave the location of production at an angle relative to the direction of incident electrons. At low electron energies, the mean angle of emission $\langle \phi \rangle$ is large. As the energy E of the incident electrons increases, the $\langle \phi \rangle$ decreases so that at megavoltage energies the x rays are emitted predominantly in the forward direction. Consequently, a reflection target of the type used in lower-energy x-ray tubes is not used in a linear accelerator. Instead, a thin transmission target is used.

The *radiation length* is the thickness of a material that attenuates an electron beam to 1/e of its incident intensity.

Today's medical linac requires a flattening filter so that the x-ray beam reaching the patient is as uniform as possible. Treatment techniques recently introduced, such as intensity-modulated radiation therapy (IMRT), do not require a uniform beam and may allow the production of machines without flattening filters.

Accelerator engineers use the term *raw lobe* to describe the profile of the x-ray beam before it is modulated by the flattening filter.

Today, most clinics refer to the digital display of an accelerator output as "monitor units" but accepted terminology in the past included "clicks" and "riddles," among others.

beam without generating an unacceptable quantity of bremsstrahlung radiation or degrading the beam energy by too great an amount.

Monitor Ionization Chamber

In contrast to ^{60}Co units, in which the source decays predictably to furnish a beam of slowly decreasing intensity, the dose rate of an accelerator beam may vary unpredictably or by design. Consequently, it is not possible to rely on the elapsed time to control the dose delivered to a patient. Instead the radiation leaving the target or scattering foil passes through a *monitor ionization chamber* (Figure 4-12), where it produces an ionization current that is proportional to the beam intensity. The ionization current is conducted to the control panel, where it is converted to a digital display of *monitor units*. The dose delivered to the patient is controlled by programming the accelerator to deliver a prescribed number of monitor units, often referred to as the "meter setting."

Collimator

The final control over the beam, before it is delivered to the patient, is exerted by the collimator. In contrast to ^{60}Co sources, which are often several centimeters in diameter, the source of x rays in a linac is only 1 or 2 mm in diameter. As a result, the collimator can be of simpler design because the geometric penumbra is smaller. For x-ray beams, the collimator consists of jaws made of a high atomic number material such as lead or tungsten. In most cases, the jaws are adjusted under motor control to create rectangular beams of almost any size. Most modern accelerators can deliver beams up to 40×40 cm^2.

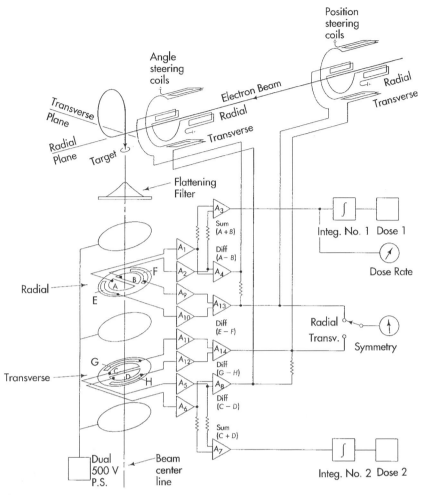

FIGURE 4-12

A modern multisegment monitor ion chamber showing the role of each segment in measuring the beam flatness and symmetry as well as the dose rate. (Used with permission from Karzmark, C. J., Nunan, C. S., and Tanabe, E. *Medical Electron Accelerators*, New York, McGraw-Hill, 1993.)

Because electrons can be scattered easily by the intervening air between the scattering foil and the patient, the final stage of collimation of an electron beam must be close to the skin surface. An *electron applicator* or *cone*, such as those shown in Margin Figure 4-20, is used to shape electron beams. Although the cone is rectangular, a slot is often provided to place a shaped insert to customize the field shape to the patient' s target volume.

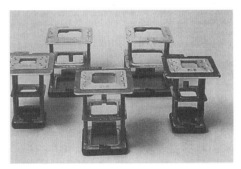

MARGIN FIGURE 4-20
Representative electron applicators. (Courtesy of Varian Associates, Inc.)

Treatment Couch

To support the patient during treatment, a treatment couch is provided as part of a linear accelerator. The couch is usually mounted isocentrically, so that it pivots about an axis that passes through the gantry isocenter. Sometimes an eccentric axis of rotation is provided to provide greater convenience for patients or to permit extended lateral movement of the couch. Most couch motions are motorized.

■ OTHER MEDICAL ACCELERATORS

Van de Graaff Generators

The first particle accelerator developed by Van de Graaff was described in 1931.[18] Van de Graaff generators used in research provide beams of positively charged particles

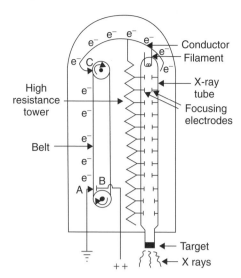

MARGIN FIGURE 4-21

Diagram of a Van de Graaff generator for the production of high-energy x rays. (Used with permission from Karzmark, C. J., Nunan, C. S., and Tanabe, E. *Medical Electron Accelerators*, New York, McGraw-Hill, 1993.)

Although Van de Graaff generators are no longer used in medicine, a few may still be found in research and industrial settings. The Physics Department at the University of Kentucky uses a 7-MeV Van de Graaff generator to accelerate protons which are used to generate a neutron beam. The neutron beam has been used for radiation-hardening experiments.

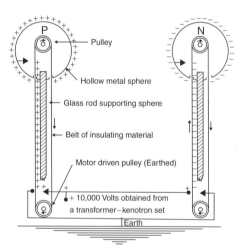

MARGIN FIGURE 4-22

Van de Graaff's supervoltage unit. *P*, Positive spherical terminal; *N*, negative spherical terminal. (Van de Graaff, R. J. A 1,500,000-volt electrostatic generator. *Phys. Rev.* 1931; **38**:1919–1920.

One of the generators constructed by Van de Graaff required an airship hangar 140 ft × 75 ft × 75 ft high.

with energies of 20 MeV and higher. In radiation therapy, Van de Graaff generators have been used to accelerate electrons to energies of up to 3 MeV. A Van de Graaff generator is diagrammed in Margin Figure 4-21. Electrons are attracted from ground to point *A* by the large positive potential (e.g., +20 kV) of point *B*. Electrons are sprayed from electrode *A* toward electrode *B* and are intercepted by the belt moving between the electrodes. The belt is usually composed of layers of cotton webbing impregnated with a neoprene compound. The electron collector *C* removes electrons carried toward the hollow conductor by the belt. These electrons are transferred from the electron collector to the hollow conductor, lowering the electrical potential of the conductor. The potential is lowered until the charge leaks from the conductor as rapidly as it is collected.

An x-ray tube and high-resistance "tower" are connected between the negatively charged hollow conductor and ground. Aluminum electrodes inside the x-ray tube are connected to the high-resistance tower. Electrons liberated by the heated filament of the accelerator tube are accelerated through the electrodes and focused onto a water-cooled transmission target. The length of the accelerator tube and the spacing of the focusing electrodes are designed to prevent arcing between elements of the tube.

Van de Graaff generators are usually housed within an insulating atmosphere of 80% nitrogen and 20% carbon dioxide at a pressure of up to 20 atm. In some units, this mixture of gases is replaced by sulfur hexafluoride at a pressure of up to 6 atm. A typical Van de Graaff generator provides a focal spot of less than 3 mm. The dose rate varies from 80 to 250 cGy/min at 1 m and is relatively stable.

Betatrons

Betatrons have largely been replaced in the clinic by linear accelerators, but for several decades after their introduction they enjoyed considerable popularity. None is presently in clinical operation in the United States. The first betatron, constructed by Kerst[19] in 1941, accelerated electrons to an energy of 2 MeV. In later years, electrons and x rays with energies up to 45 MeV were available from betatrons. A cross section of a betatron is shown in Margin Figure 4-23A. Electrons from a tungsten filament are injected with an energy of about 50 keV into a hollow, evacuated annulus or "donut" composed of glass or porcelain (Margin Figure 4-24). The donut is mounted between the poles of an electromagnet, which is energized by an alternating voltage oscillating at a frequency between 50 and 180 Hz. The magnetic field forces the injected electrons into an equilibrium orbit of constant radius. The radius of the equilibrium orbit varies from a few centimeters to a meter or more, depending on the maximum energy desired for electrons revolving in the donut. The radius *r* of the equilibrium orbit in meters is computed with the equation

$$r = \frac{mv}{Bq} \qquad (4\text{-}5)$$

In Equation (4-5), *m* represents the mass of an electron in kilograms, *v* is the velocity in meters per second, *q* represents the charge of an electron in coulombs, and *B* is the intensity of the magnetic field in webers per square meter. Note that this equation is identical to the equation that describes the radius of curvature of electrons passing through a bending magnet in a linear accelerator.

Cyclotrons

The first cyclotron, developed by Lawrence and Livingston in 1932,[20] provided the background for modern orbital accelerators. Electrons are not accelerated in cyclotrons, and these machines are used for radiation therapy in only a few institutions in which the therapeutic applications of neutrons or positive ions are being investigated. Cyclotrons are also used extensively to produce radioactive nuclides, including positron emitters that are useful in nuclear imaging and medical research.

The operation of a cyclotron is outlined in Margin Figure 4-25. Two hollow, semicircular electrodes or "dees" are mounted between the poles of an electromagnet and separated from each other by a gap of 2–5 cm. The electromagnet is energized by direct current and furnishes a magnetic field of constant intensity across the dees. An alternating voltage applied to the dees oscillates with a frequency that is chosen with consideration for the intensity of the magnetic field and the type of particle being accelerated. For most cyclotrons available commercially, the frequency is between 10 and 40 MHz.

Positive ions (e.g., $^1H^+$, $^2H^+$, $^3He^{2+}$, or $^4He^{2+}$) are released by a cathode-arc source in the gap between the dees and are accelerated in bunches toward the negative dee. After the ions enter the dee, they are shielded from the electric field. The magnetic field forces the particles into a circular path, which the particles follow with constant speed. Just as the polarity reverses across the dees, the ions emerge from the first dee and accelerate across the gap toward the second dee. The ions follow a circular orbit in the second dee and emerge as the polarity reverses again. In this manner, the particles are accelerated each time they cross the dee aperture until they attain the desired energy.

The radius of the orbit followed by ions within a dee is described by Equation (4-5):

$$r = \frac{mv}{Bq} \qquad (4\text{-}5)$$

where r is the radius in meters, m is the mass of the accelerated particles in kilograms, v is the velocity of the particles in meters per second, q is the charge of the particles in coulombs, and B is the magnetic field intensity in webers per square meter. This equation is identical to the equation that describes the equilibrium orbit of electrons in a betatron and within a bending magnet. If the magnetic field intensity B and the mass m are constant, the radius of the orbit increases linearly with the velocity of the accelerated particles.

The time T for a half-revolution of the particles in a dee is

$$T = \frac{\pi m}{Bq}$$

If the mass of the particles remains constant, the time for a half-revolution is also constant, and the emergence of the particles from the dees is synchronized easily with changes in the dee polarity. However, the relativistic mass m of a particle moving with velocity v is

$$m = \frac{m_0}{\sqrt{1 - \dfrac{v^2}{c^2}}} \qquad (4\text{-}6)$$

When the velocity of particles in a cyclotron reaches about $0.2c$, the increased mass of the particles disturbs the synchronization between the emergence of particles from the dees and the changing polarity across the dees. For example, deuterons may be accelerated in a cyclotron to a maximum energy of about 35 MeV. Above 35 MeV, the relativistic increase in mass causes the deuterons to emerge from the dees out of phase with the changing polarity of the dees.

To maintain the synchronization between particle emergence from the dees and changing polarity of the dees, the frequency of the alternating voltage applied to the dees may be reduced as the particles gain energy. This approach is used in the synchrocyclotron, and deuterons have been accelerated to energies up to 200 MeV in these machines.

For experimental studies, a beam of heavy particles may be extracted from a cyclotron. Additionally, radioactive nuclides may be produced in a cyclotron by directing accelerated particles onto a target. For example, the radioactive nuclides listed in Table 4-1 are produced in a cyclotron by the reactions described in the table. An increasing number of medical institutions are using a cyclotron to produce short-lived,

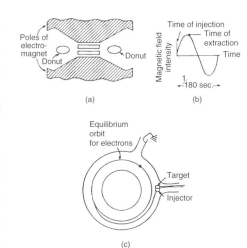

MARGIN FIGURE 4-23
Principles of a betatron. **A:** Cross section illustrating the electromagnet and the donut. **B:** Graph of the intensity of the magnetic field across the electron orbit as a function of time. Times of injection and extraction of electrons are denoted. The power supply oscillates at a frequency of 180 Hz. **C:** Path of electrons in a betatron donut. The electron injector and x-ray target are indicated. (Used with permission from Karzmark, C. J., Nunan, C. S., and Tanabe, E. *Medical Electron Accelerators*, New York, McGraw-Hill, 1993.)

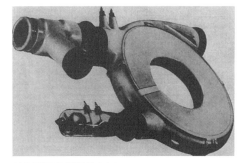

MARGIN FIGURE 4-24
A typical betatron donut.

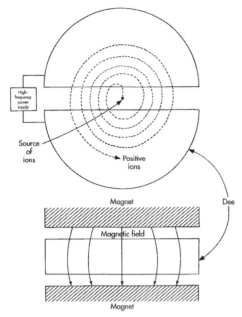

MARGIN FIGURE 4-25

Conventional two-dee cyclotron. The path of positively charged particles is denoted by the *dashed curve*. The particles are accelerated each time they cross the gap between the dees.

TABLE 4-1 Representative Radioactive Nuclides Produced in a Cyclotron and Used in Medicine

Radioactive Nuclide	Reaction[a]	Half-Life	Medical Uses
^{11}C	^{10}Ba (d, n)^{11}C	20 min	PET imaging of lung function, blood circulation
^{15}O	^{14}N (d, n)^{15}O	2 min	PET imaging of lung function, blood circulation
^{18}F	^{16}O (α, pn)^{18}F	110 min	PET imaging of epileptogenic foci, differentiation between tumor and necrosis
^{67}Ga	^{68}Zn (p, 2n)^{67}Ga	78 hr	Imaging of tumors and abscesses
^{123}I	^{127}I (p, 5n)^{123}Xe $\xrightarrow{EC}$ ^{123}I or ^{124}Xe(p, 2n)^{123}Cs $\xrightarrow{EC+\beta^+}$ ^{123}Xe $\xrightarrow{EC}$ ^{123}I	13.3 hr	Evaluation of thyroid function and morphology
^{111}In	^{109}Ag (α, 2n) ^{111}In[b]	2.8 days	Imaging of occult inflammatory lesions
^{57}Co	^{56}Fe(d, n)^{57}Co or ^{56}Fe (p, 8)^{57}Co	270 days	Diagnosis of intestinal absorption deficiencies; substitute for ^{99m}Tc for some QA procedures
^{201}Tl	^{203}Tl (p, 3n)^{201}Pb $\xrightarrow{EC+\beta^+}$ ^{201}Tl	73 hr	Assessment of myocardial function

[a] The nuclear reactions are indicated by the symbols in parentheses. For example, (d, n) describes a reaction in which a target nucleus is bombarded by a deuteron, and a neutron is emitted. The target nucleus thus contains one additional proton following the reaction.

[b] Several alternate reactions exist for producing this nuclide.

Some cyclotrons use one or three dees rather than two. These units differ from cyclotrons with two dees primarily in the high-frequency power supply required for the dees.

The mass of a moving particle is greater than the mass of the same particle when stationary. This change in mass is described as the relativistic increase in mass with velocity.

Electrons reach the limiting velocity of $0.2c$ when their kinetic energy is only about 10 keV. Consequently, electrons are not accelerated in cyclotrons.

positron-emitting radioactive nuclides (^{11}C, ^{13}N, ^{15}O, ^{18}F) useful in nuclear medicine. These nuclides are used in combination with a positron-emission tomographic unit (PET).

Microtrons

With the availability of microwave accelerator cavities came the development of another device for accelerating electrons in circular or elliptical orbits. This device, called the *microtron*, combines the static magnetic field of the cyclotron with the accelerating cavity of the linear accelerator.[21] In contrast to the linear accelerator, electrons pass through the accelerating cavity multiple times, gaining energy each time (Figure 4-13). The path of the electron bunch is bent by the static magnetic field in a circular or racetrack shape, bringing the electrons back to the cavity.

As electrons reach velocities close to the speed of light, they can be considered to be traveling at constant velocity during the entire acceleration process. As their energy increases, however, their momentum increases proportionately, and their bending radius increases as well:

$$r = \frac{mv}{Bq} \tag{4-5}$$

In a circular microtron, the electron's energy increases in equal increments, and therefore the circumference of the path increases by corresponding increments. Consequently, the electron bunch arrives at the accelerating cavity at the correct moment to be accelerated again.

The maximum energy of electrons in a microtron is essentially limited only by the dimensions and strength of the static magnetic field. In practice, microtrons can accelerate electrons to energies up to 50 MeV.[21] Difficulties with the stability of

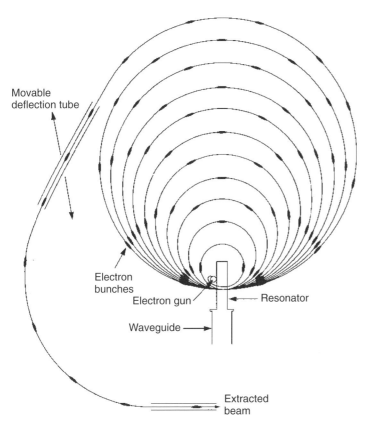

FIGURE 4-13
The design of a circular microtron, showing electron bunches spaced throughout several orbits. A movable magnetic shunt permits extraction of electrons of a selected energy. (Redrawn with permission from Brahme, A., and Svensson, H. Radiation beam characteristics of a 22 MeV microtron, *Acta Radiat. Oncol.* **18**:244–272; copyright 1979, Munksgaard International Publishers, Ltd., Copenhagen, Denmark.)

operation have made microtrons unreliable in the clinic, and pursuit of their clinical application has been discontinued.

▤ SIMULATORS

Basic Design

Delivery of radiation therapy requires high accuracy in the placement of treatment fields. Small errors can result in a recurrence or in a serious complication. Placement of radiation fields, however, is complicated by the inability of the physician to see inside the patient. It is common to make use of *port films*, or radiographs taken with a small radiation exposure from the treatment unit. However, these films have relatively poor contrast because of the predominance of Compton interactions (see Chapter 3). Consequently a technique is needed to take diagnostic-quality radiographs using the geometry of the treatment unit.

A simulator is essentially a conventional radiographic/fluoroscopic x-ray unit mounted in a manner that allows the x-ray beam to mimic the high-energy beam from a treatment unit. This configuration enables the acquisition of diagnostic-quality radiographs, while maintaining the geometry of a conventional treatment unit. Because many departments have a single simulator to service several treatment machines with different geometries, most simulators permit adjustments to several parameters (such as target-to-axis distance) over the range commonly found in practice. A representative radiation therapy simulator is shown in Figure 4-14, and it is shown in schematic form in Figure 4-15.

In many clinics, conventional radiation therapy simulators are being replaced by CT simulators. These devices are conventional CT scanners equipped with software to produce *digitally reconstructed radiographs* (DRRs) and to permit *segmentation*, or outlining of anatomical structures. The resulting CT data set can often be exported to a treatment planning system.

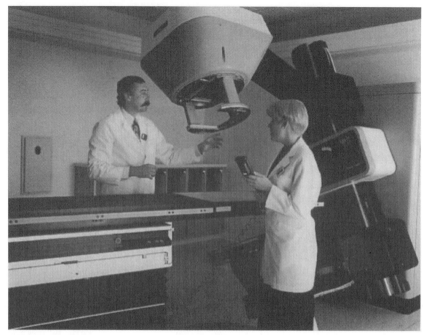

FIGURE 4-14
A typical radiation therapy simulator, showing the treatment couch, the gantry, and the radiation head. (Courtesy of Varian Associates, Inc.)

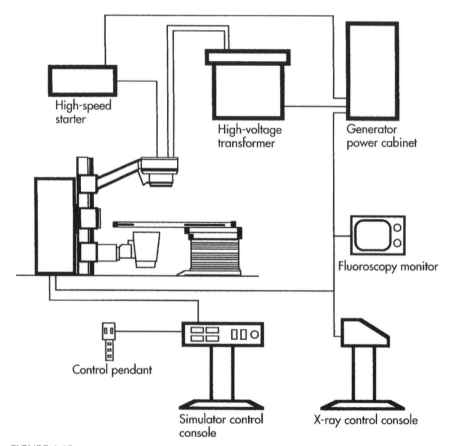

FIGURE 4-15
A block diagram of a simulator showing the control console, generator, stand, gantry, x-ray tube, collimator, image intensifier, and treatment couch.

Most simulators are equipped with an image intensifier, so that the patient's anatomy can be visualized under fluoroscopy before radiographs are taken. Most mechanical parameters can be adjusted under remote control, including the treatment couch position, gantry angle, and collimator settings.

Generator

The generator of a simulator, similar to that of a conventional diagnostic x-ray unit, should deliver voltages over the range of 40–150 kVp and should supply tube currents between 50 and 600 mA. Exposure times as short as a few milliseconds, and as long as several seconds, are required. Generators that provide less than the full range of voltage and tube current may still be adequate for many patients. A three-phase generator is preferred for a simulator because it permits shorter exposure times and provides x rays with greater penetrating power for examining thick body sections.

X-Ray Tube

A tube of the type referred to as "general purpose" is appropriate for simulators. It should have two focal spots, nominally 0.6 and 1.2 mm, and should have a heat capacity of at least 2 million heat units.

Image Intensifier

Most radiation oncologists prefer an image intensifier of at least 12 inches (30 cm) diameter for treatment simulation. A smaller-diameter intensifier is more maneuverable, however. Different magnification modes are useful on occasion and are commonly available. A collision-detection device is useful because serious and expensive damage can result from a collision.

Mechanical Subsystems: Collimator

The collimator of a simulator is generally a two-component device. A conventional diagnostic collimator, equipped with lead *blades*, is provided to limit the radiation to the patient. Often the blades can be controlled independently to mimic the motion of a treatment unit collimator. During fluoroscopy, the blades in some units can be adjusted automatically to follow the position of the image intensifier. This practice limits the radiation beam to the volume of tissue being imaged.

This collimator is followed by two pairs of *delineator wires* that can be adjusted under remote control. Their purpose is to allow the operator to indicate the location of the treatment field without obscuring the radiation beam. Similarly to the blades, the delineator wires often can be adjusted independently to simulate the treatment unit collimator jaws. The shadow of the delineator wires is visible on the fluoroscopic image as well as on the radiograph (Margin Figure 4-26).

The appearance of the delineator wires on the radiograph depends both on their construction and on their location. As shown in Margin Figure 4-27, the width of the penumbra of the shadow cast by the delineator wires changes from one side of the image to the other. This is a consequence of the difference in apparent focal spot size on the anode and cathode sides of the image. Delineator wires constructed from material of too large a diameter can cast objectionably broad shadows and introduce uncertainty over the location of the intended field edge. The delineator wires must be of adequate thickness, however, to attenuate the beam sufficiently to cast a visible shadow.

To simulate treatment, the simulator must also mimic blocked radiation fields. The collimator must therefore be constructed with a slot for a *beam-shaping platform* or blocking tray. Ideally the construction of the simulator should permit the use of full-thickness cast blocks, so that the blocks constructed for a patient's treatment can

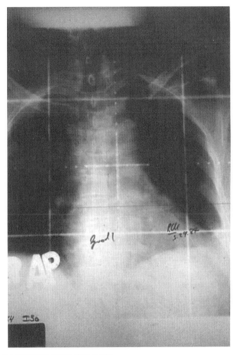

MARGIN FIGURE 4-26
A representative radiograph made with a radiation therapy simulator.

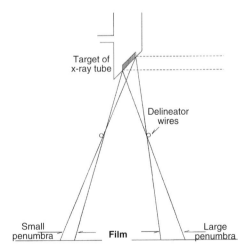

MARGIN FIGURE 4-27
The delineator wires of a radiation therapy simulator cast shadows of different widths, owing to their location relative to the x-ray target. Note the similarity with Figure 4-6.

be placed on the beam-shaping platform during simulation. Should the design of the simulator not permit the additional weight, blocks can be simulated by dipping Styrofoam blocks (such as the material removed when Styrofoam is used to cast metal blocks) into a contrast agent. This alternative, however, is decidedly inferior to the use of actual cast blocks.

See Chapter 9 for additional information regarding imaging devices in radiation therapy.

■ SUMMARY

- Radiation treatment unit design has evolved significantly since the first x-ray tubes became available in 1896.
- The use of x rays for radiation therapy began within months of their discovery.
- Low-energy x-ray units are in use in many clinics for treatment of superficial disease.
- The introduction of the ^{60}Co teletherapy unit made "megavoltage" radiation therapy affordable and practical.
- The development of the side-coupled standing-wave electron linear accelerator allowed the construction of a 4-MV linac that is physically no larger than a ^{60}Co unit.
- Refinements have made dual-photon energy linacs practical and affordable for many radiation therapy departments.
- ^{60}Co units remain a practical and economic alternative in countries where accelerator service capabilities are limited.

PROBLEMS

4-1. The source-to-collimator distance is 62 cm for a particular ^{60}Co unit. The ^{60}Co source has a diameter of 2 cm. What are the widths of the geometric penumbra at the skin and at 15 cm below the skin when the source-skin distance is 80 cm?

4-2. **A.** The beam penumbra of a linac is measured at the surface of a phantom at 100 cm SSD and found to be 8 mm. The source-to-collimator distance is 55 cm. If the measured penumbra equals the geometric penumbra, what must the effective source diameter be? **B.** How much smaller would the penumbra be if tapered blocks were positioned in the beam at 65 cm from the source?

4-3. What is the maximum specific activity for ^{60}Co?

4-4. What minimum value of shunt impedance must an accelerator

waveguide have to develop a potential difference of 18 MV over a distance of 1 m and consume no more than 2 MW of power?

4-5. What is the fractional increase in mass of a particle moving with a velocity of $0.1c$? $0.5c$? $0.99c$?

4-6. 15-MeV electrons enter a bending magnet with a magnetic field strength of 0.7 tesla. What is the radius of the path of the electrons? What range of energies could electrons have and still be confined to orbits with radii within 5% of the 15-MeV electrons?

4-7. Distinguish between the operation of magnetron and klystron microwave tubes.

4-8. Distinguish between a standing wave and a traveling wave linear accelerator.

REFERENCES

1. Ewing, J. Early experience in radiation therapy. *AJR* 1934; **31**:153–163.
2. Lederman, M. The early history of radiotherapy: 1895–1939. *Int. J. Radiat. Oncol. Biol. Phys.* 1981; **7**:639–648.
3. Lauritsen, C. C., and Bennett, R. D. A new high potential x ray tube. *Phys. Rev.* 1928; **32**:850–857.
4. Mayneord, W. V., and Roberts, J. E. Measurements of high-voltage x rays. *Br. J. Radiol.* 1933; **6**:321–341.
5. Johns, H., Bates, L., and Watson, T. 1000 curie cobalt units for radiation therapy: I. The Saskatchewan cobalt-60 unit. *Br. J. Radiol.* 1952; **25**:296–302.
6. Johns, H. E., Epp, E. R., Cormack, D. V., and Fedoruk, S. O. Depth dose data and diaphragm design for the Saskatchewan 1000 curie cobalt unit. *Br. J. Radiol.* 1952; **25**:302–308.
7. Johns, H., et al. Physical characteristics of the radiation in cobalt-60 beam therapy. *J. Can. Assoc. Radiol.* 1952; **3**:2.
8. Ibbott, G., and Hendee, W. Beam-shaping platforms and the skin-sparing advantage of ^{60}Co radiation. *AJR* 1970; **108**:193–196.
9. Debois, J. The determination of the penumbra at different depths. *J. Belg. Radiol.* 1966; **49**:200–205.

10. Brucer, M. An automatic controlled pattern cesium-137 teletherapy machine. *AJR* 1956; **75:**49–55.

11. Wideröe, R. Uber ein neues prinzip zur Herstellung hohen Spannungen, *Arch. Elektrotech.* 1928; **21:**387.

12. Cutler, C. C. Bell Telephone Laboratories Report MN-44-160-218, 1944, as described by Karzmark, C. J., Nunan, C. S., Tanabe, E. *Medical Electron Accelerators.* New York, McGraw-Hill, 1993.

13. Fry, D. W., Harvie, S.-R. B. R., Mullet, L. B., Walkinshaw, W. Traveling-wave linear accelerator for electrons. *Nature* 1947; **160:**351–352.

14. Ginzton, E. L., Hansen, W. W., and Kennedy, W. R. A linear electron accelerator. *Rev. Sci. Instr.* 1948; **19:**89–108.

15. Chodorow, M., Ginzton, E. L., and Hansen, W. W. Design and performance of a high-power pulsed klystron. *Proc. IRE,* 1953; **41:**1584.

16. Knapp, E. A., Knapp, B. C., and Potter, I. M. Standing wave high energy linear accelerator structures. *Rev. Sci. Instr.* 1968; **39:**979–991.

17. Karzmark, C. J., Nunan, C. S., and Tanabe, E. *Medical Electron Accelerators.* New York, McGraw-Hill, 1993.

18. Van de Graaff, R. A 1,500,000 volt electrostatic generator. *Phys. Rev.* 1931; **348:**1919–1920.

19. Kerst, D. Acceleration of electrons by magnetic induction. *Phys. Rev.* 1941; **60:**47–53.

20. Lawrence, E., and Livingston, M. The production of high speed light ions without the use of high voltages. *Phys. Rev.* 1932; **40:**19–35.

21. Brahme, A., and Svensson, H. Radiation beam characteristics of a 22 MeV microtron. *Acta Radiol. Oncol.* 1979; **18:**244–272.

MEASUREMENT OF IONIZING RADIATION

OBJECTIVES 80

INTRODUCTION 80

RADIATION INTENSITY 80

RADIATION EXPOSURE 82

Energy and Photon Fluence per Unit Exposure 82

MEASUREMENT OF RADIATION EXPOSURE 84

Free-Air Ionization Chamber 85
Thimble Chambers 87
Condenser Chambers 88
Correction Factors 90
Extrapolation and Parallel-Plate Chambers 92

RADIATION DOSE 92

MEASUREMENT OF RADIATION DOSE 94

Calorimetric Dosimetry 95

Photographic Dosimetry 95
Chemical Dosimetry 96
Scintillation and Semiconductor Dosimetry 97
Thermoluminescence Dosimetry 97
Other Solid-State Dosimeters 98

ABSORBED DOSE MEASUREMENTS WITH
AN IONIZATION CHAMBER 99

Bragg–Gray Principle 99

DOSE EQUIVALENT 100

RADIATION QUALITY 102

Spectral Distributions 103

SUMMARY 105

PROBLEMS 105

REFERENCES 106

Radiation Therapy Physics, Third Edition, by William R. Hendee, Geoffrey S. Ibbott, and Eric G. Hendee
ISBN 0-471-39493-9 Copyright © 2005 John Wiley & Sons, Inc.

■ OBJECTIVES

After studying this chapter, the reader should be able to:

- Define and apply various concepts used to describe radiation quantity, including
  - Radiation intensity (photon and energy fluence and flux density), exposure, kerma dose, dose equivalent
  - Mean dose equivalent and effective dose equivalent
- Explain the concepts of electron equilibrium, effective atomic number, mass stopping power, and the Bragg–Gray principle.
- Describe the purpose and operation of the free air ionization chamber; and why it is limited to exposure measurements for photons with energy less than about 3 MeV.
- Distinguish among a Bragg–Gray cavity, thimble chamber and condenser chamber.
- Identify the correction factors necessary for measurements of exposure (or dose) with an ionization chamber.
- Delineate the principles of radiation dose measurements by calorimetry, photography, and chemical, scintillation and thermoluminescence dosimetry.
- Articulate an understanding of radiation quality and factors that influence it.

■ INTRODUCTION

The term *radiation* refers to energy in transit from one location to another. *Radiation quantity* describes an amount of energy measured in some fashion at a specific position in space over a prescribed period of time. The method of measurement defines the unit employed to describe radiation quantity. Common units of radiation quantity are described in this chapter. The term *radiation intensity* is used generically in the literature to describe radiation quantity. In this text, radiation intensity is given a specific definition.

The term "ionizing radiation" encompasses directly ionizing charged particles, indirectly ionizing uncharged particles (e.g., neutrons), and electromagnetic photons (x and γ rays).

■ RADIATION INTENSITY

The number N of x or γ rays (electromagnetic photons, hereafter referred to simply as photons), crossing a unit area A at a location in a beam of radiation is known as the *photon fluence* Φ ($\Phi = N/A$) at the specific location. The rate at which the photons cross the area is termed the photon flux ϕ (or *photon flux density*) ($\phi = \Phi/t = N/At$, where t represents time). If the fluence varies with time, the flux must be specified at a particular moment or expressed as an average over time.

The flux density is occasionally referred to as the "fluence rate."

If the photons in the beam all possess the same energy, the *energy fluence* Ψ is simply the product of the photon fluence and the energy per photon ($\psi = \Phi E = NE/A$). The *energy flux* ψ (or *energy flux density*, often termed the *radiation intensity*) is the photon flux multiplied by the energy per photon ($\psi = \phi E = NE/At$). If the radiation beam contains photons of different energies ($E_1, E_2, \ldots, E_m$), the intensity or energy flux is expressed as

In some texts the rate of change of a variable with time is denoted by placing a dot over the variable. That is, the energy flux density would be designated as $\dot{\Phi}$, where Φ is the symbol for the energy fluence. This convention is followed in subsequent chapters of this text.

$$\psi = \sum_{i=1}^{m} f_i \phi_i E_i$$

where f_i represents the fraction of photons with energy E_i and the symbol $\sum_{i=1}^{m}$ reveals that the intensity is determined by summing the components of the beam at each of the "m" energies.

Example 5-1

A 6-MV x-ray port film requires 10^{16} x rays over an exposure time of 2 seconds to expose a film with an area of 1500 cm^2. With the assumption that the average photon energy is 2 MeV, determine the photon flux ϕ, photon fluence Φ, energy flux ψ, and energy fluence Ψ.

$$\text{Photon fluence } \Phi = \frac{N}{A} = \frac{10^{16} \text{ photons}}{1.5 \times 10^{-1} \text{ m}^2} = 6.7 \times 10^{16} \text{ photons/m}^2$$

$$\text{Photon flux } \phi = \frac{N}{At} = \frac{\Phi}{t} = \frac{6.7 \times 10^{16} \text{ photons/m}^2}{2 \text{ sec}}$$

$$= 3.4 \times 10^{16} \text{ photons/m}^2\text{-sec}$$

$$\text{Energy fluence } \Psi = \frac{NE}{A} = \Phi E = (6.7 \times 10^{16} \text{ photons/m}^2)\,(2 \text{ MeV/photon})$$

$$= 1.3 \times 10^{17} \text{ MeV/m}^2$$

$$\text{Energy flux } \psi = \frac{NE}{At} = \frac{\Psi}{t} = \frac{1.3 \times 10^{17} \text{ MeV/m}^2}{2 \text{ sec}} = 6.7 \times 10^{16} \text{ MeV/m}^2\text{-sec}$$

An x-ray beam actually contains a spectrum of energies. A more exact computation of Ψ and ψ would involve a weighted sum of the contributions of the various photon energies. This procedure is illustrated in Example 5-2.

Example 5-2

Gamma rays of 1.7 and 1.33 MeV are released each time a ^{60}Co atom decays. What are the photon and energy fluence per m^2 at 1 m from a ^{60}Co source in which 10^6 atoms decay?

The surface area of a sphere of radius r is $4\pi r^2$. The surface area of a sphere of 1-m radius is $4\pi (1 \text{ m})^2$. Because gamma rays are emitted isotropically (equal numbers in all directions) from a radioactive source, the photon fluence is equal at all locations on the sphere surface if the source is positioned at the center of the sphere. The fraction of the photons intercepted by a 1-m^2 area on the sphere surface is

$$\text{Fraction of total emissions} = \frac{1 \text{ m}^2}{4\pi (1 \text{ m})^2} = 7.96 \times 10^{-2}$$

Because 2 photons are released per decay, 2×10^6 photons are released during 10^6 decays:

$$\text{Photon fluence} = \Phi = (2 \times 10^6 \text{ photons})(7.96 \times 10^{-2}) \cong 16 \times 10^4 \text{ photons/m}^2$$

The energy fluence is

$$\Psi = \sum_{i=1}^{2} f_i \Phi E_i = (0.5)(16 \times 10^4)(1.17 \text{ MeV}) + (0.5)(16 \times 10^4)(1.33 \text{ MeV})$$

where the photon fluence of 16×10^4 photons/m^2 is composed of equal numbers of photons (8×10^4 photons/m^2) of 1.17 and 1.33 MeV:

$$\Psi = (9.36 \text{ MeV/m}^2 + 10.64 \text{ MeV/m}^2) \times 10^4 = 20 \times 10^4 \text{ MeV/m}^2$$

Although photon and energy fluences and fluxes are important in many computations, these quantities are not easily measured. Usually, radiation quantity is expressed in units that are related directly to common methods of radiation measurement. Several units of radiation quantity (e.g., roentgen, rad, and rem) have been used over the years. Today the preferred units of radiation (e.g., coulombs/kg, gray and sievert)

TABLE 5-1 Traditional (T) and Système International (SI) Units

Unit Quantity	To Convert from T to SI		Multiply by
	T	SI	
Exposure	roentgen(R)	coulomb/kg	2.58×10^{-4}
Absorbed dose (kerma)	rad	gray (Gy)	0.01
Dose equivalent	rem	sievert (Sv)	0.01

rad is an acronym for radiation absorbed dose; rem is an acronym for roentgen equivalent man.

The unit gray honors the English physicist L. H. Gray; the unit sievert honors the Swedish physicist Rolf Sievert.

In some texts the exposure X is defined as $X = \Delta Q/\Delta m$, where the delta (Δ) signifies a very small amount of charge produced in a very small volume of air.

The definition of the roentgen is ascribed to the French physicist Villard, who first defined it in 1908. Twenty years later (1928) the Second International Congress of Radiology adopted a modified version of Villard's definition as the first official unit of radiation quantity, described in terms of the unit "roentgen."

STP = 0°C temperature and 1 atmosphere (760 mm Hg) pressure. Under these conditions, 1 m³ of air has a mass of 1.293 kg.

are part of the Système International definition of units (SI units). Conversions from traditional to SI units are shown in Table 5-1.

■ RADIATION EXPOSURE

Primary ion pairs (electrons and positive ions) are produced as ionizing radiation interacts in a medium. These ion pairs (IP) produce additional ionization (secondary IP) as they dissipate their energy by interacting with nearby atoms. The total number of IP produced is proportional to the energy absorbed as the radiation interacts in the medium. If the medium is air, the total charge Q (negative or positive) of the ionization produced as the radiation interacts with a unit mass m of air is known as the *radiation exposure* X ($X = Q/m$). The charge Q includes both primary and secondary IP, with the secondary IP produced both inside and outside of the volume of air of mass m. The SI unit of radiation exposure is coulombs/kg, and the earlier unit of exposure is the roentgen (R), defined as 1 R = 2.58×10^{-4} coulomb/kg of air. This definition is numerically equivalent to an older description of the roentgen that states that 1 roentgen equals 1 electrostatic unit of charge (esu) released per cubic centimeter (cm³) of air at standard temperature and pressure (STP). The unit roentgen has virtually disappeared from use as the SI unit of coulombs/kg has become accepted.

The roentgen is applicable only to x radiation and gamma radiation less than about 3 MeV, and it cannot be used for beams of particles or high-energy photons. At photon energies above 3 MeV, it is difficult to determine how many secondary IP are produced outside the measurement volume by ionization originating inside the volume (and vice versa). This problem restricts the roentgen to x- and γ-ray beams of relatively low energy.

Energy and Photon Fluence per Unit Exposure

The energy E_a absorbed per unit mass of air during an exposure of X coulombs/kg is

$$E_a = \frac{(X \text{ coulombs/kg})(33.97 \text{ eV/IP})(1.6 \times 10^{-19} \text{ J/eV})}{(1.6 \times 10^{-19} \text{ coulombs/IP})}$$

$$= 33.97 \cdot X \, [(\text{J/kg})]$$

where 33.97 eV/IP is the work function defined as the average energy expended per IP produced by ionizing radiation in air. The absorbed energy E_a is also the product of the energy fluence and the total mass energy absorption coefficient $(\mu_{en})_m$ for the x or γ rays that contribute to the energy fluence.

$$E_a = \Psi(\text{J/m}^2) \cdot (\mu_{en})_m \, [(\text{m}^2/\text{kg})]$$

$$= \Psi(\mu_{en})_m \, [(\text{J/kg})]$$

The coefficient $(\mu_{en})_m$ is $\mu_m (E_a/h\nu)$, where μ_m is the total mass attenuation coefficient of air for photons of energy $h\nu$, and E_a represents the average energy transformed into kinetic energy of electrons and positive ions per photon absorbed or scattered from the x- or γ-ray beam, corrected for energy released as characteristic radiation

TABLE 5-2 Mass Energy-Absorption Coefficient $(\mu_{en})_m$, $m^2/kg \times 10^3$

Photon Energy (MeV)	Water	Air	Compact Bone	Muscle
0.010	489	466	1900	496
0.015	132	129	589	136
0.020	52.3	51.6	251	54.4
0.030	14.7	14.7	74.3	15.4
0.040	6.47	6.40	30.5	6.77
0.050	3.94	3.84	15.8	4.09
0.060	3.04	2.92	9.79	3.12
0.080	2.53	2.36	5.20	2.55
0.10	2.52	2.31	3.86	2.52
0.15	2.78	2.51	3.04	2.76
0.20	3.00	2.68	3.02	2.97
0.30	3.20	2.88	3.11	3.17
0.40	3.29	2.96	3.16	3.25
0.50	3.30	2.97	3.16	3.27
0.60	3.29	2.96	3.15	3.26
0.80	3.21	2.89	3.06	3.18
1.0	3.11	2.80	2.97	3.08
1.5	2.83	2.55	2.70	2.81
2.0	2.60	2.34	2.48	2.57
3.0	2.27	2.05	2.19	2.25
4.0	2.05	1.86	1.99	2.03
5.0	1.90	1.73	1.86	1.88
6.0	1.80	1.63	1.78	1.78
8.0	1.65	1.50	1.65	1.63
10.0	1.55	1.44	1.59	1.54

Source: International Commission on Radiation Units and Measurements: Physical Aspects of Irradiation, National Bureau of Standards Handbook 85.

and bremsstrahlung as electrons interact with electrons and nuclei in the medium. Mass energy absorption coefficients for a few selected media, including air, are listed in Table 5-2.

By combining the equations for $E_a = (\mu_{en})_m \Psi = 33.97\,(X)$, the energy fluence per unit exposure (Ψ/X) is

The mass energy absorption coefficient can be defined as the fractional energy absorption from a beam of x or γ rays.

$$\Psi/X = 33.97/(\mu_{en})_m$$

where $(\mu_{en})_m$ is expressed in units of m^2 per kg, Ψ in J/m^2, and X in C/kg. For monoenergetic photons, the photon fluence per unit exposure Φ/X is the quotient of the energy fluence per unit exposure divided by the energy per photon:

$$\Phi/X = \Psi X [1/(h\nu \cdot 1.6 \times 10^{-13}\,J/MeV)]$$

with $h\nu$ expressed in MeV and in Φ units of photons per m^2.

The photon and energy fluence per unit exposure are plotted in Figure 5-1 as a function of photon energy. At lower energies, the large influence of photon energy on the energy absorption coefficient of air is reflected in the rapid change in the energy and photon fluence per unit exposure. Above 100 keV, the energy absorption coefficient is relatively constant, and the energy fluence per unit exposure does not vary greatly. However, the photon fluence per unit exposure decreases steadily as the energy per photon increases.

Example 5-3

Determine the energy and photon fluence per unit exposure in C/kg for ^{60}Co gamma rays. The average energy of the gamma rays is 1.25 MeV, and the total energy

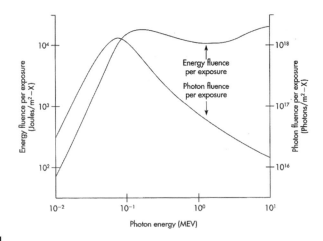

FIGURE 5-1
Photon and energy fluence per unit exposure, plotted as a function of the photon energy in MeV. To convert the vertical axis to exposure in roentgens, multiply the vertical scale by 2.58×10^{-4}.

absorption coefficient is 2.67×10^{-3} m²/kg (Table 5-2).

$$\Psi/X = 33.97/(\mu_{en})_m = 33.97/2.67 \times 10^{-3} \text{ m}^2/\text{kg}$$

$$\cong 12,600 \text{ J/m}^2$$

$$\Phi/X = 12,600 \frac{J}{m^2}[1/(1.6 \times 10^{-13} \text{ J/MeV})(1.25 \text{ MeV})]$$

$$= 6.4 \times 10^{16} \text{ photons/m}^2$$

◼ MEASUREMENT OF RADIATION EXPOSURE

By rearranging one of the previous equations, the energy fluence can be expressed as $\Psi = E_a/(\mu_{en})_m$. However, $E_a = E/\rho$, where E is the energy absorbed per unit volume and ρ is the density of air (1.29 kg/m³ at STP). If J_g is the number of primary and secondary IP produced by this energy deposition, then $E = J_g \overline{W}/e$, where $\overline{W}/e = 33.97$ eV/IP. The energy fluence is

$$\Psi = J_g \frac{\overline{W}/e}{\rho}\Bigg/(\mu_{en})_m$$

Example 5-4

A 1-cm³ volume of air is exposed to a photon fluence of 10^{15} photons/m². Each photon has an energy of 1 MeV, and the total mass energy absorption coefficient of air is 2.80×10^{-3} m²/kg for photons of this energy. How many IP are produced inside the 1-cm³ volume? How much charge of either sign is measured if all of the IP are collected?

$$\Psi = \Phi h\nu = (10^{15} \text{ photons/m}^2)(1 \text{ MeV/photon})(1.6 \times 10^{-13} \text{ J/MeV})$$

$$= 1.6 \times 10^2 \text{ J/m}^2$$

But

$$\Psi = J_g \frac{\overline{W}/e}{\rho}\Bigg/(\mu_{en})_m \quad \text{and} \quad J_g = \frac{\Psi \rho (\mu_{en})_m}{\overline{W}/e}$$

$$J_g = \frac{(1.6 \times 10^2 \text{ J/m}^2)(1.29 \text{ kg/m}^3)(2.8 \times 10^{-3} \text{ m}^2/\text{kg})(10^{-6} \text{ m}^3/\text{cm}^3)(1 \text{ cm}^3)}{(33.97 \text{ eV/IP})(1.6 \times 10^{-19} \text{ J/eV})}$$

$$= 10.7 \times 10^{10} \text{ IP}$$

The charge Q collected is

$$Q = (10.7 \times 10^{10} \text{ IP})(1.6 \times 10^{-19} \text{ coulomb/IP})$$

$$\cong 17 \times 10^{-9} \text{ coulombs}$$

When energy is deposited in a small *collecting volume* of air, some secondary electrons are produced outside the collecting volume by primary IPs (particularly electrons) that escape the collecting volume. It is not possible to collect and measure all of these secondary electrons. However, the collecting volume may be chosen so that ionization produced outside the volume by IP originating inside of the collecting volume is balanced by ionization produced inside the volume by IP that originate outside. This condition, known as *electron equilibrium*, results in the collection of a number of IP inside the volume equal to the total ionization J_g. The principle of electron equilibrium is fundamental to the measurements of radiation exposure and is employed in the *free-air ionization chamber*.

Free-Air Ionization Chamber

Fundamental measurements of radiation exposure are achieved in standards laboratories with an instrument known as the free-air ionization chamber. These measurements form the standard against which measurements obtained with simpler instruments are compared to yield calibration factors for the simpler instruments. The simpler instruments can then be used in the clinical setting to measure radiation exposures from sources of x and γ rays employed clinically.

X or γ rays incident on a free-air chamber are collimated into a beam with a cross-sectional area A at the center of the chamber (Figure 5-2). Inside the chamber, the beam traverses an electrical field between parallel electrodes A and B, with electrode A at ground potential and the potential of electrode B highly negative. The collecting volume of air inside the chamber has an area A and a length L. The charge Q (positive or negative) collected by the chamber is $Q = N$ (1.6 × 10⁻¹⁹ coulomb/IP), where N is the total number of IPs collected. For an accurate measurement of N, the range of electrons liberated by the incident radiation must be less than the distance between each electrode and the collecting volume. Also the photon flux must remain constant across the chamber, and the distance from the collimator to the border of the collecting volume must exceed the electron range. If these requirements are satisfied, electron equilibrium is achieved in the collecting volume, and the number of ion pairs liberated by the incident photons per unit volume of air is N/AL.

Electron equilibrium exists in a volume when the energy deposited outside the volume by ionization created within equals the energy deposited in the volume by ionization created outside.

The physical basis of the ionization chamber for measurement of radiation quantity was first explored in 1896 by Rutherford and co-workers at the Cavendish Laboratory in Cambridge, England.

The principle of the free-air chamber was developed by the American physicist William Duane.

In the free-air chamber, the voltage between electrodes A and B must be large enough to collect all of the ionization without significant recombination, yet not so large that the ions are accelerated to an energy where they create additional ionization on their way to the electrodes.

The length L of the collecting volume is defined by guard electrodes positioned adjacent to the collecting electrodes.

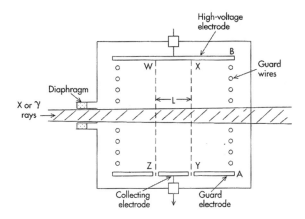

FIGURE 5-2
A free-air ionization chamber. The collecting volume of length L is enclosed within the region WXYZ. The air volume exposed directly to the x-ray and gamma ray beam is depicted by the hatched area.

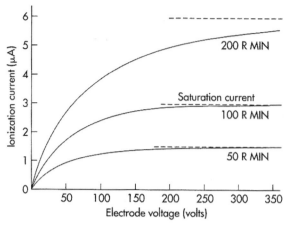

FIGURE 5-3

Current in a free-air ionization chamber as a function of the potential difference across the electrodes of the chamber. Saturation currents are shown for different exposure rates. Data were obtained from a chamber with electrodes 1 cm apart. (From H. Johns and J. Cunningham.[2])

Because 1 R = 2.58 × 10⁻⁴ coulomb/kg, the number of roentgens X corresponding to a charge Q in coulombs collected in a free-air ionization chamber is

$$X = Q/[AL\rho(2.58 \times 10^{-4} \text{ coulomb/kg-R})]$$

where ρ is the density of air in kg/m³ and AL is expressed in m³. As mentioned earlier, the preferred unit of radiation exposure is coulombs/kilogram rather than roentgen, so the conversion factor of 2.58 × 10⁻⁴ coulombs/(kg-R) is no longer needed in exposure measurements with a free-air chamber.

To prevent IP from recombining before expending all their energy by producing secondary ionization, the potential difference between the electrodes in a free-air chamber must be sufficient to attract all ion pairs to the electrodes. This potential difference is referred to as a *saturation voltage*. As shown in Figure 5-3, the saturation voltage increases with exposure rate. A potential difference between the electrodes below the saturation voltage permits IP to recombine before they are collected. Measurements obtained at a potential difference below the saturation voltage underestimate the true exposure. Errors caused by IP recombination can be especially severe during measurements of x-ray beams in which the x rays are furnished in short pulses of high intensity. Such beams are commonly furnished by linear accelerators employed in radiation therapy. Recombination errors must be guarded against when measurements are obtained with conventional ionization chambers used in the clinical setting. When recombination cannot be prevented in a pulsed x-ray beam, a correction factor must be applied to correct the chamber response for a decrease in collection efficiency caused by IP recombination.

The range of released electrons in air increases rapidly with the energy of incident x or γ rays (Table 5-3). Electrodes in a free-air chamber used to measure 1-MV x rays would have to be separated by about 4 m. A chamber this large is impractical, particularly since a uniform electrical field would be difficult to maintain over such a distance. Other problems, such as reduced efficiency of IP collection, would also be encountered. Free-air chambers operated at elevated air pressures permit extension of their use to photon energies as high as 3 MeV. This energy is an upper limit to the use of free-air chambers as well as to the definition of the roentgen. At lower energies, free-air ionization chambers can achieve accuracies to within ± 0.5% for measurements of x- and γ-ray beams under carefully controlled conditions. Free-air chambers are too fragile and bulky to be used routinely in the clinical setting. Hence, their application is limited to use as a standard against which the response of more useful chambers can be compared.

All ionization chambers, including free-air chambers, operate at or near the saturation voltage.

Factors applied to free-air ionization measurements usually include corrections for:

- Air attenuation
- Ion pair recombination
- Temperature, pressure, humidity
- Ionization produced by scattered photons

The international standard for exposure measurements is maintained by the Bureau International des Poids et des Mesures (BIPM) in Sevres, France.

TABLE 5-3 Range and Percent of Total Ionization Produced by Photoelectrons and Compton Electrons for X Rays Generated at 100, 200, and 1000 kVp

X-Ray Tube Voltage (kVp)	Photoelectrons Range in Air (cm)	% of Total Ionization	Compton Electrons Range in Air (cm)	% of Total Ionization	Electrode Separation in Free-Air Ionization Chamber at STP[a]
100	12	10	0.5	90	12 cm
200	37	0.4	4.6	99.6	
1000	290	0	220	100	4 m

[a] STP, standard temperature and pressure; defined as 273°K (0°C) and 760 mm Hg.
Source: W. Meredith and J. Massey.[3]

Thimble Chambers

The amount of ionization collected in a small volume of air is not influenced by the physical density of the medium surrounding the collecting volume of air, provided that the medium has an atomic number equal to the effective atomic number of air. Consequently, the large volume of air surrounding the collecting volume in a free-air chamber may be replaced by a lesser thickness of a more dense material with an effective atomic number equal to that of air. That is, the large distances in air required for electron equilibrium in a free-air chamber may be replaced by smaller thicknesses of a more dense *air-equivalent* material with an effective atomic number close to 7.64, the effective atomic number of air.

The *effective atomic number* $\overline{Z}$ of a material is the atomic number of a hypothetical single element that attenuates photons at the same rate as the material. When photoelectric and Compton interactions are the dominant processes of photon attenuation, the $\overline{Z}$ of a mixture of element is

Chambers with air-equivalent walls are known as *thimble chambers* because they resemble a sewing thimble.

$$\overline{Z} = \left(a_1 Z_1^{2.94} + a_2 Z_2^{2.94} + \cdots + a_n Z_n^{2.94}\right)^{1/2.94}$$

where $Z_1, Z_2, \ldots, Z_n$ are the atomic numbers of elements in the mixture and $a_1, a_2, \ldots, a_n$ are the fractional contributions of each element to the total number of electrons in the mixture. A reasonable approximation for $\overline{Z}$ may be obtained by rounding 2.94 to 3. The $\overline{Z}$ of air is 7.64, as computed in Example 5-5.

Example 5-5

Calculate $\overline{Z}$ for air. Air contains 75.5% nitrogen, 23.2% oxygen, and 1.3% argon. Gram-atomic masses are nitrogen, 14.007; oxygen, 15.999; and argon, 39.948.

The number of electrons contributed to 1 g of air is as follows:

For nitrogen:
$$\frac{(1 \text{ g})(0.755)(6.02 \times 10^{23} \text{ atoms/g-atomic mass})(7 \text{ electrons/atom})}{(14.007 \text{ g/g-atomic mass})}$$

$$= 2.27 \times 10^{23} \text{ electrons}$$

For oxygen:
$$\frac{(1 \text{ g})(0.232)(6.02 \times 10^{23} \text{ atoms/g-atomic mass})(8 \text{ electrons/atom})}{(15.999 \text{ g/g-atomic mass})}$$

$$= 0.70 \times 10^{23} \text{ electrons}$$

For argon:
$$\frac{(1 \text{ g})(0.013)(6.02 \times 10^{23} \text{ atoms/g-atomic mass})(18 \text{ electrons/atom})}{(39.948 \text{ g/g-atomic mass})}$$

$$= 0.04 \times 10^{23} \text{ electrons}$$

Total electrons $= (2.27 + 0.70 + 0.04) \times 10^{23} = 3.01 \times 10^{23}$ electrons

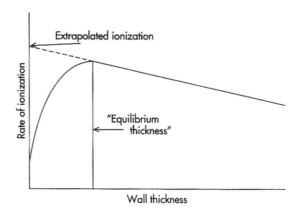

FIGURE 5-4
Ionization in an air-filled cavity exposed to x or γ radiation is expressed as a function of the thickness of the air-equivalent wall surrounding the cavity.

The fractional contributions of electrons are

$$\alpha_N = \frac{2.27 \times 10^{23}}{3.01 \times 10^{23}} = 0.753$$

$$\alpha_O = \frac{0.70 \times 10^{23}}{3.01 \times 10^{23}} = 0.233$$

$$\alpha_A = \frac{0.04 \times 10^{23}}{3.01 \times 10^{23}} = 0.013$$

$$\overline{Z}_{air} = \left[\alpha_N Z_N^{2.94} + \alpha_O Z_O^{2.94} + \alpha_A Z_A^{2.94}\right]^{1/2.94}$$

$$= [(0.753)(7)^{2.94} + (0.233)(8)^{2.94} + (0.013)(18)^{2.94}]^{1/2.94}$$

$$= 7.64$$

The first thimble chamber was developed by Otto Glasser of the Cleveland Clinic in the early 1920s.

A thin-wall thimble chamber designed for measurement of low-energy photons can be used at higher energies by placing a cap around the chamber to produce a wall of adequate thickness. Such a cap is called a "buildup cap."

Carbon-coated bakelite

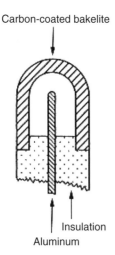

Insulation
Aluminum

MARGIN FIGURE 5-1
Diagram of a thimble chamber with an air-equivalent wall.

In a thimble chamber, most of the ionization collected in the air volume originates during interactions of photons in the air-equivalent wall of the chamber. The ionization in an air-filled cavity is shown in Figure 5-4 as a function of the thickness of the wall surrounding the cavity. The ionization increases with wall thickness until the thickness equals the range of electrons liberated by the incident photons. At this thickness, electrons from the outer portion of the wall just reach the cavity, and the ionization inside the cavity is maximum. A thinner wall would not provide electron equilibrium, and a thicker wall would attenuate the photons unnecessarily, as reflected in the slow decline in ionization beyond the equilibrium thickness. The wall thickness required for electron equilibrium increases with photon energy. Extrapolation of the curve in Figure 5-4 to zero wall thickness denotes the ionization that would occur in the cavity if photons were not attenuated at all in the surrounding wall.

A thimble chamber is diagrammed in the margin. The inside of the chamber is coated with a conducting material (e.g., carbon), and the central positive electrode is a conductor such as aluminum. The chamber response may be varied by changing the size of the collecting volume of air, the thickness of the chamber coating, or the length of the central electrode. The response of the chamber can be calibrated at several photon energies to provide accurate measurements of radiation exposure over a range of photon energies.

Condenser Chambers

The ratio of the charge Q in coulombs collected by an ionization chamber to the voltage reduction ΔV in volts across the chamber caused by the collected charge is known as the *chamber capacitance* C expressed in units of farads. That is, $C = Q/\Delta V$. If a chamber of volume v is exposed to X coulombs/kg, the charge Q collected is

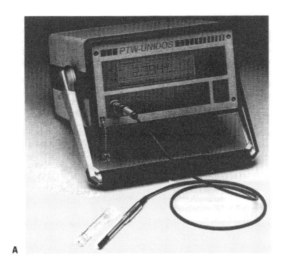

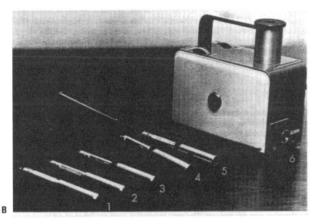

FIGURE 5-5
A: Integrated ionization chamber and electrometer used for radiation measurements in radiation therapy. (Courtesy of P. T. W. Freiburg). **B:** Detachable ionization chambers and charger-reader previously used for radiation measurements in radiation therapy. (Courtesy of Victoreen Inc., Cleveland, Ohio.)

$Q = X(C/\text{kg}) \cdot \rho(\text{kg/m}^3) \cdot v(\text{m}^3) = X\rho v$. For an air density of 1.29 kg/m^3 at STP, $Q = 1.29Xv$. The reduction in voltage ΔV is $Q/C = (1.29Xv)/C$, and the voltage reduction per unit exposure $\Delta V/X = 1.29$ v/C, where v is the volume of the chamber in m^3 and C is the capacitance of the chamber in farads. The voltage reduction per unit exposure, termed the *sensitivity* of the chamber, can be decreased by reducing the volume or increasing the capacitance of the chamber.

Most ionization chambers used for radiation measurements consist of a thimble chamber connected to a capacitor (sometimes called a condenser) to reduce the sensitivity to a value appropriate for routine clinical use. The total capacitance C of the resulting *condenser chamber* is $C = C_t + C_s$, where C_t and C_s are the capacitance of the thimble and condenser stem and cable. Usually, $C_s \gg C_t$. The sensitivity $\Delta V/X$ of a condenser chamber is $\Delta V/X = 1.29V/(C_t + C_s)$.

Various instruments are available commercially for measuring radiation exposure with a condenser chamber. In most of these devices, the chamber is connected during exposure to an electrometer used to measure the small electrical charge or current generated during the exposure. While in the x- or γ-ray beam, the chamber is made sensitive to radiation for a selected interval of time, and the exposure rate or cumulative exposure is determined. A typical exposure-measuring device is shown in Figure 5-5A. If the electrometer has a capacitance C_e, the sensitivity $\Delta V/X$ of the entire device is $\Delta V/X = 1.29V/(C_t + C_s + C_e)$.

The chamber shown in Figure 5-5A is often referred to as a "Farmer chamber," because it was originally designed by the physicists Aird and Farmer.

Example 5-6

The capacitance $(C_t + C_s)$ of a condenser chamber is 100 picofarads, and the capacitance of the charger-reader is 15 picofarads. The air volume of the chamber is 0.46 cm^3. What is the sensitivity of the chamber? What voltage reduction occurs across the chamber following an exposure of 0.015 coulombs/kg?

$$\text{Sensitivity} = \frac{\Delta V}{X} = 1.29V/(C_t + C_s)$$

$$= \frac{1.29(0.46 \text{ cm}^3)(10^{-6} \text{ m}^3/\text{cm}^3)}{(100 + 15) \times 10^{-12} \text{ farads}}$$

$$= 5.2 \times 10^3 \text{ volts/coulomb/kg}$$

The reduction in voltage following an exposure of 0.015 coulombs/kg is
$$\Delta V = (5.2 \times 10^3 \text{ volts/coulomb/kg}) \cdot (0.015 \text{ coulombs/kg}) = 78.0 \text{ volts}$$

In a different approach to the design of an instrument to measure radiation exposure, the condenser chamber is charged to a prescribed voltage then disconnected from the electrometer (called a charger-reader) before being placed in the radiation beam. After exposure, the chamber is reinserted into the electrometer, and the reduction in voltage is determined. Chambers with different air volumes are available to yield different sensitivities, and chambers with different wall thicknesses are provided so that the device can be used to measure exposures for beams of different energies. The most common instrument of this type is the condenser "R meter" shown in Figure 5-5B. Widely used in the past, this type of radiation detector is seldom used today for calibration of radiation beams.

The Victoreen condenser "R meter" was for many years the standard measuring instrument for calibration of x- and γ-ray beams in radiation therapy.

Correction Factors

When a condenser chamber is exposed to a radiation beam, all of the thimble must be irradiated to yield an accurate measurement of radiation exposure. Usually, part or all of the stem also is exposed. Additional ionization may be produced in the stem itself and in the case of a detachable chamber, in air trapped between the end of the stem and a metal cap placed around the stem to reduce the radiation penetrating the stem. This extraneous ionization can produce slight differences in the measured exposure depending on how much of the stem is irradiated. These differences must be accounted for with a *stem correction factor*. This correction factor is obtained by measuring the response of the chamber with different amounts of stem exposed, and comparing this response with that measured under conditions (usually full stem irradiation) employed when the calibration factor for the chamber is determined. The stem correction factor can be obtained by making several measurements with the chamber positioned at one end of a rectangular field, with the chamber oriented differently for each measurement so that different amounts of stem are exposed.[4]

In some applications of condenser chambers, the efficiency of IP collection differs slightly, depending on whether the chamber wall is negative and the central electrode positive, or vice versa. This *polarity effect*, noticed most often when electron or high-energy photon beams are measured with an ionization chamber, is usually caused by slight differences in the collection efficiency of ionization originating outside the collecting volume of air.[5] It can be minimized by averaging measurements obtained with normal and reversed polarities across the chamber. Measurements obtained with opposite polarities should not differ by more than 0.5% to ensure that the averaging procedure yields a reasonable correction for the polarity effect. The polarity effect is a result of several processes, including:

- The "Compton current" created by high-energy Compton electrons ejected during interactions of energetic photons
- Ionization collected outside the collecting volume ("extracameral current")

The polarity effect is typically more significant for electron beams than for photon beams.

Most condenser chambers are not sealed and therefore are open to the atmosphere. In these chambers, the number of air molecules in the collecting volume varies with the air density, which, in turn, is affected by the ambient temperature and atmospheric pressure. The response of an unsealed chamber must be normalized to the atmospheric conditions existing when the chamber calibration factor was determined. In the United States, these conditions are 1 atmosphere (760 mm Hg) of barometric pressure and 22°C (295 K) temperature. The *pressure-temperature correction factor* $C_{p,t}$ for a chamber calibrated in the United States is

$$C_{p,t} = [760/P(\text{mm Hg})] \cdot [(273 + T(°C))/295]$$

where P is the atmospheric pressure in mm Hg, and the factor 273 corrects the ambient temperature T in degrees Celsius to absolute degrees (Kelvin). An all-too-common error in exposure measurements is use of an ambient pressure obtained from a weather station in which a correction has been applied to convert the pressure to an equivalent pressure at sea level. At an elevation of 1 mile above sea level, the use of ambient pressure "corrected to sea level" can produce an error of more than 20% in exposure measurements. When ambient pressure is obtained from a local weather station, it is advisable to request the uncorrected *station pressure* and to be aware of differences in elevation between the location of the station and the site of exposure measurements.

Example 5-7

Determine $C_{p,t}$ for an ambient temperature of 25°C and an atmospheric pressure of 630 mm Hg at 1 mile (1609 m) elevation above sea level:

$$C_{p,t} = (760/P) \cdot [(273 + T)/295]$$
$$= (760/630) \cdot [(273 + 25)/295]$$
$$= (1.21)(1.01) = 1.22$$

In measurements of radiation exposure with a condenser chamber, the readings M should be corrected by the following expression to obtain true measurements of exposure X:

$$X = M \cdot N_c \cdot C_{p,t} \cdot C_i \cdot C_s$$

where N_c is the chamber calibration factor, $C_{p,t}$ is the pressure–temperature correction factor, C_i is the correction for collection efficiency loss caused by recombination, and C_s is the stem correction factor. The exposure X obtained by this procedure represents the true exposure at the location of measurement in the absence of the chamber because any perturbation of the radiation caused by the presence of the chamber, including attenuation of photons in the chamber wall, is included in the chamber calibration factor N_c.

Example 5-8

A reading of 68 coulombs/kg (uncorrected) is obtained in air with a condenser chamber with a calibration factor of 1.03 at full-stem irradiation for the average energy of x rays in the x-ray beam. The pressure-temperature correction is 1.22; the ionization collection efficiency is 100% when the entire stem of the chamber is exposed. What is the corrected exposure?

$$X = M \cdot N_c \cdot C_{p,t} \cdot C_i \cdot C_s$$
$$= (68) \cdot (1.03) \cdot (1.22) \cdot (1.0) \cdot (1.0)$$
$$= 85.4 \text{ coulombs/kg}$$

Several instances of miscalibration of a radiation therapy unit have occurred because of the failure to correct for reduced atmospheric pressure at higher elevations.

In the United States, chamber calibration factors are acquired by sending the chamber and associated electrometer to an Accredited Dosimetry Calibration Laboratory (ADCL).

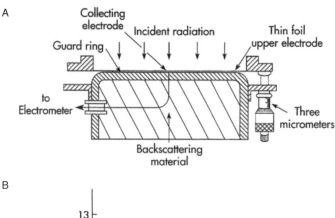

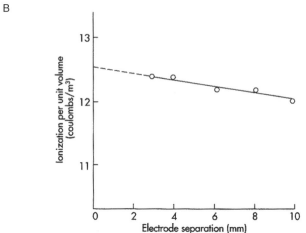

FIGURE 5-6
A: Failla extrapolation chamber. (From F. M. Khan. *The Physics of Radiation Therapy*. Baltimore, Williams & Wilkins, 1984. As redrawn from J. W. Boag,[5] used with permission). **B:** Ionization current per unit chamber volume as a function of electrode spacing in an extrapolation chamber. (From L. Stanton.[6])

Favorable characteristics of ion chambers used for routine clinical measurements include:

- Minimum variation in sensitivity with photon energy
- Minimum variation in response with the direction of incident radiation
- Linear response over the expected range of exposures
- Minimum stem correction
- Minimum ion pair recombination

The first extrapolation chamber was designed by G. Failla in 1937.

Parallel-plate ionization chambers are sometimes referred to as "pancake" chambers.

1 centigray equals 1 rad.

Extrapolation and Parallel-Plate Chambers

At times, a measurement of exposure is desired at the surface of a medium. This measurement can be obtained with an extrapolation chamber such as that described in Figure 5-6A. The radiation beam enters the chamber through a thin foil that serves as the upper electrode. The lower electrode is backed by the medium. The thickness of the electrode spacing (and therefore the collecting volume) can be varied by micrometer screws that cause the upper electrode to descend toward the lower electrode. The ionization per unit collection volume is plotted against electrode spacing and extrapolated to zero spacing to yield a measure of the exposure at the surface of the medium (Figure 5-6B).

The parallel-plate ionization chamber is similar to an extrapolation chamber except that the electrodes are immobile. Ionization between the closely spaced electrodes is measured as the thickness of the medium above the upper electrode is increased. In this manner, the exposure can be measured as a function of depth at shallow depths where a cylindrical thimble chamber would perturb the radiation field.

■ RADIATION DOSE

Chemical and biologic changes in tissue exposed to ionizing radiation are caused by the deposition of energy from the radiation into the tissue. This deposition is described by two closely related quantities, kerma and absorbed dose. Both quantities are described in units of gray or, formerly, rads. One rad equals 10^{-2} joule of energy per kilogram (or 100 ergs per gram) of irradiated medium. The SI unit for kerma and absorbed dose is the gray (Gy), defined as 1 joule/kg of irradiated medium. The centigray (cGy) is 1/100 gray.

The *kerma* (an acronym for kinetic energy released in matter) is the sum of the initial kinetic energies of all IP liberated in a volume element of matter, divided by the mass of matter in the volume element. The *absorbed dose* is the energy actually absorbed per unit mass in the volume element. If ion pairs escape the volume element without depositing all of their energy, and if they are not compensated by ion pairs originating outside the volume element but depositing energy within it (electron equilibrium), the kerma exceeds the absorbed dose. The kerma also is greater than the absorbed dose when energy is radiated from the volume element as bremsstrahlung or characteristic radiation. Under conditions in which electron equilibrium is achieved and the radiative energy loss is negligible, the kerma and absorbed dose are identical. The output of x-ray tubes is sometimes described in terms of *air kerma* expressed as the energy released per unit mass of air.

Example 5-9

A dose of 2 Gy (200 cGy or 200 rad) is delivered to a 1000-g tumor during a single radiation therapy session. How much energy is delivered to each gram of tumor and to the entire tumor?

$$\frac{\text{Energy absorbed}}{\text{per gram}} = 2 \text{ Gy} \left(1\frac{J}{\text{kg-Gy}}\right)\left(10^{-3}\frac{\text{kg}}{\text{g}}\right)$$

$$= 2 \times 10^{-3} \text{ J/g}$$

$$\frac{\text{Energy absorbed}}{\text{in 1000 gram}} = 2 \times 10^{-3} \frac{J}{G}(1000 \text{ g})$$

$$= 2 \text{ J}$$

The difference between kerma and absorbed dose is useful in explaining the skin-sparing effect of high-energy photons such as multi-MV x rays used in radiation therapy. As shown in Figure 5-7, the kerma is greatest at the surface of irradiated tissue because the photon intensity is highest at the surface and causes the greatest number of interactions with the medium. The photon intensity diminishes gradually as the photons interact on their way through the medium. The electrons set into motion during the photon interactions at the surface travel several millimeters in depth before their energy is completely dissipated (Figure 5-8). These electrons add to the ionization produced by photon interactions occurring at greater depths. Hence, the absorbed dose increases over the first few millimeters below the surface to reach the greatest dose at the depth of maximum dose (d_{max}) several millimeters below the

The absorbed dose is a measure of the energy absorbed per unit mass of irradiated material. The total energy absorbed is termed the integral dose in the irradiated material.

Kerma k may be defined as

$$k = \frac{\Delta E_{tr}}{\Delta m}$$

and absorbed dose D may be defined as

$$D = \frac{\Delta E_{ab}}{\Delta m}$$

where E_{tr} is the energy transferred, E_{ab} is the energy absorbed, m is the mass of the irradiated material, and Δ represents an infinitesimal quantity.

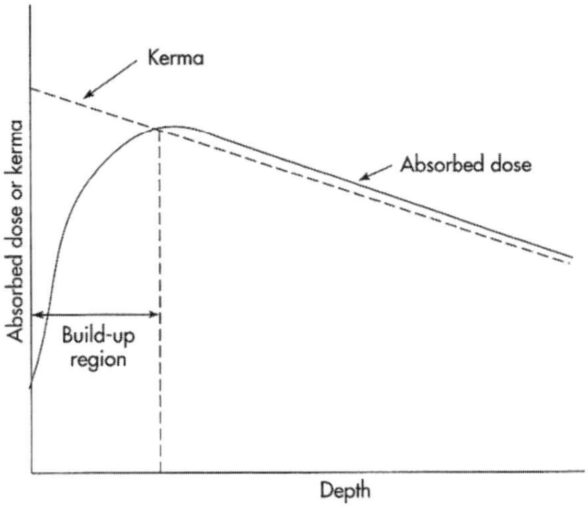

FIGURE 5-7
Kerma and absorbed dose as a function of depth in an irradiated medium.

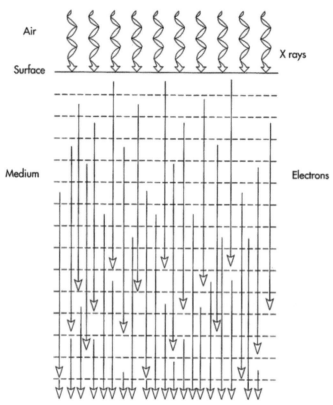

FIGURE 5-8
Dose buildup below the surface of a medium irradiated with high-energy photons as liberated electrons travel several millimeters before dissipating their energy.

The skin-sparing effect of high-energy photons was one of the major advances introduced by ^{60}Co teletherapy units after World War II.

surface. This buildup of absorbed dose over the first few millimeters below the skin is responsible for the clinically important skin-sparing effect of high-energy x and γ rays. Beyond d_{max}, the absorbed dose also decreases gradually as the photons are attenuated. At depths greater than d_{max}, the kerma curve falls below that for absorbed dose because kerma reflects the photon intensity at each depth, whereas absorbed dose reflects in part the photon intensity at shallower depths that sets electrons into motion that penetrate to the depth.

The absorbed dose D in Gy delivered to a small mass m in kg is D (Gy) $= E/m \cdot$ (1 J/kg-Gy), where E is the energy in joules absorbed in the small mass. The energy E is the total energy deposited in the small volume, corrected for energy removed from the volume in any way (loss of ionization and radiative energy loss caused by bremsstrahlung and characteristic radiation) that is not compensated by energy entering the volume from outside. During an exposure of 1 coulomb per kilogram, the energy absorbed in air is 33.97 J/kg (or 33.97 Gy), as demonstrated earlier. An exposure of 1 R corresponds to an absorbed dose of (1 R) (33.97 J/kg/C/kg) (1 Gy/J/kg) $\cdot$ 2.58 $\times$ 10^{-4} C/kg-R = 87.6 $\times$ 10^{-4} Gy (or 0.876 rads) in air. The determination of absorbed dose from measurements of exposure for x- and γ-ray beams is explained in greater detail later in this chapter.

■ MEASUREMENT OF RADIATION DOSE

A radiation dosimeter provides a measurable response to the energy absorbed in a medium from incident radiation. To be most useful, the dosimeter should absorb an amount of energy equal to that which would be absorbed in the medium displaced by the dosimeter. A dosimeter used to measure absorbed dose in soft tissue should absorb an amount of energy equal to that absorbed by the same mass of soft tissue.

Such a dosimeter is said to be *tissue equivalent*. Few dosimeters are exactly tissue equivalent, and corrections usually are required to determine the soft tissue dose when a radiation dosimeter is used.

Calorimetric Dosimetry

Almost all of the energy absorbed from radiation is eventually degraded to heat. If an absorbing medium is insulated from its environment, the rise in temperature of the medium is proportional to the absorbed energy. The temperature rise ΔT may be measured with a temperature-measuring device such as a thermocouple or thermistor.

In a calorimeter insulated from its environment, the absorbed dose D in Gy is

$$D \text{ (Gy)} = E/m = [4.186 \text{ (J/calorie)} \cdot s \cdot \Delta T](1/1 \text{ J/kg-Gy})$$

where E is the energy absorbed in joules, m is the mass in kg, s is the specific heat of the absorber in calories per kg-°C, and is the ΔT temperature rise in °C. For a calorimetric measurement of dose to mimic the absorbed dose in soft tissue, the absorbing medium must resemble soft tissue. Graphite is often used as the absorbing medium in a *tissue dose* calorimeter, although water has been used with some success.

If the medium in a calorimeter is thick and dense enough to absorb all of the incident radiation, the increase in temperature reflects the total energy in the radiation beam. A measurement of this type, referred to as absolute calorimetry, usually employs a massive lead block as the absorbing medium.

Photographic Dosimetry

The emulsion of a photographic film contains crystals of a silver halide (e.g., AgBr) embedded in a gelatin matrix. When the film is developed, metallic silver is deposited in regions that have been exposed to radiation. Unaffected crystals of silver halide are removed during fixation of the film. The transmission of light through a region of the processed film varies with the amount of deposited silver and therefore with the energy absorbed from the radiation incident on the region of film. The transmittance T is usually expressed as the optical density OD of the film, where $OD = \log(1/T) = \log(I_0/I)$ and I and I_0 are the light intensity measured with and without the film in place. In Figure 5-9 the curve of OD versus log (exposure) is called the H–D *curve* of a film after the inventors Hurter and Driffield, who in 1890 developed this approach to describing the characteristics of photographic film. An H–D curve is sometimes referred to as a *characteristic* or *sensitometric curve*. This curve is discussed further in Chapter 9.

An instrument that measures absorbed dose by detecting the temperature rise in a medium is known as a calorimeter, and the technique is referred to as *calorimetric dosimetry* or *calorimetry*.

The first portable calorimeter for measuring radiation dose was built in the late 1960s by Steve Domen of the U.S. National Bureau of Standards (NBS), now renamed the National Institute of Standards and Technology (NIST).

Calorimetry is the most direct approach to measuring absorbed dose, because it does not rely on conversion factors such as $\overline{W}/e$ or a G value (see chemical dosimetry). However, it is a very insensitive technique; doses of several hundred gray are required to yield a temperature increase of a fraction of a degree. Hence, absorbed dose measurements by calorimetry are largely restricted to standards laboratories.

The logarithmic nature of optical density corresponds well with the logarithmic response of the human eye to light of varying intensity.

Much of the definitive work in film dosimetry was done by Margarete Ehrlich, a physicist at the National Bureau of Standards (now NIST).

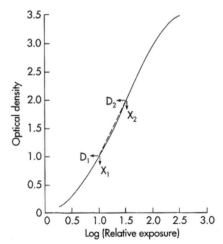

FIGURE 5-9
Characteristic curve for an x-ray film.

Photographic dosimetry is subject to severe errors for several reasons. The optical density of a film depends not only on the radiation exposure to the emulsion, but also on variables such as the type and energy of the radiation and the conditions under which the film is developed. Photographic film has several high-Z components and interacts with photons in ways different from soft tissue, especially when the photons are relatively low in energy and interact by Z-dependent photoelectric interactions. Photographic dosimetry is said to be *energy dependent* because photographic film responds to x rays and gamma rays differently from the response of air or soft tissue. The OD measured for an exposed film must be interpreted by comparison with a calibration H–D curve obtained under identical conditions of exposure. This requirement is often difficult to satisfy, especially when films are exposed in a medium in which a large amount of scattered radiation is present. Other problems of photographic dosimetry include the rapid attenuation of photons in a dense, high-Z film emulsion and variations in the thickness and composition of the photographic emulsion from one film or film batch to the next.

Because of its many variables, film should be considered a "radiation sensor" rather than a "radiation dosimeter."

Chemical Dosimetry

Oxidation and reduction reactions may be initiated when chemical solutions are exposed to ionizing radiation. The number of molecules affected in a solution depends on the energy absorbed in the solution. Measuring the extent of oxidation or reduction is the technical basis of *chemistry dosimetry*.

The solution used most often to measure radiation dose is ferrous sulfate ($FeSO_4$), sometimes referred to as a Fricke dosimeter.[7] For high-energy photons that interact primarily by Compton scattering, the ratio of the energy absorbed in $FeSO_4$ to that absorbed in soft tissue is 1:1.024, the ratio of the electron densities (electrons/m^3) in the two media. Although the Fricke dosimeter is reasonably accurate ($\pm 3\%$), it is relatively insensitive, and doses of 50–500 Gy are required before the oxidation of Fe^{2+} to Fe^{3+} is measurable. The Fricke dosimeter is sometimes used to measure absorbed doses from beams of electrons and other charged particles.[8]

The Fricke dosimeter is named after the Cleveland physicist Hugo Fricke, who for many years collaborated with Glasser in the development of ionization chambers.

Other chemical dosimeters that are occasionally used include ceric sulfate, oxalic acid and benzene.

The yield of a chemical dosimeter such as $FeSO_4$ is described by its G value, defined as the number of molecules affected per 100 eV of energy absorbed. The G value for the Fricke dosimeter varies from 15.3 to 15.7 molecules/100 eV over a range of photon energies from ^{137}Cs (662 keV) to 30-MV x rays. For electrons from 1 to 30 MeV, the G value for $FeSO_4$ is often taken as 15.4 molecules/100 eV. After exposure, the amount of Fe^{3+} in the solution is determined by measuring the transmission of ultraviolet light of 305-nm wavelength through the solution. Once the number of affected molecules is known, the absorbed dose can be computed by dividing the number of affected molecules per unit mass of solution by the G value and converting energy units appropriately.

The G value for chemical dosimetry is similar in concept to the work function $\overline{W}/e$ for ionization dosimetry.

Example 5-10

A solution of ferrous sulfate is exposed to 6-MV x rays. Measurement of the ultraviolet light (305 nm) transmitted through the solution reveals the presence of Fe^{3+} at a concentration of 0.00008 g-molecular weight/L. What was the absorbed dose in the solution, and what would the equivalent dose have been to soft tissue?

$$\text{Number of } Fe^{3+} \text{ ions/kg} = \frac{(0.00008 \text{ g-mol wt/L})(6.02 \times 10^{23} \text{ molecules/g-mol wt})}{(1 \text{ kg/L})}$$

$$= 4.82 \times 10^{19} \text{ molecules/kg}$$

For a G value of 15.6 molecules per 100 ev for $FeSO_4$, the absorbed dose in the solution is

$$D(Gy) = \frac{(4.82 \times 10^{19} \text{ molecules/kg})(1.6 \times 10^{-19} \text{ J/eV})}{(15.6 \text{ molecules/100 eV})(1 \text{ J/kg-Gy})}$$

$$= 49.4 \text{ Gy}$$

The equivalent dose to soft tissue is

$$D(Gy) = (49.4 \text{ Gy})(1.024)$$

$$= 50.6 \text{ Gy}$$

where 1.024 is the ratio of electron densities in tissue compared with $FeSO_4$.

Scintillation and Semiconductor Dosimetry

Certain materials fluoresce or "scintillate" during exposure to ionizing radiation. The intensity of emitted light depends on the rate of absorption of energy in the scintillator. With a solid scintillation detector such as thallium-activated sodium iodide (NaI(T1)), a light guide directs the emitted light onto a photomultiplier tube (pmt). The pmt releases electrons in proportion to the intensity of the received light. The number of electrons is multiplied at each of several dynodes in the pmt to yield an electrical signal at the final electrode (the anode) that is proportional to the energy deposited in the scintillator by the incident radiation.

Scintillation detectors furnish a measurable response at low dose rates and respond linearly over a wide range of radiation intensities. However, most scintillators contain high-Z atoms, and their response is strongly energy dependent compared with air or soft tissue. The energy dependence of scintillators such as NaI(T1) is the major limitation in using these detectors for measurement of absorbed dose in soft tissue.

Semiconductors are materials with properties for electrical conduction that are intermediate between conductors and insulators. Semiconductor materials can be intentionally modified with impurities to yield an excess of electrons (n-type) or electron "holes" (p-type). When a voltage is applied with "reverse bias" across a junction between n-type and p-type semiconductors, a depletion zone devoid of excess electrons or holes is created. Radiation interacting in the depletion zone of the semiconductor diode can induce a current proportional to the dose delivered by incident radiation. Measurement of this current constitutes use of the semiconductor diode as a radiation dosimeter.

Thermoluminescence Dosimetry

A thermoluminescent dosimeter (TLD) is a device that releases light when it is heated following exposure to ionizing radiation. Shown in Figure 5-10 are electron levels in crystals of a thermoluminescent material such as LiF or $Li_2B_4O_7$. When energy is absorbed from incident radiation, electrons are raised from the valence to the conduction band. Some of the electrons return instantly to the valence band, but others are "trapped" in intermediate energy levels supplied by impurities in the crystals. The number of trapped electrons is proportional to the energy absorbed from the radiation. Unless energy is supplied to the crystals, most of the trapped electrons remain in the intermediate energy levels for an indefinite period. If the crystals are heated, however, the trapped electrons are released and return to the conduction band. These electrons then fall to the valence band, releasing light in the process. The light is directed onto a pmt to generate an electrical signal proportional to the energy originally deposited in the crystals by the radiation. Detection of this signal yields a measure of the absorbed dose in the crystals. Because the $\overline{Z}$ of LiF (8.18) and $Li_2B_4O_7$ (7.4) are close to that of air (7.64) and soft tissue (7.4), the energy absorbed by these materials

Rutherford was the first investigator who is known to have used a scintillation detector. He employed a thin layer of zinc sulfide to observe the scintillations produced when alpha particles interacted in the zinc sulfide.

The first scintillation detector, consisting of a calcium tungstate crystal mounted to a photomultiplier tube, was constructed by Cassen and Curtis in the late 1940s at the University of California—Los Angeles.

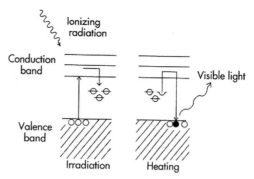

FIGURE 5-10
Electron transitions occurring when a thermoluminescent material is irradiated and heated.

The amount of light released when TLD crystals are heated depends on several factors in addition to the energy absorbed in the TLDs from the radiation. The factors include the temperature to which the crystals are heated, the reflectivity of the heating pan, and the time over which the crystals are heated. Hence, TLD measurements must be calibrated against the light from crystals receiving a known dose of radiation.

Light from thermoluminescent dosimeters is measured under carefully controlled conditions, including exacting requirements for the temperature of the heating pan for the crystals, heating cycle, position of the PMT, and amplification in the PMT itself.

Thermoluminescence in LiF was discovered in the 1950s by the chemist Farrington Daniels and was applied to radiation dosimetry by the physicist John Cameron; both of these scientists were at the University of Wisconsin.

is close to that absorbed by an equal mass of air or soft tissue. Small differences in the energy absorption are reflected in the *energy-dependence* curves for LiF and $Li_2B_4O_7$ shown in Figure 5-11. CaF_2:Mn is an especially sensitive thermoluminescent material and is often used in personnel monitors. The presence of high-Z components makes this material more energy dependent than LiF or $Li_2B_4O_7$ (Figure 5-11).

LiF is frequently used for measurement of absorbed dose in patients and soft-tissue-equivalent media (phantoms). Dosimetric LiF may be purchased as loose crystals, solid extruded rods, pressed pellets, or crystals embedded in a Teflon matrix. Dosimetric LiF contains selected impurities to provide the electron traps required for the thermoluminescent process. Pure LiF is useless as a radiation dosimeter.

Other Solid-State Dosimeters

Photoluminescent dosimeters are similar to TLDs except that ultraviolet light rather than heat is used to free trapped electrons, resulting in the emission of light. Most photoluminescent dosimeters are composed of Ag-activated metaphosphate glass of either high-Z or low-Z composition. Both types of dosimeter are strongly energy dependent but yield a response that is independent of dose rate up to at least 10^6 Gy/sec. Photoluminescent dosimeters are now frequently used for personnel monitoring, and efforts are promising to produce a photoluminescent personnel dosimeter that is an order of magnitude more radiation-sensitive than either film or TLD.

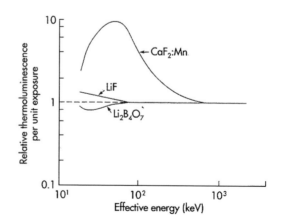

FIGURE 5-11
Relative thermoluminescence from various materials per unit exposure plotted as a function of the effective energy of incident x rays or gamma rays. Data are normalized to the response per unit exposure for [1] ^{60}Co gamma rays.[1]

ABSORBED DOSE MEASUREMENTS WITH AN IONIZATION CHAMBER

Estimates of absorbed dose in soft tissue or any other medium can be obtained by measurements of ionization in a small gas-filled cavity in the medium. The conversion of ionization in the gas-filled cavity to absorbed dose in the medium is accomplished by application of the *Bragg–Gray relationship*. This principle underlies many of the dosimetric measurements made in routine clinical dosimetry important to radiation oncology.

Bragg–Gray Principle

Suppose that a small gas-filled cavity is suspended in a homogeneous medium exposed to a beam of x or γ rays. As the photons interact in the medium, high-energy electrons are released that penetrate the gas-filled cavity and produce ionization in it. If the cavity is small, its presence does not influence the number or energy of primary and secondary electrons that traverse the medium at the location of the cavity. The energy E_g absorbed in eV per unit mass (kg) of gas in the cavity is $E_g = J_g \cdot \overline{W}/e$, where J_g is the ionization in IP/kg in the gas, and $\overline{W}/e$ is the average energy expended per ion pair produced in the gas (33.97 eV/IP if the gas is air). E_g, which is the absorbed dose to the gas in units of eV/kg, can be rewritten as $E_g = Q[\overline{W}/e/m]$, where J_g has been replaced by Q/m. This expression is often stated as E_g (or $D_g) = Q N_{gas}$, where $N_{gas} = (\overline{W}/e)_{gas}/m_{gas}$. N_{gas} is called the *cavity gas calibration factor*.

A Bragg–Gray cavity in a medium is a gas-filled cavity that is so small that (a) the direct interaction of photons with the cavity gas is negligible; (b) the ionization in the cavity is attributable entirely to particles that originate in the medium and cross the cavity; and (c) the range of the particles is much greater than the cavity dimensions.

If the cavity described in the paragraph above were replaced by an equal amount of medium, the energy E_m that would be absorbed per unit mass of medium would be $E_m = \overline{s}_m \cdot E_g$, where $\overline{s}_m$ is the ratio of the average mass stopping powers of the medium and the gas for the electrons traversing the cavity. The dose D_m in gray to the medium at the location of the cavity is

$$D_m = E_m(1.6 \times 10^{-19} \text{ J/eV})/[(1 \text{ J/kg-Gy})(1.6 \times 10^{-19} \text{ coulombs/IP})]$$

$$= (\overline{s}_m \cdot J_g \cdot \overline{W}/e)$$

$$= (\overline{s}_m Q N_{gas})$$

where $\overline{W}/e$ is expressed in units of eV/IP, J_g is described in units of C/kg, Q is measured in C, and N_{gas} has units of (eV/IP-kg). These expressions are known as the Bragg–Gray relationship.

The *mass stopping power* s_m of a medium describes the rate of energy loss of electrons traversing the medium, divided by the density of the medium. *The mass stopping power ratio* $\overline{s}_m$ describes the rate of energy loss of electrons in one medium compared with another. Stopping power ratios are computed with the Bethe–Block formula and corrected for the density (polarization) effect.[9,10] The density effect accounts for a reduction in the influence of a charged particle on a distant atom caused by polarization of the atoms between the particle and the distant atom. Listed in Table 5-4 are average mass stopping power ratios relative to air in a few materials for electrons set into motion by high-energy x rays and ^{60}Co γ rays ($E_{avg} = 1.25$ MeV). Tables of mass stopping power ratios are available in the literature.[11,12]

For measurement of absorbed dose in a medium according to the Bragg–Gray relationship, the gas-filled cavity should be so small (<1 cm in diameter) that its presence does not affect the electrons set into motion as photons interact in the surrounding medium. That is, none of the high-energy electrons traversing the cavity should originate or terminate in the cavity. In actual practice, the gas-filled cavity is part of a thimble chamber with a wall that separates the cavity from the surrounding medium. The chamber wall should be infinitestimally thin so that all electrons traversing the cavity originate in the medium and none are released from the wall.

TABLE 5-4 Average Mass Stopping Power $\bar{s}_m$ Relative to Air for Photon Beams in Selected Materials

Nominal Accelerating Potential (MV)	Water	Polyethylene	Acrylic	Graphite	Bakelite	Nylon
2	1.135	1.114	1.104	1.015	1.084	1.146
^{60}Co	1.134	1.113	1.103	1.012	1.081	1.142
4	1.131	1.108	1.099	1.007	1.075	1.136
6	1.127	1.103	1.093	1.002	1.070	1.129
8	1.121	1.097	1.088	0.995	1.063	1.120
10	1.117	1.094	1.085	0.992	1.060	1.114
15	1.106	1.083	1.074	0.982	1.051	1.097
20	1.096	1.074	1.065	0.977	1.042	1.087
25	1.093	1.071	1.062	0.068	1.038	1.084
35	1.084	1.062	1.053	0.958	1.027	1.074
45	1.070	1.048	1.041	0.939	1.006	1.061

Source: Task Group 21. Radiation Therapy Committee, American Association of Physicists in Medicine: A protocol for the determination of absorbed dose from high energy photons and electron beams. *Med. Phys.* 1983; **10**:741. Used with permission.

Alternatively, the chamber wall may have a finite thickness, provided that the wall composition is identical to the surrounding medium. Often, these conditions are not satisfied, and the ionization chamber slightly disturbs the distribution of absorbed dose in the medium. This disturbing influence is accounted for by introducing a *perturbation correction p* into the Bragg–Gray relationship:

$$D_m = (p \cdot \bar{s}_m \cdot J_g \cdot \overline{W}/e)$$

The Bragg–Gray relationship is essential to the calibration of radiation beams from high-energy accelerators employed for radiation therapy in clinical radiation oncology. Its applications to the calibration of these beams are discussed in Chapter 6.

■ DOSE EQUIVALENT

Most chemical and biological effects of radiation depend not only on the amount, but also on the distribution, of energy absorbed in an irradiated medium. That is, various types and energies of radiation may elicit different chemical and biological responses even though the absorbed doses delivered by the radiations are identical. The *relative biological effectiveness* (RBE) of a particular type or energy of radiation describes the efficiency with which the radiation evokes a particular response. The RBE is determined by comparing chemical or biological results produced by a particular radiation with those obtained with a reference radiation, usually medium-energy x rays or ^{60}Co gamma rays:

$$\text{RBE} = \frac{\text{Dose of reference radiation required to produce a particular response}}{\text{Dose of radiation in question required to produce the same response}}$$

For a particular type of radiation, the RBE may vary from one chemical or biologic response to another, as well as from one biological system or organism to another. Shown in Table 5-5 are the results of investigations into the RBE of ^{60}Co for eliciting a variety of biological effects. For these data, the reference radiation is medium-energy x rays.

TABLE 5-5 Relative Biologic Effectiveness of ^{60}Co gammas, with Different Biologic Effects Used as a Criterion for Measurement

Effects	RBE of ^{60}Co Gammas	Source
30-day lethality and testicular atrophy in mice	0.77	Storer et al.[13]
Splenic and thymic atrophy in mice	1	Storer et al.[13]
Inhibition of growth in Vicia faba	0.84	Hall[14]
LD$_{50}$ in mice, rat, chick embryo, and yeast	0.82–0.93	Sinclair[15]
Hatchability of chicken eggs	0.81	Loken et al.[16]
HeLa cell survial	0.90	Krohmer[17]
Lens opacity in mice	0.8	Upton et al.[18]
Cataract induction in rates	1	Focht et al.[19]
L cell survival	0.76	Till and Cunningham[20]

The relative biologic effectiveness of 200-kV x rays is taken as 1.
LD$_{50}$ = median lethal dose.

The RBE-dose expressed in SI units of sievert (Sv) is the product of the absorbed dose in gray (Gy) and the RBE appropriate for the particular biological response under study. That is, RBE-dose (Sv) = [absorbed dose (Gy)] · RBE. The RBE-dose should be limited to descriptions of specific radiation effects in experimental radiation biology. The traditional unit of RBE-dose is the rem (acronym for roentgen-equivalent-man), where RBE-dose (rem) = [absorbed dose (rads)] RBE. 1 Sv = 100 rems.

Often the effectiveness with which different types of radiation produce a particular chemical or biological effect varies with the linear energy transfer (LET) of the radiation. The dose equivalent H in Sv is the product of the absorbed dose in Gy and a quality factor Q that varies with the LET of the radiation. That is, $H(\text{Sv}) = D(\text{Gy}) \cdot Q$. In traditional units, the dose equivalent H in rems is H (rems) = D (rads) · Q. Quality factors are listed in Table 5-6 as a function of LET and in Table 5-7 for different types of radiation. The dose equivalent reflects differences in the effectiveness of different radiations to elicit a biological response from a small region of irradiated tissue as a reflection of the LET of the radiation.

For a particular response in a specific biological system, the RBE may vary with several factors, including dose rate, fractionation schedule, temperature, degree of oxygenation, spatial distribution of dose, and sample volume.

The quality factor varies with a physical property of the radiation (LET) rather than with the response of a biological system. Consequently, it has a fixed value for a particular radiation.

Although Q is not related to any particular biological result, its use in radiation protection is directed primarily to the carcinogenic and mutagenic effects of radiation.

Example 5-11

A person received an average whole-body x-ray dose of 0.8 mGy and 0.6 mGy from 10-MeV neutrons. What is the whole-body dose equivalent in mSv?

TABLE 5-6 Relation Between Specific Ionization, Linear Energy Transfer, and Quality Factor

Average Specific Ionization (IP/μm) in Water	Average Linear Energy Transfer (keV/μm) in Water	Quality Factor
100 or less	2.5 or less	1
100–200	2.5–7.0	1–2
200–650	7.0–23	2–5
650–1500	23–53	5–10
1500–5000	53–175	10–20

Source: Recommendations of the ICRP.[21]

TABLE 5-7 Quality Factors for Different Radiations[a]

Type of Radiation	Quality Factor
X rays, gamma rays, and beta particles	1.0
Thermal neutrons	5
Neutrons and protons	20
Particles from natural radionuclides	20
Heavy recoil nuclei	20

[a] These data should be used only for purposes of radiation protection. NCRP Report 91.[22]

$$H \text{ (mSv)} = \sum_{i=1}^{2} D_i \text{ (mGy)} \cdot Q_i$$
$$= (0.8 \text{ mGy})(1) + (0.6 \text{ mGy})(20)$$
$$= 12.8 \text{ mSv}$$

Example 5-12

A person accidentally ingests a small amount of ^{32}P (β particle $E_{max} = 1.7$ MeV). The average dose to the gastrointestinal tract is estimated to be 10 mGy. What is the dose equivalent to the gastrointestinal tract in mSv?

$$H \text{ (mSv)} = D \text{ (mGy)} \cdot Q$$
$$= (10 \text{ mGy}) \cdot (1.0)$$
$$= 10 \text{ mSv}$$

Factors other than the LET may influence the biologic effectiveness of radiations. For example, a distribution factor DF may be included to account for changes in the radiation response caused by the nonuniform distribution of radioactivity in a region of tissue. In this case, the expression for H is written as $H \text{ (Sv)} = D \text{ (Gy)} \cdot Q \cdot DF$.

Often the region of tissue of interest is sufficiently large that the absorbed dose and LET vary across the region. The mean dose equivalent (sometimes called the equivalent dose) $\overline{H}$ is defined as the average absorbed dose in a region of tissue multiplied by an effective quality factor $\overline{Q}$ (more commonly referred to as a radiation weighting factor w_r) that depends on the LET of the radiation averaged over the region of exposed tissue. Also, different organs in the body vary in terms of their radiation sensitivity and relative importance to the overall well-being of the individual. These variations are reflected in the effective dose equivalent H_e, in which doses of different tissues are adjusted by a tissue weighting factor, w_t. The mean and effective dose equivalent are discussed further in Chapter 14.

In some publications, effective dose equivalent is referred to simply as "effective dose."

■ RADIATION QUALITY

An x-ray beam is not described completely by stating the exposure or dose it delivers to a region within an irradiated medium. The penetrating ability of the radiation, termed the *quality* of the radiation, must also be known before estimates can be made of the exposure or dose at other locations in the medium; the differences in energy absorption between regions of different composition; and the biological effectiveness or quality factor of the radiation.

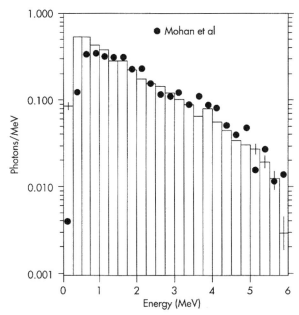

FIGURE 5-12
Energy distribution of x-ray photons in a beam generated at 6 MV. (From E. L. Chaney and T. J. Cullip,[25] used with permission.)

Spectral Distributions

The spectral distribution of an x-ray beam depicts the relative number of photons of different energies in the beam. The quality of an x-ray beam is described explicitly by the spectral distribution. The spectral distribution of an x-ray beam may be computed from an attenuation curve for the beam measured under conditions in which the area of the beam is small and the measurements are obtained at a considerable distance from the location where attenuating materials are placed in the beam. A variety of curve-fitting techniques may be applied to the attenuation curve to obtain equations used to compute the spectral distribution.[23, 24]

Most measurements of x-ray spectra are obtained with a scintillation or semiconductor detector. The height of a voltage pulse (i.e., the size of the electrical signal) from the detector varies with the energy deposited in the detector during interaction of an x-ray photon. The voltage pulses are sorted by height in a pulse-height analyzer and counted in a scaler. The recorded counts are plotted as a function of pulse height to furnish a pulse-height distribution that reflects the energy distribution of photons impinging on the detector. The pulse-height distribution must be corrected for statistical fluctuations in the energy distribution, incomplete absorption of photons in the detector, and selective absorption of lower-energy photons in the detector (i.e., the detector's energy dependence). A measured x-ray spectrum with appropriate corrections applied is shown in Figure 5-12.

The *half-value layer* (HVL), sometimes called the half-value thickness, of an x-ray beam is the thickness of a material (usually in units of mm) that reduces the exposure rate of the beam to half. The HVL may be expressed as mm Al, mm Cu, or mm Pb. Although the HVL alone furnishes a description of radiation quality that is adequate for most clinical situations, a second parameter such as the kVP or the homogeneity coefficient is sometimes stated with the HVL. The homogeneity coefficient is the quotient of the thickness of attenuator required to reduce the exposure to half, divided by the thickness of attenuator required to reduce the exposure further from half to a fourth. The homogeneity coefficient is the ratio of the first and second HVLs.

The tenth-value layer (TVL) is the thickness of a material that reduces the exposure rate of an x-ray beam to 1/10th. TVL = 3.32 (HVL).

Example 5-13

The following attenuation data are measured for a therapy x-ray beam. What are the first and second HVLs and the homogeneity coefficient?

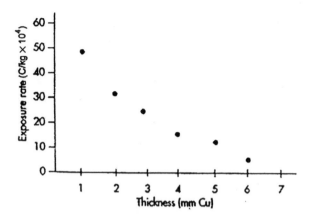

From the curve, the first HVL is approximately 1.9 mm Cu, and the second HVL is approximately 2.1 mm Cu. The homogeneity coefficient is

$$\text{Homogeneity coefficient} = \frac{(\text{HVL})_1}{(\text{HVL})_2} = \frac{1.9 \text{ mm Cu}}{2.1 \text{ mm Cu}}$$
$$= 0.90$$

HVLs are measured with solid attenuators, such as thin sheets of aluminum, copper, or lead of uniform thickness. The attenuators are placed between the x-ray source and an ionization chamber, and measurements of exposure are obtained as the total thickness of attenuator is increased. Measurements of HVL should always be made under conditions of narrow-beam ("good") geometry so that only primary and not scattered photons enter the chamber. Narrow-beam geometry requires that the measuring chamber be positioned far from the attenuators and that an x-ray beam of small cross-sectional area be used. Conditions of narrow-beam ("good") and broad-beam ("poor") geometry are depicted in Figure 3-1. Measurements of HVL under these conditions are compared in Figure 5-13. With broad-beam geometry, increasing numbers of photons are scattered into the detector as additional attenuators are added to the beam. Consequently, broad-beam conditions yield inappropriately

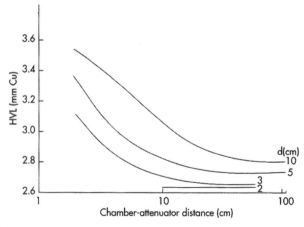

FIGURE 5-13
Variation of the HVL with the diameter d of an x-ray beam at the attenuator for various distances between the attenuator and the radiation detector. (From NCRP Report 85,[26] used with permission.)

high values of the HVL. Such values, however, are useful in the computation of shielding requirements for walls surrounding sources of radiation.

■ SUMMARY

- Radiation quantity may be described explicitly by the concepts of photon and energy fluence and flux density. The energy flux density is often referred to as radiation intensity.
- Radiation exposure (in units of coulombs/kilogram or, formerly, roentgens (R)) is defined in terms of the ionization that radiation produces in air.
- Measurements of radiation exposure with a free-air, thimble or condenser chamber require that electron equilibrium is established in the collecting volume of air.
- The effective atomic number of a material is the atomic number of a hypothetical element that attenuates x and γ rays at the same rate as the material.
- The sensitivity of air ionization chambers is the voltage reduction across the chamber per unit exposure to radiation.
- Ionization chamber readings may need correction for several influences, including a calibration factor, temperature and pressure (if the chamber is open to the atmosphere), stem irradiation, polarity effect, and collection efficiency.
- Extrapolation and parallel-plate ionization chambers are used for exposure measurements at or slightly below the surface of an irradiated material.
- Kerma is a measure of the energy deposited per unit mass of irradiated material.
- Absorbed dose is a measure of the energy absorbed per unit mass of irradiated material. Absorbed dose is the kerma corrected for energy lost by bremsstrahlung and characteristic radiation.
- Absorbed dose can be determined from ionization measurements through the application of the Bragg–Gray principle.
- Methods for measurement of absorbed dose include calorimetry and ionization, photographic, chemical, scintillation, and thermoluminescence dosimetry.
- The dose equivalent in sieverts is a product of the absorbed dose in gray multiplied by a quality factor (also called the radiation weighting factor) that varies with the LET of the radiation.
- The effective dose equivalent, also known as the effective dose, is the absorbed dose to a tissue multiplied by radiation and tissue weighting factors.
- Radiation quality is a measure of the penetrating ability of an x-ray beam.
- Radiation quality is often described in terms of the half-value layer (HVL), defined as the thickness of attenuation required to reduce the radiation exposure to half.

PROBLEMS

5-1. For an exposure of 43 R, what are the number of ion pairs and the charge in coulombs liberated per kilogram of air? How much energy is absorbed per cubic meter and per kilogram of air? What is the absorbed dose in air?

5-2. For a ^{60}Co beam, a deflection of 57 scale divisions/min is recorded with a 100-R condenser chamber (full-scale deflection = 100 divisions). The chamber has a calibration factor of 0.95 for ^{60}Co gamma rays determined at 22°C. The temperature and pressure are 24°C and 645 mm Hg. For 100% collection efficiency and a stem correction factor of 1.02, what is the exposure rate in R/min?

5-3. The photon flux is 10^{11} photons/m^2-sec for a beam of photons. Two-thirds of the photons have an energy of 600 keV, and one-third have an energy of 1.15 MeV. What is the energy flux of the beam? If the photon flux is constant over time, what is the energy fluence over a 20-second interval?

5-4. The total energy absorption coefficient of air is 2.8×10^{-3} m^2/kg for photons of 1.0 MeV. What are the energy and photon fluence required for an exposure of 0.03 coulomb/kg?

5-5. Water is 89% oxygen (gram-atomic mass 15.999) and 11% hydrogen (gram-atomic mass 1.008) by weight. Compute the effective atomic number of water.

5-6. A thimble chamber with an air-equivalent wall receives an exposure of 0.025 coulomb/kg in 1 minute. The volume of the chamber is 0.52 cm^3. What is the ionization current from the chamber?

5-7. A condenser chamber has a sensitivity of 1.43×10^4 volts/coulomb/kg and a volume of 0.52 cm³. The capacitance of the chamber is 5 times that of the electrometer. What is the capacitance of the chamber?

5-8. A miniature ionization chamber has a sensitivity of 1 V/R. The chamber is discharged by 300 V during an exposure to x rays. What exposure in roentgens did the chamber receive?

5-9. An 800-g organ receives a uniform absorbed dose of 10 Gy. How much energy is absorbed per gram, and what is the total energy absorbed in the organ?

5-10. A particular type of lesion recedes satisfactorily after receiving a dose of 55 Gy from ^{60}Co γ rays. When the lesion is treated with 10 MV x rays, a dose of 65 Gy is required to obtain the same response. Relative to ^{60}Co γ rays, what is the RBE of 10 MV x rays for treating this lesion?

5-11. A patient undergoing a nuclear medicine procedure receives a dose of 2.5 cGy to the thyroid. A total of 2.1 cGy is delivered by beta particles and 0.4 cGy is contributed by gamma rays. What is the dose equivalent in cSv to the thyroid?

5-12. The specific heat of graphite is 170 cal/(kg°C). A uniform dose of 10 Gy is delivered to a graphite block that is insulated from its environment. What is the temperature rise of the block?

5-13. With $G = 15.4$ molecules/100 eV, how many Fe^{2+} ions are oxidized to Fe^{3+} when a dose of 100 Gy is delivered to a 10-mL solution of $FeSO_4$? (Assume that the density of $FeSO_4$ is 1 kg/L.)

5-14. Attenuation measures for a diagnostic x-ray beam yield the following results:

Added Filtration (mm Al)	Percent Transmission
1.0	60.2
2.0	41.4
3.0	30.0
4.0	22.4
5.0	16.9

Plot the data on semilogarithmic graph paper, and determine the first and second HVL and the homogeneity coefficient.

REFERENCES

1. Hendee, W. R., and Ritenour, E. R. *Medical Imaging Physics,* 4th edition. New York, John Wiley & Sons, 2001.
2. Johns, H., and Cunningham, J. *The Physics of Radiology,* 3rd edition. Springfield, IL, Charles C Thomas, 1969.
3. Meredith, W., and Massey, J. *Fundamental Physics of Radiology.* Baltimore, MD, Williams & Wilkins, 1968.
4. Ibbott, G. S., et al. Stem correction for ion chambers. *Med. Phys.* 1975; **2**:328–330.
5. Boag, J. W. Ionization chambers. In *Radiation Dosimetry,* vol. II, 2nd edition, F. H. Attix and W. C. Roesch (eds). New York, Academic Press, 1969.
6. Stanton, L. *Basic Medical Radiation Physics.* New York, Appleton-Century-Crofts, 1968.
7. Fricke, H., and Morse, S. The action of x rays on ferrous sulfate solutions. *Philos. Mag.* 1929; **7**:129–141.
8. ICRU Report 21. *Radiation Dosimetry: Electrons with Initial Energies Between 1 and 50 MeV.* Washington, DC, International Commission on Radiological Units and Measurements, 1972.
9. Bethe, H. Quanten mechanik der ein- and zwei-elektronen problems. In *Hanbuch der Physik,* vol. 24, part 1, 2nd edition, G. Geiger and K. Scheel (eds.). Berlin, Julius Springer, 1933, pp. 273–551.
10. Sternheimer, R. The density effect for the ionization loss in various materials. *Phys. Rev.* 1957; **88**:851–859.
11. Berger, M. J., and Seltzern, S. M. *Stopping Powers and Ranges of Electrons and Positrons,* 2nd edition. Washington, DC, National Bureau of Standards, 1983.
12. Burlin, T. Cavity chamber theory. In *Radiation Dosimetry,* vol. 1, 2nd edition, F. H. Attix and W. C. Roesch (eds). New York, Academic Press, 1968.
13. Storer, J. B., Harris, P. S., Furchner, J. E., and Langham, W. H. Relative biological effectiveness of various ionizing radiations in mammalian systems. *Radiat. Res.* 1957; **6**:188.
14. Hall, E. Relative biological efficiency of x rays generated at 200 kVp and gamma radiation from cobalt 50 therapy unit. *Br. J. Radiol.* 1961; **34**:313.
15. Sinclair, W. Relative biological effectiveness of 22-MeVp x-rays, cobalt 60 gamma rays and 200 kVp rays: 1. General introduction and physical aspects. *Radiat. Res.* 1962; **16**:336.
16. Loken, M. K., Beisang, A. A., Johnson, E. A., and Mosser, D. G. Relative biological effectiveness of ^{60}Co gamma rays and 220 kVp x-rays on viability of chicken eggs. *Radiat. Res.* 1960; **12**:202.
17. Krohmer, J. RBE and quality of electromagnetic radiation at depths in water phantom. *Radiat. Res.* 1965; **24**:547.
18. Upton, A. C., and Odell, T. T., Jr. Relative biological effectiveness of neutrons, x-rays, and gamma rays for production of lens opacities: Observations on mice, rats guinea pigs and rabbits. *Radiology* 1956; **67**:686.
19. Focht, E. F., Merriam, G. R., Jr., Schwartz, M. S., and Parsons, R. W. The relative biological effectiveness of cobalt 60 gamma and 200 kV x radiation for cataract induction. *Am. J. Roentgenol.* 1968; **102**:71.
20. Till, J., and Cunningham J. Unpublished data. In *The Physics of Radiology,* 3rd edition, H. Johns and J. Cunningham. Springfield, IL, Charles C Thomas, 1969, p. 720.
21. International Commission on Radiological Protection. Recommendations of the ICRP. *Br. J. Radiol.* 1955; **28**(Suppl. 6).
22. National Council on Radiation Protection and Measurements. *Recommendations on Limits for Exposure to Ionizing Radiation,* Report 91. Washington, DC, NCRP, 1991.
23. Kramers, H. A. On the theory of x-ray absorption and the continuous x-ray spectrum. *Philos. Mag.* 1923; **46**(series 6): 836–871.
24. Schiff, LI. Energy-angle distribution of thin target bremsstrahlung. *Phys. Rev.* 1951; **83**:252–253.
25. Chaney, E. L., and Cullip, T. J. A Monte Carlo study of accelerator head scatter. *Med. Phys.* 1994; **21**:1383–1390.
26. NCRP Report 85. *Physical Aspects of Irradiation.* Washington, DC, National Bureau of Standards Handbook 85, 1964.

CALIBRATION OF MEGAVOLTAGE BEAMS OF X RAYS AND ELECTRONS

OBJECTIVES   108

CALIBRATION STANDARDS AND LABORATORIES   108

Calibration Coefficient as a Function of Energy   109
Estimation of Dose to a Medium from a Calibration in Air   109
Measurement in a Phantom   113

CALIBRATION OF LOW-ENERGY X-RAY BEAMS   114

Beam Quality   114
In-Air Calibrations   116
In-Phantom Calibrations   116

CALIBRATION OF MEGAVOLTAGE BEAMS—THE AAPM PROTOCOL   117

Calibration of Photon Beams Versus Electron Beams   117
Calibration with an Ionization Chamber in a Medium   118
Dose to Water from a Measurement of Ionization   118
Dose to Water Calibration Coefficient ($N_{D,w}$)   120
Effective Point of Measurement   121
Beam Quality Specification   122
Calibration of Photon Beams   123
Calibration of Electron Beams   124

THE IAEA CALIBRATION PROTOCOL   126

SUMMARY   127

PROBLEMS   127

REFERENCES   127

■ OBJECTIVES

By studying this chapter, the reader should be able to:

- Describe the procedures for calibrating beams of x and γ rays and electrons.
- Discuss the pathways by which exposure, air kerma, and dose calibration standards are promulgated in the United States.
- Explain the similarities and differences among past and current U.S. calibration protocols and among international protocols.
- Describe the influences on the response of an ionization chamber and the procedures for correcting for these influences.
- Compare the calibration protocols recommended in the United States with those published by international agencies.

Determination of the dose delivered at a reference point in a beam of radiation is termed *calibration*. Calibration must be performed before a radiation beam can be used for the treatment of patients and is generally repeated on a regular basis to ensure constancy in dose delivery (see Chapter 15). Most often, calibration involves a measurement of ionization, followed by calculations to estimate the dose at the location of measurement. Alternate methods of measuring dose have been described (e.g., calorimetry), but these are inconvenient for regular use. Methods for measuring exposure are described in Chapter 5. The relationship between exposure and dose has also been discussed. The procedures that must be used to calibrate radiation beams in practice are described in this chapter.

■ CALIBRATION STANDARDS AND LABORATORIES

Many of the ionization measurement procedures described in Chapter 5 require knowledge of the mass of air inside an ionization chamber. Determination of the exact mass of air inside the collecting volume of a thimble chamber is beyond the capabilities of the practicing physicist. Instead, the instrument is submitted to a calibration laboratory, where its response is determined in relation to one or more radiation quantities. This relationship is called a *calibration coefficient*. In the United States, instruments are calibrated by AAPM—Accredited Dosimetry Calibration Laboratories (ADCLs).[1]

An ADCL provides the practicing physicist with the ratio of the known exposure, air kerma, or dose at the location of the chamber (with the chamber removed from the beam) to the response of the chamber in coulombs. For example, the ratio of exposure to chamber response is termed the *exposure calibration coefficient*, N_X. When the instrument is placed in the customer's beam, the product of chamber signal in coulombs and the coefficient N_X yields the exposure at the location of measurement. The user must specify the energy or quality of the beam in which the calibration is to be performed. ADCLs generally provide chamber calibrations in x-ray beams with half-value layers (HVLs) from about 0.1 mm Al to 3 mm Cu, as well as in ^{60}Co γ-ray beams. Calibrations are not provided in accelerator-produced x-ray or electron beams, because of the expense and impracticality of maintaining modern linear accelerators at NIST and at the ADCLs. Instead, calibration protocols provide mathematical corrections to account for the change in ionization chamber response with energy.

The ADCLs possess ionization chambers that are periodically submitted for calibration by the National Institute of Standards and Technology (NIST, formerly the National Bureau of Standards). The ADCL must also participate in periodic *measurement quality assurance* (MQA) tests to verify constancy of calibrations. The NIST-calibrated instruments are used to calibrate x- and γ-ray beams at the ADCL, under carefully controlled conditions. The instruments submitted by clinical medical physicists are

---

The National Institute of Standards and Technology maintains the U.S. dosimetry standards and is therefore the U.S. Primary Standard Dosimetry Laboratory (PSDL). Most developed countries have a PSDL, and these trace their dosimetry standards to the Bureau Internationale des Poids et Mesures, or BIPM, located in Paris.

The American Association of Physicists in Medicine (AAPM) supervises the promulgation of dosimetry standards in the United States. The AAPM-accredited dosimetry calibration laboratories (ADCLs) calibrate radiation dosimetry instruments primarily for medical physicists working in the United States. Elsewhere in the world, a network of Secondary Standard Dosimetry Laboratories (SSDLs) provides a similar function. The SSDLs are supervised by the International Atomic Energy Agency (IAEA), in Vienna, Austria.

NIST recently adopted terminology in general use throughout the world.[2] The term calibration *coefficient* is used for parameters with dimensions such as Gy/C, whereas a calibration *factor* is dimensionless. A calibration factor would be used to correct an instrument reading that is already in desired units, such as cGy.

The *exposure calibration coefficient* N_x is the ratio of exposure at the location of the chamber to the chamber signal.

The *air-kerma calibration coefficient*, N_k, is the ratio of the air kerma at the location of chamber to the chamber signal.

The *dose-to-water calibration coefficient*, $N_{D,w}$, is the ratio of the dose to water at the chamber location in a water phantom to the chamber signal.

placed in the same beams, and calibration coefficients are thus derived. The customers' instruments are said to be *directly traceable* to NIST because they are no more than one step removed from a NIST calibration.

Example 6-1

An ion chamber has an exposure calibration coefficient N_X of 4.0×10^9 R/C determined by an ADCL in a ^{60}Co beam. During exposure in air in the user's ^{60}Co beam, an electrometer connected to the chamber records a signal of 1.5×10^{-8} C. What is the exposure in the beam at the location of the chamber?

$$\text{Exposure} = 4.0 \times 10^9 \, \text{R/C} \cdot 1.5 \times 10^{-8} \, \text{C}$$

$$\text{Exposure} = 60.0 \, \text{R}$$

ADCLs offer their customers the choice of calibrating an ionization chamber by itself or together with an electrometer as a system. If only the chamber is to be calibrated, the calibration laboratory substitutes the customer's chamber for its own and uses the ADCL electrometer to obtain the reading. In this way, the calibration coefficient of the customer's chamber is determined by direct comparison with the ADCL instrument. If a chamber is submitted with an electrometer with which it is to be calibrated as a system, the ADCL may use the customer's electrometer to determine the chamber response. Alternatively, the ADCL may determine a calibration coefficient for the customer's electrometer independently. The *system calibration coefficient* may be reported in terms of exposure per unit electrometer reading, which often is described in "roentgens." Consequently, the calibration coefficient is dimensionless (and is called the calibration factor) or has the units R/reading.

The quality of calibrations at NIST and at the ADCLs is very high. Estimates of the calibration uncertainty introduced by these facilities indicate that a customer's instrument, such as a cable-connected ionization chamber of good quality, can be calibrated with an *overall uncertainty* of 1.5%. (expressed at the 2 standard deviation level, or 95% confidence level).[4,5]

Calibration Coefficient as a Function of Energy

The value of N_X or N_K for an ionization chamber generally varies with photon beam energy. ($N_{D,w}$ is not determined at energies other than ^{60}Co at NIST or the ADCLs). The N_X values for a representative ionization chamber are shown in Margin Figure 6-1 as a function of HVL. In general, the calibration coefficient increases as the beam energy decreases, reflecting increased attenuation of lower-energy radiation in the wall of the chamber. An ionization chamber intended for use with superficial or orthovoltage x-ray beams would generally be submitted to an ADCL for calibration in beams of similar energies. The N_X for the user's beam might be determined by interpolation between the N_X values assigned by the ADCL.

The response of any chamber depends on its design. For example, a thin-window chamber exhibits less attenuation at low photon energies, whereas a *buildup-up cap* is often required at higher energies to provide sufficient wall thickness to achieve *electron equilibrium*.

Estimation of Dose to a Medium from a Calibration in Air

Once the exposure calibration coefficient N_X for an ionization chamber is known for the beam energy to be measured, a measurement of exposure is straightforward, as described previously and in Chapter 5. Determination of the dose at the location of measurement requires several additional steps. If, as is often the case, the chamber wall is made from an air-equivalent material such as graphite or air equivalent plastic, the dose in gray to the air in the chamber or to the chamber wall material is computed

The world's PSDLs work hard to ensure that their dosimetry standards are accurate and in good agreement. An international comparison, conducted by circulating a set of ionization chambers, revealed that each PSDL assigned calibration coefficients to the instruments that were within 0.5% of the mean value, and that most were within 0.2% of the mean.[3]

Directly traceable means that an instrument has been calibrated at NIST or an ADCL.

Indirectly traceable means that an instrument has been calibrated by comparison with an instrument having a directly traceable calibration coefficient.

Obtaining a system calibration factor for an ion chamber and electrometer that are used together is convenient, because only one factor must be obtained and documented. However, it also means that if either component fails or is damaged, the system is rendered unusable. By obtaining a calibration coefficient for each component, any calibrated chamber can be used with any calibrated electrometer.

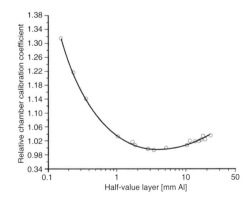

MARGIN FIGURE 6-1
A graph of N_X as a function of photon beam HVL. The data are for an Exradin A-2 chamber.

The special unit of absorbed dose is the gray, Gy. A dose of 1 Gy corresponds to 1 joule of energy absorbed per kilogram of medium.

Ionizations tend to occur in clusters of three.[8]

When exposures are expressed in units of roentgens, the definition of the roentgen, $k = 2.58 \times 10^{-4}$ C/kg · R, is needed. The product of $\overline{W}/e \cdot k$ is 0.876×10^{-2} J/kg · R.

by multiplying the exposure in C/kg by the *work function*, the energy absorbed by air per unit ionization.

Work Function

The determination of dose from a measurement of ionization is accomplished through knowledge of the energy absorbed by the air to produce the ionization. It is generally accepted that the *work function* (alternately known as the *W*-quantity), the average energy required to ionize dry air, has the value 33.97 electron volts/ion pair.[6,7] This does not mean that the binding energy for an electron in a typical air atom is 33.97 eV. Instead, it means that, on average, 33.97 eV are expended for every atom ionized. For each ion pair produced, several atoms are excited but not ionized.

For convenience, the work function can be described in SI units as 33.97 joules/coulomb, and the symbol $\overline{W}/e$ is used. When the total charge (in coulombs) produced by ionization (of either sign) per unit mass of dry air is known, multiplying the value by $\overline{W}/e$ yields the energy absorbed by the medium in joules. A small correction must be applied for laboratory air with about 50% humidity.[6] In this case, $\overline{W}/e = 33.77$ J/C. A humidity correction to N_X is applied by the ADCLs, so $\overline{W}/e = 33.97$ J/C should be used in calculations of the type described here.

Example 6-2

An ionization chamber filled with dry air records a charge of 1.5×10^{-8} coulombs during irradiation with a 4-MV x-ray beam. How much energy was deposited in the air by the beam?

$$1.5 \times 10^{-8}\,\text{C} \cdot 33.97\,\text{J/C} = 5.10 \times 10^{-7}\,\text{J}$$

Dose to Air

The dose (in J/kg or Gy) absorbed by air is therefore determined as follows:

$$D_{\text{air}} = M \cdot N_X \cdot 0.876 \times 10^{-2}\,[\text{J/kg}]$$

where the product of the chamber reading M and the exposure calibration coefficient N_X yields the exposure X in air. When X is expressed in roentgens, the dose to air is

$$D_{\text{air}} = X \cdot 0.876 \times 10^{-2}\left[\frac{\text{Gy}}{\text{R}}\right] \tag{6-1}$$

ADCLs provide the calibration coefficient for an ionization chamber in terms of the *air kerma*, as well as the exposure. As discussed in Chapter 5, the term *air kerma* describes the energy transferred from the beam to the medium, in this case air, without correction for energy reradiated from the local area of absorption.

Air kerma K_{air} is related to exposure X by

$$K_{\text{air}} = \frac{X \cdot \overline{W}/e \cdot k}{(1 - G)} \tag{6-2}$$

where G is a correction for energy dissipated as bremsstrahlung outside the volume of interest. For ^{60}Co gamma rays, the value of G is 0.003.[6] The *air-kerma calibration coefficient*, N_K, is the ratio of the air-kerma to the chamber signal. The air-kerma and exposure calibration coefficients are related by

$$N_K = \frac{N_X \cdot \overline{W}/e \cdot k}{(1 - G)}$$

Comparing the above formula with Equation (6-1) reveals that air kerma is closely related, but not equal to, the dose to air. The air-kerma calibration coefficient may not be substituted directly for the exposure calibration coefficient, and caution must be exercised when values of air kerma are available.

Higher-energy photons, such as gamma rays from a ^{60}Co source, furnish a dose buildup region of significant thickness. Measurements in these beams require use of a buildup cap over the chamber, unless the chamber wall is of adequate thickness to provide maximum dose buildup.

Example 6-3

An ionization chamber/electrometer system has a system calibration factor $N_X = 0.94$, determined in a beam of HVL = 0.5 mm Cu (effective energy = 55 keV). Following a 1-minute exposure in a beam of x rays of the same quality, the electrometer reads 213 R. What is the dose to air at the location of the chamber (when the chamber is removed)?

$$D_{air} = M \cdot N_X \cdot 0.876 \times 10^{-2} \, [J/kg]$$

$$D_{air} = 213\,R \cdot 0.94 \cdot 2.58 \times 10^{-4} \, C/kg\text{-}R$$

$$\cdot 33.97 \, J/C \cdot 1 \, Gy/J/kg$$

$$D_{air} = 175 \times 10^{-2} \, Gy$$

Dose to Another Medium

The dose to air is rarely of great interest. Instead, we usually wish to know the dose to tissue or tissue-equivalent material. As described in Chapter 3, the mass energy absorption coefficient $(\mu_{en})_m$ [also written (μ_{en}/ρ)] describes the rate at which energy is absorbed in an irradiated medium.[9] To determine the energy-absorption characteristics of a medium such as tissue, the ratio of its mass energy absorption coefficient to that of air may be determined at the energy of interest:

$$D_{tissue} = D_{air} \cdot \frac{(\mu_{en}/\rho)_{tissue}}{(\mu_{en}/\rho)_{air}} \qquad (6\text{-}3)$$

This calculation yields the dose to an infinitesimal mass of tissue suspended in air at the location of the ionization chamber, with the chamber removed. The mass of tissue must be only large enough to provide electron equilibrium. For convenience, the ratio in Equation (6-3) is often written $(\mu_{en}/\rho)_{air}^{tissue}$. A correction A_{eq} must be included to correct for attenuation of photons in the equilibrium thickness. Values of A_{eq} vary from unity for photons less than 400 keV to 0.985 for ^{60}Co gamma rays.

Equations (6-1) and (6-3) may be combined.

$$D_{tissue} = X \cdot 0.876 \times 10^{-2} \frac{Gy}{R} \cdot (\mu_{en}/\rho)_{air}^{tissue} \cdot A_{eq} \qquad (6\text{-}4)$$

The product of 2.58×10^{-4} C/kg-R $\cdot 33.97$ J/C $\cdot (\mu_{en}/\rho)_{air}^{tissue} \cdot 100$ has been named the f factor, yielding

$$D_{tissue} = X \cdot f_{tissue} \cdot A_{eq} \qquad (6\text{-}5)$$

When the f factor is used and exposure is expressed in R, the dose to tissue is expressed in cGy (rads). Values of absorption coefficients and f factors are found in Tables 6-1 and 6-2. Use of Equation (6-5) is not recommended; instead, a calibration protocol such as one described later in this chapter should be used for calibration of x- and γ-ray beams.

Example 6-4

Referring to Example 6-3, determine the dose to a small mass of muscle tissue in air at the location of the chamber.

ADCLs routinely provide the air-kerma calibration coefficient N_k for thimble and parallel plate ionization chambers. However, N_k is not used in all calibration protocols recommended for use in the United States. A significant error would result if N_k were to be used inappropriately.

At this point, the reader may question the value of the discussion of f factor and its derivation. It must be emphasized that while the use of f factor for calibration of therapeutic x- and γ-ray beams is not recommended, the principles described up to this point are important to establish the foundation for modern calibration procedures.

TABLE 6-1 Photon Mass Attenuation Coefficients, μ/ρ, and Mass Energy-Absorption Coefficients, μ_{en}/ρ, in m²/kg for Energies 1 keV to 20 MeV[a]

Photon Energy (eV)	Air, Dry $\overline{Z} = 7.78$ $\rho = 1.205\ kg/m^3(20°C)$ $3.006 \times 10^{26}\ e/kg$		Water $\overline{Z} = 7.51$ $\rho = 1000\ kg/m^3$ $3.343 \times 10^{26}\ e/kg$		Muscle $\overline{Z} = 7.64$ $\rho = 1040\ kg/m^3$ $3.312 \times 10^{26}\ e/kg$	
	μ/ρ	μ_{en}/ρ	μ/ρ	μ_{en}/ρ	μ/ρ	μ_{en}/ρ
1.0 + 03	3.617 + 02	3.616 + 02	4.091 + 02	4.089 + 02	3.774 + 02	3.772 + 02
1.5 + 03	1.202 + 02	1.201 + 02	1.390 + 02	1.388 + 02	1.275 + 02	1.273 + 02
2.0 + 03	5.303 + 01	5.291 + 01	6.187 + 01	6.175 + 01	5.663 + 01	5.651 + 01
3.0 + 03	1.617 + 01	1.608 + 01	1.913 + 01	1.903 + 01	1.828 + 01	1.813 + 01
4.0 + 03	7.751 + 00	7.597 + 00	8.174 + 00	8.094 + 00	8.085 + 00	7.963 + 00
5.0 + 03	3.994 + 00	3.896 + 00	4.196 + 00	4.129 + 00	4.174 + 00	4.090 + 00
6.0 + 03	2.312 + 00	2.242 + 00	2.421 + 00	2.363 + 00	2.421 + 00	2.354 + 00
8.0 + 03	9.721 − 01	9.246 − 01	1.018 + 00	9.726 − 01	1.024 + 00	9.770 − 01
1.0 + 04	5.016 − 01	4.640 − 01	5.223 − 01	4.840 − 01	5.284 − 01	4.895 − 01
1.5 + 04	1.581 − 01	1.300 − 01	1.639 − 01	1.340 − 01	1.668 − 01	1.371 − 01
2.0 + 04	7.643 − 02	5.255 − 02	7.958 − 02	5.367 − 02	8.099 − 02	5.531 − 02
3.0 + 04	3.501 − 02	1.501 − 02	3.718 − 02	1.520 − 02	3.754 − 02	1.579 − 02
4.0 + 04	2.471 − 02	6.691 − 03	2.668 − 02	6.803 − 03	2.674 − 02	7.067 − 03
5.0 + 04	2.073 − 02	4.031 − 03	2.262 − 02	4.155 − 03	2.257 − 02	4.288 − 03
6.0 + 04	1.871 − 02	3.004 − 03	2.055 − 02	3.152 − 03	2.045 − 02	3.224 − 03
8.0 + 04	1.661 − 02	2.393 − 03	1.835 − 02	2.583 − 03	1.822 − 02	2.601 − 03
1.0 + 05	1.541 − 02	2.318 − 03	1.707 − 02	2.539 − 03	1.693 − 02	2.538 − 03
1.5 + 05	1.356 − 02	2.494 − 03	1.504 − 02	2.762 − 03	1.491 − 02	2.743 − 03
2.0 + 05	1.234 − 02	2.672 − 03	1.370 − 02	2.966 − 03	1.358 − 02	2.942 − 03
3.0 + 05	1.068 − 02	2.872 − 03	1.187 − 02	3.192 − 03	1.176 − 02	3.164 − 03
4.0 + 05	9.548 − 03	2.949 − 03	1.061 − 02	3.279 − 03	1.052 − 02	3.250 − 03
5.0 + 05	8.712 − 03	2.966 − 03	9.687 − 03	3.299 − 03	9.599 − 03	3.269 − 03
6.0 + 05	8.056 − 03	2.953 − 03	8.957 − 03	3.284 − 03	8.876 − 03	3.254 − 03
8.0 + 05	7.075 − 03	2.882 − 03	7.866 − 03	3.205 − 03	7.795 − 03	3.176 − 03
1.0 + 06	6.359 − 03	2.787 − 03	7.070 − 03	3.100 − 03	7.006 − 03	3.072 − 03
1.5 + 06	5.176 − 03	2.545 − 03	5.755 − 03	2.831 − 03	5.702 − 03	2.805 − 03
2.0 + 06	4.447 − 03	2.342 − 03	4.940 − 03	2.604 − 03	4.895 − 03	2.580 − 03
3.0 + 06	3.581 − 03	2.054 − 03	3.969 − 03	2.278 − 03	3.932 − 03	2.257 − 03
4.0 + 06	3.079 − 03	1.866 − 03	3.403 − 03	2.063 − 03	3.370 − 03	2.043 − 03
5.0 + 06	2.751 − 03	1.737 − 03	3.031 − 03	1.913 − 03	3.001 − 03	1.894 − 03
6.0 + 06	2.523 − 03	1.644 − 03	2.771 − 03	1.804 − 03	2.743 − 03	1.785 − 03
8.0 + 06	2.225 − 03	1.521 − 03	2.429 − 03	1.657 − 03	2.403 − 03	1.639 − 03
1.0 + 07	2.045 − 03	1.446 − 03	2.219 − 03	1.566 − 03	2.195 − 03	1.548 − 03
1.5 + 07	1.810 − 03	1.349 − 03	1.941 − 03	1.442 − 03	1.918 − 03	1.424 − 03
2.0 + 07	1.705 − 03	1.308 − 03	1.813 − 03	1.386 − 03	1.790 − 03	1.367 − 03

Photon Energy (eV)	Fat $\overline{Z} = 6.46$ $\rho = 920\ kg/m^3$ $3.192 \times 10^{26}\ e/kg$		Bone $\overline{Z} = 12.31$ $\rho = 1850\ kg/m^3$ $3.192 \times 10^{26}\ e/kg$		Polystrene $\overline{Z} = 5.74$ $\rho = 1046\ kg/m^3$ $3.238 \times 10^{26}\ e/kg$	
	μ/ρ	μ_{en}/ρ	μ/ρ	μ_{en}/ρ	μ/ρ	μ_{en}/ρ
1.0 + 03	2.517 + 02	2.516 + 02	3.394 + 02	3.392 + 02	2.047 + 02	2.046 + 02
1.5 + 03	8.066 + 01	8.055 + 01	1.148 + 02	1.146 + 02	6.227 + 01	6.219 + 01
2.0 + 03	3.535 + 01	3.526 + 01	5.148 + 01	5.133 + 01	2.692 + 01	2.683 + 01
3.0 + 03	1.100 + 01	1.090 + 01	2.347 + 01	2.303 + 01	8.041 + 00	7.976 + 00
4.0 + 03	4.691 + 00	4.621 + 00	1.045 + 01	1.025 + 01	3.364 + 00	3.312 + 00
5.0 + 03	2.401 + 00	2.345 + 00	1.335 + 01	1.227 + 01	1.704 + 00	1.659 + 00
6.0 + 03	1.386 + 00	1.338 + 00	8.129 + 00	7.531 + 00	9.783 − 01	9.375 − 01
8.0 + 03	5.853 − 01	5.474 − 01	3.676 + 00	3.435 + 00	4.110 − 01	3.773 − 01
1.0 + 04	3.048 − 01	2.716 − 01	1.966 + 00	1.841 + 00	2.150 − 01	1.849 − 01
1.5 + 04	1.022 − 01	7.499 − 02	6.243 − 01	5.726 − 01	7.551 − 02	5.014 − 02

(continued)

TABLE 6-1 (*Continued*)

Photon Energy (eV)	Fat $\overline{Z} = 6.46$ $\rho = 920 \ kg/m^3$ $3.192 \times 10^{26} \ e/kg$		Bone $\overline{Z} = 12.31$ $\rho = 1850 \ kg/m^3$ $3.192 \times 10^{26} \ e/kg$		Polystrene $\overline{Z} = 5.74$ $\rho = 1046 \ kg/m^3$ $3.238 \times 10^{26} \ e/kg$	
	μ/ρ	μ_{en}/ρ	μ/ρ	μ_{en}/ρ	μ/ρ	μ_{en}/ρ
2.0 + 04	5.437 − 02	3.014 − 02	2.797 − 01	2.450 − 01	4.290 − 02	2.002 − 02
3.0 + 04	3.004 − 02	8.881 − 03	9.724 − 02	7.290 − 02	2.621 − 02	6.059 − 03
4.0 + 04	2.377 − 02	4.344 − 03	5.168 − 02	3.088 − 02	2.177 − 02	3.191 − 03
5.0 ± 04	2.118 − 02	2.980 − 03	3.504 − 02	1.625 − 02	1.982 − 02	2.387 − 03
6.0 + 04	1.974 − 02	2.514 − 03	2.741 − 02	9.988 − 03	1.868 − 02	2.153 − 03
8.0 + 04	1.805 − 02	2.344 − 03	2.083 − 02	5.309 − 03	1.724 − 02	2.152 − 03
1.0 + 05	1.694 − 02	2.434 − 03	1.800 − 02	3.838 − 03	1.624 − 02	2.293 − 03
1.5 ± 05	1.506 − 02	2.747 − 03	1.490 − 02	3.032 − 03	1.448 − 02	2.631 − 03
2.0 + 05	1.374 − 02	2.972 − 03	1.332 − 02	2.994 − 03	1.322 − 02	2.856 − 03
3.0 + 05	1.192 − 02	3.209 − 03	1.141 − 02	3.095 − 03	1.147 − 02	3.088 − 03
4.0 + 05	1.067 − 02	3.298 − 03	1.018 − 02	3.151 − 03	1.027 − 02	3.174 − 03
5.0 + 05	9.740 − 03	3.318 − 03	9.274 − 03	3.159 − 03	9.376 − 03	3.194 − 03
6.0 + 05	9.008 − 03	3.304 − 03	8.570 − 03	3.140 − 03	8.672 − 03	3.181 − 03
8.0 + 05	7.912 − 03	3.226 − 03	7.520 − 03	3.061 − 03	7.617 − 03	3.106 − 03
1.0 + 06	7.112 − 03	3.121 − 03	6.758 − 03	2.959 − 03	6.847 − 03	3.005 − 03
1.5 + 06	5.787 − 03	2.850 − 03	5.501 − 03	2.700 − 03	5.571 − 03	2.744 − 03
2.0 + 06	4.963 − 03	2.619 − 03	4.732 − 03	2.487 − 03	4.778 − 03	2.522 − 03
3.0 + 06	3.972 − 03	2.282 − 03	3.826 − 03	2.191 − 03	3.822 − 03	2.196 − 03
4.0 + 06	3.390 − 03	2.055 − 03	3.307 − 03	2.002 − 03	3.261 − 03	1.977 − 03
5.0 + 06	3.005 − 03	1.894 − 03	2.970 − 03	1.874 − 03	2.889 − 03	1.820 − 03
6.0 + 06	2.732 − 03	1.775 − 03	2.738 − 03	1.784 − 03	2.626 − 03	1.706 − 03
8.0 + 06	2.371 − 03	1.613 − 03	2.440 − 03	1.667 − 03	2.227 − 03	1.548 − 03
1.0 + 07	2.147 − 03	1.508 − 03	2.263 − 03	1.598 − 03	2.060 − 03	1.446 − 03
1.5 + 07	1.840 − 03	1.361 − 03	2.040 − 03	1.508 − 03	1.763 − 03	1.304 − 03
2.0 + 07	1.693 − 03	1.290 − 03	1.948 − 03	1.474 − 03	1.620 − 03	1.234 − 03

^{a} Multiply m^2/kg by 10 to convert to cm^2/g. The numbers following + or − refer to the power of 10; for example, 3.617 + 02 should be read as 3.617×10^2.
Source: Hubbell, J. H. Photon mass attenuation and energy-absorption coefficients from 1 keV to MeV. *Int. J. Appl. Radiat. Isot.* 1982;**33**:1269–1290. Used with permission.

The dose to muscle is determined from Equation (6-4) or (6-5):

$$D_{muscle} = X[R] \cdot 0.876 \times 10^{-2} \frac{Gy}{R} \cdot (\mu_{en}/\rho)_{air}^{muscle} \cdot A_{eq}$$

$$D_{muscle} = 213 \ R \cdot 0.94 \cdot 0.876 \times 10^{-2} \frac{Gy}{R} \cdot 1.068 \cdot 1.00$$

$$D_{muscle} = 1.87 \ Gy$$

Alternatively,

$$D_{tissue} = X[R] \cdot f_{tissue} \cdot A_{eq}$$

$$D_{tissue} = 213 \cdot 0.94 \cdot 0.936 \cdot 1.00$$

$$D_{muscle} = 187 \ cGy$$

Measurement in a Phantom

It is recommended by modern calibration protocols that calibrations of megavoltage beams be performed in tissue-equivalent phantoms rather than in air.[10–13] This practice reduces the risk that scatter from the collimator or devices in the beam might influence the measurement. At low photon energies (below about 400 kVp), procedures for measurement in air, similar to those described previously, are generally used. At higher energies, however, the chamber is placed in the phantom at the desired depth and with its long axis oriented perpendicular to the beam (Margin Figure 6-2).

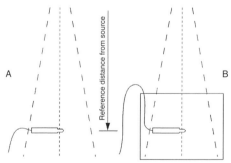

MARGIN FIGURE 6-2
Positioning of an ionization chamber, in air (A) and in a water phantom (B), for measurements of absorbed dose.

TABLE 6-2 Exposure-to-Dose Conversion Factor

Energy (keV)	ƒ-Factors				
	Water	Muscle	Bone	Fat	Polystyrene
10	0.914	0.925	3.477	0.513	0.349
15	0.903	0.924	3.860	0.506	0.338
20	0.895	0.922	4.086	0.503	0.334
30	0.888	0.922	4.257	0.519	0.354
40	0.891	0.926	4.045	0.569	0.418
50	0.903	0.932	3.533	0.648	0.519
60	0.920	0.941	2.914	0.733	0.628
80	0.946	0.953	1.944	0.858	0.788
100	0.960	0.960	1.451	0.920	0.867
150	0.971	0.964	1.065	0.965	0.925
200	0.973	0.965	0.982	0.975	0.934
300	0.974	0.966	0.944	0.979	0.942
400	0.975	0.966	0.936	0.980	0.943
500	0.975	0.966	0.933	0.980	0.944
600	0.975	0.966	0.932	0.981	0.944
800	0.975	0.966	0.931	0.981	0.945
1000	0.975	0.966	0.931	0.981	0.945
1500	0.945	0.966	0.930	0.981	0.945
2000	0.974	0.965	0.931	0.980	0.944
3000	0.972	0.963	0.935	0.974	0.937

$$f_{\text{med}} = 0.876 \frac{(\mu_{\text{en}}/\rho)_{\text{med}}}{(\mu_{\text{en}}/\rho)_{\text{air}}} \text{ for several materials expressed in [cGy/R]}.$$

The phantom material most recommended by calibration protocols is water. This is because water is readily available, practical, and does not vary in composition. Water- and tissue-equivalent plastics, on the other hand, are generally expensive and may vary in composition from one manufacturer or batch to another. Plastic phantoms are recommended for frequent quality assurance checks because they are convenient to use.

A listing of x-ray beam qualities provided by NIST and the ADCLs for calibration at low-energies.

		First HVL		
Beam Code	kVp	(mm Al)	(mm Cu)	Homogeneity Coefficient (Al)
L40	40	0.50		0.59
L50	50	0.76		0.60
L80	80	1.83		0.57
L100	100	2.77		0.57
M20	20	0.15		0.69
M30	30	0.36		0.65
M40	40	0.73		0.69
M50	50	1.02		0.66
M60	60	1.68		0.66
M80	80	2.97		0.67
M100	100	5.02		0.73
M120	120	6.79		0.77
M150	150	10.2	0.67	0.87
M200	200	14.9	1.69	0.95
M250	250	18.5	3.2	0.98
M300	300	22.0	5.3	1.00

The homogeneity coefficient (HC) is the ratio of the first half-value layer to the second half-value layer. A HC with a value close to 1.00 indicates that the beam has a spectrum that is nearly monoenergetic.

Most often, a depth of 2 cm to 10 cm is used. This procedure yields the dose to tissue or tissue-equivalent material that is immersed in a large volume of the same material.

■ CALIBRATION OF LOW-ENERGY X-RAY BEAMS

Calibration procedures for low-energy x-ray beams (those from superficial and orthovoltage x-ray generators) are relatively straightforward. In part, this is because instruments used for calibration can be compared with other calibrated instruments in beams whose energies are comparable to the beam to be calibrated. A calibration procedure recommended by the AAPM states that calibrations should be performed with instruments having air-kerma calibration coefficients directly traceable to NIST.[14] The dose to a medium is then determined by

$$D_{\text{med}} = MN_k \, (\mu_{\text{en}}/\rho)_{\text{air}}^{\text{med}} \qquad (6\text{-}6)$$

where M is the instrument reading.

When the relationship between the exposure calibration coefficient and the air-kerma calibration coefficient is considered, it can be seen that Equation (6-6) is equivalent to Equation (6-4).

Beam Quality

The instrument to be used to calibrate a low-energy x-ray beam should itself have a NIST-traceable calibration coefficient. It is recommended that instruments be calibrated over a range of x-ray energies spanning those of the beams to be calibrated. The half-value layer (HVL) is generally used as a specification of beam quality. However, HVL alone is insufficient because beams having considerably different spectra may have the same first HVL. Therefore, calibration laboratories provide exposure and air-kerma calibration coefficients as a function of HVL and kVp, to minimize this ambiguity.

Ionization Chamber

The instrument to be used for low energy x-ray calibration should be chosen carefully. In general, air-filled ionization chambers are used for reference dosimetry in such beams. For the most part, cylindrical ionization chambers are used, but parallel plate chambers with thin entrance windows are recommended for x-ray beams generated at tube potentials below 70 kV. When thin-window parallel-plate chambers are used, it may be necessary to add thin plastic foils or plates to the entrance window to remove electron contamination and provide full buildup.

Ionization chambers must be corrected for environmental conditions and instrument characteristics as described earlier. The correction takes the form

$$M = M_{raw} \cdot P_{tp} \cdot P_{ion} \cdot P_{pol} \cdot P_{elec} \qquad (6\text{-}7)$$

where M_{raw} is the ionization reading in coulombs/minute obtained with the ionization chamber. The ionization reading, M_{raw}, is determined by dividing the electrometer reading by the exposure time. A correction for *end effect* may be needed if the output does not reach the steady-state value simultaneously with the starting of the timer and return to zero instantaneously when the timer turns off. The end effect δt may be determined by (a) plotting the electrometer reading against exposure time for several different values of exposure time and (b) extrapolating to zero reading. The end effect may also be measured by

$$\delta t = \frac{M_2 \Delta t_1 - M_1 \Delta t_2}{M_1 - M_2}$$

where M_1 and M_2 are the electrometer readings from exposure times Δt_1 and Δt_2, respectively.[15] P_{tp} is the correction for temperature and pressure, while P_{ion} is the correction for ionic recombination. Some of the ions formed by the radiation recombine with ions of the opposite sign before reaching the collecting electrode, and are not measured. Several procedures have been described to estimate the actual number of ions formed by taking measurements at two voltages.[16,17] The AAPM protocol recommends that measurements be made at the normal collecting voltage and at one-half that voltage. The measured values are then compared using an expression that, for continuous beams, such as those from an orthovoltage machine or a ^{60}Co unit, assumes a nonlinear relationship between P_{ion} and voltage. P_{ion} is thus

$$P_{ion} = \frac{1 - (V_H/V_L)^2}{\left(M_{raw}^H/M_{raw}^L\right) - (V_H/V_L)^2}$$

where M_{raw}^H and M_{raw}^L are ionization readings taken with bias voltages V_H and V_L, respectively, and $V_L \leq 0.5\,V_H$. When measuring P_{ion}, care should be taken to allow sufficient time for the instrument to stabilize at each bias voltage. It is not generally necessary to measure P_{ion} each time a beam is calibrated; it is better to measure it very carefully at the time of annual calibration.

P_{ion} has also been fitted to a polynomial expression for several ratios of V_H/V_L.[18] It should be noted that P_{ion} and A_{ion} (recombination measured by an ADCL) are determined under different conditions and will not have the same value. In addition, P_{ion} is a *correction* for collection efficiency and is therefore always greater than 1. If an ion chamber exhibits P_{ion} greater than 1.05, the uncertainty of the measurement becomes unacceptably large. Another ion chamber with P_{ion} closer to 1.0 should be used instead.

P_{pol} is to be used if the instrument was calibrated by the ADCL using a different polarity of bias than is used to calibrate the user's x-ray beam. This is usually not the case with low-energy x rays, and P_{pol} is generally equal to 1.0. P_{elec} is the electrometer calibration coefficient, as determined by the calibration laboratory.

Total wall thickness required to provide full buildup and eliminate electron contamination when using thin-window parallel-plate chambers.

Tube Potential (kV)	Total Wall Thickness (mg cm^{-2})
40	3.0
50	4.0
60	5.5
70	7.3
80	9.1
90	11.2
100	13.4

For pulsed beams, such as those from a linear accelerator, and for values of $P_{ion} < 1.05$, P_{ion} varies linearly with voltage ratio. The appropriate expression is

$$P_{ion} = \frac{1 - (V_H/V_L)}{\left(M_{raw}^H/M_{raw}^L\right) - (V_H/V_L)}$$

Example 6-5

Ionization measurements are made in an orthovoltage beam. With a bias voltage of 300 V the reading is 1.875×10^{-8} C/min, but when the bias is reduced to 150 V the reading decreases to 1.865×10^{-8} C/min. What is the ionization recombination correction factor?

For a continuous beam, the nonlinear form of the expression must be used:

$$P_{ion} = \frac{1 - (V_H/V_L)^2}{\left(M_{raw}^H/M_{raw}^L\right) - (V_H/V_L)^2}$$

$$P_{ion} = \frac{1 - (2)^2}{(1.875/1.865) - (2)^2}$$

$$P_{ion} = 1.002$$

In-Air Calibrations

It is recommended by the AAPM that low energy x-ray beams be calibrated in air (Margin Figure 6-2). This recommendation is consistent with historical practice and represents a practical and straight forward approach to calibration. Equation (6-6) can then be used to determine the dose to an infinitesimal volume of medium suspended in air. Equation (6-6) must be modified slightly to permit determination of the dose at the surface of a phantom or patient. Regardless of whether a cylindrical or parallel plate ionization chamber is used, the AAPM protocol stipulates that the effective point of measurement is the center of the air cavity of the ionization chamber. Therefore, when calibrating a low-energy x-ray beam, the center of the ionization chamber air volume must be placed at the point of interest. This is normally the nominal treatment distance, which may also be at the end of a treatment cone. If it is not possible to position the ionization chamber at the intended reference point, an inverse-square correction may be made from the point of measurement to the reference point. When this is done, it is necessary to recognize that the inverse-square variation in beam intensity may be influenced by scattering from the cone and may not correspond to the actual distance from the x-ray target to the point of measurement.

The dose determined from a measurement of ionization in air is

$$D_{w,0} = MN_K \, BSF \, P_{stem} \, (\mu_{en}/\rho)_{air}^w \tag{6-8}$$

where $D_{w,0}$ is the dose to water at the surface of a phantom. M is determined according to Equation (6-7). BSF is the backscatter factor for the beam quality being calibrated. BSF relates the dose at the surface of a medium to the dose to a small mass of medium suspended in air (see Chapter 7). The parameter P_{stem} is applied if the field size being calibrated is different from the field size in which the instrument itself was calibrated. The change in field size results in a different length of chamber stem or cable being irradiated, which may change the response of the instrument. The determination of stem correction factors is discussed in Chapter 5. The ratio of energy absorption coefficients is used to relate the dose in water to the dose determined in air at the location of the instrument. This ratio must be chosen from Table 6-1 for the energy spectrum of the beam being calibrated at the position of the ionization chamber in air. Note that Equation (6-8), in accordance with the AAPM protocol, determines the dose to water at the surface of a water phantom. The dose to tissue may be determined by substituting the energy absorption coefficient ratios for tissue and air in Equation (6-8).

In-Phantom Calibrations

The AAPM protocol recommends that, as an alternative, calibrations may be performed in a water phantom for beam energies >100 kV. The recommended calibration depth is 2 cm. As indicated in Margin Figure 6-2, the center of the ionization chamber collecting volume should be placed at 2 cm depth in the water phantom. It is recommended that a 10- × 10-cm field be used for calibrations in a water phantom.

TABLE 6-3   Correction Factor, P_{chbr}^Q, for Several Common Chamber Models and Beam Qualities[19]

	Chamber Type					
HVL (mm Cu)	NE2571	Capintec PR06C	PTW N30001	Exradin A12	NE2581	NE2611 or NE2561
0.10	1.008	0.992	1.004	1.002	0.991	0.995
0.15	1.015	1.000	1.013	1.009	1.007	1.007
0.20	1.019	1.004	1.017	1.013	1.017	1.012
0.30	1.023	1.008	1.021	1.016	1.028	1.017
0.40	1.025	1.009	1.023	1.017	1.033	1.019
0.50	1.025	1.010	1.023	1.017	1.036	1.019
0.60	1.025	1.010	1.023	1.017	1.037	1.019
0.80	1.024	1.010	1.022	1.017	1.037	1.018
1.0	1.023	1.010	1.021	1.016	1.035	1.017
1.5	1.019	1.008	1.018	1.013	1.028	1.014
2.0	1.016	1.007	1.015	1.011	1.022	1.011
2.5	1.012	1.006	1.012	1.010	1.017	1.009
3.0	1.009	1.005	1.010	1.008	1.012	1.006
4.0	1.004	1.003	1.006	1.005	1.004	1.003

Under these conditions, the dose to water at 2-cm depth is

$$D_{w,2} = MN_K P_{chbr}^Q P_{sheath} (\mu_{en}/\rho)_{air}^w \qquad (6\text{-}9)$$

where $D_{w,2}$ is the dose at 2-cm depth in the water phantom. P_{chbr}^Q is a chamber correction factor that accounts for displacement of water by the ionization chamber and the chamber stem, as well as the effects of changes in energy spectrum and angular distribution of the photon beam in the phantom compared to calibration of the chamber in air.[19] Values of P_{chbr}^Q are given in Table 6-3. P_{sheath} is a correction for photon absorption and scattering in a waterproof sleeve, if used. The ratio of mass energy absorption coefficients must be chosen for the energy spectrum of the beam at the position of the ionization chamber in the water phantom. This may be different from the value that will be used for an in-air calibration of the same beam.

■ CALIBRATION OF MEGAVOLTAGE BEAMS—THE AAPM PROTOCOL

Calibration of megavoltage radiation beams involves the application of a ^{60}Co calibration coefficient to measurements in photon or electron beams of higher energies. In materials from which ionization chambers are constructed, high-energy radiations interact differently than do ^{60}Co γ rays, and corrections are required to determine the dose accurately. In 1971, the American Association of Physicists in Medicine (AAPM) Subcommittee on Radiation Dosimetry (SCRAD) published a protocol describing procedures for calibrating photon and electron beams.[20] The protocol recommended the use of factors called C_λ (for photons) and C_E (for electrons) in place of the f factor and A_{eq} used in Equation (6-4). The SCRAD protocol has since been superseded and is no longer in widespread use. In 1983, AAPM Task Group 21 published a protocol that, until recently, enjoyed widespread use within the United States.[11] In 1999, it was replaced by a protocol written by AAPM Task Group 51.[10] The current AAPM protocol is described below.

Calibration of Photon Beams Versus Electron Beams

Previous texts have addressed the calibration of high-energy photon beams separately from the calibration of electron beams. This was because the procedures for calibration

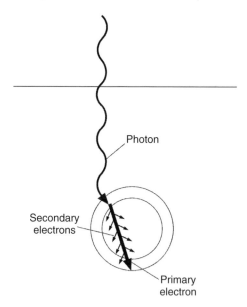

MARGIN FIGURE 6-3

The interactions of photons and electrons in the materials surrounding the air cavity of an ionization chamber.

Unlike low-energy x-ray beams, megavoltage x-ray beams of energies greater than ^{60}Co cannot realistically be calibrated in air. The chamber wall thickness required for full buildup and the removal of contaminant electrons requires a buildup cap at least 3 cm and as much as 8 cm in diameter. The attenuation and scattering of radiation by such a large mass approaches that of a water phantom. Therefore, the use of a water phantom is preferred.

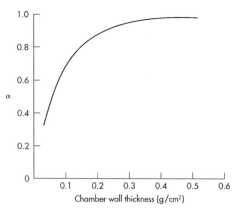

MARGIN FIGURE 6-4

When determining the characteristics of specific ionization chambers, the spectrum of electrons passing through the air volume is important. This figure shows the fraction of electrons depositing energy in the sensitive volume of the chamber that arise in the chamber wall, during irradiation with ^{60}Co gamma rays. The remaining electrons originate in the phantom material outside the chamber.[11] Used with permission.

were different. However, recent protocols for megavoltage calibrations address both photons and electrons, and the procedures are essentially identical. Therefore, this text addresses both together.

Calibration with an Ionization Chamber in a Medium

When high-energy photons interact in a medium, they set in motion high-speed *primary* electrons (Margin Figure 6-3). These electrons ionize the surrounding medium and generate *secondary* electrons. (When a phantom is irradiated with an electron beam, the incident electrons may be considered the primary electrons.) These electrons ionize the medium at a much higher rate than do the photons. In fact, the contribution of photons to the ion pairs produced in the air inside an ion chamber may be neglected. It is customary to think of the photons as interacting only outside the chamber, in the medium surrounding the chamber, or in the wall of the chamber itself. The electrons set in motion by these interactions penetrate the ion chamber's air volume and produce the ionization that ultimately is measured.

Dose to Water from a Measurement of Ionization

For calibrating megavoltage beams of radiation, the point of interest is generally located within a water or tissue-equivalent phantom. The measurement is made with an ion chamber immersed in the phantom. A first step in the use of the Bragg–Gray relation is to determine the dose to the air inside the chamber. As discussed in Chapter 5, the Bragg–Gray relation requires that several assumptions are satisfied. First, the cavity (the ionization chamber) must be sufficiently small to have a negligible influence on the electron energy spectrum and fluence at the point of measurement. Second, the wall of the chamber either must be constructed of material effectively identical to the medium (i.e., having the same effective atomic number) or must be sufficiently thin that an insignificant number of photon interactions take place in the wall. A third important assumption is that the energy of a secondary electron must be deposited at the site of origin.

Few ionization chambers in use fulfill these criteria exactly (see Table 6-4). To enable the collection of enough ion pairs to create a measurable signal, the chamber's collecting volume must be of at least modest size. Volumes of 0.1 to 1.0 cm^3 are most common. However, the diameter of a cylindrical chamber should not exceed 1 cm. The wall thickness must be sufficiently robust for mechanical rigidity and to withstand handling. The wall material is often graphite, nylon, a plastic such as A-150 (a tissue-equivalent plastic) or C-552 (an air-equivalent plastic). The phantoms used by most physicists are composed either of water, polystyrene, or a water-equivalent plastic, and therefore the chamber wall is unlikely to be identical to the phantom material. Consequently the flux of electrons passing through the chamber is not identical to the flux that occurs in the absence of the chamber, and corrections must be applied. Finally, secondary electrons generated inside the air cavity may have sufficient energy to escape the cavity and deposit some of their energy in the medium. This has the effect of reducing the energy absorbed by the air in the chamber.

These failures of the chamber to meet the Bragg–Gray criteria mean that the Bragg–Gray relation $D_{\text{medium}} = D_{\text{gas}} \cdot (\bar{s}/\rho)_{\text{gas}}^{\text{medium}}$ cannot be used without modification. The AAPM protocol relies on the Spencer–Attix formulation,[21] which can be expressed

$$D_{\text{medium}} = D_{\text{gas}} \cdot (\overline{L}/\rho)_{\text{gas}}^{\text{medium}} \qquad (6\text{-}10)$$

where $(\overline{L}/\rho)_{\text{gas}}^{\text{medium}}$ represents the restricted mean mass collisional stopping power, averaged over the electron slowing-down spectrum in the wall material. Values of $\overline{L}/\rho$ are provided in Table 6-5. The electron slowing-down spectrum includes primary and secondary electrons with a spectrum of energies, and the restricted stopping powers include only energy losses less than Δ. The formulation includes track-end corrections that account for secondary electrons that undergo inelastic collisions in which both

TABLE 6-4   Physical Characteristics of Thimble Ionization Chambers Commonly Used for Radiation Therapy Calibrations[a]

Chamber Manufacturer Description (Wall Material/Cap Material)	Thimble Wall Dimensions (cm)	Thimble Wall Dimensions (g/cm²)	Inner Axial[b] Length (cm)	Inner Diameter (cm)	Buildup Cap Thickness (cm)	Buildup Cap Thickness (g/cm²)	A_{wall}	α	$(L/\rho)_{air}^{wall} \cdot (\mu_{en}/\rho)_{wall}^{cap}$	$(L/\rho)_{air}^{wall} \cdot (\mu_{en}/\rho)_{wall}^{air}$	$N_{gas}/N_X A_{ion}$ (Gy/R)
Capintec PR-06C, PR-06G: 0.6-cm³ Farmer-type, with BC-06F cap (AE plastic/polystyrene)	0.028	0.050	2.30	0.64	0.516	0.539	0.991	0.46	1.000	1.032	8.51×10^{-3}
Exradin A1 Spokas: 0.5 cm³, air-equivalent, with 4-mm cap (AE plastic/AE plastic)	0.102	0.182	0.97	0.94	0.40	0.712	0.976	0.86	1.000	1.00	8.53×10^{-3}
Exradin T2 Spokas: 0.5-cm³, tissue-equivalent, with 4-mm cap (TE plastic/TE plastic)	0.102	0.115	0.97	0.94	0.40	0.450	0.985	0.73	1.037	1.037	8.30×10^{-3}
NEL 2505/3,3B: 0.6-cm³ Farmer (since 1974), with 2507/3, 3A cap (Nylon 66/acrylic)	0.036	0.041	2.25	0.63	0.465	0.551	0.990	0.40	1.038	1.020	8.42×10^{-3}
NEL 2571 guarded: 0.6-cm³ Farmer (since 1979), with 2571 cap (graphite/Delrin)	0.036	0.065	2.25	0.63	0.387	0.551	0.990	0.54	1.009	1.019	8.54×10^{-3}
NEL 2581 robust: 0.6-cm³ Farmer (since 1980), with 2581 cap (TE plastic/Lucentine)	0.036	0.040	2.25	0.63	0.551	0.584	0.990	0.39	1.037	1.032	8.37×10^{-3}
PTW N23333: 0.6-cm³ Farmer-type, with NA30-387 cap (acrylic/acrylic)	0.045	0.053	2.19	0.61	0.465	0.551	0.990	0.48	1.020	1.020	8.48×10^{-3}

[a]It should be noted that there are discrepancies between the chamber data published in the AAPM protocol and those presented here. In some cases, the data given differ from the nominal values listed by the manufacturers in certain advertising brochures, but each manufacturer has confirmed these data. In many cases, the least significant digit is uncertain but is given as the best estimate, and appropriate rounding off is left to the user.

[b]The axial length listed is the average of the volume axial length and the central electrode length, in an attempt to account for conically or spherically tipped chambers. Although the length chosen is not critical to the calculation, this convention has been adopted for consistency.

Source: Gastorf, R., Humphries, L. and Rozenfeld, M. Cylindrical chamber dimensions and the corresponding values of A_{wall} and $N_{gas}/(N_X A_{ion})$. *Med. Phys.* 1986;**13**:751–754. Used with permission.

The concept of restricted stopping powers is rather complicated. Consider a photon that interacts with an atom in a chamber wall, releasing an electron with several hundred keV of energy. This "primary" electron crosses the chamber air cavity and interacts multiple times with air atoms. If collisions with electrons result in the transfer of more than about 10 keV, the probability is high that the electron receiving the energy will also cross the cavity and deposit its energy in the chamber wall.

Because the energy lost in the interaction is carried out of the collecting volume, it is not measured. The probability of the interaction is not relevant when comparing the rate of local energy deposition in air to that in tissue. Therefore, only the stopping powers for interactions in which less than 10 keV (or another appropriate value, designated Δ) is transferred are considered when calculating mean restricted stopping powers.

TABLE 6-5   Ratio of Average, Restricted Collisional Mass Stopping Powers for Photon Spectra, $\Delta = 10$ keV

Nominal Accelerating Potential (MV)	$(\overline{L}/\rho)_{air}^{medium}$							
	Water	Polystyrene	Acrylic	Graphite	A-150	C-552	Bakelite	Nylon
2	1.135	1.114	1.104	1.015	1.154	1.003	1.084	1.146
^{60}Co	1.134	1.113	1.103	1.012	1.151	1.000	1.081	1.142
4	1.131	1.108	1.099	1.007	1.146	0.996	1.075	1.136
6	1.127	1.103	1.093	1.002	1.141	0.992	1.070	1.129
8	1.121	1.097	1.088	0.995	1.135	0.987	1.063	1.120
10	1.117	1.094	1.085	0.992	1.130	0.983	1.060	1.114
15	1.106	1.083	1.074	0.982	1.119	0.972	1.051	1.097
20	1.096	1.074	1.065	0.977	1.109	0.963	1.042	1.087
25	1.093	1.071	1.062	0.968	1.106	0.960	1.038	1.084
35	1.084	1.062	1.053	0.958	1.098	0.952	1.027	1.074
45	1.071	1.048	1.041	0.939	1.087	0.942	1.006	1.061

Source: Cunningham, J. R., and Schultz, R. J. On the selection of stopping-power and mass energy-absorption coefficient ratios for high-energy x-ray dosimetry. *Med. Phys.* 1984;**11**:618–623. Used with permission.

ejected electrons have less than Δ in energy. The cutoff energy Δ is chosen to take account of the size of practical ionization chambers.

Example 6-6

The dose to air in an ionization chamber irradiated by a 6-MV photon beam is determined to be 1 Gy. Calculate the dose to water replacing the air.

Using Equation (6-10), the dose to water is determined by multiplying the dose to air by the ratio of restricted mean mass collisional stopping powers (see Table 6-5):

$$D_{medium} = D_{gas} \cdot (\overline{L}/\rho)_{gas}^{medium}$$
$$D_{medium} = 1 \text{ Gy} \cdot 1.127 = 1.127 \text{ Gy}$$

The AAPM protocol provides further corrections and procedures to account for other perturbations of the photon and electron fluence.

Dose to Water Calibration Coefficient ($N_{D,w}$)

The AAPM TG-21 protocol defined a cavity-gas calibration factor

$$N_{gas} = \frac{D_{gas} \cdot A_{ion}}{M}$$

which related the chamber signal M to the dose D_{gas} to the air inside the collecting volume and a correction for ionic recombination. N_{gas} was determined from N_x through the use of stopping power ratios and mass-energy absorption coefficient ratios. The dose to a medium was then related to the dose to the chamber air by the Bragg–Gray relation and corrections for the effects of the chamber wall and the displacement of the medium.

The AAPM calibration protocol is based upon the relationship between the dose to water at the location of the ionization chamber and the chamber's signal:

$$D_w^Q = M \cdot N_{D,w}^Q \qquad (6-11)$$

where D_w^Q is the dose to water at the point of measurement in a beam whose quality is Q. The dose to water calibration coefficient, $N_{D,w}^Q$ is determined by the calibration laboratory and is directly traceable to NIST. The corrected instrument signal M is determined as

$$M = M_{raw} \cdot P_{tp} \cdot P_{ion} \cdot P_{pol} \cdot P_{elec} \qquad (6-7)$$

The parameters in Equation (6-7) have been described earlier. P_{ion} must be calculated using an appropriate expression for a continuous or pulsed beam (see margin note on page 115; also see Example 6-7). P_{pol} takes on greater significance for megavoltage calibrations, as the chamber sensitivity may change with bias polarity. In this case, P_{pol} is calculated as

$$P_{pol} = \left| \frac{M_{raw}^+ - M_{raw}^-}{2M_{raw}} \right|$$

where the superscript indicates the polarity of the charge being collected. The denominator includes either M_{raw}^+ or M_{raw}^-, whichever polarity signal was be used for calibration. M_{raw}^+ and M_{raw}^- generally have opposite signs; these signs must be used when calculating P_{pol}. Measurement of P_{pol} is not necessary each time a beam is calibrated, but when measured, it must be done carefully with sufficient time allowed after changing the bias polarity for the instrument to stabilize.

P_{pol} should be 1.0 ± 0.02. Values significantly different from unity most likely indicate an error in calculation.

Example 6-7

The ionization recombination correction is determined in an accelerator beam in the manner described in Example 6-5. At 300 V, the reading is 1.624×10^{-8} C for an exposure of 100 monitor units, and at 150 V the reading is 1.615×10^{-8} C. What is P_{ion}?

For pulsed beams, the linear form of the equation is used:

$$P_{ion} = \frac{1 - (V_H/V_L)}{\left(M_{raw}^H/M_{raw}^L\right) - (V_H/V_L)}$$

$$P_{ion} = \frac{-1}{(1.624/1.615) - (2)}$$

$$P_{ion} = 1.002$$

Compare the ratio of ionization measurements with those given in Example 6-5.

The dose to water calibration coefficient, $N_{D,w}^Q$ must be appropriate for the beam energy, Q, being calibrated. However, it is rarely practical for calibration laboratories to attempt to provide calibrations over a range of megavoltage beam energies. Instead, NIST and the ADCLs provide dose to water calibration coefficients determined in a ^{60}Co beam. The ^{60}Co calibration coefficient is then related to the calibration coefficient at beam quality Q by a quality conversion factor, k_Q,

$$N_{D,w}^Q = N_{D,w}^{^{60}Co} \cdot k_Q \qquad (6\text{-}12)$$

The quality conversion factor may be calculated as the ratio of energy-dependent chamber characteristics for the user's beam energy and for ^{60}Co. Specifically,

$$k_Q = \left[(\bar{L}/\rho)_{air}^{water} \cdot P_{repl} \cdot P_{wall} \cdot P_{cel} \right]_{^{60}Co}^Q$$

where P_{repl}, P_{wall} and P_{cel} are the chamber's replacement correction, wall correction, and central electrode correction, respectively. These parameters are defined in the AAPM TG-21 calibration protocol.[11]

For x-ray beams, the quality conversion factor is a function of beam quality and varies smoothly over a small range for a wide variety of ionization chambers. Values of k_Q are provided in Table 6-6.

It is possible to estimate a value for k_Q for a chamber that is not listed by selecting a listed chamber that has (1) the same wall material, (2) the same central electrode material, and (3) approximately the same wall thickness. In addition, the listed chamber should have a collecting volume with similar length and diameter as the user's instrument, although the dependence of k_Q on these parameters is weak.

Effective Point of Measurement

Cylindrical Chambers

As discussed at the beginning of this chapter, the effective point of measurement of an ionization chamber used in air is considered to be its axis (see Margin Figure 6-2). When used in a phantom, however, the effective point of measurement may move upstream from the axis of the chamber. As shown in Margin Figure 6-5, a beam of electrons traveling along parallel paths strikes the wall of a cylindrical ion chamber at different distances upstream from the chamber center. Through an averaging procedure, the effective point of interaction can be found. In a phantom, scattering of electrons modifies the calculations. As a result, the AAPM[10,17] has recommended that the effective point of measurement be located 0.6 of the inner radius r_{cav} upstream

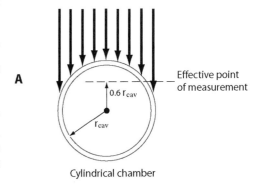

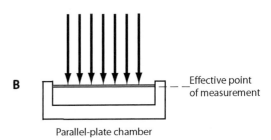

MARGIN FIGURE 6-5
Location of the effective point for (**A**) a cylindrical ionization chamber and (**B**) a parallel-plate ionization chamber.

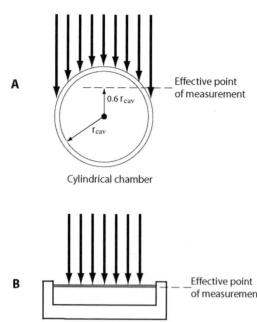

A

Effective point
of measurement

$0.6\, r_{cav}$

r_{cav}

Cylindrical chamber

B

Effective point
of measurement

Parallel-plate chamber

MARGIN FIGURE 6-6

Effect of shifting depth ionization data. Measurements were made with a cylindrical chamber.[10] Data were shifted upstream by $0.6\, r_{cav}$ for photon beams (**upper figure**) and $0.5\, r_{cav}$ for electron beams (**lower figure**). In both figures, curve I (dashed) indicates raw data while curve II (solid) indicates shifted data. The short-dashed line in the lower figure indicates percentage depth dose. From Reference 10, by permission.

Measurements show that calibration of low-energy electron beams can be made accurately with cylindrical ion chambers.[22] At 6 MeV, the output measured with a 0.6-cm[3] chamber differed by less than 0.5% from that measured with a parallel-plate chamber. At 4 MeV, the difference was less than 2%.

TABLE 6-6   Values of the Quality Conversion Factor k_Q for Commonly Used Cylindrical Ionization Chambers[10]

	k_Q %dd (10)$_x$					
Ion Chamber	58.0	63.0	66.0	71.0	81.0	93.0
Capintec PR-05/PR-05P	0.999	0.997	0.995	0.990	0.972	0.948
Capintec PR-06C/G 0.6-cm[3] Farmer	1.000	0.998	0.994	0.987	0.968	0.944
Exradin A1 Shonka[a]	0.999	0.998	0.996	0.990	0.972	0.948
Exradin A12 Farmer	1.000	0.999	0.996	0.990	0.972	0.948
NE2505/3,3A 0.6-cm[3] Farmer	1.000	0.998	0.995	0.988	0.972	0.951
NE2561 0.3-cm[3] NPL Sec. Std[b]	1.000	0.998	0.995	0.989	0.974	0.953
NE2571 0.6-cm[3] Farmer	1.000	0.998	0.995	0.988	0.972	0.951
NE2577 0.2-cm[3]	1.000	0.998	0.995	0.988	0.972	0.951
NE2581 0.6-cm[3] robust Farmer	1.000	0.994	0.988	0.979	0.960	0.937
PTW N30001 0.6-cm[3] Farmer[c]	1.000	0.996	0.992	0.984	0.967	0.945
PTW N30002 0.6-cm[3] all graphite	1.000	0.997	0.994	0.987	0.970	0.948
PTW N30004 0.6-cm[3] graphite	1.000	0.998	0.995	0.988	0.973	0.952
PTW N31003 0.3-cm[3] waterproof[d]	1.000	0.996	0.992	0.984	0.967	0.946
Wellhofer IC-10/IC-5	1.000	0.999	0.996	0.989	0.971	0.946

The cavity radius of the A1 here is 2 mm, although in the past Exradin has designated chambers with another radius as A1.

[b] The NE2611 has replaced the equivalent NE2561.

[c] PTW N30001 is equivalent to the PTW N23333 it replaced.

[d] PTW N31003 is equivalent to the PTW N233641 it replaced.

from the chamber axis when measuring in megavoltage photon beams, and $0.5\, r_{cav}$ for electron beams. Note that the correction for the location of the effective point of measurement is to be used only when determining relative depth doses. The correction is not to be applied during calibration measurements in either photon beams or electron beams.

Parallel-Plate Chambers

The depth dose in low-energy ($\leq$6 MeV) electron beams changes rapidly. The use of a cylindrical ionization chamber is not recommended by the AAPM because the size of the cavity of many chambers is large relative to the dose gradient.[10] Instead, the AAPM recommends the use of a parallel-plate chamber.

As shown in Margin Figure 6-5, the effective point of measurement of a parallel-plate chamber is at the inside surface of the entrance window, when the chamber is used in a phantom. No adjustment of depth for parallel-plate chambers is required.

Beam Quality Specification

For photon beams, the quality Q of the beam is determined from the percent depth dose (%D_n) at 10-cm depth in a 10- $\times$ 10-cm field. This is a departure from the earlier AAPM calibration protocol, and also from several international protocols, in which the beam quality is related to a ratio of percent depth dose values or tissue maximum ratios. The AAPM protocol recognizes that measurement of percent depth dose is complicated by the possibility that electron contamination will influence the measurements at the depth of maximum dose, d_{max}. Therefore, the AAPM protocol specifies that, at energies of 10 MV or above, the percent depth dose must be measured using a technique that removes contaminant electrons originating in the accelerator head and that introduces a known quantity of contaminant electrons for which mathematical corrections may be made. The procedure involves inserting a lead foil 1 mm in thickness into the beam and making measurements of percent depth dose at 100-cm SSD. Through a mathematical manipulation described in the protocol (see margin note on this page), the percent depth dose due to x rays alone, $\%D(10)_X$, is determined. For x-ray energies below 10 MV, $\%D(10)_X$ is simply the $\%D_n$ at 10-cm depth in a 10- × 10-cm field at 100-cm SSD. The values of k_Q that are reproduced in Table 6-6 are related to $\%D(10)_X$.[23]

Example 6-8

Determine the beam quality Q for an x-ray beam of nominal energy 18 MV. A lead foil 1 mm thick is placed at 50 cm from the water surface, and ionization measurements are made at 100-cm SSD in a 10- × 10-cm field. At the depth of maximum ionization, an exposure of 100 MU yields an electrometer reading of 1.901. At 10-cm depth (with the axis of the chamber positioned at 10 cm + 0.6 r_{cav}) the reading is 1.498.

Under these circumstances,

$$\%D(10)_x = [0.8905 + 0.00150\%D(10)_{Pb}]\%D(10)_{Pb}$$

where

$$\%D(10)_{Pb} = 1.498/1.901 \times 100$$

$$= 78.8\%$$

Then

$$\%D(10)_x = 79.5\%$$

For electron beams, k_Q is likewise related to the beam quality. Electron beam quality is characterized by a parameter, R_{50}, the depth at which the dose falls to 50% of the maximum dose. R_{50} is measured in a field large enough to provide full side scatter. For $R_{50} \le 8.5$ cm, a 10- × 10-cm field is used; for $R_{50} > 8.5$ cm, a 20- × 20-cm field is used.

R_{50} is actually determined from a measurement of I_{50}, the depth at which the measured ionization falls to 50% of the maximum ionization value. If the ionization is measured with a cylindrical chamber, the depth must be adjusted by 0.5 r_{cav}.

For electron beams in which I_{50} is ≤10 cm, R_{50} is calculated as follows:

$$R_{50} = 1.029 \cdot I_{50} - 0.06$$

where R_{50} and I_{50} are expressed in cm.

The determination of k_Q for electron beams is addressed later in this chapter.

Calibration of Photon Beams

The dose to water in a photon beam is determined through a measurement of ionization under reference conditions. Reference conditions recommended by the AAPM protocol are at 10-cm depth in a 10- × 10-cm field. Calibration may be performed for either an SSD setup (nominally 100 cm to the surface of the water phantom) or an SAD set up (normally 90 cm from the source to the surface of the water phantom, so that the ionization chamber at 10-cm depth is positioned at the accelerator axis of rotation.) Under these circumstances, the dose to water D_W^Q at the position of measurement is determined by combining Equations (6-11) and (6-12):

$$D_w^Q = M \cdot N_{D,w}^{^{60}Co} \cdot k_Q \qquad (6\text{-}13)$$

The parameters in Equation (6-12) have been defined earlier. Equation (6-13) yields the dose to water at the location of measurement. The AAPM protocol recommends that the measurement be transferred to d_{max} by dividing by the $\%D_n$ (or the TMR if calibration is performed at the isocenter). In this manner, the accelerator output is described in terms of cGy at d_{max} per MU. The $\%D_n$ used in this step must be the *clinical* $\%D(10)$, taken from data tables used for treatment planning. It should not be the $\%D(10)$ measured at the time of calibration and *must not* be $\%D(10)_x$ or $\%D(10)_{Pb}$.

A number of calibration protocols, including the previous AAPM protocol known as TG-21,[11] describe beam quality by a parameter called the ionization ratio, IR. IR is calculated from the ratio of TMRs at 20-cm and 10-cm depth, for a 10- × 10-cm field.

At x-ray energies ≥10 MV, $\%D(10)_x$ is determined from a measurement in water of $\%D(10)_{Pb}$, made with a 1-mm-thick lead foil in the beam. The field size must be 10 × 10 cm, the SSD must be 100 cm, and the depth (corrected by 0.6 r_{cav}) must be 10 cm. If the lead foil is 50 cm ± 5 cm from the water phantom surface, then

$$\%D(10)_x = [0.8905 + 0.00150\%D(10)_{Pb}]$$
$$\times \%D(10)_{Pb}$$

If the lead foil is at 30 cm ± 1 cm from the water phantom surface, then

$$\%D(10)_x = [0.8116 + 0.00264\%D(10)_{Pb}]$$
$$\times \%D(10)_{Pb}$$

If the lead foil is not available, then $\%D(10)$ is measured and $\%D(10)_x$ is

$$\%D(10)_x = [1.267\%D(10)] - 20.0$$

When calculating $\%D(10)_x$ from $\%D(10)_{Pb}$, it is essential to use values of *percent* depth dose. The use of *fractional* depth dose will lead to large errors. $\%D(10)_x$ should be between 0% and 2.5% larger than $\%D(10)_{Pb}$.[24]

In many clinics, the calibrated dose rate determined in water is corrected to yield the dose rate in muscle. In an x-ray beam, this correction is $(\mu_{en}/\rho)_{water}^{muscle}$. Table 6-1 indicates that over the range of photon energies used in radiation therapy, the correction is approximately 0.99.

Example 6-9

Determine k_Q for an Exradin model A-12 ionization chamber used in the x-ray beam described by Example 6-8.

In Example 6-8, $\%D(10)_x$ was determined to be 79.5%. Linear interpolation in Table 6-6 yields $k_Q = 0.975$.

Calibration of Electron Beams

The AAPM recommends that electron beams be calibrated at an energy-dependent reference depth. The reference depth d_{ref} may not be precisely at d_{max}, and a $\%D_n$ correction is made to relate the calibrated dose rate to d_{max}. d_{ref} is calculated from the electron beam quality as follows:

$$d_{ref} = 0.6\,R_{50} - 0.1\ \text{cm}$$

where R_{50} was described earlier. d_{ref} should be close to d_{max} for beam energies below 10 MeV, but will be deeper for higher energies.

The choice of an energy-dependent reference depth for calibrating electron beams simplifies the protocol by permitting the use of stopping-power ratios computed as a function of R_{50}.[25]

As was the case with photon beams, the effective point of measurement of a cylindrical chamber is located upstream from the axis of the chamber. For electron beams, the AAPM recommends a shift of $0.5\,r_{cav}$. The shift in chamber depth is used only for measurements of relative ionization, not for calibrations or determination of other dosimetric parameters.

The determination of k_Q is slightly more complicated for electron beams than for x-ray beams. k_Q may be separated into a chamber-specific energy-dependent component, $k_{R_{50}}$, and for cylindrical chambers, a correction for gradient effects at the reference depth, P_{gr}^Q. Then,

$$k_Q = P_{gr}^Q \cdot k_{R_{50}}$$

P_{gr}^Q is determined by the user at the time of calibration, and it is the ratio of ionization measurements made with the chamber axis at $(d_{ref} + 0.5\,r_{cav})$ and at d_{ref}. $k_{R_{50}}$ may be further separated into a chamber-specific component and an energy-dependent component,

P_{gr}^Q is typically less than 1.0 for electron beams of energy greater than 10 MeV. At lower beam energies, P_{gr}^Q may equal 1.0 or even be slightly above unity.

$$k_{R_{50}} = k_{ecal} \cdot k'_{R_{50}}$$

k_{ecal} is almost independent of chamber model. For most commonly used ionization chambers, k_{ecal} is within 1% of 0.9.

k_{ecal} is the photon-electron conversion factor. For an electron beam energy of Q_{ecal}, k_{ecal} converts $N_{D,w}^{60Co}$ into $N_{D,w}^{Q_{ecal}}$. The AAPM protocol defines Q_{ecal} as $R_{50} = 7.5$ cm. As will be seen later, the decision to separate k_Q in this manner facilitates the development and application of absorbed dose standards for electrons, and it simplifies the determination of $N_{D,w}^{60Co}$ for parallel plate chambers. Values of k_{ecal} for commonly used cylindrical chambers are given in Table 6-7.

$k'_{R_{50}}$ is dependent on both R_{50} and chamber model. Graphs of $k'_{R_{50}}$ are provided by the AAPM protocol[10] but selected values for a few commonly used chamber are given in Table 6-8.

Combining the equations above yields, for electron beams,

$$k_Q = P_{gr}^Q \cdot k_{ecal} \cdot k'_{R_{50}} \tag{6-14}$$

The dose at d_{ref} is therefore

$$D_w^Q = M \cdot P_{gr}^Q \cdot k_{ecal} \cdot k'_{R_{50}} \cdot N_{D,w}^{60Co}\ (\text{Gy}) \tag{6-15}$$

The use of parallel-plate chambers is recommended by the AAPM, especially for low-energy electron beams.[10] However, experience has shown that the use of cylindrical chambers yields errors of less than 0.5% at energies as low as 6 MeV.[24] When parallel-plate chambers are used, an alternate procedure for determining calibration coefficient has been recommended.[10,11,26] The product of $k_{ecal} \cdot N_{D,w}^{60Co}$ is evaluated by comparison with an ADCL calibrated cylindrical ionization chamber as follows:

$$\left(k_{ecal} \cdot N_{D,w}^{60Co}\right)^{pp} = \left(D_w^Q\right)^{cyl} / \left(M \cdot k'_{R_{50}}\right)^{pp}$$

TABLE 6-7 Values of the Photon-Electron Conversion factor, k_{ecal}, for Commercial Cylindrical Chambers, Based on a Reference Beam Quality Q_{ecal} of $R'_{50} = 7.5$ cm[10]

| Chamber | k_{ecal} | Wall | | Cavity Radius r_{cav}(cm) | Al Electrode Diameter (mm) |
		Material	Thickness g/cm²		
Farmer-like					
Exradin A12	0.906	C-552	0.088	0.305	
NE2505/3,3A	0.903	Graphite	0.065	0.315	1.0
NE2561[a]	0.904	Graphite	0.090	0.370[e]	1.0
NE2571	0.903	Graphite	0.065	0.315	1.0
NE2577	0.903	Graphite	0.065	0.315	1.0
NE2581	0.885	A-150	0.041	0.315	
Capintec PR-06C/G	0.900	C-552	0.050	0.320	
PTW N23331	0.896	Graphite	0.012	0.395[e]	1.0
		PMMA	0.048		
PTW N30001[b]	0.897	Graphite	0.012	0.305	1.0
		PMMA	0.033		
PTW N30002	0.900	Graphite	0.079	0.305	
PTW N30004	0.905	Graphite	0.079	0.305	1.0
PTW N31003[c]	0.898	Graphite	0.012	0.275	1.0[f]
		PMMA	0.066		
Other cylindrical					
Exradin A1[d]	0.915	C-552	0.176	0.200	
Capintec PR-05/PR-05P	0.916	C-552	0.210	0.200	
Wellhofer IC-10/IC-5	0.904	C-552	0.070	0.300	

[a] the NE2611 has replaced the equivalent NE2561.

[b] PTW N30001 is equivalent to the PTW N23333 it replaced.

[c] PTW N31003 is equivalent to the PTW N233641 it replaced.

[d] The cavity radius of the A1 here is 2 mm although in the past Exradin has designated chambers with another radius as A1.

[e] In electron beams there are only data for cavity radii up to 0.35 cm, and so 0.35 cm is used rather than the real cavity radius shown here.

[f] Electrode diameter is actually 1.5 mm, but only data for 1.0 mm are available.

TABLE 6-8 Values of $k'_{R_{50}}$ for Selected Values of R_{50} and a Few Commonly Used Ionization Chambers

R_{50} (cm)	Exradin A1, Capintec PR-05, Capintec PR-05P	NE 2505-3, -3A, 2571, 2577, 2581 Capintec PR-06C, -0G, PTW N30001	PTW N31003	Exradin A12, PTW N30002, N30004 Wellhofer IC 10/5	Exradin P11, Holt MPPK, PTB Roos, NACP	Markus PTW N23343	Capintec PS O33
2.0	1.039	1.033	1.035	1.032	1.055	1.041	1.016
2.5	1.032	1.027	1.030	1.026	1.047	1.036	1.014
3.0	1.027	1.022	1.025	1.021	1.040	1.032	1.012
3.5	1.022	1.018	1.020	1.017	1.034	1.028	1.011
4.0	1.018	1.015	1.017	1.013	1.028	1.024	1.010
4.5	1.015	1.012	1.014	1.011	1.023	1.020	1.009
5.0	1.012	1.010	1.011	1.009	1.019	1.016	1.008
5.5	1.009	1.007	1.008	1.006	1.012	1.013	1.006
6.0	1.007	1.005	1.006	1.005	1.011	1.010	1.005
6.5	1.004	1.003	1.003	1.003	1.007	1.006	1.004
7.0	1.002	1.001	1.001	1.002	1.003	1.003	1.001
7.5	1.000	1.000	1.000	1.000	1.000	1.000	1.000
8.0	0.998	0.999	0.999	0.999	0.997	0.997	0.998
8.5	0.996	0.997	0.997	0.998	0.994	0.994	0.996
9.0	0.994	0.996	0.995	0.996	0.991	0.992	0.994
9.5	0.992	0.994	0.993	0.994	0.988	0.990	0.992
10.0	0.990	0.993	0.992	0.993	0.986	0.988	0.990

An exposure or dose-to-water calibration coefficient assigned to a parallel-plate chamber by an ADCL is valuable for verifying the constancy of chamber response, and for satisfying state and federal regulations, but should not be used for calibration.

The effective point of measurement of a parallel-plate ionization chamber is the inside surface of the entrance window. There is no adjustment to the depth, and therefore no calculation of P_{gr}^Q is required.

When calibrating a linear accelerator, it is customary to adjust the sensitivity of the monitor chamber to yield the desired dose rate. In most clinics, the output is adjusted to 1.000 cGy/MU at d_{max} in a 10- × 10-cm field at 100-cm SSD (or SAD).

The calibrated dose rate determined in water in an electron beam can be corrected to provide the dose rate to muscle. The correction is $(S/\rho)_{water}^{muscle}$. Stopping power ratios published by the ICRU indicate that this ratio is approximately 0.99 over the clinically useful range of energies.[27]

where the superscripts "pp" and "cyl" refer to parallel-plate and cylindrical chambers, respectively. $(D_w^Q)^{cyl}$ is obtained from Equation (6-15). The comparison should be performed in a beam with R_{50} as close to 7.5 cm possible, so that $k'_{R_{50}}$ is nearly unity.

The procedures described above for both cylindrical and parallel-plate chambers yield D_w^Q, the dose to water at the reference depth, d_{ref}. To determine the dose at d_{max}, the dose at d_{ref} must be divided by the percent depth dose at d_{ref}. The value of $\%D_n$ should be taken from the clinic's treatment-planning data, to ensure that patient dose calculations are consistent with calibration procedures.

Example 6-10

Determine k_Q for an Exradin model A-12 cylindrical ionization chamber when used to calibrate a 12-MeV electron beam. Measurements are as follows: $R_{50} = 4.67$ cm, $d_{ref} = 2.70$ cm, a measurement at d_{ref} yields a reading of 4.478×10^{-8} C per 200 MU, while a measurement at $(d_{ref} + 0.5\,r_{cav})$ yields 4.457×10^{-8} C.

$$P_{gr}^Q = M_{raw}(d_{ref} + 0.5\,r_{cav})/M_{raw}(d_{ref})$$

$$= 4.457/4.478$$

$$= 0.995$$

k_{ecal} (from Table 6-7) = 0.906
$k'_{R_{50}}$ (from Table 6-8) = 1.010

$$k_Q = P_{gr}^Q \cdot k_{ecal} \cdot k'_{R_{50}}$$

$$k_Q = 0.995 \cdot 0.906 \cdot 1.010$$

$$k_Q = 0.910$$

■ THE IAEA CALIBRATION PROTOCOL

In 2000, the International Atomic Energy Agency (IAEA) published a calibration protocol based on dose-to-water standards.[28] The protocol, known as TRS-398, is similar in many ways to the AAPM TG-51 protocol. A comprehensive comparison of TRS-398 with TG-51 indicates that, with few exceptions, the two protocols yield nearly identical results.[29]

The TRS-398 protocol determines dose in a beam of quality Q as

$$D_{w,Q} = M_Q \cdot N_{D,w,Q_0} \cdot k_{Q,Q_0} \qquad (6\text{-}16)$$

where Q_0 indicates a reference beam quality. When the reference beam quality is ^{60}Co, the subscript Q_0 is dropped. TRS-398, unlike TG-51, permits the use of reference beam qualities other than ^{60}Co. Some primary standard dosimetry laboratories (PSDLs) have developed dose-to-water calibration standards in accelerator beams. In rare cases, ionization chambers are calibrated in a reference beam quality Q_0 equivalent to the user's beam quality Q. In this circumstance, $k_{Q,Q_0} = 1.0$ and Equation (6-16) is simplified. Otherwise, k_{Q,Q_0} is calculated in a similar fashion as k_Q (see margine note on page 121).

$$k_{Q,Q_0} = \left(S_{air}^w\right)_{Q_0}^Q (W_{air})_{Q_0}^Q \frac{P_Q}{P_{Q_0}} \qquad (6\text{-}17)$$

The superscript Q and subscript Q_0 indicate that the stopping-power ratio, the work function, and a perturbation correction are to be evaluated at Q and Q_0 and the ratios of the quantities determined. W_{air} has generally been assumed to be independent of beam quality, but TRS-398 leaves open the possibility that this is not the case. TRS-398 uses the symbol S to represent the mean restricted collisional mass stopping power, a quantity for which TG-51 uses the symbol $\overline{L}/\rho$.

The perturbation correction P_Q is

$$P_Q = [P_{dis} P_{wall} P_{cav} P_{cel}]_Q$$

where P_{wall} and P_{cel} are correction factors for the chamber wall and central electrode material, respectively, as described in the AAPM TG-21 protocol.[11] (see margin note on page 121). P_{dis} corrects for the displacement of the effective point of measurement upstream from the axis of a cylindrical chamber. P_{cav} corrects for the perturbation of electron fluence due to differences between air and the water medium, and it is equivalent to P_{repl} used in TG-51.

TRS-398 describes the quality Q of a photon beam in terms of the ionization ratio, or the ratio of TMR_{20}/TMR_{10}. For electron beams, TRS-398 describes Q in terms of R_{50} in exactly the same fashion as TG-51. Both protocols accommodate the use of parallel plate chambers, but TRS-398 requires their use at below 10 MeV.

■ SUMMARY

- Instruments used to calibrate clinical x- and γ-ray beams in the U.S. are assigned calibration coefficients by an ADCL.
- The dose to tissue is related to the dose to air by the ratio of the mass-energy absorption coefficients.
- Measurements with an ionization chamber must be corrected for environmental conditions, electrical effects, and recombination of ions.
- The effective point of measurement of a cylindrical ionization chamber is displaced a small distance toward the source from the chamber axis.
- The effective point of measurement is considered for relative measurements of beam characteristics, such as percent depth dose.
- The chamber axis is used as the reference point for radiation beam calibrations.

PROBLEMS

6-1. An ADCL-calibrated chamber has an air-kerma calibration coefficient $N_K = 4.33 \times 10^7$ Gy/C, and it is used with an electrometer whose correction factor is 1.006. This system is used to measure the dose rate to water in a 250-kVp orthovoltage x-ray beam (HVL = 1.0 mm Cu) for which this value of N_K is appropriate. A 10- × 10-cm field at 50-cm SSD is used. An exposure of 1 minute yields an electrometer reading of 1.517×10^{-8}. What is the exposure rate at the location of the chamber? What is the dose rate to water at the surface of a patient or phantom?

6-2. Compare the dose to bone with the dose to muscle for 250-kVp x-rays. For 100-kVp x rays. For ^{60}Co gamma rays.

6-3. The depth of 50% ionization R_{50} in an electron beam of nominal energy 9 MeV is 3.8 cm of water. How much uncertainty is there in the determination of k_Q for an Exradin P11 chamber, if R_{50} is known with an uncertainty of 1 mm?

6-4. An ionization chamber was calibrated by an ADCL with negative bias, but measurements are made in the user's electron beam with both positive and negative bias settings. Positive bias yielded a reading of 4.45×10^{-8} C, while negative bias gave -4.49×10^{-8} C. Determine P_{pol}.

6-5. Determine P_{ion} for an ionization chamber that gives the following readings in a 6-MeV electron beam: At 300 V, 4.442×10^{-8} C; and at 150 V, 4.403×10^{-8} C.

6-6. Depth dose measurements are made in a 10- × 10-cm photon beam at 100-cm SSD with a 1-mm-thick lead sheet at 30 cm above the water phantom surface. The reading at d_m is 0.953×10^{-8} C; and with the chamber at 10 cm + 0.6 r_{cav}, it is 0.754×10^{-8} C. Determine $\%D(10)_X$ and k_Q for a NE model 2571 chamber.

REFERENCES

1. Criteria for accreditation of dosimetry calibration laboratories by the American Association of Physicists in Medicine, AAPM, January 2002.
2. I.S.O. Report 31-0: Quantities and units—Part O: General Principles. International Organization for Standardization, Geneva, 1992. Amendment 1, 1998.
3. Report of the 17th Meeting of the Consultative Committee for Ionizing Radiation (CCRI). Published by the Bureau International des Poids et Mesures at http://www.bipm.org.
4. Ibbott G. S., Attix F. H., Slowey, T. W., Fontenla, D. P., Rozenfeld, M. Uncertainty of calibrations at the Accredited Dosimetry Calibration Laboratories. Med. Phys. 1997; 24(8):1249–1254.

5. Blackwell, C. R., and McCullough, E. C. A chamber and electrometer calibration factor as determined by each of the five AAPM accredited dosimetry calibration laboratories. *Med. Phys.* 1993; **19**:207–208.

6. International Commission on Radiation Units and Measurements. *Average Energy Required to Produce an Ion Pair,* Report no. 31. Washington, DC, ICRU, 1979.

7. Niatel, M. T., Perroche Roux, A. M., and Boutillon, M. Two determinations of W for electrons in dry air. *Phys. Med. Biol.* 1985; **30**:67–75.

8. Johns, H., and Cunningham, J. *The Physics of Radiology*, 3rd edition. Springfield, Il, Charles C Thomas, 1969.

9. Hubbell, J. H. Photon mass attenuation and energy-absorption coefficients from l keV to 20 MeV. *Int. J. Appl. Radiat. Isot.* 1982; **33**:1269–1290.

10. Almond, P. R., Biggs, P. J., Coursey, B. M., Hanson, W. F., Huq, M. S., Nath, R., and Rogers, D. W. O. AAPM's TG-51 protocol for clinical reference dosimetry of high-energy photon and electron beams. *Med. Phys.* 1999; **26**:1847–1870.

11. Schulz, R. J., Almond, P. R., Cunningham, J. R., Holt, J. G., Loevinger, R., Suntharalingam, N., Wright, K. A., Nath, R., and Lempert, G. A protocol for the determination of absorbed dose from high-energy photons and electron beams. *Med. Phys.* 1983; **10**:741–771.

12. International Atomic Energy Agency, *Absorbed dose determination in external beam radiotherapy: An International Code of Practice for Dosimetry Based on Standards of Absorbed Dose to Water*, Technical Reports series no. 398, Vienna, 2000.

13. Hospital Physicists Association Protocol: Code of practice for high-energy photon therapy dosimetry based on the NPL absorbed dose calibration service. *Phys. Med. Biol.* 1990; **35**:1355–1360.

14. Ma, C.-M., Coffey, C. W., DeWerd, L. A., Liu, C., Nath, R., Seltzer, S. M., Seuntjens, J. P., AAPM Protocol for 40–300 kV x-ray beam dosimetry in radiotherapy and radiobiology. *Med. Phys.* 2001; **28**(6).

15. Attix, F. H., *Introduction to Radiological Physics and Radiation Dosimetry*. New York, Wiley & Sons, 1986, pp. 358–360.

16. Boag, J. W. The recombination correction for an ionisation chamber exposed to pulsed radiation in a 'swept beam' technique. I. Theory. *Phys. Med. Biol.* 1983; **27**:201–211.

17. Boag, J. W., and Curran, J. Current collection and ionic recombination in small cylindrical ionization chambers exposed to pulsed radiation. *Br. J. Radiol.* 1980; **53**:471–478.

18. Weinhous, M. S., and Meli, J. A. Determining P_{ion}, the correction factor for recombination losses in an ionization chamber. *Med. Phys.* 1984; **11**:846–849.

19. Seuntjens, J. P., Van der Zwan, L., and Ma, C. M. Type dependent correction factors for cylindrical chambers for in-phantom dosimetry in medium-energy x-ray beams. *Proceedings Kilovoltage X-Ray Beam Dosimetry for Radiotherapy and Radiobiology*, C. M. Ma, and J. P. Seuntjens, (eds.). Madison, MPP, 1999, pp. 159–174.

20. SCRAD. Protocol for the dosimetry of x- and gamma-ray beams with maximum energies between 0.6 and 50 MeV. *Phys. Med. Biol.* 1971; **16**:379–396.

21. Burlin, T. E., *Radiation Dosimetry*, vol. 1. New York, Academic Press, 1968.

22. Rogers, D. W. O. Fundamentals of dosimetry based on absorbed-dose standards. In *Teletherapy Physics, Present and Future*, J. R. Palta and T. R. Mackie (eds.). Washington, DC, AAPM, 1966, pp. 319–356.

23. Rogers, D. W. O., and Lang, C. L. Corrected relationship between $\%dd(10)_x$ and stopping-power ratios. *Med. Phys.* 1999; **26**:538–540.

24. Tailor, R. C., Hanson, W. F., and Ibbott, G. S., TG-51 Experience from 150 institutions, common errors, and helpful hints. *J. Appl. Clin. Med. Phys.*, 2003; **4**:102–111.

25. Burns, D. T., Ding, G. X., and Rogers, D. W. O. R50 as a beam quality specifier for selecting stopping-power ratios and reference depths for electron dosimetry. *Med. Phys.* 1996; **23**:383–388.

26. Almond, P. R., Attix, F. H., Goetsch, S., Humphries, L. J., Kubo, H., Nath, R., and Rogers, D. W. O., The calibration and use of plane-parallel ionization chambers for dosimetry of electron beams: An extension of the 1983 AAPM protocol, Report of AAPM Radiation Therapy Committee Task Group 39. *Med. Phys.* 1994; **21**:1251–1260.

27. ICRU. *Stopping powers for electrons and positrons*. ICRU Report 37. Washington, DC, ICRU, 1984.

28. International Atomic Energy Agency. *Absorbed dose determination in external beam radiotherapy*. IAEA Technical Report Series No. 398. Vienna, 2000.

29. Andreo, P., Huq, M. S., Westermark, M., Song, H., Tilikidis, A., DeWerd, L., and Shortt, K. Protocols for the dosimetry of high-energy photon and electron beams: A comparison of the IAEA TRS-398 and previous International Codes of Practice. *Phys. Med. Biol.* 2002; **47**:3033–3053.

DOSIMETRY OF RADIATION FIELDS

OBJECTIVES   130

PERCENT DEPTH DOSE   130

Influence of Depth and Radiation Quality   131
Effect of Field Size and Shape   131
Effect of Distance from Source to Surface   133
Effect of Depth of Underlying Tissue   134

TABLES OF PERCENT DEPTH DOSE   135

TISSUE/AIR RATIO   139

Computing Tissue/Air Ratio from Percent Depth Dose   140
Influence of Field Size and Source-Axis Distance on Tissue/Air Ratio   141
Influence of Radiation Energy and Depth   141

DOSE COMPUTATIONS FOR ROTATIONAL THERAPY   142

BACKSCATTER   143

SCATTER/AIR RATIO   144

TISSUE/PHANTOM RATIO   144

ISODOSE CURVES   145

Decrement Lines   148
Dose Gradients   148
Polar Coordinates   148
Ray Lines   149
Wedge Isodose Curves   149
Comparison of Isodose Curves   150
Influence of Field Size   151
Electron Depth Dose and Isodose Curves   151
Measuring X-Ray and γ-Ray Isodose Curves   152

SUMMARY   154

PROBLEMS   154

REFERENCES   155

Radiation Therapy Physics, Third Edition, by William R. Hendee, Geoffrey S. Ibbott, and Eric G. Hendee
ISBN 0-471-39493-9 Copyright © 2005 John Wiley & Sons, Inc.

The use of the word "phantom," meaning phantom patient, may have developed from a definition of the word phantom: a representation of an ideal.

Perhaps the earliest recorded use of a water phantom as a substitute for human tissue is by Krönig and Friedrick in 1918.[1]

Quimby referred to measurement in "....something of similar size and density, a so-called 'phantom'."[2]

Some researchers chose materials obviously similar to human tissue for the measurements. Failla and his collegues in 1922 reported measuring depth dose data in "beef muscle."[3]

Water was used as a phantom material for some time before its suitability was confirmed. Failla and Quimby described measurements with a small bakelite chamber in a water phantom in 1923.[4] Mayneord also reported using a water phantom in 1929.[5]

The tissue-equivalence of a material is established by comparing its mass energy absorption coefficients with those of water at different photon energies.

The tissue-equivalence of water was finally established by Quimby[2] in 1934 by comparing measurements in a cadaver with those made in water, beeswax, paraffin, wood, "pressed wood", rice and other grains. Quimby concluded that water was a satisfactory substitute for all soft tissues except for the lungs and intraoral region.

When detectors other than ionization chambers are used for measurements in phantoms, a correction for energy dependence may be required.

Perhaps the first documented use of the term "percentage depth dose" was by Wintz in Germany, before 1922.[7]

OBJECTIVES

By studying this chapter, the reader should be able to:

- Compare and contrast parameters describing radiation dose distributions.
- Explain the influence of radiation energy, depth, field size, and SSD on percent depth dose and related parameters.
- Calculate radiation beam parameters from measured or tabulated data.
- Use radiation beam parameters to determine patient treatment time for stationary and moving beams.
- Discuss and compare isodose distributions for radiation beams of different modalities and a range of energies.
- Use tabulated dosimetry parameters to determine the relative contributions of primary and scattered radiation.

The amount of radiation delivered to a location of interest in a patient by a radiation beam traversing the patient often is estimated from radiation doses measured with the radiation beam incident on a device filled with a homogeneous medium such as water. The device is referred to as a *patient-simulating (tissue-equivalent) phantom*. Measurements are usually made with a small ionization chamber, although semiconductor diodes, thermoluminescence dosimeters, other small point detectors, or x-ray film can be used.[6] Often the measurements are obtained at incremental depths along the central axis of the radiation beam and expressed as fractions of the amount of radiation measured at a reference location, also on the beam axis. Depending on the location of the reference dose, these fractions are described as fractional (or percent) depth doses, tissue/air ratios, tissue/phantom ratios, or tissue/maximum ratios.

PERCENT DEPTH DOSE

The central-axis depth dose D_n is the absorbed dose along the central axis of the radiation beam at some depth in the medium. The ratio of D_n to the maximum dose D_0 along the central axis is termed the *fractional depth dose*, or the *percent depth dose* $\%D_n$ if the ratio is multiplied by 100 (Margin Figure 7-1):

$$\%D_n = (D_n/D_0) \times 100$$

For x rays generated at voltages below 400 kVp, the maximum dose occurs at the surface of the phantom, and the reference dose is measured on the central axis at the phantom surface. For higher-energy photons, the reference dose is determined on the central axis at the depth of maximum dose below the surface.

Example 7-1

An absorbed dose of 2 Gy is desired each day at a depth of 7 cm below the surface. An 8- × 8-cm 6-MV x-ray beam is used at 100-cm source-skin distance (SSD). With $\%D_n = 77.7\%$, what is the dose per treatment at the depth of maximum dose 1.5 cm below the surface?

$$\%D_n = (D_n/D_0) \times 100$$
$$D_0 = (D_n/\%D_n) \times 100$$
$$= (2\,\text{Gy}/77.7) \times 100$$
$$= 2.57\,\text{Gy}$$

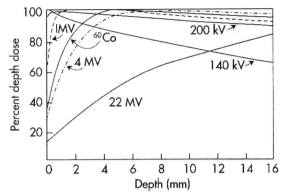

FIGURE 7-1
Percent depth dose for different x-ray and γ-ray beams over the first few millimeters below the surface of a tissue-equivalent phantom. All fields are 10×10 cm^2. For photons of higher energy, %D_n is 100 at the depth of maximum dose below the surface. (From Johns, H. E., Cunningham, J. R. *The Physics of Radiology*, 4th edition, *Springfield, Il., Charles C Thomas, 1983*. Used by permission.)

Influence of Depth and Radiation Quality

Percent depth doses of x- and γ-ray beams of various energies are plotted in Figure 7-1 as a function of depth in millimeters below the surface of a tissue-equivalent phantom. For lower-energy x-ray beams, %D_n decreases rapidly with depth because the lower-energy x rays are rapidly attenuated in the medium. For photons of higher energy, %D_n initially increases rapidly below the surface until the depth of maximum dose is attained. Beyond this depth, the dose decreases slowly with depth. The region between the surface and the depth of maximum dose is termed the *region of dose buildup*.

For a beam of high-energy x or γ rays, the region of dose buildup provides a *skin-sparing advantage* that should be preserved in all therapeutic applications of high-energy photons except when the skin or superficial tissues are to be treated. To retain the skin-sparing advantage, the surface of the patient should be uncovered at the beam-entrance port (i.e., where the radiation beam enters the patient). Any material (e.g., clothing; bolus, satellite collimators, or beam-shaping blocks) on or near the beam entrance surface increases the skin dose and compromises the skin-sparing advantage. To prevent this problem, materials used to shape the radiation beam or flatten the beam-entrance port should be placed several centimeters above the skin rather than on the patient.

Percent depth doses for x- and γ-ray beams of different energies are shown in Figure 7-2 as a function of depth in water. Beyond the region of dose buildup, %D_n falls at a rate that varies inversely with the beam energy. Each %D_n curve reflects the contributions of (1) the inverse square decrease in dose with distance from the radiation source, (2) the attenuation of primary photons in the medium, and (3) the presence of scattered photons in the medium.

Effect of Field Size and Shape

For an x- or γ-ray beam with small area, the central-axis depth dose is delivered almost entirely by primary photons that have traversed the overlying medium without interacting. For larger radiation fields, photons are scattered to every location on and below the surface, including those along the central axis. The relative contribution of scattered radiation to the absorbed dose increases more rapidly at depth than at locations on or near the surface because photons used in radiation therapy tend to be scattered in the forward direction. At any particular depth, the contribution of primary photons does not change with field size. Therefore, D_n increases more rapidly than

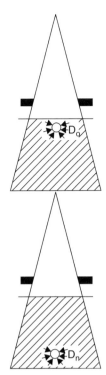

MARGIN FIGURE 7-1
Percent depth dose. D_n is the central axis absorbed dose delivered at some depth within a patient or tissue-equivalent phantom. D_0 is the central axis absorbed dose at the depth of maximum dose. The percent depth dose is $(D_n / D_0) \times 100$.

Measurement of percent depth dose at energies below ^{60}Co is beyond the capabilities of most institutions. Generally, tables from sources such as the *British Journal of Radiology* are used.

The *buildup factor* is the ratio of the absorbed dose at the depth of maximum dose to that at the surface.

Before the introduction of megavoltage treatment units such as ^{60}Co teletherapy units and linear accelerators, physicians were able to gauge patient doses by the appearance of *erythema*, or reddening of the skin.

In 1922, the unit of radiation dose in Germany was known as the "skin standard dose" while in the United States it was called the "erythema dose," or the exposure time required to produce erythema. Therapeutic doses were related to erythema dose. According to Holfelder ". . . carcinoma dose lies between 90 and 125 percent of erythema dose."[7]

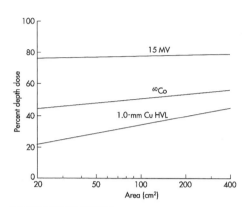

MARGIN FIGURE 7-2

Percent depth dose at 10-cm depth as a function of field size for various x-ray and γ-ray beams with circular cross section. SSD = 100 cm for the 15-MV x-ray beam. (From Hendee, W. R. *Medical Radiation Physics,* 1st edition. Chicago, Mosby—Year Book, 1970.)

The introduction of megavoltage treatment units with the corresponding skin-sparing advantage meant that physicians could no longer prescribe erythema doses. Instead, they were forced to depend on dosimetric measurements in tissue equivalent materials. The role of the medical physicist was thus enhanced and secured for the future.

Variation in percent depth dose with field asymmetry.

Field Size (cm²)	⁶⁰Co	18 MV
20 × 20	63.3	79.0
20 × 10	60.3	79.9
20 × 5	56.8	80.4

HVLs of megavoltage beams have been measured in water. Representative HVLs are listed below.[9]

Energy (MV)	HVL (cm of water)
4	12.8
6	15.5
10	20.4
18	24.3

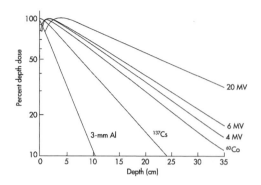

FIGURE 7-2

Percent depth dose for 100 cm² area x-ray and γ-ray beams of different energies as a function of depth in water. The SSD is 100 cm for all beams except the 3.0-mm Al. (SSD = 15 cm) x-ray beam and the ¹³⁷Cs beam (SSD = 35 cm). (From Hendee, W. R. *Medical Radiation Physics,* 1st edition. Chicago, Mosby–Year Book, 1970.)

D_0 as the size of the radiation field is increased, and $\%D_n$ increases with field size. This effect is demonstrated in Margin Figure 7-2.

As the photon energy increases, the increase in $\%D_n$ with field size becomes less pronounced because higher-energy photons are scattered increasingly sharply in the forward direction, and photons scattered near the periphery of the radiation field do not reach the central axis. For example, scattered radiation contributes about 71% of the central axis dose at 10 cm depth for an x-ray beam of 2.0-mm Cu half-value layer (HVL), 100-cm² area, and 50-cm SSD (Example 7-2). For a ⁶⁰Co beam of similar area and 80-cm SSD, scattered radiation contributes only about 26% to the central axis dose at 10-cm depth. At 6 MV, for a 10- × 10-cm field at 100-cm SSD, the contribution from scatter at 10-cm depth is only about 22%. For fields of 100-cm² cross-sectional area, scattered radiation contributes 3.6% to the dose at the depth of maximum dose for ⁶⁰Co γ rays and 29% to the surface dose for x rays of 2.0-mm Cu HVL. The $\%D_n$ for very high-energy photons (e.g., 18-MV x rays) is virtually unaffected by field size because the photons are scattered forward in a direction almost parallel to the primary photons.

For any x- or γ-ray beam of specific cross-sectional area, the $\%D_n$ decreases with increasing asymmetry of the field. Although the volume of irradiated medium may remain constant, fewer scattered photons reach the central axis of an asymmetric beam because the average distance is greater between the origin of the scattered photons and the central axis.

As an x-ray beam penetrates a medium, lower-energy photons are selectively attenuated, and the average energy of the primary beam increases (i.e., the beam is "hardened"). Except for beams of small area, however, the presence of lower-energy scattered photons more than compensates for the hardening effect, and the HVL of the beam decreases with depth. The HVL of a monoenergetic beam (e.g., ⁶⁰Co) also decreases with depth because the primary beam cannot be hardened, and the contribution of scattered radiation increases with depth. The reduction in HVL with depth is more pronounced for x- and γ-ray beams of large cross-sectional area because more scattered photons reach the central axis. Because of the forward direction of photons scattered from high-energy x-ray beams, the reduction in HVL with depth is less noticeable.

Example 7-2

Find the contribution of scattered radiation to the total dose at 10-cm depth for a 10- × 10-cm x-ray beam of 2.0-mm Cu HVL at 50-cm SSD. The $\%D_n$ at 10-cm depth is 35.5% for a 10- × 10-cm field and 13.4% for a field of 0-cm² cross-sectional area. The backscatter factors are 1.286 for the 10- × 10-cm field and 1.000 for the 0-cm² field.

The $\%D_n$ for a field of 0-cm^2 reflects the contribution of primary photons only. For a dose D_{air} of 1 Gy (100 cGy) delivered to a small mass of tissue in air at the SSD, the absorbed dose is 0.134 Gy (13.4 cGy) at a depth of 10 cm for a field of 0-cm^2 area:

$$D_n = (D_{air}) (BSF) (\%D_n/100)$$

$$= (100 \text{ cGy})(1.000)(13.4/100)$$

$$= 13.4 \text{ cGy}$$

For the same absorbed dose to a small mass of tissue in air, the absorbed dose is 45.6 cGy [(100cGy)(1.286)(35.5/100)] at a depth of 10 cm for a 10- × 10-cm field:

Primary radiation contributes 13.4 cGy, and scattered radiation contributes $(45.7 - 13.4) = 32.3$ cGy to the absorbed dose at 10-cm depth. The percent contributions of primary and scattered radiation to the total absorbed dose at 10-cm depth for a 10- × 10-cm x-ray beam of 2.0-mm Cu HVL at 50-cm SSD are

$$\% \text{ Contribution of primary radiation}$$

$$= (13.4/45.7) = 29\%$$

$$\% \text{ Contribution of scattered radiation}$$

$$= (32.3/45.7) = 71\%$$

Example 7-3

Repeat Example 7-2 at 10-cm depth for a ^{60}Co gamma-ray beam of 10- × 10-cm area and 80-cm SSD. The $\%D_n$ is 42.7%, and the backscatter factor is 1.000 for a field of 0 cm^2, whereas the same variables have values of 55.6% and 1.036 for a 10- × 10-cm field.

For a dose of 100 cGy to a small mass of tissue, the 0-cm^2 field yields

$$D_n = (D_{air}) (BSF)(\%D_n/100)$$

$$= (100 \text{ cGy})(1.000)(42.7/100)$$

$$= 42.7 \text{ cGy}$$

and the 10- × 10-cm field yields

$$D_n = (D_{air}) (BSF)(\%D_n/100)$$

$$= (100 \text{ cGy})(1.036)(55.6/100)$$

$$= 57.6 \text{ cGy}$$

The percent contributions to the total dose at 10-cm depth are

$$\% \text{ Contribution of primary radiation}$$

$$= (100)(42.7 \text{ cGy}/57.6 \text{ cGy}) = 74\%$$

$$\% \text{ Contribution of scattered radiation}$$

$$= (100)[(57.6 - 42.7) \text{ cGy}/57.6 \text{ cGy}] = 26\%$$

Effect of Distance from Source to Surface

At any location in an irradiated medium, the rate of delivery of radiation is reduced by increasing the distance between the medium and the radiation source. If the radiation is emitted by a point source and attenuation of the radiation in air is ignored, the dose rate varies inversely as the distance squared. This relationship between

Backscatter factor BSF is defined as $BSF = D_0/D_{air}$: D_0 is the central axis dose at the depth of maximum dose, and D_{air} is the dose at the same location to a small mass of tissue in air (or in *free space*). Backscatter factors are discussed in greater detail later in this chapter.

The percent backscatter factor %BSF is defined as

$$\%BSF = 100(D_0 - D_{air})/D_{air}$$

$$= 100(BSF - 1)$$

The $\%D_n$ for a field of 0 cm^2 is determined by extrapolation and is therefore an approximation.

The x-ray target of a linear accelerator behaves almost as a point source of radiation, unlike the larger source of a ^{60}Co unit. In both types of equipment, the scattering of radiation high in the collimator has the effect of broadening the source. When the divergence of the beam is measured, the radiation appears to be diverging from a "virtual source," a point sometimes located several centimeters from the actual source. The distance from the virtual source, or "effective SSD," should be used for inverse-square calculations. The location of the virtual source may be determined by extrapolation from a plot of $1/\sqrt{R}$ versus distance, where R is the reading from an ionization chamber with buildup in air.

Caution must be applied when using the inverse square relationship to determine dose rates from megavoltage photon beams at large distances. Scattered radiation from the walls, floor or ceiling may influence the result.

Extended treatment distances of 3 m or more are used for total body irradiation (TBI) for ablation of bone marrow prior to transplantation. Reliance on the inverse-square law over long distances is unwise. Instead, measurements are generally made in a water phantom at the actual treatment distance. The maximum field size is generally used, and the water phantom is chosen to mimic the dimensions of a patient.

Modern linear accelerators can achieve higher dose rates than older machines, allowing both shorter treatment times and treatments at extended distances to permit larger field dimensions. The choice of treatment distance is also influenced by practical limits on the size of the equipment.

A "build-down" region exists near the exit surface of a radiation beam, if there is no backscattering medium present.

Measurements with a parallel-plate ion chamber indicate that standard depth dose tables overestimate the exit dose by approximately 20% at 6 MV and 15% at 18 MV.[11]

dose rate and distance is described as an *inverse-square relationship*. For a source of finite size, the decrease in dose rate with increase in distance does not obey an inverse square relationship exactly. Except at short distances from the radiation source, however, the dose rate delivered by most photon sources used in radiation therapy may be estimated with the inverse square relationship to an accuracy of a least a few percent.

Example 7-4

Estimate the improvement in $\%D_n$ at a depth of 10 cm if the SSD is increased from 100 to 150 cm for an x-ray beam with the maximum dose at 1.5 cm below the surface

$$(\%D_n)_{150} = (150 + 1.5 \text{ cm})^2/[(150 + 10)\text{cm}]^2 e^{-\mu(10 \text{ cm})}(100)$$

$$(\%D_n)_{100} = (100 + 1.5 \text{ cm})^2/[(100 + 10)\text{cm}]^2 e^{-\mu(10 \text{ cm})}(100)$$

The term $e^{-\mu(10 \text{ cm})}$ describes the attenuation of the x rays in 10 cm of medium, and the squared ratio of distances represents the inverse square falloff of radiation intensity with distance. The improvement in $\%D_n$ is described by the ratio

$$\frac{(\%D_n)_{150}}{(\%D_n)_{100}} = \left[\frac{(151.5 \text{ cm}/160 \text{ cm})}{(101.5 \text{ cm}/110 \text{ cm})}\right]^2$$
$$= 1.053$$

where the expressions $e^{-\mu(10 \text{ cm})}$ and (100) cancel in numerator and denominator. The $\%D_n$ at 10-cm depth is increased by the factor 1.053 (i.e., by 5.3%) in shifting the SSD from 100 to 150 cm.

As the distance increases between a radiation source and an absorbing medium, the dose rate decreases, but the $\%D_n$ increases at every location below the depth of maximum dose in the medium. The $\%D_n$ increases because the reduction in dose rate is less severe for locations farther from the source. That is, the dose rate reduction at depths below the depth of maximum dose is less than the reduction in dose rate at d_{max}, and the ratio $\%D_n$ increases.

The ratio of percent depth doses at a particular depth for two SSDs is called the *F-factor* and was originally described by Mayneord.[10] The increase in $\%D_n$ with increasing SSD is accompanied by a reduction in the actual dose rate delivered to any location within the medium. In Example 7-4, for example, the dose rate at d_{max} decreases to less than half $[(101.5 \text{ cm}/151.5 \text{ cm})^2 = 0.45]$ as the SSD is increased from 100 to 150 cm. The distance from the radiation source to the patient in radiation therapy sometimes is influenced by a compromise between an increase in $\%D_n$ and a reduction in dose rate as the distance is increased.

Effect of Depth of Underlying Tissue

The $\%D_n$ usually is measured with a thickness of underlying tissue sufficient to provide complete scatter of photons in the backward direction (backscatter). If these measurements are used to estimate the absorbed dose at locations near the beam exit surface of a patient treated with low-energy photons, the computed dose may require a correction for the absence of underlying tissue. The *exit dose* D_e is the absorbed dose delivered to a surface where the central axis of a radiation beam emerges from the patient. The exit dose usually is estimated from central axis depth dose data or from isodose distributions. If a scattering medium (e.g., a treatment table) is not present beyond the patient, this estimate may overestimate the actual exit dose. For high-energy radiation, corrections are rarely required because most of the scatter occurs in the forward direction.

TABLE 7-1 Central Axis Percent Depth Dose for X-Ray Beam of 2.0-mm Cu HVL and 50-cm Source-Skin Distance[a]

Depth (cm)	Field Size (cm × cm)						
	0 × 0 B = 1.000	4 × 4 B = 1.144	6 × 6 B = 1.201	8 × 8 B = 1.248	10 × 10 B = 1.286	15 × 15 B = 1.358	20 × 20 B = 1.415
0	100.0	100.0	100.0	100.0	100.0	100.0	100.0
2	66.5	83.9	88.4	91.4	93.6	96.9	98.9
4	44.2	62.1	68.7	73.6	77.4	83.4	86.8
6	29.6	44.9	51.3	56.5	60.6	67.3	71.6
8	19.9	32.1	37.8	42.7	46.6	53.5	58.1
10	13.4	22.9	27.7	32.0	35.5	42.0	46.5
12	9.1	16.5	20.2	23.8	26.9	32.7	36.7
14	6.2	11.9	14.8	17.6	20.3	25.2	28.7
16	4.2	8.5	10.9	13.1	15.2	19.5	22.5
18	2.9	6.1	7.9	9.8	11.5	15.2	17.6
20	2.0	4.4	5.7	7.2	8.7	11.7	13.7

[a] The beam was collimated with an open-end applicator. B represents the backscatter factor. HVL, half-value layer.
Source: Johns, H., and Cunningham, J. *The Physics of Radiology,* 1st edition. Springfield, IL, Charles C Thomas, 1983. Used by permission.

TABLES OF PERCENT DEPTH DOSE

Tables of central axis percent depth dose are available from several sources, including Supplements 11, 17, and 25 of the *British Journal of Radiology,*[12] texts by Johns and Cunningham[13] and Khan,[14] and sources cited in ICRU Report 24.[15] Selected tabulations of $\%D_n$ are shown in Tables 7-1 to 7-5. Published data are generally not used for patient dose calculations because the likelihood is too great that the treatment beam characteristics are significantly different from the published data. However, published data may be valuable for comparison with measurements or to validate patient dose calculations.

Percent depth doses may not always be available for the particular radiation energy, field size, or SSD to be used. For an x-ray beam with an energy between those for which published data are available, the $\%D_n$ can be interpolated to a value

Mayneord and Lamerton published a comprehensive survey of percent depth dose data in 1941.[10] The survey covered x-ray beam qualities from 1 mm to 5 mm Cu HVL and treatment distances from 40 cm to 100 cm SSD. Additional limited data were presented for x-ray beam qualities up to 17 mm Cu HVL. The data were obtained by averaging measured data sets submitted in response to a survey. In later years, updated compilations became so voluminous that they were published as supplements to the *British Journal of Radiology*.

TABLE 7-2 Central Axis Percent Depth Dose for a ^{60}Co Gamma-Ray Beam with Skin-Source Distance of 80 cm[a]

Depth (cm)	Field Size (cm × cm)						
	0 × 0 B = 1.000	4 × 4 B = 1.015	6 × 6 B = 1.022	8 × 8 B = 1.029	10 × 10 B = 1.035	15 × 15 B = 1.051	20 × 20 B = 1.063
0.5	100.0	100.0	100.0	100.0	100.0	100.0	100.0
2	87.1	90.6	91.9	92.7	93.3	93.9	94.0
4	72.7	79.0	81.1	82.5	83.4	84.7	85.2
6	60.8	68.1	70.7	72.4	73.6	75.4	76.4
8	50.9	58.0	60.8	62.7	64.1	66.5	68.0
10	42.7	49.3	52.0	54.0	55.6	58.4	60.2
12	35.9	41.9	44.5	46.5	48.1	51.2	53.2
14	30.2	35.6	38.0	40.1	41.8	44.9	47.0
16	25.4	30.4	32.6	34.5	36.2	39.3	41.5
18	21.4	26.0	28.0	29.8	31.4	34.5	36.7
20	18.0	22.1	24.0	25.7	27.2	30.3	32.6

[a] The beam was collimated with an open-end applicator. B represents the backscatter factor. HVL, half-value layer.
Source: Johns, H., and Cunningham, J. *The Physics of Radiology,* 4th edition. Springfield, IL, Charles C Thomas, 1983. Used by permission.

TABLE 7-3 Central Axis Percent Depth Dose for a 6-MV X-Ray Beam

	Field Size (cm²)											
	4 × 4	5 × 5	6 × 6	7 × 7	8 × 8	10 × 10	12 × 12	15 × 15	20 × 20	25 × 25	30 × 30	40 × 40
NPSF	0.981	0.984	0.988	0.991	0.994	1.000	1.005	1.013	1.023	1.030	1.035	1.037
Depth												
1.5	100	100	100	100	100	100	100	100	100	100	100	100
2.0	97.8	97.8	97.9	97.9	97.9	98.0	98.1	98.1	98.2	98.2	98.2	98.3
3.0	93.6	93.7	93.7	93.8	93.9	94.1	94.3	94.4	94.6	94.7	94.8	95.0
4.0	89.5	89.6	89.8	89.9	90.1	90.4	90.6	90.9	91.1	91.3	91.5	91.9
5.0	85.5	85.7	85.9	86.1	86.3	86.8	87.1	87.4	87.8	88.1	88.3	88.8
6.0	80.8	81.1	81.4	81.6	81.9	82.5	83.0	83.5	84.0	84.4	84.7	85.3
7.0	76.2	76.6	77.0	77.3	77.7	78.4	79.0	79.6	80.4	80.8	81.2	81.8
8.0	71.8	72.2	72.7	73.2	73.6	74.5	75.2	75.9	76.8	77.3	77.0	78.5
9.0	67.5	68.1	68.6	69.2	69.7	70.7	71.5	72.4	73.4	74.0	74.5	75.3
10.0	63.4	64.1	64.7	65.3	65.9	67.0	67.9	68.9	70.1	78.8	71.3	72.2
11.0	59.9	60.6	61.3	62.8	62.6	63.7	64.6	65.7	66.9	67.6	68.2	69.2
12.0	56.5	57.3	58.0	58.7	59.3	60.5	61.4	62.5	63.8	64.5	65.2	66.2
13.0	53.3	54.0	54.8	55.5	56.2	57.4	58.4	59.4	60.7	61.6	62.3	63.4
14.0	50.1	50.9	51.7	52.5	53.2	54.4	55.4	56.4	57.8	58.7	59.5	60.6
15.0	47.1	47.9	48.7	49.5	50.3	51.6	52.5	53.6	55.0	56.0	56.7	58.0
16.0	44.6	45.3	46.1	46.9	47.6	48.8	49.8	50.9	52.4	53.4	54.2	55.5
17.0	42.2	42.9	43.6	44.3	45.0	46.2	47.2	48.4	49.8	50.9	51.7	53.1
18.0	39.8	40.5	41.1	41.8	42.4	43.6	44.7	45.9	47.4	48.5	49.3	50.7
19.0	37.5	38.1	38.7	39.3	40.0	41.2	42.2	43.5	45.0	46.1	47.0	40.4
20.0	35.3	35.9	36.4	37.0	37.6	38.0	39.8	41.2	42.7	43.9	44.0	46.2
21.0	33.4	34.0	34.5	35.1	35.6	36.8	37.9	39.2	40.7	41.8	42.7	44.2
22.0	31.7	32.2	32.7	33.2	33.8	34.9	35.9	37.2	38.7	39.8	40.7	42.2
23.0	29.9	30.4	30.9	31.4	31.9	33.2	34.1	35.3	36.8	37.9	38.7	40.2
24.0	28.2	28.7	29.2	29.7	30.2	31.3	32.3	33.5	34.9	36.0	36.8	38.3
25.0	26.6	27.1	27.5	28.0	29.5	29.5	30.5	31.7	33.1	34.2	35.0	36.5

Source: Barnes, W. H, Hammond, D. B., Janik, G. G. Beam characteristics of the Clinac 2500. Presented at Varian Users Group Meeting (1983).

intermediate between those in the published data. Usually, however, the %D_n for a particular photon beam and a particular depth is selected from data tabulated for the nearest energy, and a value is not interpolated between tables for x rays of different energies. This procedure is acceptable for validating clinical dosimetry calculations, provided that a table is available for a beam energy near that to be used clinically, because %D_n changes only gradually with photon energy.

Burns[16] has developed a set of expressions to convert %D_n from one SSD to another. These equations may be used to compute the %D_n at any SSD for which published data are not available. Burns' expression is

$$\%D_n(d, r, f_2) = [\%D_n(d, r/F, f_1)][\text{PSF}(r/F)/\text{PSF}(r)](F^2)$$

where r is the field size at the surface, f_1 is the SSD at which %D_n is known, f_2 is the SSD at which %D_n is desired, d is the depth, PSF is the peakscatter factor (see next section) for the selected area and beam energy, and F is the Mayneord F factor defined as (with d_m = depth of maximum dose)

$$F = [(f_1 + d)/(f_2 + d)] \times [(f_2 + d_m)/(f_1 + d_m)]$$

For high-energy x rays, the variation in %D_n with field size is small and *PSF* is essentially unity. In this case, the Burns conversion of %D_n from one SSD to another simplifies to the square of the Mayneord F factor.

Percent depth doses usually are compiled for square fields. However, most radiation fields employed clinically are rectangular or irregularly shaped, and a method is needed to convert %D_n for square fields into values for fields of other shapes. Clarkson's method for irregular fields is discussed later in this chapter. To find the

TABLE 7-4 Central Axis Percent Depth Dose for a 10-MV X-Ray Beam

Depth (cm)	A/P and Field Size (cm²)									
	0 $\times$ 0	1.00 4 $\times$ 4	1.50 6 $\times$ 6	2.00 8 $\times$ 8	2.50 10 $\times$ 10	3.00 12 $\times$ 12	3.75 15 $\times$ 15	5.00 20 $\times$ 20	6.25 25 $\times$ 25	7.50 30 $\times$ 30
0	5.0	6.5	8.5	10.7	12.5	14.5	17.0	21.0	24.5	28.0
0.2	37.0	40.0	43.0	45.0	46.5	48.0	50.0	52.5	54.0	56.0
0.5	65.0	67.0	69.0	70.5	72.0	73.0	74.0	76.0	77.0	79.0
1.0	86.0	88.0	89.0	90.0	91.0	91.5	92.0	93.0	94.0	95.0
1.5	94.5	95.5	96.0	96.5	97.0	97.0	97.5	98.0	98.0	98.5
2.0	96.5	97.5	98.0	98.0	98.0	98.5	99.0	99.0	99.5	99.5
2.5	100.0	100.0	100.0	100.0	100.0	100.0	100.0	100.0	100.0	100.0
3.0	97.4	99.0	99.0	99.0	99.0	99.0	99.0	99.0	99.0	99.0
4.0	92.3	96.4	96.4	96.4	96.4	96.5	96.5	96.5	96.5	96.5
5.0	87.5	91.6	91.8	91.9	92.1	92.2	92.3	92.5	92.6	92.7
6.0	83.0	87.0	87.4	87.7	87.9	88.1	88.3	88.6	88.8	89.0
7.0	78.7	82.6	83.2	83.6	83.9	84.2	84.5	84.9	85.2	85.5
8.0	74.7	78.5	79.2	79.7	80.1	80.4	80.8	81.4	81.8	82.1
9.0	70.8	74.6	75.4	76.0	76.5	76.9	77.3	78.0	78.4	78.8
10.0	67.2	70.8	71.8	72.5	73.0	73.5	74.0	74.7	75.3	75.7
11.0	63.8	67.3	68.4	69.1	69.7	70.2	70.8	71.6	72.2	72.7
12.0	60.6	63.9	65.1	65.9	66.6	67.1	67.7	68.6	69.3	69.8
13.0	57.5	60.7	62.0	62.8	63.5	64.1	64.8	65.7	66.5	67.1
14.0	54.6	57.7	59.0	59.9	60.7	61.3	62.0	63.0	63.8	64.4
15.0	51.9	54.8	56.2	57.1	57.9	58.5	59.3	60.4	61.2	61.8
16.0	49.3	52.1	53.5	54.5	55.3	55.9	56.8	57.8	58.7	59.4
17.0	46.8	49.5	50.9	52.0	52.8	53.5	54.3	55.4	56.3	57.0
18.0	44.5	47.0	48.5	49.5	50.4	51.1	52.0	53.1	54.0	54.8
19.0	42.3	44.7	46.1	47.2	48.1	48.8	49.7	50.9	51.8	52.6
20.0	40.2	42.4	43.9	45.0	45.9	46.7	47.6	48.8	49.7	50.5
22.0	36.3	38.3	39.8	41.0	41.9	42.6	43.5	44.8	45.8	46.6
24.0	32.8	34.6	36.1	37.2	38.2	38.9	39.9	41.1	42.1	43.0
26.0	29.7	31.2	32.7	33.9	34.8	35.5	36.5	37.8	38.8	39.6
28.0	26.9	28.1	29.7	30.8	31.7	32.5	33.4	34.7	35.7	36.5
30.0	24.3	25.4	26.9	28.0	28.9	29.6	30.6	31.8	32.9	33.7

Source: Khan, F. M., Moore, V. C., and Sato, S. Depth dose and scatter analysis of 10 MV X-rays. *Radiology* 1973; **106**:662. Used by permission.

equivalent square of a rectangular field, the data developed originally by Day[17] and shown in Table 7-6 may be employed. In this table, a rectangular field of 15 $\times$ 8 cm is shown to be equivalent to a square field 10.3 cm on a side.

Another approach to determining the equivalent square of a rectangular field is the use of Sterling's rule.[8] This rule states that a rectangular field is equivalent to a square field if both have the same ratio of area/perimeter (A/P). For example, a 15- $\times$ 8-cm field has an A/P of 2.61. A square field 10.3 cm on a side has an A/P of 2.59, a value close to 2.61. The A/P of a rectangular field is $(a \times b)/2(a + b)$, and the A/P of a square field is $a/4$, where a and b are the sides of the rectangular field, and $a = b$ for the square field. Because Sterling's rule equates the A/P ratios, $a = 4A/P$. For a 15- $\times$ 8-cm field, the equivalent square is $4 \times 2.61 = 10.4$ cm on a side, a value close to the 10.3 cm computed previously.

Example 7-5

An orthovoltage x-ray beam with an HVL of 2.0-mm Cu is calibrated in units of exposure rate (R/min) in air. Determine the treatment time to deliver a dose of 200 cGy to a tumor at 8 cm depth for the following data: exposure rate 80 R/min at 50-cm SSD, field size = 6 $\times$ 6 cm, %D_n = 37.8 at 8 cm, BSF = 1.201, and f-factor (cGy/R

To facilitate calculations in rectangular, or slightly irregular fields, some institutions tabulate percent depth dose by A/P. Interpolation to find a specific A/P is then somewhat simplified.

TABLE 7-5 Central Axis Percent Depth Dose for an 18-MV X-Ray Beam

Depth (cm)	Field Size (cm²)												
	5 × 5	6 × 6	7 × 7	8 × 8	9 × 9	10 × 10	12 × 12	14 × 14	15 × 15	20 × 20	25 × 25	30 × 30	35 × 35
2.0	89.0	91.2	93.3	94.9	96.1	97.4	98.2	98.7	98.9	99.3	99.7	99.8	100.0
3.0	100.0	100.0	100.0	100.0	100.0	100.0	100.0	100.0	100.0	100.0	100.0	100.0	100.0
4.0	99.7	99.5	99.4	99.2	99.0	98.9	98.4	98.0	97.8	96.8	96.0	95.8	95.6
5.0	98.0	97.4	97.1	96.8	96.5	96.2	95.6	95.0	94.7	93.3	92.7	92.6	92.4
6.0	94.3	94.0	93.6	93.4	93.1	93.0	92.3	91.7	91.5	90.3	89.4	89.2	89.0
7.0	90.1	89.8	89.7	89.5	89.4	89.0	88.8	88.1	87.8	87.0	86.0	86.0	86.0
8.0	86.5	86.1	86.0	85.9	85.8	85.5	85.0	84.3	83.9	83.5	83.1	83.0	83.0
9.0	83.0	82.6	82.5	82.3	82.2	82.2	82.0	81.8	81.5	81.0	80.5	80.0	80.0
10.0	79.7	79.6	79.4	79.2	79.1	78.9	78.7	78.4	78.3	77.6	77.3	77.2	77.1
11.0	76.0	75.8	75.7	75.5	75.5	75.5	75.5	75.3	75.1	74.5	74.2	74.2	74.2
12.0	73.1	73.1	73.0	73.0	72.9	72.9	72.7	72.6	72.5	72.2	71.9	71.9	71.9
13.0	69.7	69.7	69.7	69.6	69.7	69.5	69.7	69.5	69.5	69.0	69.0	69.0	69.0
14.0	66.8	66.8	66.8	66.8	66.8	66.8	66.8	66.8	66.8	66.8	66.8	66.8	66.8
15.0	64.0	64.0	64.0	64.0	64.0	64.0	64.0	64.0	64.0	64.1	64.2	64.3	64.4
16.0	61.2	61.6	61.6	61.7	61.7	61.7	61.7	61.8	61.9	61.9	62.0	62.2	62.4
17.0	58.4	58.8	58.8	58.8	58.8	59.0	59.1	59.2	59.2	59.3	59.3	59.5	59.7
18.0	55.8	55.9	56.1	56.4	56.6	56.9	57.0	57.1	57.2	57.3	57.4	57.8	57.6
19.0	53.5	54.0	54.1	54.2	54.3	54.4	54.6	54.7	54.8	55.0	55.1	55.2	55.5
20.0	51.0	51.4	51.6	51.9	52.2	52.3	52.5	52.6	52.7	52.8	53.0	53.2	53.5
22.0	47.0	47.7	47.9	48.0	48.2	48.3	48.4	48.5	48.7	48.9	49.2	49.4	49.8
24.0	42.8	43.8	43.9	44.0	44.1	44.2	44.4	44.6	44.8	45.0	45.6	45.8	46.0
26.0	39.4	40.2	40.4	40.5	40.6	40.7	40.9	41.2	41.5	41.8	42.3	42.5	42.9
28.0	36.2	37.0	37.2	37.3	37.4	37.5	37.7	38.0	38.2	38.4	39.2	39.4	39.8
30.0	33.7	33.9	34.1	34.2	34.4	34.6	34.7	35.0	35.2	35.8	36.4	36.6	36.9

Source: British Journal of Radiology, Supplement 17, Central axis depth dose data for use in radiotherapy. British Institute of Radiology, London, 1983.

conversion) = 0.957:

$$\text{Dose rate at tumor} = (\text{R/min})(\text{BSF})(\%D_n/100)(f\text{-factor})$$

$$= (80\ \text{R/min})(1.201)(37.8/100)(0.957)$$

$$= 34.8\ \text{cGy/min}$$

$$\text{Treatment time} = \frac{\text{Dose desired to tumor}}{\text{Dose rate at tumor}}$$

$$= \frac{200\ \text{cGy}}{34.8\ \text{cGy/min}} = 5.75\ \text{min}$$

Sterling's rule is widely used in radiation therapy to find the equivalent square of a rectangular field. It is an empiric rule, however, and does not apply to irregular (nonrectangular) or circular fields. To find the radius r of a circular field equivalent to a rectangular field (see Table 7-6), the following expression may be used[12]:

$$r = (4/\sqrt{\pi})(A/P)$$

Example 7-6

The tumor described in Example 7-5 is to be treated with ^{60}Co gamma rays. The dose rate to a small mass of tissue is 80 cGy/min at a distance of 80-cm SSD + 0.5-cm d_m.

The output of orthovoltage and cobalt units is generally expressed in terms of exposure rate (R/min) or dose rate (cGy/min) in air. X-ray beams from linear accelerators are calibrated at depth in tissue or tissue-equivalent material, in terms of dose rate (see Chapter 6). Because the output of an accelerator can vary, it is monitored continuously, and the integrated output is reported in *monitor units*. The dose rate is therefore described in terms of dose per monitor unit or cGy/MU.

TABLE 7-6 Equivalent Squares of Rectangular Fields

Long Axis (cm)	Short Axis (cm)																												
	1	2	3	4	5	6	7	8	9	10	11	12	13	14	15	16	17	18	19	20	22	24	26	28	30
1	1.0																								
2	1.4	2.0																							
3	1.6	2.4	3.0																						
4	1.7	2.7	3.4	4.0																					
5	1.8	3.0	3.8	4.5	5.0																				
6	1.9	3.1	4.1	4.8	5.5	6.0																			
7	2.0	3.3	4.3	5.1	5.8	6.5	7.0																		
8	2.1	3.4	4.5	5.4	6.2	6.9	7.5	8.0																	
9	2.1	3.5	4.6	5.6	6.5	7.2	7.9	8.5	9.0																
10	2.2	3.6	4.8	5.8	6.7	7.5	8.2	8.9	9.5	10.0															
11	2.2	3.7	4.9	5.9	6.9	7.8	8.6	9.3	9.9	10.5	11.0														
12	2.2	3.7	5.0	6.1	7.1	8.0	8.8	9.6	10.3	10.9	11.5	12.0													
13	2.2	3.8	5.1	6.2	7.2	8.2	9.1	9.9	10.6	11.3	11.9	12.5	13.0												
14	2.3	3.8	5.1	6.3	7.4	8.4	9.3	10.1	10.9	11.6	12.3	12.9	13.5	14.0											
15	2.3	3.9	5.2	6.4	7.5	8.5	9.5	10.3	11.2	11.9	12.6	13.3	13.9	14.5	15.0										
16	2.3	3.9	5.2	6.5	7.6	8.6	9.6	10.5	11.4	12.2	13.0	13.7	14.3	14.9	15.5	16.0									
17	2.3	3.9	5.3	6.5	7.7	8.8	9.8	10.7	11.6	12.4	13.2	14.0	14.7	15.3	15.9	16.5	17.0								
18	2.3	4.0	5.3	6.6	7.8	8.9	9.9	10.8	11.8	12.7	13.5	14.3	15.0	15.7	16.3	16.9	17.5	18.0							
19	2.3	4.0	5.4	6.6	7.8	8.9	10.0	11.0	11.9	12.8	13.7	14.5	15.3	16.0	16.7	17.3	17.9	18.5	19.0						
20	2.3	4.0	5.4	6.7	7.9	9.0	10.1	11.1	12.1	13.0	13.9	14.7	15.5	16.3	17.0	17.7	18.3	18.9	19.5	20.0					
22	2.3	4.0	5.5	6.8	8.0	9.1	10.3	11.3	12.3	13.3	14.2	15.1	16.0	16.8	17.6	18.3	19.0	19.7	20.3	20.9	22.0				
24	2.3	4.1	5.5	6.8	8.1	9.2	10.4	11.5	12.5	13.5	14.5	15.4	16.3	17.2	18.0	18.8	19.6	20.3	21.0	21.7	22.9	24.0			
26	2.3	4.1	5.6	6.9	8.1	9.3	10.5	11.6	12.6	13.7	14.7	15.7	16.6	17.5	18.4	19.2	20.1	20.9	21.6	22.4	23.7	24.9	25.0		
28	2.4	4.1	5.6	6.9	8.2	9.4	10.5	11.7	12.8	13.8	14.8	15.9	16.8	17.8	18.7	19.6	20.5	21.3	22.1	22.9	24.4	25.7	27.0	28.0	
30	2.4	4.1	5.6	6.9	8.2	9.4	10.6	11.7	12.8	13.9	15.0	16.0	17.0	18.0	18.9	19.9	20.8	21.7	22.5	23.3	24.9	26.4	27.7	29.0	30.0

Source: Day, M. The equivalent field method for axial dose dose determinations in rectangular fields. *Br. J. Radiol.* 1972; **99** (suppl. 11). used by permission.

The $\%D_n$ for a 6- $\times$ 6-cm field is 60.8%, and the backscatter factor is 1.022. What is the treatment time required to deliver 200 cGy to the tumor?

$$\text{Dose rate at tumor} = (\text{cGy/min})(\text{BSF})(\%D_n/100)$$

$$= (80 \text{ cGy/min})(1.022)(60.8/100)$$

$$= 49.7 \text{ cGy/min}$$

$$\text{Treatment time} = \frac{\text{Dose desired to tumor}}{\text{Dose rate at tumor}}$$

$$= \frac{200 \text{ cGy}}{49.7 \text{ cGy/min}}$$

$$= 4.02 \text{ min}$$

D_{air} is sometimes described as the "dose to air." This description is incorrect; D_{air} is properly defined as the absorbed dose to a small ("equilibrium") mass of tissue suspended in air.

■ TISSUE/AIR RATIO

A somewhat simpler quantity than $\%D_n$ is the tissue/air ratio TAR, defined as

$$\text{TAR} = D_d/D_{\text{air}}$$

where D_d is the absorbed dose at some location in a medium and D_{air} is the absorbed dose to a small mass of tissue suspended in air at the same location. D_{air} is sometimes described as the dose in free space D_{fs}. The TAR is usually determined at the depth along the central axis where the rotational axis of the treatment unit is centered (i.e., the *isocenter*).

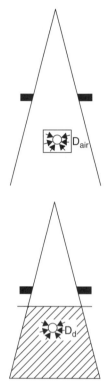

MARGIN FIGURE 7-3
The tissue/air ratio (TAR). Both D_d and D_{air} are measured at the same distance from the source. However, the conditions for absorption and scattering differ.

When obese patients are treated using isocentric techniques, the distance from the blocking tray to the skin surface may be reduced to 10 cm or less. Erythema and desquamation have been observed in these circumstances.

The relationship between D_d and D_{air} is illustrated in Margin Figure 7-3. Because the doses are measured at the same distance from the radiation source, the TAR is independent of SSD, and corrections are not required for varying SSD during therapy with multiple fields, provided that the point of calculation remains positioned at the axis of rotation of the therapy unit. The definition of TAR is essential to treatment planning in *isocentric radiation therapy*, in which the doses are measured and the target volume is positioned at the axis of rotation. Isocentric radiation therapy is used not only for rotation therapy, but also for treatment with multiple stationary fields.

Computing Tissue/Air Ratio from Percent Depth Dose

The tissue/air ratio is similar to the fractional depth dose except that the reference absorbed dose is determined in air at the location of interest instead of at the depth of maximum dose in the medium. The location of interest usually is the axis of rotation (the *isocenter*) of the treatment unit, and it is at this location that the region to be treated is centered. The procedure for computing tissue/air ratios from fractional depth doses is described below.

The cross-sectional area A of a beam of radiation impinging on the surface of a medium is

$$A = A_I \, (SSD/SAD)^2$$

where A_I is the cross-sectional area of the beam at the axis of rotation (the *isocenter*), SAD is the constant source-axis distance, and SSD is the variable distance from source to surface. The absorbed dose D_0 at the depth of maximum dose is

$$D_0 = D_{air}[SAD/(SSD + d_m)]^2 \, BSF$$

where BSF is the backscatter factor for the size and shape of the radiation field at the surface, and the term $[SAD/(SSD + d_m)]^2$ corrects for the inverse square decrease in dose rate with increasing distance from a point source of radiation. The absorbed dose D_d in a medium at the axis of rotation (where d = depth of isocenter) is

$$D_d = D_{air}[SAD/(SSD + d_m)]^2 \, BSF \, (\%D_n/100)$$

The ratio D_d/D_{air} is the tissue/air ratio TAR. Hence,

$$TAR = [SAD/(SSD + d_m)]^2 \, BSF \, (\%D_n/100)$$

The tissue/air ratios in Table 7-7 were computed with this equation. Tables of tissue/air ratios are available in the literature.[12–14,18]

TABLE 7-7 Tissue/Air Ratios for ^{60}Co Gamma Rays

Depth of Overlying Tissue (cm)	Field Size (cm)						
	0×0	4×4	6×6	8×8	10×10	15×15	20×20
0.5[a]	1.000	1.015	1.022	1.029	1.035	1.051	1.063
1	0.965	0.996	1.009	1.021	1.031	1.048	1.062
2	0.905	0.956	0.976	0.992	1.004	1.025	1.040
4	0.792	0.872	0.902	0.924	0.940	0.968	0.987
6	0.694	0.786	0.821	0.847	0.867	0.902	0.925
8	0.608	0.700	0.736	0.765	0.787	0.830	0.859
10	0.534	0.620	0.655	0.685	0.709	0.756	0.790
12	0.469	0.546	0.580	0.611	0.636	0.685	0.722
14	0.412	0.482	0.515	0.545	0.571	0.622	0.660
16	0.361	0.427	0.458	0.485	0.510	0.564	0.605
18	0.317	0.378	0.406	0.433	0.457	0.509	0.551
20	0.278	0.333	0.361	0.386	0.410	0.461	0.502

[a]This entry is also the backscatter factor (BSF).
Source: Johns, H., and Cunningham, J. R. *The Physics of Radiology,* 4th edition. Springfield, Il., Charles C Thomas, 1983. Used by permission.

Example 7-7

Determine the tissue/air ratio for a 10- × 10-cm beam of 6-MV x rays at 100-cm SAD, with 15 cm of tissue between the axis of rotation and the surface, and a d_m of 1.5 cm.

Notice that while the length of the field edge varies linearly with distance, the field area varies with the square of the distance. The field area A at the surface is

$$A = A_I \left(\frac{SSD}{SAD} \right)^2$$

$$= (10 \text{ cm})^2 \left[\frac{100 \text{ cm} - 15 \text{ cm}}{100 \text{ cm}} \right]^2$$

$$= 72.3 \text{ cm}^2 \text{ or } 8.5 \text{ cm} \times 8.5 \text{ cm}$$

From the literature, the $\%D_n$ at 15 cm depth is 48.3 for an 8.5- × 8.5-cm field of 6-MV x rays at 80-cm SSD and 48.9 when corrected to an SSD of 85 cm by the procedure illustrated earlier. The backscatter factor is 1.01. The tissue/air ratio is

$$TAR = \left(\frac{SAD}{SSD + d_m} \right)^2 (BSF)(\%D_n/100)$$

$$= \left(\frac{100 \text{ cm}}{(85 + 1.5) \text{ cm}} \right)^2 (1.01)(48.9/100)$$

$$= 0.660$$

Influence of Field Size and Source-Axis Distance on Tissue/Air Ratio

The absorbed dose D_{air} measured in air increases slowly with the size of the radiation field at the axis of rotation. The dose D_d measured in a medium increases more rapidly because more radiation is scattered in the medium than in air. Consequently the ratio D_d/D_{air} (the tissue/air ratio) increases with field size. The absorbed doses D_d and D_{air} are measured at the same distance from the radiation source, and the TAR is independent of SAD for all practical purposes.

Because it is essentially independent of distance, TAR (or a similar parameter) is often used for calculations of dose at extended distances.

Influence of Radiation Energy and Depth

Beams of x and γ rays are attenuated by tissue between the surface of the patient and the axis of rotation. Hence the dose rate D_d at the axis decreases with increasing thickness of overlying tissue. Because D_{air} is constant, TAR also decreases with increasing thickness of overlying tissue (Margin Figure 7-4).

Example 7-8

Determine the treatment time to deliver 200 cGy to a tumor placed at the isocenter (100-cm SAD) of a rotational ^{60}Co unit. The field size is 6 × 6 cm^2 at the isocenter, the thickness of overlying tissue is 8 cm, and the corresponding tissue/air ratio is 0.736. The dose rate is 80 cGy/min to a small of tissue at the isocenter:

$$TAR = \dot{D}_d/\dot{D}_{air}$$

$$\dot{D}_d = (\dot{D}_{air})(TAR)$$

$$= (80 \text{ cGy/min})(0.736)$$

$$= 58.9 \text{ cGy/min}$$

$$\text{Treatment time} = \frac{\text{Dose desired to tumor}}{\text{Dose rate at tumor}}$$

$$= \frac{200 \text{ cGy}}{58.9 \text{ cGy/min}}$$

$$= 3.40 \text{ min}$$

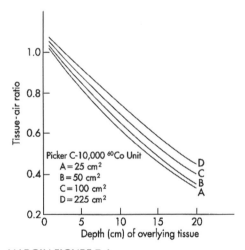

MARGIN FIGURE 7-4
Influence of the depth of overlying tissue on the tissue/air ratio for ^{60}Co γ-ray beams of various sizes at the isocenter. (From Hendee, W. R. *Medical Radiation Physics*, 1st edition. Chicago, Mosby—Year Book, 1970.)

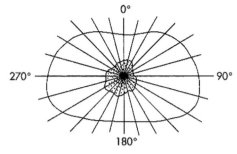

MARGIN FIGURE 7-5
Contour of patient superimposed on grid with radius at 15° increments. Tumor is indicated by the dotted region. Depths of overlying tissue are measured along each radius from the axis of rotation to the surface.

Many radiation therapy departments have installed dedicated CT scanners. Mechanical techniques for obtaining patient contours are rarely used today.

It is tempting to average the radial distances rather than the tissue/air ratios and use the average radial distance to look up the corresponding tissue/air ratio. This approximate method works reasonably well for relatively cylindrical volumes of tissue but can lead to substantial error with elliptical contours. As a general rule, the approach is not recommended.

The introduction of accelerators with x-ray beams of higher energies has made conventional rotational therapy largely obsolete. Some intensity-modulated treatment techniques have been introduced that employ gantry rotation (see Chapter 16).

■ DOSE COMPUTATIONS FOR ROTATIONAL THERAPY

To use manual techniques to compute the dose rate at the axis of rotation for an x-ray or γ-ray beam rotating around a patient, the contour of the patient is outlined in a plane containing the rotational axis. To obtain the contour outline, a mechanical,[19,20] optical,[21] ultrasonic,[22,23] or computed tomographic[24] technique may be employed. The outline is superimposed on a grid with radii extending outward from the rotational axis at selected angular increments (e.g., 10, 15, or 20 degrees) (Margin Figure 7-5). If the radiation source is rotated through 360 degrees, the center of the tumor is placed at the axis. The depth of overlying tissue between the axis and the surface is measured along each radius (see Example 7-9). For the field size and radiation energy used, the tissue/air ratio is determined for each depth of overlying tissue. The ratios are averaged to yield TAR$_{avg}$, and the dose rate at the axis is computed as

$$\text{Dose rate at axis of rotation} = (\text{Dose rate at axis in air})(\text{TAR}_{avg})$$

A representative calculation is shown in Example 7-9.

Example 7-9

Sample computation for dose rate at the center of a tumor treated by a 360-degree rotation of a ^{60}Co beam of 6 × 6 cm at the rotational axis:

Angle	Depth of Overlying Tissue (cm)	TAR	Angle	Depth of Overlying Tissue (cm)	TAR
0	9.3	0.683	180	9.3	0.683
20	7.9	0.740	200	7.8	0.744
40	8.4	0.719	220	8.0	0.724
60	7.8	0.744	240	7.7	0.749
80	8.5	0.716	260	8.4	0.719
100	8.2	0.728	280	8.1	0.732
120	8.0	0.736	300	8.0	0.736
140	8.4	0.719	320	8.4	0.719
160	9.3	0.683	340	9.3	0.683

$$\text{Average tissue/air ratio (TAR}_{avg}) = 0.72$$

$$\text{Dose rate at axis}(D_{air}) = 127 \text{ cGy/min}$$

$$\text{Dose rate at tumor} = (D_{air})(\text{TAR}_{avg})$$

$$= (127 \text{ cGy/min})(0.72)$$

$$= 91.4 \text{ cGy/min}$$

To use the method outlined in Example 7-9, the radiation source must rotate uniformly around the patient during the entire course of treatment. With cobalt units, if a whole number of revolutions is not achieved during each treatment, rotation should be started each day at the angle at which the most recent treatment was suspended. Modern linear accelerators generally control the dose rate or gantry speed of rotation to ensure that the full dose is delivered simultaneously with completion of the intended arc of rotation. Failure to complete the arc may change the shape of the dose distribution. In such cases, treatment should be delivered clockwise on alternating days and counterclockwise on the remaining days.

For many of the depths of overlying tissue shown in Example 7-9, the tissue/air ratios are interpolated from data published for centimeter intervals. The interpolation of tabulated data may be eliminated by constructing rulers, or algorithms when computerized treatment planning is employed, that are scaled in units of the tissue/air ratio. A ruler or algorithm must be developed for each field size and radiation energy used for therapy.

BACKSCATTER

When the axis of rotation is positioned at the depth of maximum dose, $D_d = D_0$ and the tissue/air ratio is defined as the backscatter factor BSF:

$$BSF = D_0/D_{air}$$

The percent backscatter %BSF is

$$\%BSF = 100(D_0 - D_{air})/D_{air}$$
$$= 100(BSF - 1)$$

The number of photons scattered at the depth of maximum dose d_m in a medium depends on the amount of underlying medium and the size, shape, and quality of the x- or γ-ray beam. Because D_0 and D_{air} are measured at the same location when the axis of rotation is placed at the depth of maximum dose, BSF is essentially independent of the distance from the radiation source to the surface (SSD). As the depth of underlying tissue increases, BSF also increases until a depth is attained from which a negligible number of scattered photons reaches d_m. Photons are scattered with increased energy as the quality of the incident radiation increases, and greater depths are required to provide an infinite thickness. The thickness of most patients is adequate to provide an infinite thickness and maximum backscatter. In certain treatment situations, however (e.g., treatment of head and neck tumors), an infinite thickness may not be present, and the dose computed for the tumor may be lower than that estimated with the assumption of infinite thickness.

For high-energy photons that yield a maximum dose below rather than on or near the surface, the increase in dose as the field size expands is due to forwardscatter and sidescatter as well as backscatter. In this case, the term *backscatter factor* is inappropriate and is replaced by the expression *peak scatter factor* PSF. Note that the PSF, like the BSF, has a value of unity at a field size of 0 × 0. The PSF is most often normalized to its value at a 10- × 10-cm field size and referred to as the normalized peak scatter factor, NPSF. The dependence of BSF (or PSF) on the quality of incident radiation is illustrated in Figure 7-3. Initially, BSF increases with HVL because more

The thickness of tissue required to furnish at least 99% of all backscattered radiation is termed an *infinite thickness*.

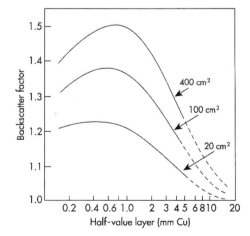

FIGURE 7-3
Influence of quality and field size on backscatter. (From Hendee, W. R. *Medical Radiation Physics*, 1st edition. Chicago, Mosby–Year Book, 1970.)

scattered photons are produced and the scattered photons are more energetic. Hence, more photons are scattered to d_m from greater depths. As the energy of incident photons continues to increase, however, photons are scattered increasingly in the forward direction, and BSF decreases as shown in the illustration. Maximum backscatter is achieved at a HVL between 0.4- and 0.8-mm Cu, depending on the area of the radiation field. For photons of very high energy (e.g., 18-MV x rays), almost all of the scatter is in the forward direction, and the value of the backscatter factor is close to unity.

The backscatter factor increases with the area of the radiation field because photons are scattered toward the surface from larger volumes of tissue (Figure 7-3). For a given area, BSF decreases with increasing asymmetry of the field because scattered photons must travel, on the average, greater distances to reach d_m on the central axis.

Backscatter factors for x-ray and γ-ray beams of different quality and field size are available in the literature.[12–14] Values of the BSF may be interpolated for photon beams with dimensions and HVLs between those listed in the literature. Backscatter factors for locations away from the central axis may be computed by a method described by Johns and Cunningham.[13]

SCATTER/AIR RATIO

For a beam of zero field size, no scattered radiation is produced in a medium, and the value of TAR at any depth is solely a measure of the primary radiation reaching the depth. At any depth, the difference between TAR for a field of finite size compared with that for zero field size reflects the contribution of scattered radiation at the depth. This difference is called the scatter/air ratio SAR:

$$SAR = TAR(\text{finite field size}) - TAR(\text{zero field size})$$

At any location in a medium, the SAR is the dose contribution by the scattered radiation at the location expressed as a fraction of the dose delivered to a small mass of tissue in air at the same location. The value of SAR varies with the depth of overlying tissue, beam energy, and field size and shape in the same manner as the tissue/air ratio.

Scatter/air ratios are used to calculate the dose caused by scattered radiation in a medium. They are especially useful in dose computations for irregularly shaped fields. Scatter/air ratios are derived from tissue/air ratios and compiled as a function of depth and radius of circular fields. Compilations are available in the literature.[12,13]

TISSUE/PHANTOM RATIO

The tissue/phantom (TPR) is the ratio of the dose at a given depth in a phantom to the dose at a reference point depth, with both points equidistant from the radiation source and exposed to the same area field (Margin Figure 7-6). The scatter/phantom ratio (SPR) is the ratio of the dose contribution solely by scattered radiation at a given point divided by the reference dose at a selected depth in the phantom. Although no universal agreement has been reached about the desired depth for the reference dose, a depth of 10 cm is often used in the determination of TPR and SPR.

If the reference dose is measured at the depth of maximum dose d_m rather than at another depth, the quantity TPR can be described as the tissue/maximum ratio (TMR). That is, TMR is a special case of TPR equal to the ratio of the dose at depth in a phantom divided by the maximum dose D_0. The scatter-maximum ratio (SMR) is defined similarly as the ratio of the dose caused solely by scattered radiation at a given point divided by the maximum dose measured at the same distance from the radiation source. Values of TMR for 6-MV x rays are shown in Table 7-8. Values of TMR and SMR for 10-MV x rays are shown in Tables 7-9 and 7-10. Because the doses are measured at identical distances from the radiation source, they are essentially

The normalized peak scatter factor NPSF is also known as the phantom scatter factor S_p and is useful when separating the influence of collimation and field blocking on the depth dose and dose rate.

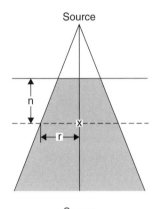

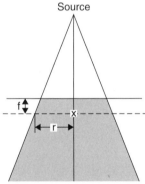

MARGIN FIGURE 7-6
The tissue/phantom ratio is the ratio of the central axis dose D_n at given depth n in a tissue-equivalent phantom to the dose delivered to the same location with the same area beam but with a reference thickness t of overlying tissue (reference depth). If the thickness of overlying tissue equals the buildup thickness required to deliver the maximum dose, the tissue/phantom ratio is termed the tissue/maximum ratio.

The use of tissue/phantom ratio as an alternative to percent depth dose was proposed by Karzmark et al.[25] in 1965.

TABLE 7-8 Tissue/Maximum Ratios for 6-MV X Rays

Depth (cm)	Field Size (cm) at Depth d												
	0 × 0	4 × 4	5 × 5	6 × 6	8 × 8	10 × 10	12 × 12	15 × 15	18 × 18	20 × 20	25 × 25	30 × 30	35 × 35
Output	0.895	0.941	0.951	0.961	0.979	0.996	1.012	1.032	1.048	1.057	1.073	1.078	1.074
1.5	1.000	1.000	1.000	1.000	1.000	1.000	1.000	1.000	1.000	1.000	1.000	1.000	1.000
2.0	0.977	0.983	0.984	0.985	0.987	0.988	0.990	0.992	0.994	0.994	0.994	0.995	0.996
3.0	0.932	0.956	0.960	0.963	0.967	0.970	0.971	0.972	0.976	0.976	0.976	0.977	0.978
4.0	0.889	0.923	0.929	0.934	0.940	0.945	0.948	0.951	0.955	0.955	0.956	0.957	0.960
5.0	0.848	0.889	0.895	0.902	0.910	0.917	0.922	0.926	0.930	0.931	0.934	0.936	0.941
6.0	0.809	0.856	0.864	0.870	0.882	0.891	0.897	0.903	0.910	0.910	0.915	0.918	0.922
7.0	0.772	0.823	0.832	0.847	0.853	0.862	0.870	0.877	0.885	0.885	0.893	0.900	0.904
8.0	0.737	0.787	0.796	0.805	0.820	0.832	0.842	0.852	0.864	0.864	0.782	0.877	0.880
9.0	0.703	0.756	0.765	0.774	0.788	0.800	0.811	0.823	0.839	0.839	0.849	0.854	0.858
10.0	0.671	0.721	0.731	0.740	0.756	0.770	0.782	0.796	0.814	0.814	0.827	0.832	0.836
11.0	0.640	0.691	0.701	0.712	0.724	0.743	0.756	0.775	0.791	0.791	0.803	0.809	0.815
12.0	0.610	0.666	0.676	0.686	0.704	0.719	0.732	0.747	0.767	0.767	0.778	0.788	0.794
13.0	0.582	0.637	0.648	0.658	0.675	0.690	0.702	0.718	0.741	0.741	0.757	0.765	0.773
14.0	0.556	0.607	0.614	0.628	0.647	0.663	0.676	0.694	0.716	0.716	0.730	0.743	0.751
15.0	0.530	0.582	0.593	0.604	0.623	0.639	0.653	0.670	0.691	0.691	0.706	0.719	0.729
16.0	0.506	0.556	0.566	0.576	0.594	0.612	0.626	0.642	0.669	0.669	0.686	0.699	0.708
17.0	0.483	0.531	0.542	0.552	0.571	0.587	0.603	0.622	0.647	0.647	0.666	0.680	0.688
18.0	0.460	0.508	0.519	0.529	0.549	0.564	0.589	0.602	0.626	0.626	0.644	0.657	0.666
19.0	0.439	0.484	0.499	0.509	0.527	0.544	0.560	0.580	0.602	0.602	0.621	0.635	0.648
20.0	0.419	0.466	0.476	0.487	0.506	0.522	0.537	0.557	0.582	0.582	0.600	0.615	0.628
21.0	0.400	0.447	0.458	0.467	0.486	0.502	0.518	0.537	0.561	0.561	0.580	0.596	0.607
22.0	0.381	0.426	0.436	0.446	0.464	0.480	0.494	0.514	0.542	0.542	0.560	0.575	0.587
23.0	0.364	0.408	0.418	0.428	0.446	0.463	0.477	0.497	0.522	0.522	0.542	0.557	0.568
24.0	0.347	0.391	0.400	0.410	0.426	0.444	0.458	0.479	0.504	0.504	0.524	0.538	0.549
25.0	0.331	0.373	0.382	0.391	0.409	0.425	0.440	0.459	0.485	0.485	0.505	0.517	0.530

Source: Jani, S. K. *Handbook of Dosimetry Data for Radiotherapy*, Boca Raton, FL, CRC Press, 1993. Used by permission.

independent of distance and vary only with beam energy, field size and shape, and depth of overlying tissue.

The TMR differs from the tissue/air ratio TAR because the reference dose in the TMR is measured in an extended tissue-equivalent medium, whereas the reference dose in TAR is measured to a small mass of tissue in air. Hence, the two reference doses differ by the backscatter factor BSF. The TMR is related to the tissue/air ratio by

$$\text{TMR}(d, r) = \text{TAR}(d, r)/\text{BSF}(r)$$

where the field size r is determined at depth d.

■ ISODOSE CURVES

The absorbed dose in tissue along the central axis of an x-ray or γ-ray beam may be depicted by tabular or graphic displays of data, such as central axis percent depth doses, tissue/air ratios, or TMRs. However, the dose to tissue away from the central axis cannot be determined from these data. To estimate the absorbed dose to off-axis locations, isodose curves for the x-ray or γ-ray beam should be consulted.

Figure 7-4 shows isodose curves for a 10- × 10-cm beam of 10-MV x rays at 100-cm SSD. Each isodose curve defines locations in a homogeneous, tissue-equivalent medium at which the absorbed dose is a prescribed percent of the dose on the central axis at the depth d_m of maximum dose. For x-ray beams of less than 400 kVp, doses in the phantom are compared with the dose on the central axis at the surface, because the maximum dose occurs on the surface. The field size of an x- or γ-ray beam is

The identification of tissue/maximum ratio as a special case of TPR was proposed by Holt et al.[26] in 1970.

Calculation of treatment time (meter setting) for isocentric treatment with megavoltage beams is most easily done using TMRs. Repeat Example 7-8 for 6-MV x rays with SAD = 100 cm: The dose rate at isocenter in a 6- × 6-cm field under d_{max} thickness of tissue is 0.961 cGy/MU. The TMR at 8-cm depth is 0.805.

$$\text{TMR} = \dot{D}_d / \dot{D}_0$$

$$\dot{D}_d = \dot{D}_0 \text{TMR}$$

$$= (0.961)(0.805)$$

$$= 0.774 \text{ cGy/MU}$$

$$\text{Treatment time} = \frac{\text{Dose desired to tumor}}{\text{Dose rate to tumor}}$$

$$= \frac{200 \text{ cGy}}{0.774 \text{ cGy/MU}}$$

$$= 258 \text{ MU}$$

TABLE 7-9   Tissue/Maximum Ratios for 10-MV X Rays[a]

Depth d (cm)	0 × 0	1.00 / 4 × 4	1.50 / 6 × 6	2.00 / 8 × 8	2.50 / 10 × 10	3.00 / 12 × 12	3.75 / 15 × 15	5.00 / 20 × 20	6.25 / 25 × 25	7.50 / 30 × 30
0	0.048	0.062	0.081	0.102	0.119	0.138	0.162	0.200	0.233	0.267
0.2	0.354	0.382	0.411	0.430	0.444	0.459	0.478	0.502	0.516	0.535
0.5	0.625	0.644	0.663	0.678	0.692	0.702	0.711	0.731	0.740	0.759
1.0	0.835	0.854	0.864	0.874	0.884	0.888	0.893	0.903	0.913	0.922
1.5	0.927	0.936	0.941	0.946	0.951	0.951	0.956	0.961	0.961	0.966
2.0	0.956	0.966	0.970	0.970	0.970	0.975	0.980	0.980	0.985	0.985
2.5	1.000	1.000	1.000	1.000	1.000	1.000	1.000	1.000	1.000	1.000
3.0	0.983	1.000	1.000	1.000	1.000	1.000	1.000	1.000	1.000	1.000
4.0	0.950	0.992	0.992	0.993	0.993	0.993	0.993	0.993	0.993	0.994
5.0	0.918	0.960	0.963	0.965	0.966	0.967	0.968	0.970	0.971	0.972
6.0	0.887	0.930	0.934	0.937	0.939	0.941	0.944	0.947	0.949	0.951
7.0	0.858	0.899	0.906	0.910	0.913	0.916	0.920	0.924	0.928	0.931
8.0	0.829	0.870	0.878	0.884	0.888	0.892	0.896	0.902	0.906	0.910
9.0	0.801	0.841	0.851	0.858	0.863	0.867	0.873	0.880	0.885	0.889
10.0	0.774	0.813	0.824	0.832	0.838	0.843	0.850	0.858	0.864	0.869
11.0	0.748	0.786	0.798	0.807	0.814	0.820	0.827	0.836	0.843	0.849
12.0	0.723	0.760	0.773	0.783	0.791	0.797	0.805	0.815	0.823	0.830
13.0	0.699	0.734	0.749	0.759	0.768	0.774	0.783	0.794	0.803	0.810
14.0	0.676	0.709	0.725	0.736	0.745	0.752	0.762	0.774	0.783	0.791
15.0	0.653	0.684	0.701	0.713	0.723	0.731	0.741	0.753	0.764	0.772
16.0	0.631	0.661	0.678	0.791	0.701	0.710	0.720	0.734	0.744	0.753
17.0	0.610	0.638	0.656	0.669	0.680	0.689	0.700	0.714	0.727	0.735
18.0	0.589	0.615	0.634	0.648	0.659	0.669	0.680	0.695	0.707	0.717
19.0	0.570	0.593	0.613	0.628	0.639	0.649	0.661	0.676	0.689	0.699
20.0	0.551	0.572	0.593	0.608	0.620	0.629	0.642	0.658	0.671	0.681
22.0	0.514	0.532	0.553	0.569	0.582	0.592	0.605	0.622	0.636	0.647
24.0	0.480	0.494	0.516	0.533	0.546	0.556	0.570	0.588	0.602	0.614
26.0	0.449	0.458	0.481	0.498	0.511	0.522	0.536	0.555	0.570	0.583
28.0	0.419	0.425	0.448	0.465	0.479	0.490	0.505	0.524	0.539	0.552
30.0	0.392	0.394	0.417	0.434	0.448	0.459	0.474	0.494	0.509	0.523

[a] Projected at depth d.

Source: Khan, F. M. Depth dose and scatter analysis of 10 MV x rays. *Radiology* 1973; **106**:662 (letter to editor). Used by permission.

TABLE 7-10   Scatter/Maximum Ratios for 10-MV X Rays

| Depth d (cm) | Field Radius (cm) at Depth d | | | | | | | | | | | | |
	2	4	6	8	10	12	14	16	18	20	22	24	26
2.5	0	0	0	0	0	0	0	0	0	0	0	0	0
3.0	0.017	0.017	0.017	0.017	0.017	0.017	0.017	0.017	0.017	0.017	0.017	0.017	0.017
4.0	0.042	0.042	0.043	0.043	0.043	0.043	0.043	0.043	0.044	0.044	0.044	0.044	0.044
6.0	0.043	0.048	0.053	0.056	0.058	0.060	0.062	0.063	0.065	0.066	0.067	0.068	0.069
8.0	0.041	0.052	0.060	0.066	0.070	0.074	0.077	0.080	0.082	0.084	0.086	0.088	0.090
10.0	0.039	0.055	0.066	0.074	0.080	0.085	0.089	0.093	0.097	0.100	0.102	0.105	0.107
12.0	0.037	0.056	0.070	0.080	0.087	0.094	0.099	0.104	0.109	0.112	0.116	0.119	0.122
14.0	0.033	0.056	0.072	0.084	0.093	0.101	0.107	0.113	0.118	0.123	0.127	0.130	0.134
16.0	0.030	0.055	0.073	0.086	0.097	0.106	0.113	0.119	0.125	0.130	0.135	0.140	0.144
18.0	0.026	0.053	0.073	0.088	0.099	0.109	0.117	0.124	0.131	0.137	0.142	0.147	0.151
20.0	0.021	0.051	0.072	0.088	0.101	0.111	0.120	0.128	0.135	0.141	0.147	0.152	0.157
22.0	0.018	0.048	0.071	0.087	0.101	0.112	0.121	0.129	0.137	0.144	0.150	0.155	0.161
24.0	0.014	0.045	0.069	0.086	0.100	0.112	0.121	0.130	0.138	0.145	0.152	0.158	0.163
26.0	0.009	0.042	0.066	0.084	0.098	0.110	0.121	0.130	0.138	0.145	0.152	0.158	0.164
28.0	0.006	0.039	0.063	0.082	0.096	0.109	0.119	0.129	0.137	0.145	0.152	0.158	0.164
30.0	0.002	0.035	0.060	0.079	0.094	0.106	0.117	0.127	0.136	0.143	0.151	0.157	0.163

Source: Khan, F. M. Depth dose and scatter analysis of 10 mV x-rays. *Radiology* 1973; **106**:662 (letter to editor). Used by permission.

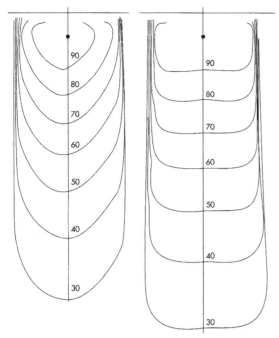

FIGURE 7-4
Isodose curves for a 10-MV x-ray beam without (**left**) and with (**right**) the beam-flattening filter in place. Lateral horns of the curves are apparent near the surface with the beam-flattening filter.

usually defined as the area enclosed within a boundary containing points where the dose is 50% of the dose on the central axis at the depth of maximum dose.

For many x- and γ-ray beams, the isodose curves attain their greatest depth along the central axis and curve toward the surface near the edges of the beam. This curvature reflects the decreased contribution of scattered radiation along the edge of the beam and the greater distance traveled by primary photons to reach a given depth along the beam edge compared with the central axis. Because the contribution of scattered photons is reduced along the beam edge, the average energy of the beam is greater at the edge than along the central axis. This effect is demonstrated in the isoenergy curves depicted in Figure 7-5.

With high-energy x-ray beams from a linear accelerator, the x rays emerging from the transmission target are strongly peaked in the forward direction, and the dose is much higher along the central axis than at the periphery of the radiation field. To improve the dose uniformity of the radiation beam, a metal flattening filter is placed in the x-ray beam. This cone-shaped filter attenuates the central portion of the beam so that at shallow depths, the x-ray intensity is greater along the beam's periphery than along the central axis. This greater intensity, referred to as the "horns" of the higher-percentage isodose curves, compensates for reduced scattered radiation at greater depths along the field edge. The flattening filter also "hardens" the x-ray beam by preferentially attenuating low energy photons. Manufacturers generally "over-flatten" the beam to compensate for the increased penetration of photons traveling along the central axis. In this manner, the isodose curves are relatively flat at usual treatment depths, as shown in Figure 7-4 for 10-MV x rays.

An alternative presentation of isodose curves is shown in Figure 7-6, in which the curves are normalized to a location beyond the depth of maximum dose. Usually, this location corresponds to the axis of rotation of a rotational therapy unit. When this isocentric representation of isodose curves is used, the SAD is fixed, whereas the SSD varies depending on the angular orientation of the incident beam of radiation. With this presentation, the field size is defined at the axis of rotation. Such a presentation is

Isodose distributions are three-dimensional, and they are described by isodose surfaces that resemble isotherms and isobars in weather maps. An isodose curve is a two-dimensional representation of the intersection of a plane with an isodose surface.

The field size of an x-ray or γ-ray beam is usually defined as the area enclosed within a boundary containing points where the dose is 50% of the dose on the central axis at the depth of maximum dose.

Flattening filters for low megavoltage energies (i.e., 4 MV) are generally made of a high-Z material such as lead or tungsten. However, to reduce the contribution of Compton-scattered photons, flattening filters for high-energy beams are usually made of aluminum or another low-Z material.

For megavoltage x rays, the flattening filter is usually designed to provide a variation in intensity of <±3% across 80% of the geometric beam width at 10 cm in water.

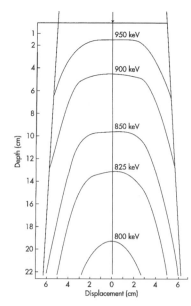

FIGURE 7-5
Isoenergy curves for a 10- × 10-cm field at 80-cm SSD for ^{60}Co γ rays from an AECL Therathon ^{60}Co unit. (From Krohmer, J., and Adamski, J. Isoenergy distribution for a typical cobalt-60 teletherapy unit. *Radiology* 1968; **91**:559. Used by permission.)

An x- and γ-ray beam can be thought of as having three zones:

- A useful inner region covering 80–90% of the beam's geometric width
- A fall-off (penumbra) region at the margins of the beam
- A distal region where the dose is contributed by leakage and scattered radiation

An ideal beam would have:

- A highly uniform intensity profile across the inner region
- A rapid fall-off at the margin
- A negligible dose in the distal region.

(Adapted from reference 27.)

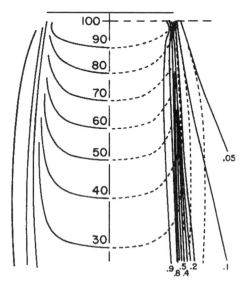

MARGIN FIGURE 7-7
Conventional (**left**) and decrement (**right**) isodose curves for a 10- × 10-cm ^{60}Co beam at 80-cm SSD.

rare today, because most clinics can measure dose distributions and prepare graphical representations that address specific clinical requirements.

On rare occasions, representations of isodose curves are encountered that differ somewhat from those described previously. Among these variations are decrement line curves, dose gradient vectors, and isodose curves displayed graphically in polar coordinates or ray lines rather than in Cartesian (*x–y*) coordinates.

Decrement Lines

In this manner of isodose presentation, data are described as a combination of central axis depth dose data and a family of lines referred to as *decrement lines*. Each decrement line contains points at which the absorbed dose is a prescribed fraction of the dose on the central axis at the same depth (Margin Figure 7-7). This method of presentation of isodose data is especially adaptable to computer computations of composite isodose distributions as described in the next chapter.[28]

Dose Gradients

In the dose gradient presentation of isodose curves,[30,31] gradients of absorbed dose are specified as vectors that vary with location in the radiation beam. The lengths of the vectors represent the rate of change of dose with position. For composite isodose distributions representing two or more radiation fields, regions where the vector sum of the dose gradient vectors equals zero are regions where the composite dose is uniform. The dose gradient method facilitates rapid examination of dose uniformity for multifield treatments and is readily adaptable to treatment planning by computer. This method is rarely seen today.

Polar Coordinates

For computation of dose curves for a rotational therapy unit, it may be convenient to describe the radiation beam in polar coordinates. An example of isodose curves in polar coordinates is shown in Margin Figure 7-8.

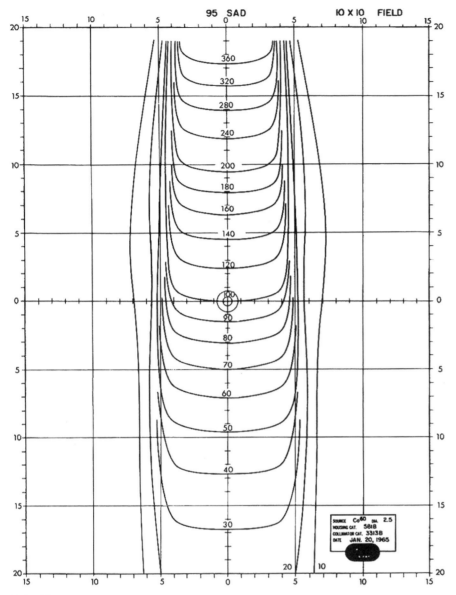

FIGURE 7-6
Isodose curves for a 10- × 10-cm ^{60}Co γ-ray beam normalized to 100% at the isocenter 95 cm from the source. (From Hendee, W. R. *Medical Radiation Physics,* 1st edition. Chicago, Mosby–Year Book, 1970.)

Ray Lines

Isodose curves may be superimposed on a graphic framework of lines perpendicular to the beam central axis and ray lines representing the path of primary photons from the radiation source. Usually the ray lines are drawn close together near the edge of the radiation field and with wider spacing in other regions. This approach facilitates correction for perturbations in the curves introduced by the patient's contour and the presence of beam modifiers, such as wedge filters. A set of ray-line isodose curves is shown in Margin Figure 7-9.

Wedge Isodose Curves

Radiation beams may be modified in various ways to furnish isodose curves useful for specific clinical applications in radiation therapy. One useful modification is

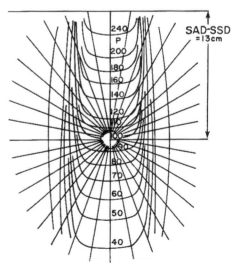

MARGIN FIGURE 7-8
Isodose curves in polar coordinates.[29]

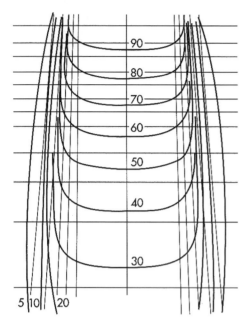

MARGIN FIGURE 7-9
Ray line isodose curves.[29]

The International Electrotechnical Commission (IEC) defines wedge angle as the angle between a line perpendicular to the central axis and a straight line connecting points at 1/4 the field width on either side of the axis, at which the dose equals the dose at 10-cm depth on the central axis.[32]

In some linear accelerators, a single 60° wedge is installed in the collimator head, above the collimator jaws, with a mechanism allowing it to be moved into the beam under operator control. This device is sometimes called an *autowedge* or *dynamic wedge*. To achieve wedge isodose angles of less than 60°, the wedge is moved into the field for a portion of the treatment and the remainder is delivered without the wedge.

placement of a wedge filter in the beam to produce isodose curves that intersect the central axis at some angle other than 90 degrees. A typical wedge filter is shown in Margin Figure 7-10 together with the resulting isodose distribution. For high-energy radiation, the wedge is constructed of high-Z material, such as lead or copper, and positioned far from the patient's skin to retain the skin-sparing advantage of high-energy photons.

The *wedge isodose angle* is defined as the angle between the isodose curve and a line perpendicular to the central axis. Because of the increasing contribution of scattered radiation, the steepness of the isodose angle decreases with depth along the central axis. For lower beam energies, the wedge isodose angle is described as the angle between the 50% isodose curve and a line perpendicular to the central axis. For high-energy x rays, the 50% isodose curve may occur at a depth greater than that of clinical interest, especially when x rays are used to treat relatively superficial tumors in the head and neck. For high-energy x rays, the wedge angle usually is defined at a depth of 10 cm along the central axis.

The presence of a wedge filter reduces the dose rate from an x-ray or γ-ray beam. Sometimes the dose rate reduction is incorporated into the isodose curves for the wedge filter. In Margin Figure 7-10, for example, the maximum dose rate in the distribution is 80% in the upper left corner and about 65% at the depth of maximum dose along the central axis. More commonly, the isodose curves are plotted with a dose of 100% at the depth of maximum dose on the central axis. With this approach, a wedge correction factor must be applied to the central axis dose rate to compensate for attenuation of radiation in the wedge filter.

For radiation therapy units such as ^{60}Co that provide low dose rates, individual wedges for different field widths are desirable to minimize attenuation of the radiation in the wedge filter. With this approach, the thin end of the wedge is aligned with one border of the radiation field, and the isodose curves are "wedged" with minimum attenuation along the central axis. With x-ray beams produced by linear accelerators, the radiation output is more intense, and a *universal wedge* can be used for all field sizes, even though the wedge attenuates the radiation more severely along the central axis.

Modern linear accelerators often provide wedged isodose distributions by manipulating the collimator jaws during irradiation, rather than through the insertion of a metal filter into the beam. In one design, one collimator jaw is moved across the field during treatment. The speed of the jaw is controlled with respect to the dose rate so that the beam intensity is modulated monotonically from one side of the beam to the other. The speed of the jaw can be selected to yield a wedge angle up to 60°. Wedged isodose distributions produced in this fashion can compensate for variations in field uniformity with field size, and provide isodose curves with more uniform slope than can metal wedges.

Comparison of Isodose Curves

Four isodose curves are compared in Margin Figures 7-11 through 7-14. The curves in Margin Figure 7-11 are for a 200-kVp, 10- × 10-cm x-ray beam, HVL 2-mm Cu, and 50-cm SSD. In this illustration, the %D_n decreases rapidly along the central axis because the SSD is relatively short and the primary x rays possess relatively little energy. At 10-cm depth, the dose is only 32% of the dose at the surface. The %D_n falls abruptly along the beam edge because the effective focal spot of the x-ray tube is small, and the collimator attenuates almost all of the photons outside the primary beam. The significant lateral extension of the 10% and 5% isodose curves outside the primary beam reflects the wide-angle scattering of the relatively low-energy x-rays during Compton interactions. These scattered photons deliver significant dose to tissue outside the treated region when an orthovoltage x-ray beam is used for therapy.

The isodose curves in Margin Figure 7-12 describe a 10- × 10-cm ^{60}Co beam at 80-cm SSD. At a depth of 10 cm along the central axis, the percent depth dose is about 56%, an increase of more than 20% in percent depth dose over that provided by the orthovoltage x-ray beam. This increase reflects the greater penetration of the higher-energy γ rays and the increased SSD. The edges of the ^{60}Co beam are defined less sharply because the radiation source and therefore the geometric penumbra are both larger and because the higher-energy γ rays are more difficult to collimate. However, the absorbed dose outside the primary beam is low, because high-energy photons are scattered predominantly in the forward direction.

The distribution in Margin Figure 7-13 represents x rays from a 6-MV linear accelerator with an SSD of 100 cm. Compared with ^{60}Co γ rays, the %D_n for 6-MV x rays is somewhat greater (67% at 10-cm depth). The dose decreases rapidly outside the primary beam because photons are scattered in the forward direction and because the focal spot is small (<2 mm). The sharp demarcation of the radiation field is one of the major advantages of x-ray beams from a linear accelerator. The depth of maximum dose for the 6-MV x-ray beam is 1.5 cm below the surface.

The isodose curves in Margin Figure 7-14 are for 20-MV x rays (10×10 cm, 100-cm SSD). The isodose curves have been flattened with a cone-shaped filter positioned in the x-ray beam. The boundaries of the field are sharp, and the dose decreases rapidly outside the primary beam. The region of dose buildup extends to a depth of about 4.5 cm, and the %D_n is 83% at 10-cm depth. With megavoltage x rays, the dose delivered to tissue near the exit surface of the patient often is greater than the dose at the beam entrance.

Influence of Field Size

Two sets of isodose curves are compared in Figure 7-7. The curves on the left represent a 5- × 5-cm ^{60}Co gamma-ray beam with an SSD of 80 cm. The curves on the right describe a similar distribution except that the dimensions of the field have been expanded to 10×10 cm^2. At any depth, the percent depth dose is greater for the larger field because a greater fraction of the dose is contributed by scattered radiation. The edge of the radiation beam is slightly less sharp with the 10×10 cm beam because more γ rays are scattered from the larger volume of irradiated medium. This effect is reduced considerably at higher energies, and is almost negligible in a beam of 18 MV x-rays.

Electron Depth Dose and Isodose Curves

Percent depth doses along the central axis of selected electron beams are compared in Figure 7-8. Although a slight reduction in surface dose is provided by a high-energy electron beam, the dose is fairly uniform from the surface to the depth of maximum dose. The depth of maximum dose increases gradually with increasing energy of the incident electrons. Beyond this depth, the dose decreases abruptly for low-energy electrons and somewhat less rapidly for electrons of higher energy. For electrons of a particular energy, the decrease in depth dose is slightly more rapid for beams of very small area. The tissue penetration depth (depth for 10% depth dose) may be estimated roughly with the expression:

$$\text{Penetration depth} = [\text{Electron energy (MeV)}]/(2 \text{ MeV/cm})$$

For example, the depth of penetration is about 3 cm for a 6-MeV electron beam, about 5 cm for a 10-MeV beam, and about 10 cm for electrons of 20 MeV.

Isodose curves for electron beams are frequently constructed from densitometric measurements of exposed x-ray film. In Figure 7-9, radiographs exposed "edge on" to electrons of 4 and 26 MeV are accompanied by isodose curves measured densitometrically. Because electrons are scattered rapidly as an electron beam penetrates a medium, the field size for an electron beam expands rapidly below the surface.

When electron-beam depth-dose and isodose curves are measured with ionization chambers, corrections must be applied for the change in stopping power with electron energy. According to the AAPM,[33] the mean incident energy $\overline{E}_0$ of an electron

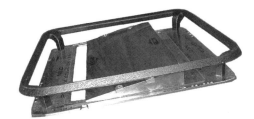
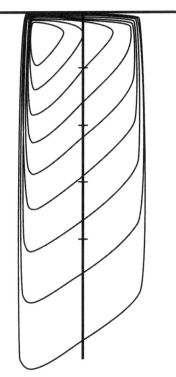

MARGIN FIGURE 7-10
A 45° wedge filter for a 6 MV x-ray beam **(above)** and a set of wedge isodose curves **(below)** for a 10- × 10-cm 6-MV x-ray beam (SSD = 100 cm). The isodose curves near 10-cm depth are angled at 45° with respect to a line perpendicular to the central axis.

An electron beam dose distribution is influenced by

- Energy loss during interaction of primary electrons
- Production and interactions of secondary electrons
- Directional changes of primary and secondary electrons
- Production of bremsstrahlung
- Beam divergence causing a fall-off of electron fluence

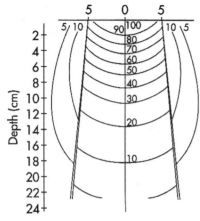

MARGIN FIGURE 7-11
Isodose curves for orthovoltage x rays (200 kVp, 10×10 cm^2, 50-cm SSD, 2.0-mm Cu HVL). (From Hendee, W. R. *Medical Radiation Physics*, 1st edition. Chicago, Mosby–Year Book, 1970.)

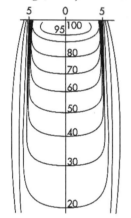

MARGIN FIGURE 7-12
Isodose curves for ^{60}Co γ rays (10×10 cm^2, 100-cm SSD). (From Hendee, W. R. *Medical Radiation Physics*, 1st edition. Chicago, Mosby–Year Book, 1970.)

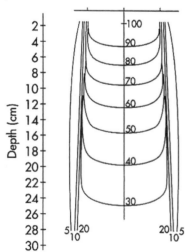

MARGIN FIGURE 7-13
Isodose curves for x rays from a 6-MV linear accelerator (10×10^2, 100-cm SSD). (From Hendee, W. R. *Medical Radiation Physics*, 1st edition. Chicago, Mosby–Year Book, 1970.)

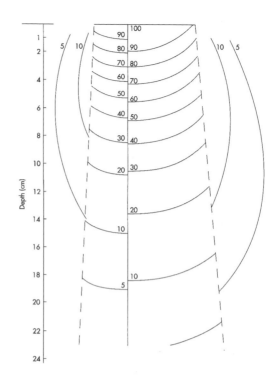

FIGURE 7-7
Influence of field size on central axis percent depth dose and on lateral scatter for ^{60}Co γ rays at 80-cm SSD. **Left:** 5- × 5-cm field. **Right:** 10- × 10-cm field. (From Hendee, W. R. *Medical Radiation Physics*, 1st edition, Chicago, Mosby–Year Book, 1970.)

beam is

$$\overline{E}_0 = 2.33 I_{50}$$

The mean energy $\overline{E}_d$ is presumed to decrease linearly with depth d to the extrapolated range, R_p, shown in Margin Figure 7-15. Therefore,

$$\overline{E}_d = \overline{E}_0(1 - d/R_p)$$

As was discussed in Chapter 6, measurements of electron beam percent depth dose should be shifted by 0.5 r_{cav}.

Measuring X-Ray and γ-Ray Isodose Curves

Isodose curves for photon beams may be constructed from data measured in a water-filled phantom by use of an ionization chamber with a tissue-equivalent wall and containing air-equivalent gas. Alternatively, thermoluminescent dosimeters, semiconductors diodes, or photographic film may be used in a water-filled or tissue-equivalent solid phantom, provided that care is taken to avoid energy dependence and other problems.[6] The ionization chamber should be less than 15 mm long, with an inside diameter of 5 mm or less. In most applications, the chamber is used with an automatic isodose plotter that causes the chamber to scan across the phantom while doses are measured at periodic intervals. Isodose data are determined with a computer that analyzes the chamber signal. When isodose curves are measured for an x-ray beam with a fluctuating output, a monitor chamber is positioned in the beam to compensate for the fluctuations. A complete set of isodose curves may include curves of, for example, 95%, 90%, 80%, 70%, 60%, 50%, 40%, 30%, and 20% and can be constructed in a few minutes.

Isodose curves for various x-ray and γ-ray beams may obtained from a number of sources, including the International Atomic Energy Agency.[34] Isodose data also may

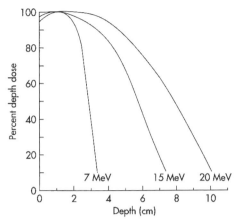

FIGURE 7-8
Central-axis depth doses for electron beams of different energies. Beams are either 10 cm in diameter (7 MeV) or 10 × 10 cm² (15 and 20 MeV). (From Hendee, W. R. *Medical Radiation Physics* 1st edition, Chicago, Mosby–Year Book, 1970.)

be obtained from manufacturers of radiation therapy units and from institutions that employ radiation units of similar manufacture. Before beam data furnished by another source are used with a particular radiation unit, percent depth doses along the central axis of the furnished data should be compared with those measured for the particular unit. The furnished data should not be used if the differences are significant (>2%). In addition, the edges of the distribution should be checked against measurements on the particular therapy unit to ensure that differences in source size and collimation do not produce significant (>2 mm) differences in the isodose distribution along the beam edge.

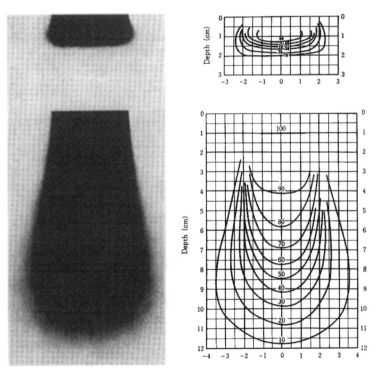

FIGURE 7-9
Photographic films (**left**) exposed "edge on" to 4- × 4-cm electron beams of a 4 MeV (**top**) and 26 MeV (**bottom**) at a source-film distance of 90 cm. Isodose curves (**right**) were measured densitometrically. The film is Sakura Konolitho contact film. (From Hendee, W. R. *Medical Radiation Physics*, 1st edition. Chicago, Mosby–Year Book, 1970. Courtesy of Shimadzu Seisakusho Ltd., an Medical Services Division, Westinghouse Electric Corp.)

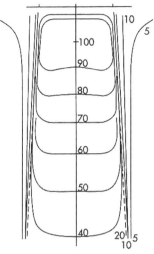

MARGIN FIGURE 7-14
Isodose curves for 20-MV x rays (10 × 10 cm², 100-cm SSD). (From Hendee, W. R. *Medical Radiation Physics,* 1st edition. Chicago, Mosby–Year Book, 1970.)

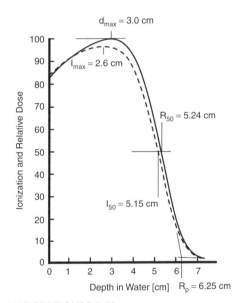

MARGIN FIGURE 7-15
Ionization and dose as a function of depth for a nominal 12-MeV electron beam. The locations of I_{50}, R_{50}, R_p, I_{max}, and d_{max} are shown. The ionization measurements incorporated a shift towards the surface of 0.5 r_{cav}.

■ SUMMARY

- Percent depth dose ($\%D_n$) is the ratio of dose at depth to dose at the surface, expressed as a percentage for a constant SSD.
- $\%D_n$ is frequently used for calculating patient treatment times for treatments at fixed SSD.
- $\%D_n$ varies with beam energy, depth, field size, and SSD.
- Tissue/air ratio (TAR) is the ratio of dose at depth in tissue to the dose to an equilibrium mass of tissue suspended in air.
- TAR can be computed from $\%D_n$.
- Backscatter factor (BSF) is equivalent to the TAR at d_{max}.
- The scatter/air ratio (SAR) is determined by subtracting the zero field size TAR from the TAR for finite field size.
- The tissue/phantom ratio (TPR) is the ratio of dose at depth to dose at a reference depth.
- The tissue/maximum ratio (TMR) is a special case of TPR where the reference depth is set equal to the depth of d_{max}.
- Treatment time calculations for isocentric treatments are most easily performed using TAR, TPR, and TMR.
- Calculations for isocentric rotational treatments can also be performed with TAR, TPR or TMR.
- Isodose curves describe the distribution of dose in two dimensions.
- Isodose charts are useful tools to describe representative dose distributions for specific combinations of beam energy and field size.

PROBLEMS

7-1. The backscatter factor is 1.282 for a 7- × 7-cm x-ray beam with an HVL of 1.0-mm Cu. What is the percent backscatter? What is the absorbed dose at the surface of a patient for an exposure to 105 R (f-factor = 0.957).

7-2. The backscatter factor is 1.256 for a 7- × 7-cm x-ray beam with an HVL of 1.5-mm Cu. Estimate the backscatter factor for a 7- × 7-cm x-ray beam with an HVL of 1.2-mm Cu.

7-3. The $\%D_n$ is 70.7 at 9-cm depth for a particular 6-MV x-ray beam. What dose is required at the 1.5-cm d_m to deliver 250 cGy to a tumor at 9-cm depth?

7-4. Determine the treatment time (MU setting) to deliver 200 cGy to a tumor 8 cm below the surface of a patient exposed to a 10- × 10-cm 6-MV field at 100-cm SSD (see Table 7-3). The accelerator is calibrated to deliver 1 cGy/MU at d_m, 10- × 10-cm, 100-cm SSD. What is the dose per treatment at d_m? Determine the exit dose for a patient thickness of 20 cm.

7-5. Using Table 7-4, determine the contributions of primary and scattered radiation at 16-cm depth for a 10- × 10-cm field of 10-MV x rays (SSD = 100 cm).

7-6. Using Table 7-6, determine the equivalent square of an 8- × 14-cm 10-MV x-ray beam. Estimate the absorbed dose delivered by this field at the depth of maximum dose and at the beam exit surface of a patient receiving 200 cGy to a tumor at 10-cm depth. The patient is 26 cm thick and the SSD is 100 cm.

7-7. At a depth of 10 cm and an SSD of 100 cm, the $\%D_n$ is 67.0 for a 10- × 10-cm beam of 6-MV x rays. The $\%D_n$ for the field increases to 70.6 if the SSD is increased to 150 cm. What change in MU setting is required to deliver the same dose at 10-cm depth with the increased SSD?

7-8. The tissue/maximum ratio is 0.756 for an 8- × 8-cm beam of 6-MV x rays with 10 cm of overlying tissue. If the dose rate at d_{max} is 1.009 cGy/mu at the axis of rotation, what is the dose rate at the rotational axis of an 8- × 8-cm beam with 10 cm of overlying tissue? Determine the meter setting to deliver 200 cGy at the rotational axis (the *isocenter*).

7-9. Determine the time required to deliver 200 cGy with a ^{60}Co γ-ray beam 6 × 6 cm^2 in area at the isocenter positioned at the center of a water-filled cylinder with a radius of 11 cm. The dose rate is 61.3 cGy/min at the isocenter in air. What speed of rotation in rpm should be selected if four complete revolutions are desired per treatment.

7-10. Determine the tissue/air ratio for a 7.5- × 7.5-cm beam of 4-MV x rays at 100-cm SAD, with 16 cm of tissue between the axis rotation and the surface. The $\%D_n$ at 16-cm depth is 37.8 for a 6- × 6-cm field at 80-cm SSD, and the backscatter factor is 1.01.

7-11. At 10-cm depth, $\%D_n = 58.5$ for a 10- × 10-cm ^{60}Co beam at 80-cm SSD. Estimate $\%D_n$ at 10-cm depth for a 10- × 10-cm ^{60}Co beam at 100-cm SSD.

REFERENCES

1. Krönig, B., and Friedrick, W. *The Principles and Physics of Radiation Therapy.* English edition by Dr. Henry Schmitz. New York, Rebman Co., 1922.

2. Quimby, E. H., Copeland, M. M., and Woods, R. C. The distribution of Roentgen rays within the human body. *Am. J. Roentgenol. Rad. Ther.* 1934; **32**:534.

3. Failla, G., Quimby, E. H., and Dean, A. Some problems of radiation therapy. *Am. J. Roentgenol.* 1922; **9**:479–497.

4. Failla, G., and Quimby, E. H. The economics of dosimetry in therapy. *Am. J. Roentgenol. Rad. Ther.* 1923; **10**:944.

5. Mayneord, W. V. Experimental and theoretical studies in x-ray intensity measurement. II. Distribution of x-rays within an irradiated medium. *Br. J. Radiol. New Ser.* 1929; **2**:267–296.

6. Ibbott, G. S., Professional Roles in Vascular Brachytherapy, AAPM Summer School Proceedings, July 2000 Madison, WI, Medical Physics Publishing Co.

7. Holfelder, H. The underlying principles in the radiotherapy of malignant tumors at the surgical clinic of Professor Schmieden of the University of Frankfort. *Am. J. Roentgenol.* 1922; **9**:341–346.

8. Sterling, T., Perry, H., and Katz, L. Automation of radiation treatment planning. IV. Derivation of a mathematical expression for the percent depth dose surface of cobalt 60 beams and visualization of multiple field dose distributions. *Br. J. Radiol.* 1964; **37**:544–550.

9. Tailor, R. C., Tello, V. M., Schroy, C. B., Vossler, M., and Hanson, W., A generic off-axis energy correction for linac photon beam dosimetry. *Med. Phys.* 1998; **25**(5):662–667.

10. Mayneord, W., and Lamerton, L. A survey of depth dose data. *Br. J. Radiol.* 1941; **14**:255–264.

11. Kron, T., and Ostwalk, P. Skin exit dose in megavoltage x-ray beams determined by means of a plane parallel ionization chamber (Attix chamber). *Med. Phys.* 1995; **22**(5):577–578.

12. Central axis depth dose data for use in radiotherapy. *Br. J. Radiol.* 1961; **34**(suppl 11):1–114. 1972; **45**(suppl 17):1–147. 1983; **56**(suppl 25):1–148.

13. Johns, H. E., and Cunningham, J. R. *The Physics of Radiology,* 4th edition. Springfield IL., Charles C Thomas, 1983.

14. Khan, F. M. *The Physics of Radiation Therapy.* Baltimore, Williams & Wilkins, 1984.

15. International Commission of Radiation Units and Measurements. *Determination of absorbed dose in a patient irradiated by beams of x- or γ rays in radiotherapy procedures,* Recommendations of ICRU, Report 24, Washington, DC, 1976.

16. Burns, J. Conversion of percentage depth doses from one FSD to another, and calculation of tissue/air ratios. *Br. J. Radiol.* 1961; **34**(suppl 10):83–85.

17. Day, M. The equivalent field method for axial dose determinations in rectangular fields, *Br. J. Radiol.* 1961; **34**(suppl 10):95–100.

18. Jani, S. K. *Handbook of Dosimetry Data for Radiotherapy,* Boca Raton, FL, CRC Press, 1993.

19. Clarke, H. C. A contouring device for use in radiation treatment planning, *Br. J. Radiol.* 1969; **42**:858–860.

20. Hills, J. F., Jr, Ibbott, G. S., Hendee, W. R. Computerized patient contours using the scanning arm of compound B-scanner, *Med. Phys.* 1979; **6**:309–311.

21. Clayton, C., and Thompson, D. An optical apparatus for reproducing surface outlines of body cross-sections, *Br. J. Radiol.* 1970; **43**:489–492.

22. Carson, P. L., Wenzel, W., Avery, P., and Hendee, W. R. Ultrasound imaging as an aid to cancer therapy—a review. Part I *Int. J. Radiat. Oncol. Biol. Phys.* 1975; **1**:119–132.

23. Carson, P. L., Wenzel, W. Avery, P., and Hendee, W. R. Ultrasound imaging as an aid to cancer therapy—a review. Part II, *Int. J. Radiat. Oncol. Biol. Phys.* 1976; **1**:335–343.

24. Khan, F. M., and Potish, R. A. *Treatment Planning in Radiation Oncology.* Baltimore, Williams & Wilkins, 1989.

25. Karzmark, C. J., Deubert, A., and Loevinger, R. Tissue phantom ratios—an aid to treatment planning. *Br. J. Radiol.* 1965; **38**:158–159.

26. Holt, J. G., Laughlin, J. S., and Moroney, J. P. The extension of the concept of tissue-air ratios (TAR) to high energy x-ray beams. *Radiology.* 1970; **96**:437–446.

27. Hope, C., and Walters, J. The computation of single and multiple field depth doses for 4 MV x-rays. *Phys. Med. Biol.* 1964; **9**:517–519.

28. Jayaraman, A., and Lanzl, L. *Clinical Radiotherapy Physics*, Vol. II. Boca Raton FL, CRC Press, 1996.

29. International Commission on Radiation Units and Measurements: *Determination of absorbed dose in a patient irradiated by beams of x- or γ rays in radiotherapy procedures,* ICRU Report 24, 1976, 11.

30. Hamilton, M., Laurie, J., and Orr, J. Dose gradient vectors in 4 MV x-ray treatment planning, *Br. J. Radiol.* 1968; **41**:687–691.

31. Hope, C., and Orr, J. Computer optimization of 4 MeV treatment planning. *Phys. Med. Biol.* 1965; **10**:365–373.

32. International Electrotechnical Commission. *Particular requirements for the safety of electron accelerators in the range 1 MeV to 50 MeV,* IEC International Standard 60601-2-1, 2nd edition, 1998.

33. AAPM TG25, Clinical electron-beam dosimetry. *Med. Phys.* 1991; **18**:73–109.

34. Webster, E., and Tsien, K. *Atlas of Isodose Distributions,* Vol. I. *Single-Isodose Charts.* Vienna, International Atomic Energy Agency, 1965.

8

TREATMENT PLANNING BY MANUAL METHODS

OBJECTIVES 158

POINT DOSE CALCULATIONS 158

Percent Depth Dose, TAR or TMR 158
Treatment Unit Calibration 159

TREATMENT AT STANDARD SSD 160

TREATMENT UNDER ISOCENTRIC CONDITIONS 161

ISODOSE DISTRIBUTIONS FOR MULTIPLE FIELDS 162

Isodose Distributions for Two Opposing Fields 162
Isodose Distributions for Isocentric Beam Arrangements 163
Isodose Distributions for Multiple Opposing Fields 163
Isodose Distributions for Fields at Angles Other than 180° 164

DOSE CALCULATIONS FOR IRREGULAR FIELDS 166

OBLIQUE INCIDENCE AND IRREGULAR BEAM SURFACE 168

Bolus 169
Compression Cones 169
Tissue-Compensating Filters 169

CORRECTIONS FOR OBLIQUE INCIDENCE
AND SURFACE IRREGULARITY 170

Effective SSD Method 170
Ratio of TARs Method 171

EFFECTS OF TISSUE INHOMOGENEITIES 172

Photon Beams 172
Electron Beams 172

CORRECTION FOR THE PRESENCE OF INHOMOGENEITIES 173

Photon Beams 173
Electron Beams 178

SEPARATION OF ADJACENT FIELDS 179

INTEGRAL DOSE 180

DOSE SPECIFICATION FOR EXTERNAL BEAM THERAPY 181

Treatment Volumes 182
Recommendations for Reporting Dose 183

SUMMARY 184

PROBLEMS 185

REFERENCES 185

Radiation Therapy Physics, Third Edition, by William R. Hendee, Geoffrey S. Ibbott, and Eric G. Hendee
ISBN 0-471-39493-9 Copyright © 2005 John Wiley & Sons, Inc.

■ OBJECTIVES

By studying this chapter, the reader will be able to:

- Identify and explain the beam parameters used for patient dose calculations.
- Perform patient dose calculations for dosimetric conditions commonly found in the clinic.
- Apply the most appropriate computational methods for each patient treatment configuration.
- Perform manual summation of isodose distributions for multiple field arrangements.
- Perform simple corrections for the presence of heterogeneities.
- Determine the separation necessary for adjacent fields.
- Calculate the integral dose.

Manual calculations fall into two broad categories: point calculations and dose distributions. Today, it is unusual for dose distributions to be prepared by manual methods, because these techniques are extremely time-consuming and computers are almost universally available. On the other hand, manual methods of point dose calculations are used frequently. Manual methods may be required when unusual calculations are necessary, such as the determination of dose at an unusual treatment distance. It is not uncommon for a dose calculation to be required quickly, and under circumstances that make "firing up" the computer impractical. For the most part, calculations of treatment time (for accelerators, *monitor units* [MU] or *meter settings*) performed by computer follow the same procedure as manual methods. Hence, an understanding of manual methods is essential.

Even in departments where computers are routinely used to calculate meter settings, manual methods must be used as part of a regular Quality Assurance program to verify the continued accuracy of computer calculations.

■ POINT DOSE CALCULATIONS

Calculations of dose at a point are performed for two purposes: to determine the meter setting to carry out a prescription and to determine the dose at points other than the location where the dose was prescribed. The calculations may consider irregularities in the field shape or tissue composition, although such corrections are often complex and time-consuming when performed manually.

The data required for point calculations depend on the complexity of the calculation being performed, the manner in which the patient is being treated, and the way in which the treatment unit was calibrated. These differences can be handled in a systematic fashion; it is not necessary or appropriate to learn a "different" method for each situation. Rather, it is preferable to learn the relationship between the different procedures and to be able to use the most convenient procedure for any clinical situation.

Dosimetric parameters such as $\%D_n$, TAR, and TMR and their interrelationships are described in Chapter 7.

Percent Depth Dose, TAR or TMR

All dose calculations require some means of describing the effect of overlying tissue above the calculation point. Unless the point of interest is at the depth of maximum dose (d_m), a method of correcting for attenuation and scatter in the overlying tissue must be used. The method chosen generally depends on the type of treatment. For treatments delivered at a customary source-to-skin distance (SSD), the use of percent depth dose ($\%D_n$) is often most convenient. If the point of interest is located at the isocenter (isocentric setup), the dose may be easily calculated with either tissue/air ratios (TARs) or tissue/maximum ratios (TMRs).

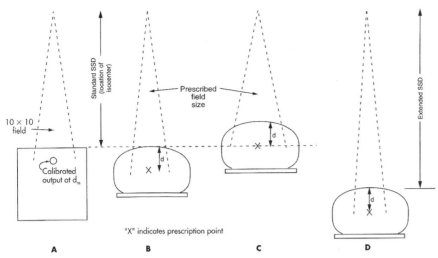

FIGURE 8-1

Comparison between calibration conditions and treatment conditions. **A:** Calibration is frequently performed to provide the machine output in terms of dose rate at d_m in water for a 10- × 10-cm field at the standard *SSD*. **B:** Treatment at the same SSD as the calibration. The depth of the prescription point is usually greater than d_m. The prescribed field size is defined at the patient's surface. **C:** Treatment using isocentric positioning. The prescribed field size is defined at the isocenter. **D:** Treatment at an extended SSD. The prescribed field size may be defined at the patient's surface or at the depth of the prescription point.

Treatment Unit Calibration

The procedure used for calibrating the treatment unit must be known before meter setting calculations can be performed. This is necessary because the prescribed dose must be related to the measured dose rate at some reference point. The calibration may consider scattered radiation from a patient or phantom, or it may be performed in a way that excludes such scatter, by measuring the dose rate in air. The location of the measurement point must also be known; it is typically located at the isocenter, or at the nominal treatment distance plus the depth d_m. Its location frequently is different for each beam energy from multimodality treatment units. Likewise, the field size in which the beam is calibrated must be known; it is usually chosen to be 10 × 10 cm.

Most megavoltage units are calibrated in accordance with one of several national or international protocols. In the United States, physicists generally follow the protocol of the American Association of Physicists in Medicine (AAPM).[1] This protocol requires that the calibration be performed in a phantom composed of water, and that the output of the treatment unit be stated in terms of the dose to water or muscle at d_m. In some institutions, cobalt units and low-energy x-ray machines are calibrated in air, and the output is stated in terms of the dose to a small mass of tissue suspended in air. The different methods of calibrating beams were discussed in Chapter 6.

Regardless of the means of calibration, and of the technique used for treatment, calculation of the meter setting requires that the intended dose at the prescription point must be related to the calibrated dose rate under *calibration conditions* (Figure 8-1). Adjustments must be made for any difference in distance from the source to the calibration point and to the prescription point, and corrections must also be made for changes in field size and depth in tissue.

The above discussion can be summarized by the following equation:

$$\text{Meter setting} = \frac{\text{Prescribed dose related to calibration conditions}}{\text{Calibration dose rate}}$$

where the *prescribed dose* is expressed in units such as cGy, and the *calibration dose rate* is expressed in cGy/MU or cGy/minute. The meter setting will be in corresponding

It is rare today for treatment units to be calibrated in air. Calibration protocols require that all but very low energy beams be calibrated in a water phantom. However, many departments convert an in-phantom measurement to an in-air dose rate, to enable the use of TARs in treatment time calculations. This facilitates the handling of scatter when calculating dose in complex field shapes.

Treatment at a standard SSD is rather unusual today, because *isocentric* techniques offer advantages when multiple fields are treated. However, standard SSD techniques are used for single field treatments with x-ray or electron beams, and extended SSDs may be used when a larger field dimension is required as for treatment of the spinal axis.

The term *given dose* is archaic but is used in many departments to describe the dose delivered to the depth of dose maximum. Its use stems from the early days of radiation therapy during which doses were customarily prescribed at the surface. It was understood that the dose to the target volume was lower, but the prescribed dose determined the treatment time and therefore was the *given dose*.

The *corrected field size* is the field size measured at the patient's surface and adjusted for the presence of shielding. A simple method of accounting for minor alterations in field shape was described in Chapter 7. The ratio of area/perimeter is calculated for the clinical field. Beam characteristics are then similar to those of a square field having the same area/perimeter.

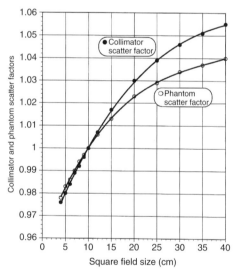

MARGIN FIGURE 8-1
Representative normalized collimator scatter factors (S_c) and normalized phantom scatter factors (S_p) plotted as a function of field edge for square fields. Data for 6-MV linac.

When field-shaping is accomplished through the use of customized or standard shielding blocks, the treated field size will generally be smaller than the collimator setting. If extended treatment distances are used, the treated field size may be larger than the collimator setting.

units (MU or minutes). Relating the prescribed dose to the calibration conditions may require the use of the inverse-square ratio, corrections for differences in field size and shape, and a correction for tissue attenuation. Examples of several situations follow.

■ TREATMENT AT STANDARD SSD

Whenever a patient is treated at a fixed *SSD* (typically 80 cm or 100 cm) the following equations can be used for calculating the meter setting:

$$\text{Meter setting} = \frac{\text{Given dose}}{\text{Dose rate at } d_m}$$

where

$$\text{Given dose} = \frac{(\text{Prescribed dose at depth})(100)}{(\% D_n)}$$

$\% D_n$ was defined in Chapter 7 and represents the percent depth dose. The percent depth dose is obtained from a table of values for the depth of interest, the SSD used for treatment, and the equivalent square of the corrected field size. Representative values of percent depth dose for 6-MV x rays are shown in Table 7-3.

From the dose specified at the prescription point, the dose at the calibration point can be computed. So long as the dose rate at the calibration point is known for the same field size and SSD, the meter setting can be determined. Changes in field size from the calibration field size require that the ratio of collimator factors and peakscatter factors be used. The nomenclature used here has evolved into widespread use in the United States.[2]

Variations in dose rate with collimator setting are described by the *normalized collimator scatter factor S_c*, and changes due to the irradiated field size at the location of the patient are described by the *normalized phantom scatter factor*, S_p. Note that S_p is also the normalized peak scatter factor (NPSF). A representative graph of S_c and S_p is shown in Margin Figure 8-1. The relationship between doses at points at equal distance from the source, but under conditions of different collimator settings or field size, is described by ratios of these parameters.

The dose rate $\dot{D}_m$ at d_m is computed as

$$\dot{D}_m = \dot{D}_c \cdot S_c \cdot S_p \cdot F$$

where:

$\dot{D}_c$ is the *calibration dose rate*, normally the dose rate at d_m in a 10- × 10-cm field at the standard treatment distance. When the conventional SSD is used for treatment, $\dot{D}_c = 1.0$ cGy/MU. An inverse square correction, or another measured value, must be used for nonstandard treatment distances (Figure 8-1).

S_c is the *collimator scatter factor*, or relative primary dose rate normalized to a 10- × 10-cm field. The collimator factor represents the effect of collimator setting (but not that of backscattered radiation) on the dose rate at d_m. The equivalent-square of the collimator setting is used. For electron beams, this term may describe the *applicator factor*, the relative dose rate as a function of electron applicator size.

S_p is the *phantom scatter factor*, or relative peakscatter factor normalized to a 10- × 10-cm field. The equivalent-square of the corrected field size at the patient surface is used. For electron beams, this term may be used to reflect changes in the dose rate due to the use of customized field shaping.

F is the product of the transmission factors of all beam-modifying devices.

Example 8-1

A patient is to receive a dose of 100 cGy at 8-cm depth through a 7- × 7-cm field of 6-MV x rays. An SSD of 100 cm will be used, and it was also used for calibration. No attenuating devices will be used. The output at d_m in a 7- × 7-cm field was measured to be 0.989 cGy/MU.

From Table 7-3 the percent depth dose at 8-cm depth in a 7- × 7-cm field is 73.2%. The product $\dot{D}_c \cdot S_c \cdot S_p$ was measured and is 0.989 cGy/MU. $F = 1.000$. Therefore,

$$\text{Meter setting} = \frac{100 \text{ cGy}\left(\dfrac{100}{73.2\%}\right)}{(0.989 \text{ cGy/MU})(1.000)} = 138 \text{ MU}$$

The expressions given above may be combined to yield an equation for meter settings:

$$\text{Meter setting} = \frac{\text{Prescribed dose at depth} \cdot 100}{\%D_n \cdot \dot{D}_c \cdot S_c \cdot S_p \cdot F} \tag{8-1}$$

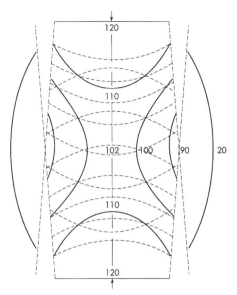

MARGIN FIGURE 8-2
Resultant isodose distribution for two opposing x-ray beams (6 × 6 cm², 3.0-mm Cu HVL, 50-cm SSD). The beam entrance surfaces are separated by 12 cm of tissue. (From Hendee, W. R. *Medical Radiation Physics*, 1ˢᵗ edition. Chicago, 1970, Mosby–Year Book. Used with permission.)

■ TREATMENT UNDER ISOCENTRIC CONDITIONS

Patients frequently are treated isocentrically, meaning that the location of interest to the physician is positioned at the axis of rotation of the treatment unit. Calculation of the meter setting for isocentric treatments is conducted according to the equation

$$\text{Meter setting} = \frac{\text{Prescribed dose at isocenter}}{\text{Dose rate at depth at isocenter}}$$

$$\text{Dose rate at depth of isocenter} = (\dot{D}_i)\,(\text{TMR})\,(S_c)\,(S_p)\,(F)$$

where

($\dot{D}_i$) is the *isocenter dose rate*. This is the *calibration dose rate* $\dot{D}_c$ adjusted from the location of d_m at the conventional SSD to the location of the isocenter, or SAD (Figure 8-1). Again, it represents the dose rate at the depth of maximum dose, in a 10- × 10-cm field. Generally,

$$\dot{D}_i = \dot{D}_c \left(\frac{\text{SSD} + d_m}{\text{SAD}}\right)^2$$

S_c is the *collimator scatter factor*, described earlier.
S_p is the *phantom scatter factor*, described earlier. However, this factor must be based on the equivalent-square of the corrected field size at the isocenter, not at the patient's surface.
TMR is the *tissue/maximum ratio*, for the depth of tissue overlying the isocenter and for the corrected field size as measured at the isocenter. Representative TMR values for 6-MV x rays are given in Table 7-8.
F is the product of the transmission factors of all beam-modifying devices.

For isocentric treatments, the corrected treatment field size is always less than or equal to the collimator setting.

These expressions may be combined as follows:

$$\text{Meter setting} = \frac{\text{Prescribed dose at isocenter}}{\dot{D}_c \cdot \left(\dfrac{\text{SSD}+d_m}{\text{SAD}}\right)^2 \cdot \text{TMR} \cdot S_c \cdot S_p \cdot F} \tag{8-2}$$

It is possible (although not always practical) to use $\%D_n$ values to compute the meter setting for isocentric treatments, or to use TMR values to compute settings for SSD treatments. One must simply ensure that (1) $\%D_n$ values are appropriate for the SSD being used for treatment and (2) an inverse-square correction is performed to relate the calibration dose rate to the proper reference point.

Example 8-2

A patient will be treated with 6-MV photons using an isocentric technique at 100-cm SAD. A dose of 90 cGy is to be delivered at the isocenter. A collimator setting of 12- ×

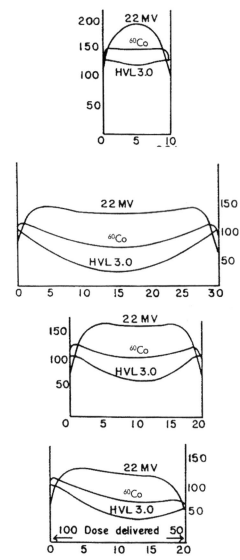

12-cm will be used, but blocking will reduce the effective field size to an equivalent-square field of 9 cm. The blocks are supported on a plastic tray with a transmission factor of 0.96. The isocenter depth will be 8 cm. Calibration was performed in a 10- × 10-cm field at 100-cm SSD, at $d_m = 1.5$ cm. The output under these conditions is 1.0 cGy/MU. Determine the meter setting.

From Margin Figure 8-1, the collimator setting of 12 × 12 cm² is used to determine $S_c = 1.004$. The blocked field size of 9 cm yields $S_p = 0.997$, and from Table 7-8 the TMR at 8 cm = 0.826. The tray transmission factor must also be placed in the denominator. Therefore,

$$\dot{D}_i = \dot{D}_c \left(\frac{100 + 1.5}{100} \right)^2 = 1.030 \text{ cGy/MU}$$

$$\text{Meter setting} = \frac{90 \text{ cGy}}{1.030 \text{ cGy/MU} \cdot 0.826 \cdot 1.004 \cdot 0.997 \cdot 0.96}$$

Meter setting = 110 MU.

◼ ISODOSE DISTRIBUTIONS FOR MULTIPLE FIELDS

Isodose distributions for single fields were described in Chapter 7. On rare occasions, a tumor may be treated adequately with radiation through a single field. More often, two or more fields are required to provide an acceptable distribution of absorbed dose within the patient. For a patient treated with multiple fields, a resultant dose distribution is constructed by adding the percent depth doses contributed to various locations by each field.

Today it is customary to use a computerized treatment planning system to calculate the dose distribution for multiple fields (Chapter 11). However, many computerized systems utilize methods essentially identical to manual techniques. Hence manual techniques can be discussed to illustrate computerized methods. As mentioned earlier, if a computer is unavailable, manual methods may be used to initiate the treatment of patients.

Isodose Distributions for Two Opposing Fields

Two x- or γ-ray beams "oppose" each other if they impinge on opposite sides of a patient and if the central axes of the beams coincide. Such field arrangements are generally called *parallel-opposed fields*. Parallel-opposed fields are diagrammed in Margin Figure 8-2. Orthovoltage beams are depicted in this figure to illustrate the superposition of parallel-opposed beams. Curves designated as 100 contain points where 100% is obtained by adding the percent depth dose contributed by each field. Tissue enclosed within these lines receives an absorbed dose at least equal to that delivered by either field at the depth of maximum dose. That is, an absorbed dose of at least 100 cGy is delivered to tissue in this region if 100 cGy is delivered by each x-ray beam at its depth of maximum dose.

An absorbed dose of at least 90 cGy is delivered to tissue enclosed within the 90% isodose curves. In this resultant isodose distribution, the central axis percent depth dose is highest at the surface and is lowest at the center of the patient. The percent depth dose decreases with depth more rapidly along the sides of the isodose distribution than along the superimposed central axes. As the energy of the radiation decreases or the thickness of the patient increases, the difference increases between the dose near the surface and that at the center of the treated volume. Depicted in Margin Figure 8-3 are the effects of radiation quality and patient thickness on the uniformity of absorbed dose along the superimposed central axes of two opposing fields.

Compared with opposing beams of orthovoltage x-rays, opposing fields of high-energy x or γ rays furnish a more uniform dose throughout the irradiated volume and

MARGIN FIGURE 8-3
Relative dose along the superimposed central axes of two opposing 6- × 8-cm fields separated by 10 cm, 20 cm, and 30 cm of tissue. Data are depicted for orthovoltage x rays (3.0-mm Cu HVL, 50-cm SSD), ^{60}Co γ rays (80-cm SSD), and 22-MV x rays (100-cm SSD). All curves except those in the bottom figure were constructed with the assumption that the percent depth dose is equal to 100 for each field at the depth of maximum dose. The distributions in the bottom figure were constructed with the assumption that the dose from the field on the right is only 50% of the dose from the field on the left. (From Johns, H., and Cunningham, J. *The Physics of Radiology,* 4th edition. Springfield, IL, Charles C. Thomas, 1983. Used with permission.)

provide an acceptable distribution of absorbed dose for patients of greater thickness. For the 6-MV beams described in Margin Figure 8-4, the percent depth dose along the common central axis does not vary greatly throughout the entire thickness of the patient. The percent depth dose along the borders of the resultant distribution is about 10% less than the relatively uniform dose along the common central axis.

Isodose distributions in Margin Figures 8-2 and 8-4 are plotted with the assumption that equal doses of radiation are delivered by each of the opposing fields (equal *given doses*) If the dose to one field is less than the dose to the opposite field, then the region of minimum dose within the patient is shifted toward the side which receives the lower dose. This shift is illustrated by the curves in the bottom panel of Margin Figure 8-3. The resultant isodose distribution for two opposing fields may be determined by manual methods even though a reduced dose is delivered to one field. Before the percent depth dose at selected points is determined, the isodose curves for the field that receives the lower dose are reduced by the quotient of the given doses. For example, if the upper field in Margin Figure 8-2 receives half the dose delivered to the lower field, then the values of the isodose curves for the upper field should be divided by two. With this method, the depth dose in the patient is expressed as a percent of the larger single field absorbed dose at the depth of maximum dose. Such an arrangement is called *unequal field weighting*. Common field weighting arrangements include 1.5:1 and 2:1.

Isodose Distributions for Isocentric Beam Arrangements

The use of isocentric positioning has been mentioned earlier (Chapter 7). Dosimetric advantages of isocentric treatment include the need for positioning the patient only once for each multiple-field treatment, and the possibility that small systematic errors in treatment distance indication are offset, particularly with parallel-opposing treatments. An example of a single-field isocentric isodose distribution was shown in Figure 7-6. When positioning a patient for an isocentric treatment using parallel-opposed fields, it is recommended that the isocenter be located at the patient's midplane.[3] The effect of offsetting the isocenter to one side is comparable to weighting the dose more heavily to that side, which distorts the dose distribution. It is tempting to position the isocenter at the center of an asymmetrically located tumor, but care should be taken to adjust the field weights if this is done.

Isodose Distributions for Multiple Opposing Fields

To increase the tumor dose relative to the dose to surrounding tissues, a patient may be treated with radiation through more than one pair of opposing fields. For example, the central areas in Margin Figure 8-5 represent regions of tissue where dose distributions from different fields add to yield a relatively uniform dose. By changing the size of the individual fields or their angle of incidence on the patient's surface, the size and shape of the region of uniform dose may be altered. An isodose distribution for two pairs of opposing fields is shown in Margin Figure 8-6. If the distances from the tumor to the beam entrance surfaces are not equal, then the radiation dose is not uniform throughout the lesion when equal doses are delivered to each surface. The uniformity of dose throughout the treated region may be improved by reducing the dose delivered to surfaces near the lesion. Care should be taken to avoid delivering unacceptably high doses near surfaces at some distance from the lesion.

To construct an isodose distribution for multiple fields by manual methods, the fields are divided into pairs and the distribution for each pair is determined. Next, distributions for paired fields are superimposed and the resultant distribution is constructed. The difficulty of this procedure increases rapidly as fields are added to the treatment plan. Fortunately, isodose distributions for multiple fields and for arc therapy may be constructed by computer. These constructions are accomplished by addition of doses from single-field isodose distributions stored in the computer as a matrix of digital dose data, or represented in the computer by mathematical formulae

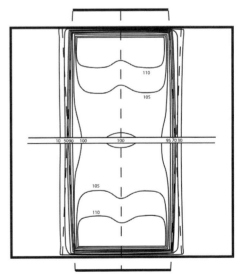

MARGIN FIGURE 8-4
Resultant isodose distribution for two opposing 6-MV x-ray fields (10- × 10-cm, 90-cm SSD). The beam entrance surfaces are separated by 20 cm of tissue. The percent depth dose is normalized to 100% at the center of the irradiated volume. Each beam delivers a dose of 94 cGy at the depth of maximum dose below the beam entrance surface.

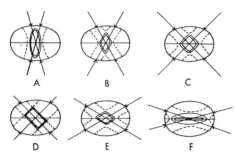

MARGIN FIGURE 8-5

Various arrangements of two opposing pairs of fields. The central area represents the region of uniform dose for each arrangement. (**A**) Two opposing pairs at 30° (**B**) two opposing pairs at 60°, (**C**) two opposing pairs at right angles; (**D**) two opposing pairs of different widths at right angles; (**E**) two opposing pairs at 120°, (**F**) two opposing pairs at 150°. (From Hendee, W. R. *Medical Radiation Physics*, 1st edition. Chicago, Mosby–Year Book, 1970. Used with permission.)

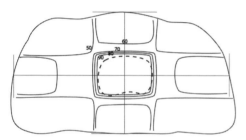

MARGIN FIGURE 8-6

Two pairs of opposing 8- × 6-cm and 6- × 6-cm 6-MV x-ray beams (SAD 100 cm) at right angles (a so-called *four-field box* plan). The percent depth dose is normalized to 100 at the intersection of the central axes. Each beam delivers a dose of 50 cGy at the isocenter.

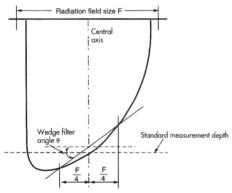

MARGIN FIGURE 8-7

Explanatory diagram for the definition of wedge filter angle indicating the location of measurement points used in the determination of wedge angle. The standard measurement depth is normally 10 cm. (Redrawn with permission from reference 4.)

which yield doses approximating the actual dose distribution (Chapter 11). Many of the multifield distributions in this chapter were constructed with a digital computer.

Composite isodose distributions such as those described in this chapter may be normalized to a dose of 100% in a variety of ways. Most often, they are normalized either to the point at which the beam central axes intersect, or at d_m for each field.

Example 8-3

Two opposing 10- × 10-cm 6-MV x-ray beams (100-cm SSD) are separated by 20 cm of tissue. The central axis percent depth dose is 67.0% at 10-cm depth and 42.4% at 18.5-cm depth for each of the x-ray beams. What is the percent variation between the dose on the central axis at the center of the irradiated volume and the central axis dose at the depth of maximum dose?

For a dose of 100 cGy from each field at the depth of maximum dose below each surface, the total dose at 1.5-cm depth is

$$\text{Total dose at depth of maximum dose} = 100 \text{ cGy} + (100 \text{ cGy})(42.4/100)$$

$$= 142.4 \text{ cGy}$$

The total dose at the center of the irradiated volume is

$$\text{Total dose at center} = 2 \cdot [(100 \text{ cGy})(67.0/100)]$$

$$= 134.0 \text{ cGy}$$

The percent variation between the dose at the center and the dose at the depth of maximum dose is

$$\% \text{ Variation} = \frac{(142.4 - 134.0) \text{ cGy}}{134.0 \text{ cGy}} \cdot 100$$

$$= 6.3\%$$

Isodose Distributions for Fields at Angles Other than 180°

If two fields are separated by an angle less than 180°, then a "hot spot" of increased dose is created in the volume of tissue irradiated by both fields (Figure 8-2, left). The uniformity of dose in the volume of interest is improved if a third field is added to the treatment plan (Figure 8-2, right). If the addition of a third field is undesirable, the fields may be aligned so that their central axes intersect slightly below the center of the target volume. By "past-pointing" the intersection of the central axes, the hot spot is moved to a position nearer to the center of the volume of interest. The percent depth dose decreases very rapidly above the hot spot. Therefore, the isodose distribution should be constructed with the axes past-pointed to verify that the distribution of radiation dose is satisfactory throughout the volume of interest.

For x- or γ-ray beams intersecting at angles less than 180°, hot spots may be reduced or eliminated by the use of wedge filters. Isodose distributions in Figure 8-3 were constructed for two 10 × 10 cm 6 MV x-ray beams separated by 60°. The improvement in dose uniformity that is achieved with wedge filters is illustrated by the distribution on the right. The hot spot has been reduced and the radiation dose is more uniform across the volume of tissue irradiated by both fields. As indicated in Figure 8-3, the thick edges (heels) of the wedges should be positioned facing each other.

As was noted in Chapter 7, the *wedge isodose angle* θ has been defined as the angle between the isodose curve passing through a selected depth (usually 10-cm depth) and a perpendicular line through the central axis. The International Electrotechnical Commission (IEC)[4] has defined the wedge angle θ as shown in Margin Figure 8-7. A measurement is made at 10-cm depth (or other appropriate depth) on the central axis, and additional measurements are made at points off axis a distance $F/4$, where F is the field width at the surface. Off-axis points at which the dose equals the dose

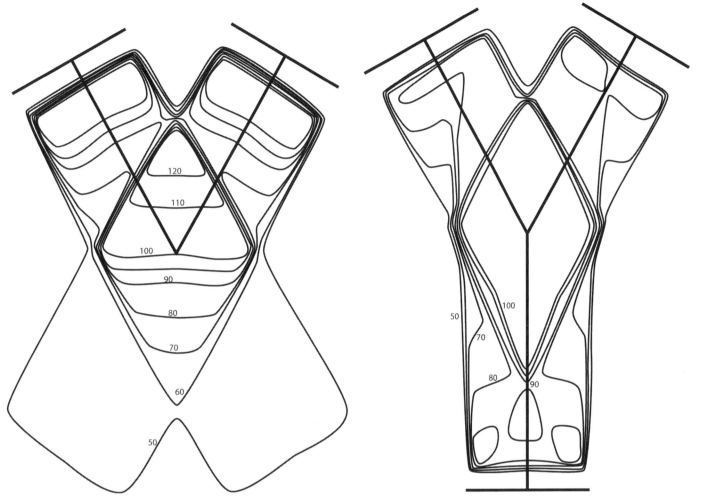

FIGURE 8-2
Left: A "hot spot" of increased dose produced by two fields which intersect at angles less than 180°. **Right:** The uniformity of dose is improved if a third field is added to the treatment plan. The hot spot created by two converging beams may be moved nearer to the center of the treated volume by past-pointing the intersection of the central axes of the converging beams. Distributions were constructed for 10- × 10-cm 6-MV x-ray beams. The percent depth dose is normalized to 100 at the location of maximum dose. In both distributions, each beam delivers a dose of 72 at the depth of maximum dose below the surface.

measured on the central axis are located. A straight line is drawn through points at $-F/4$ and $+F/4$, and its angle with a perpendicular through the central axis is the wedge angle θ. For higher energy x and γ rays, the wedge isodose angle θ that furnishes the most uniform distribution of radiation dose for two converging fields is $\theta = 90 - \phi/2$, where ϕ is the *hinge angle* between the two fields (Margin Figure 8-8).

For example, a 45° wedge filter (i.e., a wedge filter that provides an isodose distribution with a wedge isodose angle of 45°) should be used for fields separated by 90°, and 30° and 60° wedge filters should be used for fields separated by angles of 120° and 60°, respectively. Theoretically, a different wedge filter is required for every hinge angle between two converging fields. However, Sear[5] has demonstrated that a particular wedge filter usually furnishes an acceptable distribution of radiation dose over a fairly wide range of hinge angles. In the absence of more sophisticated treatment planning methods, a limited number of wedge filters may be used to satisfy the requirements of most treatment plans. Modern linear accelerators have the potential to generate wedged isodose distributions with virtually any wedge angle. However, utilizing such a variety of dose distributions effectively requires advanced treatment planning capabilities.

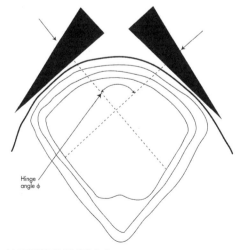

MARGIN FIGURE 8-8
Diagram of hinge angle ϕ. (From Hendee, W. R. *Medical Radiation Physics*, 1st edition. Chicago, 1970, Mosby–Year Book. Used with permission.)

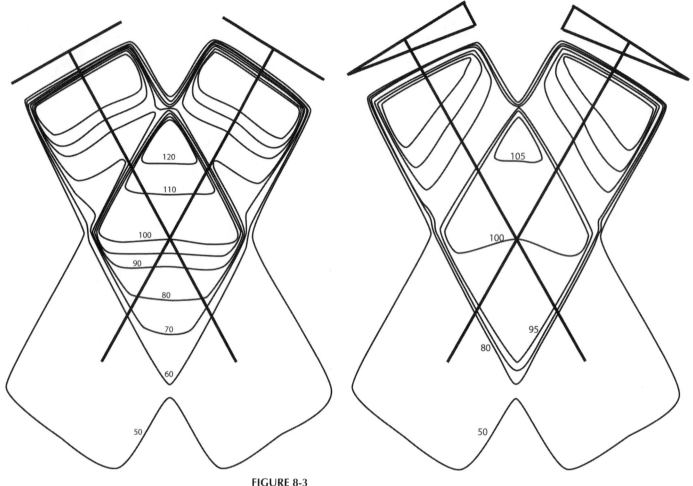

FIGURE 8-3
Two 10- × 10-cm 6-MV x-ray fields (65-cm SSD) at an angle of 60°. **Left:** The distribution exhibits a "hot spot" and a nonuniform dose across the treated volume. **Right:** In this distribution, the hot spot has been reduced with wedge filters.

The technique pioneered by Clarkson of separating the dose from primary and scattered radiation was published more than 60 years ago.[10] However, the "Clarkson scatter summation" technique is still used for manual calculations and is incorporated into several commercial treatment planning systems.

Wedge filters designed for one radiation unit should not be used with another. Wedge filters usually are not used for x rays generated below about 1 MV, because the effectiveness of a wedge filter for low-energy beams is altered greatly by slight changes in the position of the patient or the x-ray tube. Wedge filters usually are machined from brass or lead. The design and use of wedge filters are discussed extensively in the literature.[6-9]

In recent years, the use of wedge filters (now often called "hard wedges") has been discontinued in some clinics. Instead, one or both of a pair of collimator jaws is moved independently during irradiation to produce a dose distribution in which the isodose curves are tilted to a prescribed angle. This technique, called *dynamic wedge* or *virtual wedge*, eliminates the need to attach a filter to the accelerator, and it permits, in principle, the creation of dose distributions with any wedge angle.[9]

■ DOSE CALCULATIONS FOR IRREGULAR FIELDS

Large, irregularly shaped radiation fields such as mantle and inverted Y fields employed for treatment of conditions such as Hodgkin's disease present complex dosimetric problems that historically have been approached primarily with tissue/air ratios and scatter/air ratios. This approach was pioneered by Clarkson[10] and subsequently developed into the method outlined below. With this method, doses can be estimated with an accuracy of about 97% at all locations of the patient exposed to the primary beam.[11] Although the method is illustrated for a mantle field treatment of Hodgkin's disease, it is applicable to any situation requiring irregularly shaped fields. In the treatment of Hodgkin's disease, large fields (i.e., outside margins 30- × 30-cm and greater) of high-energy photons are employed in combination with shielding blocks to protect regions such as the lungs, esophagus, and gonads, where high doses are not desired. A mantle field for treatment of Hodgkin's disease above the diaphragm is illustrated in Margin Figure 8-9. In general, absorbed doses at locations of interest within a field such as that shown in Margin Figure 8-10 are computed by adding the dose contributions from scattered radiation to those from primary photons. These contributions are determined by using *zero area tissue/air ratios* to estimate the dose from primary radiation and *scatter/air ratios* to predict the dose from scattered radiation.

In many cases, the irregular-field treatment is conducted at a fixed SSD, and the calibration of the treatment beam has been conducted in a phantom. This situation therefore will be described, and common variations to the procedure will be mentioned.

Let D_c equal the central axis absorbed dose at the depth of dose maximum in a phantom for the calibration field size (normally 10×10 cm) and SSD (normally 100 cm). The in-air variation of output with field size relative to the calibration field size (described previously as the *normalized collimator scatter* factor) is S_c. The fractional transmission of photons through the tray supporting the beam-shaping blocks is F (if additional devices are present such as a wedge or compensating filter, F is the product of the fractional transmission factors of all devices). The tissue/air ratio at d_m (also the peak scatter factor) for the calibration field size is TAR_C. The normalized PSF, or S_p, cannot be used here. The product

$$D_1 = D_C \cdot S_C \cdot F \cdot \frac{1}{\text{TAR}_C}$$

represents the central axis absorbed dose D_1 for a small mass of tissue suspended in air at the source-to-calibration point distance (SCD = calibration SSD + d_m) for the field size employed for treatment, corrected for attenuation by the beam-shaping support platform or other device.

To estimate the dose D_2 in air at the distance from the source to the prescription point, an inverse-square correction must be employed:

$$D_2 = D_1 \left(\frac{\text{SCD}}{\text{SSD} + g + d} \right)^2$$

where SSD represents the source-skin distance on the central axis to be used for treatment, g is the separation between the SSD and the skin directly above the location of interest (g is negative if the skin above the location of interest is closer to the source than the skin on the central axis of the radiation beam), and d represents the depth of the prescription point within the patient. This correction may not be required if the calibration and treatment are both performed at the isocenter.

The dose at the point of interest is the sum of the dose contributions from primary and scattered radiation: $D_T = D_P + D_S$. To estimate the absorbed dose D_P in the patient due to primary radiation at the location of interest, the dose D_2 must be multiplied by

$$D_P = D_2 \cdot P \cdot \text{TAR}_{0,d}$$

where P is the *primary off-axis factor*, or the variation in the primary beam intensity away from the central axis. For calculation of dose at points under blocks, P is multiplied by the block transmission factor. $\text{TAR}_{0,d}$ is the tissue/air ratio at depth d for zero field size and is obtained by extrapolation from TAR tables. For the scatter contribution D_S to absorbed dose at the location of interest within the patient, the dose D_2 is multiplied by SAR_{avg}, the average scatter/air ratio at depth d for the treatment field involved: $D_S = D_2 \cdot \text{SAR}_{\text{avg}}$. Determination of SAR_{avg} is described below.

The total dose is determined by summing the primary and scatter components. Consequently, the entire computation for the total dose D_T delivered to the location

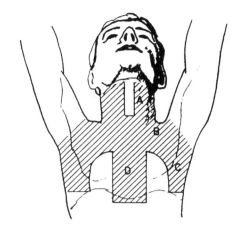

MARGIN FIGURE 8-9
Typical high-energy photon mantle field for supradiaphragmatic treatment of Hodgkin's disease. Absorbed doses usually are computed at regions A through D, corresponding to cervical, supraclavicular, axillary, and mediastinal lymph nodes, respectively. Stippled areas represent irradiated regions; clear areas designate regions (primarily the lungs and esophagus) shielded from primary radiation.

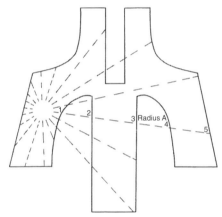

MARGIN FIGURE 8-10
Method for determining S_{avg} over all radii emanating from the location of interest. For each radius, the net scatter/air ratio is obtained by subtracting the sum of scatter/air ratios from boundaries on the far side of unshielded regions. Shielded regions are assumed to contribute no scattered radiation.

The symbols D_c and $\dot{D}_c$ are used in the text to represent the dose and dose rate, respectively, under calibration conditions. These reference conditions are typically a 10- × 10-cm field at 100-cm SSD, and depth = d_{max}. When D_c is used, the reader may mentally substitute the product of $\dot{D}_c$ and a treatment time or MU setting.

If the treatment unit is calibrated in air (a practice not recommended for energies higher than ^{60}Co), D_1 may be a measured quantity.

of interest is

$$D_T = D_C \cdot S_C \cdot F \cdot \frac{1}{\text{TAR}_C} \cdot \left(\frac{\text{SCD}}{\text{SSD} + g + d} \right)^2 \left(P \cdot \text{TAR}_{0,d} + \text{SAR}_{\text{avg}} \right) \qquad \text{(8-3)}$$

In Equation (8-3) the size of the radiation field is determined at the depth of maximum dose near the surface rather than at the depth of interest. Furthermore, the depth d is taken as a vertical depth rather than as a depth parallel to the diverging rays from the source of radiation. Each of these simplifications contributes a small error to the computation of D_T. However, the errors tend to cancel each other so that the net error is negligible in almost all situations.

The scatter-air ratio SAR is determined by extrapolating the TAR at the depth of interest to zero field size ($r = 0$). The $\text{TAR}_{0,d}$ is subtracted from the $\text{TAR}_{r,d}$ to yield the $\text{SAR}_{r,d}$.

Example 8-4

Determine the net scatter-air ratio (SAR) for radius A in Margin Figure 8-10.

Location	Distance	(+) SAR	(−) SAR
1	2.8	0.107	—
2	7.2	—	0.202
3	13.4	0.266	—
4	18.2	—	0.295
5	24.1	0.313	—
		Sum (+) SAR = 0.686	Sum (−) SAR = 0.497
			NetSAR = 0.189

To determine the average scatter/air ratio SAR_{avg}, radii at selected angular increments are drawn from the location of interest to the margins of the treatment field, as depicted in Margin Figure 8-10. Along a particular radius, distances are measured from the location of interest to intersections of the radius with boundaries separating irradiated from shielded tissue, and the scatter/air ratios are determined and summed for these distances (Margin Figure 8-10). For each radius, the sum of scatter/air ratios for unirradiated tissue is subtracted from the sum of the scatter/air ratios for irradiated tissue to yield a net scatter-air ratio for the radius. This process is repeated for each radius, and the net scatter-air ratios are then averaged over all radii. This value of SAR_{avg} is used in Equation (8-3).

The computational method for D_T is accurate to within about 3% in all anatomic regions except those in or near the shadow of shielding blocks. For these regions, more elaborate methods of dose computation are required. The approach described above for dose computations for irregularly shaped fields has been programmed for computer solution, thereby greatly simplifying its application to the complex geometric configurations often encountered in the treatment of lymphoma and other special treatment situations (see Chapter 11).[12]

◼ OBLIQUE INCIDENCE AND IRREGULAR BEAM SURFACE

Isodose curves are usually measured in a water-filled phantom with its surface perpendicular to the incident radiation. When these data are used to determine the distribution of radiation dose within a patient, corrections should be applied to compensate for differences between the water phantom and the patient. Some of the corrections used most frequently are discussed in this chapter.

Treatment planning computers are found in most radiation therapy departments today. Consequently, corrections to isodose distributions to account for patient geometry rarely are made using manual methods. However, an understanding of manual methods is valuable to appreciate the benefits, as well as the limitations, of computerized treatment planning.

In clinical practice, the radiation beam rarely impinges directly upon a flat surface. Instead, the distance from the radiation source to the beam entrance surface often varies significantly from one side of the beam to the other. This variation introduces differences in the dose delivered to locations in the patient that are equidistant from the radiation source, because the locations are below different thicknesses of overlying tissue. To eliminate distortion in an isodose distribution caused by oblique incidence of the radiation beam or by an irregular beam entrance surface, bolus or a tissue-compensating filter may be introduced into the x- or γ-ray beam.

Bolus

Today, bolus is used with megavoltage photon and electron beams to increase the surface dose or to correct for irregular surface contours. On occasion, a surgical defect such as that resulting from ophthalmic enucleation may be filled with a tissue-equivalent bolus. The bolus produces a nearly flat surface over an almost homogenous volume, greatly simplifying calculations and facilitating uniform dose delivery. This practice also ensures that superficial tissues in contact with the bolus receive a full dose, because skin-sparing is eliminated.

Bolus may be used with electron beams to raise the surface dose or to decrease the depth of penetration of the beam. Margin Figure 8-11 illustrates the depth dose curve for a 6-MeV electron beam incident upon 1 cm of bolus covering tissue. The dose at the tissue surface is increased to nearly 100%, and the depth of the 80% dose level is raised from approximately 2 cm to roughly 1 cm.

Bolus can also be used to force an isodose line to conform to patient anatomy. In Margin Figure 8-12, bolus has been placed on the chest wall to bring the 80% isodose line to the level of the chest wall.[13]

Compression Cones

With low-energy x or γ rays, which do not exhibit a skin-sparing effect, a closed-end cone sometimes is pressed against the patient's skin where the beam of x or γ rays enters. The pressure forces tissue into air gaps under the cone and provides a flat surface for the entering beam. These cones are known as compression cones and may be used when tissue is pliable under the beam entrance surface. When a *compression cone* is used, the percent depth dose should be obtained from data tabulated for a "closed-end" cone. If these data are not available, then data for an open-end applicator may be used by increasing the depth of all locations in the phantom by an amount equal to the tissue-equivalent thickness of the end of the compression cone.[14] Compression cones are rarely used today, because orthovoltage x-ray beams are generally used only for treatment of superficial diseases.

Tissue-Compensating Filters

Using bolus with high-energy x or γ radiation places the region of dose buildup in the bolus rather than in the superficial tissue of the patient. Consequently, the skin-sparing advantage of the high-energy radiation is reduced or lost. For high-energy radiation, a tissue-compensating filter may be used in place of the bolus to "flatten" the beam entrance surface.[15,16] Usually, the filter is constructed from aluminum, brass, lead, wax, or metal-impregnated rubber or gypsum mixtures.[17] To reduce the electron contamination of the x- or γ-ray beam to a negligible level, the tissue-compensating filter is positioned some distance above the patient's skin (15–20 cm or more for megavoltage radiation).[18] The procedure for constructing a tissue compensating filter includes the following steps[19]:

1. The highest point on the beam entrance surface (within the field margins) is placed at the SSD desired. In the case of isocentric treatments, the patient's position is not changed, but the SSD to the level of the highest point within the field margins is recorded.

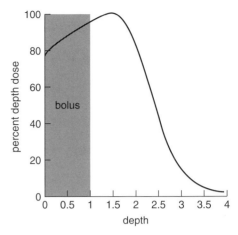

MARGIN FIGURE 8-11
Depth dose curve for a 6-MeV electron beam. Placing 1 cm of bolus on the skin surface shifts the percent depth dose towards the surface.

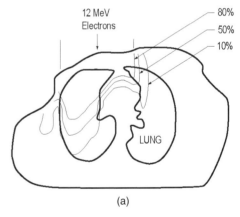

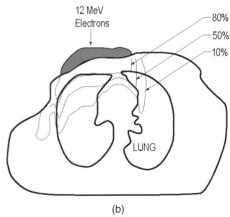

MARGIN FIGURE 8-12
The use of bolus to compensate for changing tissue thickness overlying sensitive healthy tissue. **Top:** Without bolus. **Bottom:** With bolus.

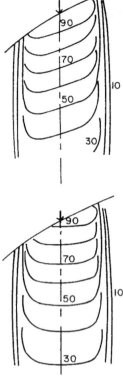

MARGIN FIGURE 8-13
Isodose distribution for a 10- × 10-cm ^{60}Co beam (80-cm SSD) measured in water-filled phantom with an irregular surface. **Top:** Without a Tissue-Compensating filter. **Bottom:** After the filter has been inserted into the beam. (From Hendee, W. R. *Medical Radiation Physics*, 1st edition. Chicago, Mosby–Year Book, 1970. Used with permission.)

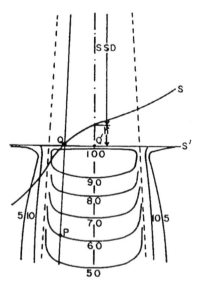

MARGIN FIGURE 8-14
The effective source-surface distance method for estimating the absorbed dose at location P in a medium with an irregular surface S. (From Hendee, W. R. *Medical Radiation Physics*, 1st edition. Chicago, Mosby–Year Book, 1970. Used with permission.)

2. All distances for which compensation is desired are measured at selected intervals across the beam entrance surface.
3. Thicknesses of compensating material, equivalent to the missing tissue, are determined. These thicknesses are slightly different from the air distances multiplied by the ratio of the linear attenuation coefficients of soft tissue to attenuator material, because scattering conditions for the compensator are different from those for the tissue which it is replacing. For this reason, the thickness of compensator material equivalent to a given thickness of tissue should be determined experimentally.[16,20] The radiation beam diverges with distance from the radiation source. Hence, the lateral dimensions of the compensating filter are shorter than the field size of the radiation beam at the patient's surface. For example, if the SSD is 80 cm and the filter is positioned 20 cm above the surface, then the lateral dimensions of the filter are three-fourths of the corresponding sides of the radiation field at the surface. In Margin Figure 8-13, isodose curves measured in a water-filled phantom with an irregular surface are shown for a ^{60}Co beam with and without a tissue-compensating filter.

■ CORRECTIONS FOR OBLIQUE INCIDENCE AND SURFACE IRREGULARITY

If the effects of surface irregularity and oblique incidence are not compensated with bolus, a compression cone, or a tissue-compensating filter, then the radiation dose to selected locations within the patient can be calculated by computer or estimated by one of the two manual methods outlined below. For ^{60}Co γ rays and megavoltage x rays, these methods are satisfactory for angles up to about 45° between the central axis of the radiation beam and a line perpendicular to the beam entrance surface. Both methods require the use of isodose charts, which are rarely found in radiation therapy departments today. The methods are presented here for historical interest, but also because they illustrate some of the simpler techniques still used by modern treatment planning systems.

Effective SSD Method

In Margin Figure 8-14, the absorbed dose delivered by primary x- or γ-ray photons at location P is essentially unchanged if the flat surface S' is substituted for the irregular surface S.

Consequently, the percent depth dose at P may be estimated from the isodose curves for a flat surface by moving the chart a distance h until the top of the chart coincides with the intersection Q of the surface and a line between P and the radiation source. When the chart is moved, the SSD is increased by a distance h. Consequently, the dose rate $D'_{o,r}$ at the location of the depth of maximum dose d_m below Q' (Margin Figure 8-14) is

$$D'_{o,r} = \left(\frac{SSD + d_m}{SSD + d_m + h} \right)^2 \cdot D_{o,r}$$

where $D_{o,r}$ is the dose rate at the location of d_m on the central axis at the SSD in a field of dimension r. The dose rate D_p at off-axis location P is

$$D_p = D'_{o,r} \, \%D_n / 100 \tag{8-4}$$

In Equation (8-4), $\%D_n$ is the percent depth dose at location P indicated by the isodose distribution. The estimated dose rate D_p at location P is approximately correct because isodose curves do not change appreciably with small changes in the *SSD*.

Example 8-5

With reference to Margin Figure 8-14, let $h = 3$ cm, and the dose rate $= 1.0$ cGy/MU at an SSD of 100 cm for a 6-MV beam. The $\%D_n$ is 67% at P when the top of the isodose chart passes through Q. What is the dose rate at P?

For a displacement h of 3 cm below the SSD, the dose rate $D'_{o,r}$ is

$$D'_{o,r} = \left(\frac{SSD + d_m}{SSD + d_m + h} \right)^2 \cdot D_{o,r}$$

$$= \left(\frac{100 + 1.5}{100 + 1.5 + 3} \right)^2 (1.0 \text{ cGy/MU})$$

$$= 0.94 \text{ cGy/MU}$$

The dose rate D_p at location P is

$$D_p = (D'_{o,r})(\%D_n/100)$$

$$= (0.94 \text{ cGy/MU})(67/100)$$

$$= 0.63 \text{ cGy/MU}$$

The percent depth dose at 10-cm depth for 6-MV x-rays changes by only 0.4% for a change in SSD from 85 to 87 cm.

Ratio of TARs Method

The Ratio of TARs method is illustrated in Margin Figure 8-15. The top of the isodose distribution is aligned with the intersection of the surface and the central axis of the x- or γ-ray beam. A thickness h of tissue is missing along the line between location P and the radiation source. Consequently, the dose at P is greater than that predicted from the isodose chart. The dose correction factor is the ratio of tissue/air ratios for the depth d of point P, divided by the TAR for a thickness $d + h$. Both TARs must be appropriate for the field size projected to the depth of point P.

$$CF = \frac{TAR(d, r)}{TAR(d + h, r)} \tag{8-5}$$

The calculation of the correction factor can be performed with TMRs as well. The correction factor is multiplied by the percent depth dose read from the unshifted isodose chart to obtain the corrected percent depth dose.

Example 8-6

With reference to Margin Figure 8-15, let $h = 3$ cm, $r = 10$ cm, $d = 7$ cm, and SSD $= 100$ cm. Determine the corrected percent depth dose at point P, assuming the treatment unit is a 6-MV linear accelerator.

From Table 7-8, TMR $(d, r) = 0.862$ and TMR $(d + h, r) = 0.770$. From Table 7-3 the percent depth dose %D $(d + h, r)$ (without correction) is 67.0%.

$$CF = \frac{TMR(d, r)}{TMR(d + h, r)}$$

$$CF = \frac{0.862}{0.770}$$

$$CF = 1.119$$

Corrected $\%D_n = $ (uncorrected $\%D_n$) (CF)

Corrected $\%D_n = (67.0\%)(1.119) = 75.0\%$

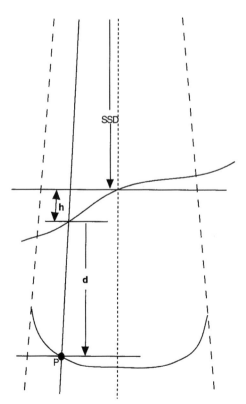

MARGIN FIGURE 8-15
The Ratio of TARs method of estimating the dose at location P in a medium with an irregular surface S.

■ EFFECTS OF TISSUE INHOMOGENEITIES

Photon Beams

If data measured in a water-filled phantom are used to compute the radiation dose delivered to a patient, then corrections should be applied for structures in the patient that are dissimilar to water. Inhomogeneities for which corrections may be necessary include bone (effective atomic number and density greater than those of water), air cavities and lung (density less than the density of water), and fat (effective atomic number and density less than those of water). The correction to be applied depends on the type and energy of the radiation, the size of the radiation field, and the size and composition of the inhomogeneity. For photons, inhomogeneities affect the distribution of radiation dose within the patient primarily in two ways:

1. Primary photons are attenuated more rapidly in bone than in an equal thickness of soft tissue. Consequently, an x- or γ-ray beam that has traversed a given thickness of bone contains fewer primary photons than a beam that has passed through an equal thickness of soft tissue. The number of primary photons transmitted by an air cavity or lung tissue exceeds the number transmitted by an equal thickness of soft tissue. The density of lung tissue ranges from 0.25 to 1 g/cm^3, depending on the amount of air in the lung tissue. Often, the density of lung is taken as 0.3 g/cm^3, unless density information can be extracted from a CT image. The major air cavities that may affect the distribution of radiation dose in a patient are the bronchus, larynx, pharynx, and maxillary sinus. Fat has a density of about 0.9 g/cm^3 and an effective atomic number of approximately 5.9 for photoelectric absorption and 5.2 for pair production.[21] The effect of fat in the dose distribution is usually neglected in treatment planning.
2. Inhomogeneities within the body influence the amount of radiation scattered to every location in the patient. The effects of inhomogeneities on the contribution of scattered radiation to absorbed dose are greatest at locations near the inhomogeneities.

Use of the often-quoted value of 1.85 g/cm^3 for the density of bone usually overestimates the attenuation of primary photons, because this density for compact bone exceeds the average density of skeletal bone.

Electron Beams

The distribution of dose in tissue irradiated with electron beams can be significantly distorted by the presence of tissue inhomogeneities such as bone, lung, and air cavities. As is the case with photon beams, electron beams are absorbed more rapidly by more dense media and are absorbed less rapidly by less dense media. The deposition of dose is related to the collisional stopping power, which varies with the electron density (electrons per gram) of the medium. However, the scattering of electrons also is affected by the medium, and under some circumstances, the dose distribution may be altered in complex ways.

In the case of broad inhomogeneities, the effects on the dose distribution may be more easily measured. Figure 8-4 is a graph of percent depth dose measured in water, as well as in a phantom composed of a layer of water above a layer of cork representing lung.[22] The increased penetration of the electron beam through the lung materials is clearly demonstrated. A small reduction in dose on the proximal side of the cork boundary is seen, resulting from reduced backscattering of electrons into the water. This small perturbation due to backscattering is generally neglected when manual heterogeneity corrections are performed, but the increased penetration through low-density material must be determined.

Sharp surface irregularities may produce localized hot and cold regions in the underlying medium due to changes in electron scattering.[23] These dose variations are demonstrated graphically in Figure 8-5. Electrons scattered from raised regions produce localized hot spots in adjacent depressed regions. Such sharp surface irregularities are occasionally found in the head and neck region of patients, but may also be caused by the use of bolus. When bolus is used with electron beams, the

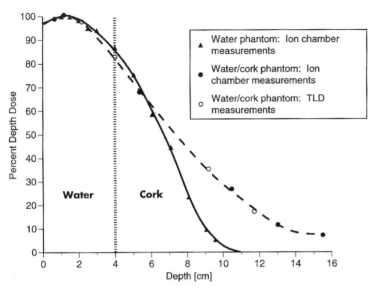

FIGURE 8-4
Electron beam depth dose curves measured in water and in a combination of water and cork. (Redrawn with permission from reference 22.)

edges should be tapered to minimize the localized hot and cold regions resulting from electron scattering.

Small inhomogeneities present a more complex problem because scattering of electrons within the heterogeneity becomes quite important. Margin Figure 8-16 indicates schematically the scattering of electrons at edges formed between high- and low-density media. As expected, absorption of electrons within a high-density heterogeneity causes a reduction in dose directly behind the heterogeneity. In addition, the increased scattering of electrons laterally from the heterogeneity causes an increase in dose beyond the edges of the heterogeneity. Conversely, the transmission of an electron beam through a low-density heterogeneity causes an increase in dose directly behind the heterogeneity but a reduction in dose laterally to the edges of the heterogeneity. This reduction is due to a lack of scattering of electrons into these regions. The presence of these hot and cold spots have important implications when small heterogeneities such as ribs and air cavities exist, or when high atomic number shielding materials are placed on or near the patient's surface.

The scattering from high-density heterogeneities has been characterized by Pohlit and Manegold.[24] In Margin Figure 8-17 the isodose distribution is shown around the edge of a lead inhomogeneity. Attenuation by the lead and scattering into regions lateral to the lead produce both hot and cold regions. Pohlit and Manegold define the angles α and β to describe the dose distribution. The angle α indicates the position of the maximum increase or decrease in the dose distribution, while β represents the extent of the perturbation. The variation of angles α and β as a function of mean electron energy is shown in Margin Figure 8-18.

■ CORRECTION FOR THE PRESENCE OF INHOMOGENEITIES

Photon Beams

The reduction in absorbed dose to tissue in the shadow of bone is greatest for low-energy photons, where the photoelectric effect is an important interaction. For x rays generated at 200 kVp, for example, the absorbed dose is reduced 10% to 30% in tissue in the shadow of a 1- to 3-cm thickness of bone. The dose reduction under bone is much less for x rays above 1 MV and reflects only the increased density of bone. For very high-energy photons, pair production interactions introduce an increased

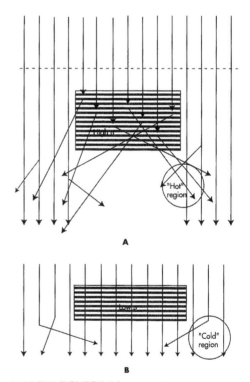

MARGIN FIGURE 8-16
A: Electrons encountering a high-density heterogeneity are scattered at a steeper angle than are electrons passing through the adjacent unit-density medium, and high-dose regions are produced. **B:** Conversely, electrons encountering a low-density heterogeneity are scatted less, resulting in low-dose regions.

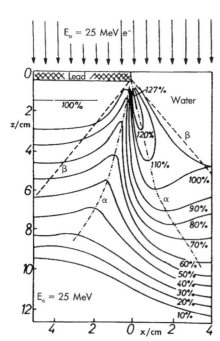

MARGIN FIGURE 8-17
Production of "hot" and "cold" spots in an electron dose distribution by a thin sheet of lead at the surface of a water phantom. (From reference 24. Used with permission.)

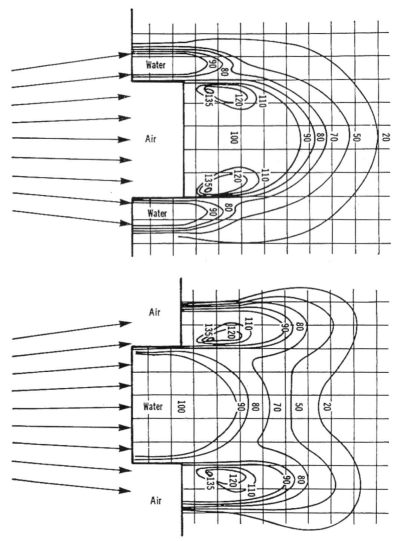

FIGURE 8-5
Influence of sharp surface irregularities on an electron beam dose distribution. (From reference 23. Used with permission.)

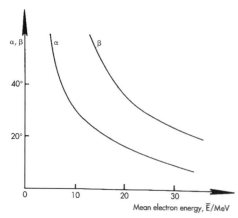

MARGIN FIGURE 8-18
Angles α and β as a function of electron beam energy. (From reference 24. Used with permission.)

attenuation in bone because of the dependence of these interactions on atomic number. Often these corrections are included in software packages for treatment planning computers. Manual methods sometimes are required, however, if only to provide an estimate of the correction.

Corrections such as those in Table 8-1 provide a crude estimate of the increase in percent depth dose caused by the increased transmission of x- and γ-ray photons through low-density lung tissue.[25,26] Because of variations among patients and among x- and γ-ray beams, the corrections in Table 8-1 are only approximate. However, percent depth doses at locations in or beyond lung tissue are estimated more accurately if these corrections are applied than if the increased transmission of lung tissue is ignored.

Example 8-7

The percent depth dose is 64.0% at 15-cm depth in a water-filled phantom exposed to a 10- × 10-cm 18-MV x-ray beam at 100-cm SSD. Using data in Table 8-1, compute the approximate percent depth dose at 15-cm depth if the beam traverses 6 cm of

TABLE 8-1 Corrections to Percent Depth Dose for X-Ray and γ-Ray Beams Passing through 5 to 8 cm of Lung Tissue

Modality	Percent
300-kVp x rays	+40
^{60}Co γ ray	+20
4-MV x rays	+15
18- to 20-MV x rays	+10

lung tissue.

$$\text{Percent } D_n = 64.0\% + (10/100)(64.0\%)$$

$$\text{Percent } D_n = 70.4\%$$

Measurements of the effects of inhomogeneities may be made by placing a small ionization chamber or thermoluminescent dosimeter at or near a location in the patient where knowledge of the absorbed dose is desired. Locations where the radiation dose may be measured directly include the skin, esophagus, trachea, oral cavity, cervix, bladder, and rectum. For example, the influence of a metal hip prosthesis on the dose to the prostate may be determined by placing a catheter containing thermoluminescent dosimeters into the patient's urethra.[27] The position of the dosimeter may be determined by attaching lead markers, which are visible during a radiographic or fluoroscopic examination. The markers should be kept at a short distance from the dosimeters. A radiograph of a tube containing LiF in the rectum is reproduced in Figure 8-6. Although the absorbed dose at specific locations within the patient may be measured with internal dosimeters, the use of these devices is restricted to situations in which the dosimeters can be placed in accessible locations and the placement of the dosimeters is not unduly uncomfortable for the patient.

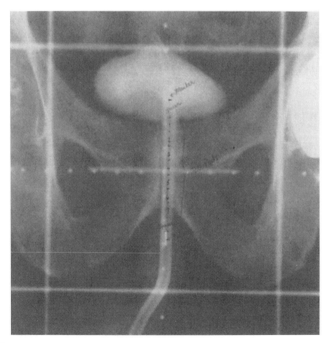

FIGURE 8-6
To measure the absorbed dose in the rectum during intracavitary therapy for carcinoma of the cervix, a tube containing LiF dosimeters may be inserted into the rectum. Lead markers in the tube indicate the position of the dosimeters in the rectum. (From reference 27. Used with permission.)

Another technique for estimating the effects of inhomogeneities is *transit dosimetry*.[2,21,28] Early implementation of this technique employed a low-activity, collimated γ-ray source (e.g., 10 mCi ^{60}Co) that was rotated in angular increments around the center of a patient whose water-equivalent thickness was to be determined. On the opposite side of the patient, a NaI (Tl) scintillation detector was moved in synchrony with the source. The ratio of the signal from the detector with the patient present to the signal measured with the patient removed from the beam was computed at each angular increment. This ratio is termed the *fractional transmission*. The water-equivalent thickness of the patient was determined at each angular increment by consulting a calibration chart relating percent transmission to depth in water. More recently, electronic portal imaging detectors (EPIDs) have been used to measure the fractional transmission of megavoltage x-rays through the patient. The water-equivalent thickness along several ray lines is combined with anatomical information to estimate the attenuating properties of tissues.[29]

In many situations, the methods described above are either considered impractical or they provide insufficient information. In these cases, the dose at points of interest within the patient can be calculated using one of several computational techniques. These calculations can be performed manually, although many have been incorporated into treatment-planning computer programs.

The influence of tissue inhomogeneities may be separated into three broad categories: (1) alterations in the primary beam intensity reaching the point of interest, (2) alterations in the radiation scattered from other locations to the point of interest, and (3) alterations in the secondary electron fluence. The degree to which each of these contributions influences the dose at the point of interest depends on the location of the point relative to the location of the inhomogeneity. At points lying behind an inhomogeneity, attenuation of the primary beam may be most important. Changes in the scattered radiation will additionally affect points lying above and to the side of a heterogeneity. Changes in electron fluence will have their greatest effect on points at interfaces between the heterogeneity and normal tissue.

Ratio of Tissue/Air Ratios Method

The ratio of tissue/air ratios method was described in the previous section, where its application to the correction of surface nonuniformities was discussed. This method is actually used more frequently to correct for the presence of tissue inhomogeneities. The dose at the point of interest is first estimated from isodose charts or depth dose tables, neglecting the presence of the inhomogeneity. A correction factor is determined as

$$CF = \frac{T(d', r_d)}{T(d, r_d)} \tag{8-6}$$

where d' is the water-equivalent depth of the point of interest. The water-equivalent depth is determined by summing the products of the thickness of each tissue layer and its electron density, as shown in Margin Figure 8-19. The corrected dose at the point of interest is the product of the dose calculated ignoring the inhomogeneity, multiplied by the correction factor.

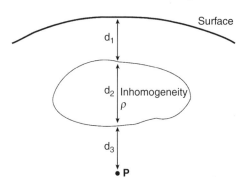

MARGIN FIGURE 8-19
Terminology and schematic representation of inhomogeneous tissues, for use with the Ratio of TARs method and the Power-Law method.

Example 8-8

In the diagram of Margin Figure 8-19, $d_1 = 2$ cm, $d_2 = 6$ cm, and $d_3 = 3$ cm. Regions 1 and 3 are unit-density tissue, while region 2 is lung tissue with density $\rho_e = 0.33$. The treatment is delivered with a 6-MV x-ray beam for which $r_d = 10$ cm. The percent depth dose at 11-cm depth is determined to be 63.7%. Determine the percent depth dose corrected for the presence of the inhomogeneity.

The water equivalent depth d' is

$$d' = d_1 + d_2\rho_e + d_3$$
$$d' = 2 \text{ cm} + 6 \text{ cm} \times 0.33 + 3 \text{ cm}$$
$$d' = 7 \text{ cm}$$

The heterogeneity correction factor [Equation (8-6) and Table 7-8] is

$$CF = \frac{TMR(d', r_d)}{TMR(d, r_d)}$$

$$CF = \frac{TMR(7, 10)}{TMR(11, 10)}$$

$$CF = \frac{0.862}{0.743} = 1.16$$

The corrected percent depth dose is $(63.7\%)(1.16) = 73.9\%$.

Power Law Tissue/Air Ratio Method

The Ratio of TARs method of heterogeneity correction described above is considered an "effective path length" method. That is, it may be used only to determine the equivalent unit-density depth of the point of interest, based on the density of the heterogeneity and the thickness of the heterogeneity measured along a line from the source to the point of interest. The method does not consider the location of the point of interest relative to the heterogeneity. It also does not consider any of the dimensions of the heterogeneity other than its thickness along the ray line to the point. Consequently, its use is limited to only "semi-infinite" slabs of inhomogeneous tissue.

In an attempt to improve the quality of inhomogeneity corrections, a technique that considers the distance from the heterogeneity to the point of interest has been developed.[30,31] The heterogeneity correction factor is expressed as

$$CF = \left[\frac{TAR(d_2 + d_3, r_d)}{TAR(d_3, r_d)}\right]^{\rho_e - 1} \tag{8-7}$$

The relative electron density ρ_e (in units of electrons/cm³) is the product of the electron content (electrons per gram) and the physical density (grams/cm³) of the heterogeneity relative to that of water. The distances d_1, d_2, and d_3 are explained in Margin Figure 8-19. r_d is the field size at depth d. The TMR can be substituted for the TAR in this method. This method applies only to the calculation of dose at points beyond a heterogeneity; it cannot be applied to points that fall inside a heterogeneity. The method can easily be extended to correct for the presence of multiple inhomogeneities.

Note that the power law method does not consider the depth of the heterogeneity below the surface of the patient.

A more general form of the power law correction method has been developed; this permits calculation at points falling within the heterogeneity.[32] The correction factor is

$$CF = \frac{[TAR(d_3, r_d)]^{\rho_3 - \rho_2}}{[TAR(d_2 + d_3, r_d)]^{1 - \rho_2}}$$

where ρ_3 is the relative electron density of the material in which point P lies, ρ_2 is the relative electron density of region 2, and d_3 is the thickness of tissue below the inhomogeneity to point P (Margin Figure 8-19). As before, TMRs can be substituted for TARs in this equation.

Example 8-9

In the absence of a heterogeneity, isodose curves for a 6-MV x-ray beam indicate that the percent depth dose at point P in Margin Figure 8-19 is 63.7%. The field size at P is 10×10 cm. If $d_1 = 2$ cm, $d_2 = 6$ cm, and $d_3 = 3$ cm, and $\rho_e = 0.33$, determine the dose at point P in the presence of the heterogeneity.

From Equation (8-7) and Table 7-8, the heterogeneity correction factor is

$$CF = \left[\frac{TMR(d_2 + d_3, r_d)}{TMR(d_3, r_d)} \right]^{\rho_e - 1} \tag{8-7}$$

$$CF = \left(\frac{0.800}{0.970} \right)^{-0.67} = 1.14$$

Therefore, the corrected percent depth dose is $(63.7\%) (1.14) = 72.6\%$.

Note the small difference between this result and that in Example 8-8.

Equivalent TAR Method

None of the heterogeneity correction methods described up to this point consider the lateral extent of the heterogeneity. Many heterogeneities of significance in radiation therapy are relatively small in size, or they may be located so that they intercept only a portion of the beam. In addition, it is important on occasion to consider heterogeneities that intercept portions of the beam that do not lie in the plane formed by the beams' central axes. As indicated, the correction techniques described previously consider only heterogeneities that fall on the line between the source and the point of interest.

A correction technique has been developed to consider the effects of scattered radiation from inhomogeneous regions of irradiated tissue. This technique, referred to as the *equivalent tissue/air ratio (ETAR) method*, requires a somewhat more complex calculation.[33] The method permits the calculation of a tissue/air ratio for an "equivalent" field size and depth that incorporates corrections for the location and extent of heterogeneities. The correction factor is computed as

$$CF = \frac{TAR(d', r_d')}{TAR(d, r_d')} \tag{8-8}$$

where d' is the water-equivalent depth of the calculation point, d is the physical depth, r_d represents the beam dimension at depth d, and r_d' is the scaled field dimension; r_d' is determined by multiplying the actual field dimension by $\tilde{\rho}$, the weighted density of the irradiated volume. The weighted density $\tilde{\rho}$ is determined by an averaging procedure:

$$\tilde{\rho} = \frac{\sum_i \sum_j \sum_k \rho_{ijk} \cdot w_{ijk}}{\sum_i \sum_j \sum_k w_{ijk}}$$

where ρ_{ijk} are the relative electron densities of scatter elements distributed throughout the irradiated volume, and w_{ijk} are the weighting factors assigned to those elements to represent their relative contribution to the scattered dose at the point of interest. The weighting factors are based on Compton scatter cross sections. This method is complex, and it is generally applied through the use of a computer program.

None of the above methods considers the contribution to the dose at interfaces from perturbations of the electron fluence. Calculations and measurements have shown that this perturbation can be considerable.[34,35] However, no straightforward calculation techniques exist for estimating this contribution. In addition, the methods described above cannot be used to estimate the loss of electronic equilibrium when high-energy photon beams pass through low-density media such as lung tissue. This effect is most noticeable at energies above 6 MV and for small field sizes. Termed "lateral disequilibrium," the effect is caused by energetic secondary electrons, which are able to scatter laterally through the lung some distance outside the beam. This scattering reduces the dose within the field margins, increases the dose outside the field, and tends to broaden the penumbra of the field.[36]

Electron Beams

CET Method

A correction for the transmission of electron beams through broad heterogeneities has been described by Laughlin and others.[22,37–39] For large and uniform thicknesses of heterogeneity, the dose distribution can be corrected by using the coefficient of equivalent thickness (CET) method.

The effective thickness of the inhomogeneity (the thickness of water to which it is equivalent) is determined by multiplying the thickness by the CET. As the point of interest generally lies behind thicknesses of normal tissue as well as behind the inhomogeneity, the effective depth is determined by

$$d_{eff} = d - z(1 - CET)$$

where d is the depth of the point of interest, and z is the thickness of inhomogeneity overlying the point of interest. For compact bone, a CET of 1.65 is recommended.[37] In lung, an average lung CET of 0.5 is suggested.[38]

Example 8-10

Determine the effective depth of a point located 2 cm into a patient's lung, along the central axis of an electron beam. A layer of unit density tissue 1 cm thick lies over the lung. An average CET of 0.5 may be used.

$$d_{eff} = d - z(1 - CET)$$

$$d_{eff} = 3 \text{ cm} - 2(1 - 0.5)$$

$$d_{eff} = 2 \text{ cm}$$

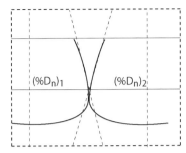

MARGIN FIGURE 8-20

Two adjacent fields separated at the surface so that the dotted lines intersect at the depth of interest. These dotted lines represent decrement lines, or points where the $\%D_n$ is half that on the central axis.

■ SEPARATION OF ADJACENT FIELDS

Frequently, two or more adjacent fields are used to irradiate large regions of tissue such as those encountered during treatment of the lymphatic chain of patients with lymphomas or testicular tumors. If the margins of adjacent fields overlap or abut on the surface of the patient, then the radiation dose may be excessive to tissue at depths below the margins. Consequently, some separation should exist between adjacent fields. However, if the distance of separation is too great, then a "cold spot" of reduced dose may occur below the surface. Often, a separation of about 1 cm is employed between adjacent fields. Although this separation may be satisfactory in many cases, a method is needed for estimating the optimum distance of separation between adjacent fields.

In Margin Figure 8-20, two adjacent fields are portrayed with a treatment depth indicated by the horizontal line. At this treatment depth, the central axis percent depth doses are $(\%D_n)_1$, and $(\%D_n)_2$. Decrement lines depicted by dotted lines contain points where the $\%D_n$ is half that on the central axis for each field. These curves are termed the 50% decrement lines. By positioning the isodose distributions so that the decrement lines are superimposed at the treatment depth, a relatively uniform dose is delivered at treatment depth across the entire treated region. The process of superimposing the isodose curves at the treatment depth in this manner defines the separation of the adjacent fields at the surface.

With modern linear accelerators, the 50% decrement line closely follows the geometric beam edge. Hence, the geometric field edge is commonly used to determine the separation of adjacent fields.

The determination of gap width can be reduced to a simple geometric calculation employing the principle of similar triangles. As shown in Margin Figure 8-21, the portion of the total gap attributed to field 1 is

$$G_1 = \left(\frac{r_1}{2}\right)\left(\frac{d}{SSD}\right) \tag{8-9}$$

where r_1 is the field width at SAD and d is the depth at which the fields are to abut. For SSD treatments, the SSD is used in place of the SAD, and the field width is determined at the surface.

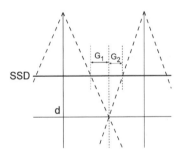

MARGIN FIGURE 8-21

An illustration of the procedure for calculating the gap between adjacent x-ray beams.

Modern linear accelerators are designed so that the nominal SSD is equal to the SAD, which is 100 cm. Consequently, the collimator setting indicates both (a) the field size at the surface for SSD treatment and (b) the field size at depth for SAD treatments.

Caution should be used when abutting fields as the overlap at depths greater than the point of abutment may lead to unacceptable doses to sensitive tissues. The field arrangement shown in Margin Figure 8-21 may be used to treat the thoracic spine from the posterior direction, but the overlapped region will then fall on structures more anterior which may include tissues such as the thyroid gland.

Careful attention should also be paid to the common practice of abutting parallel-opposed pairs of fields. As shown in Margin Figure 8-22, the use of fields of different lengths can lead to the appearance of hot and cold spots.

It is common to adjoin fields when treating large areas with electron beams. However, unlike high-energy x-ray beams, the dose distributions from electron beams do not closely follow the geometric field edges.[40] Instead, the isodose distributions tend to bulge at depth, and a hot spot may be produced when fields are abutted (Figure 8-7). When the fields are separated by 1.5 cm, as shown in the upper figure, a cold spot is produced near the surface. If the gap is eliminated or is reduced to 1.0 cm, or 0.5 cm as is shown in the lower figures, a hot spot results. To reduce the intensity of the hot spot, a wedge made of plastic can be used.[40] The wedge reduces the energy, and therefore the penetration, of electrons at the edge of the field, thereby minimizing the hot spot (Figure 8-8). However, caution must be used when placing lucite edges near the patient's surface, because scattering of electrons from the wedges can cause distortions in the dose distribution. If the wedge is in close contact with the patient's surface, it acts as bolus.

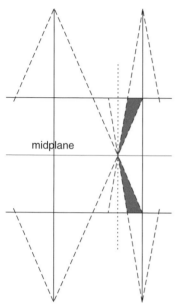

MARGIN FIGURE 8-22

Hot and cold spots can be produced when parallel-opposed pairs of fields of different lengths are abutted. The shaded regions receive dose from three of the four fields.

■ INTEGRAL DOSE

The integral dose is the total energy imparted to a medium during irradiation. The historical unit of integral dose is the gram-rad. In SI units, the unit of integral dose is the gray-kilogram, but as 1 Gy = 1 J/kg, a simpler SI unit of integral dose is the joule. If a 100-g mass of tissue is irradiated uniformly to an absorbed dose of 100 cGy, then the integral dose to the tissue is (100 cGy)(100 g) = (1 Gy)(0.1 kg) = 0.1 J.

In radiation therapy, the probability of damage to normal tissue increases with the integral dose to the patient. Consequently, the overall well-being of the patient may be expected to decrease as the integral dose is increased. The clinical significance of integral dose is related to established rules of radiation therapy, which are consulted when one treatment plan must be selected from many that are designed to provide a desired dose to a tumor. For example, a beam entrance surface near the lesion is preferred over a surface farther from the lesion. Also, a small field that just encompasses the lesion is preferred over a larger field. As a general rule, the preferred treatment plan is that which furnishes the smallest integral dose for a prescribed distribution of dose in the volume of tissue containing the lesion. The integral dose Σ delivered by an x- or γ-ray beam may be estimated with the expression[41]

$$\Sigma = 1.44 D_0 A d_{1/2} \left(1 - e^{-0.693d/d_{1/2}}\right) \left(1 + \frac{2.88 d_{1/2}}{SSD}\right) \qquad (8\text{-}10)$$

where D_0 is the dose at the depth of maximum dose, A is the area of the field, SSD is the source-surface distance for the beam, d is the total thickness of the patient, and $d_{1/2}$ is the half-value depth, or depth in tissue along the central axis where the dose rate is half the dose rate at the depth of maximum dose. The term $[1 + (2.88d_{1/2}/SSD)]$ compensates for divergence of the radiation beam. The dose computed with Equation (8-10) underestimates the integral dose slightly and should be considered as a lower limit.[42]

Effects of irradiation (e.g., blood changes) observed clinically do not correlate closely with the integral dose delivered to the patient. This lack of correlation probably reflects the omission in the concept of integral dose of a distinction between tissue components of varying sensitivity to radiation.[28]

The use of a treatment planning computer to determine integral dose is discussed in Chapter 11.

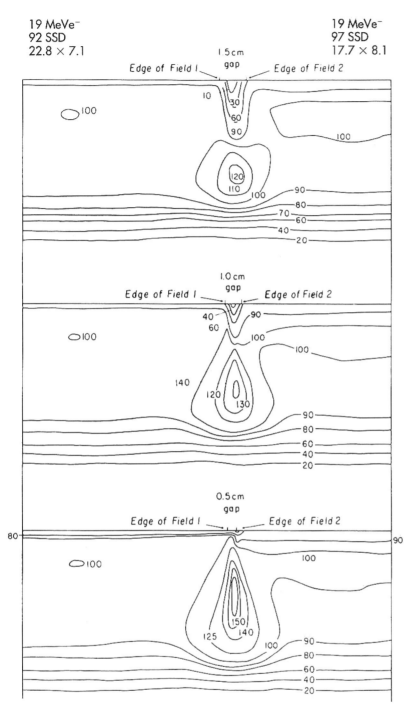

FIGURE 8-7
Isodose distributions for adjoining fields with the same electron beam energy with different gap width between the fields. (From reference 38. Used with permission.)

DOSE SPECIFICATION FOR EXTERNAL BEAM THERAPY

As the practice of radiation therapy evolves, it is important for comparisons to be made between treatment practices. In large part, the ideal dose for a particular disease is determined empirically by comparing the results in patients treated to different doses or through different fractionation schemes. However, these comparisons can only be made if the courses of treatment are reported in a consistent and meaningful fashion. Unfortunately, it is easy to overestimate the ease with which a reviewer can interpret

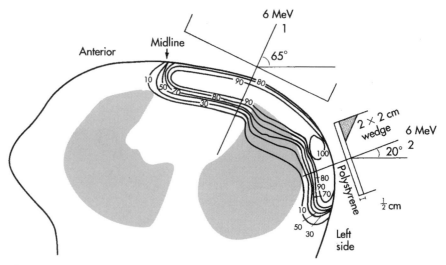

FIGURE 8-8

Case illustrating the use of a polystyrene wedge to reduce hot spots for two adjoining electron fields coming in at slight angles. The polystyrene slab is used to reduce the incident 6-MeV electrons by approximately 1 MeV so that the lung behind the chest wall will be spared. (From Chu, F. C. H., Zuppinger, A., and Poretti, G. (eds.). *Symposium on High-Energy Electrons*, Springer, Berlin, 1965, p. 347; as redrawn in Almond, P. R. Radiation physics of electron beams. In Tapley, N. D. (ed.). *Clinical Applications of the Electron Beam*, New York, John Wiley & Sons, 1976. Used with permission.)

the documentation of a particular course of treatment. Unless careful attention is paid to the way in which doses, fractionation schemes, and treated volumes are described, the results can be virtually unintelligible to an independent reviewer.

Recommendations have been made by the International Commission on Radiation Units and Measurements (ICRU) for a generalized dose-specification system. In two reports,[3,43] the ICRU has updated these recommendations. A summary of these recommendations is provided here, but the reader should refer to the original documents for complete details.

Treatment Volumes

Gross Tumor Volume

The gross tumor volume (GTV) is the demonstrable extent and location of the malignant growth. This extent can be determined by palpation or direct visualization, or indirectly through imaging techniques (Figure 8-9).

Clinical Target Volume

The gross tumor volume is generally surrounded by a region of normal tissue, which may be invaded by subclinical microscopic extensions of the tumor. Additional extension of the GTV may exist because of subclinical spread of disease, such as to regional lymph nodes.

These volumes are designated as clinical target volumes (CTVs). The CTV is an anatomic concept, representing the volume of known or suspected tumor.

Planning Target Volume

The clinical target volume is subject to changes in size and location from time to time, as a result of movements of the patient and the tissues containing the CTV. In addition, changes in size and shape of nearby tissues can change the size and location of the CTV. A margin is drawn around the CTV to accommodate these variations.

The resulting planning target volume (PTV) is a geometric concept that takes into consideration the net effect of all possible geometric variations.

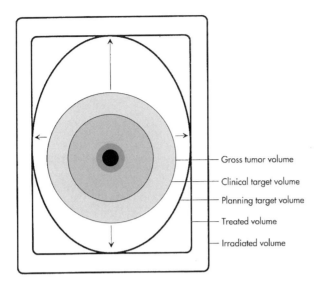

FIGURE 8-9
A schematic diagram indicating the ICRU recommendations for describing volumes and doses. (From reference 3. Used with permission.)

Treated Volume

The goal of radiation therapy is to deliver a high and uniform dose to the PTV and to limit the dose everywhere else to some minimum value. Because of practical limitations in the number and shape of the treatment fields, the treated volume is typically of some regular shape that encompasses the PTV. The treated volume is the volume of tissue enclosed by a selected isodose surface, often 95% of the dose at the prescription point.

Irradiated Volume

In the process of delivering a uniform dose throughout the PTV, surrounding normal tissues are necessarily irradiated to significant levels. The irradiated volume is defined as the volume of tissue receiving a significant dose, such as that greater than or equal to 20% of the specified target dose. A comparison between the treated volume and the irradiated volume for different beam arrangements can be used in optimizing the beam arrangement.

Organs at Risk

The ICRU defines organs at risk as normal tissues whose radiation sensitivity may significantly influence the treatment planning process.

Planning Risk Volume

ICRU Report 62[43] created the planning risk volume (PRV) in order to extend the PTV concept to organs at risk. The PRV is a geometric concept that takes into account the net effect of all possible geometric variations.

Recommendations for Reporting Dose

The ICRU recommends that the dose at or near the center of the PTV, as well as the maximum and minimum dose to the PTV, should always be reported.[3,43] When available, additional information should be provided, such as the average dose and its standard deviation, as well as dose/volume histograms (see Chapter 11). The central point at which the dose is to be reported is defined as the ICRU reference point; this location is to be selected according to the following criteria:

- The dose at this point is clinically relevant and representative of the dose throughout the PTV.
- The ICRU reference point is easy to define.
- The point is at a location at which the dose can be determined or calculated accurately.
- The dose should be selected in a region where there is no steep dose gradient.

The reference point should be located either at the center of the PTV or at the intersection of the beam central axes.

Maximum Dose

The ICRU recommends reporting the maximum dose within the PTV, and within tissues outside the PTV. To be meaningful clinically, the maximum dose must encompass at least a minimum volume. The ICRU recommends that this volume have a minimum diameter of 15 mm. A smaller volume is, in most cases, not relevant to normal tissue tolerance for large organs. However, when small organs such as the eye or optic nerve are at risk, a dimension smaller than 15 mm may be considered.

Minimum Dose

The minimum dose is the smallest dose in a defined volume. No volume limit is recommended when reporting minimum dose.

Average Dose

The average dose, or mean target dose, is determined by calculating the dose at a large number of discrete points, uniformly distributed within the PTV. The average dose is the mean of these dose values.

Median Target Dose

The median target dose is the central value of the doses at all calculation points within the volume of interest, when arranged according to magnitude.

Modal Dose

The modal dose is the dose that occurs most frequently at calculation points within the volume concerned. There may be more than one modal dose value, which then makes this concept relatively useless for reporting purposes.

Hot Spots

A hot spot is defined as a volume lying outside the PTV that receives a dose larger than 100% of the specified PTV dose or the dose at the ICRU reference point. Like the maximum target dose, a hot spot is generally considered significant only if the minimum diameter exceeds 15 mm. If the hot spot occurs in a small organ such as the eye or optic nerve, a dimension smaller than 15 mm should be considered.

■ SUMMARY

- Point dose calculations often are performed using manual techniques.
- Calculations of dose delivered during treatment at a standard SSD are conveniently performed using percent depth dose.
- When isocentric treatment is used, calculations are generally performed using tissue-maximum ratios or a similar parameter.
- Isodose distributions can be prepared manually for multiple-field treatment arrangements, by summing the doses from one pair of fields at a time.
- Wedge filters, or programmable collimators that produce wedged dose distributions, are used to provide uniform tumor doses when fields separated by angles of less than 180° are used.

- The dose in an irregular field can be determined by the Clarkson method of separating the primary and scatter contributions to the total dose.
- Corrections for surface obliquity and for the presence of heterogeneities can be performed by manual methods, and are useful for checking the results of computer calculations.

PROBLEMS

8-1. 6-MV photons are to be used to deliver a dose of 100 cGy at 9-cm depth. A 12- × 16-cm field will be used at 100-cm SSD. The accelerator has been calibrated to deliver an output of 1.00 cGy/MU at d_m in a 10- × 10-cm field at 100-cm SSD. No blocking will be used. How many monitor units will be required?

8-2. The treatment conditions described in problem 1 are changed to an isocentric technique. The field size is 12 × 16 cm at the isocenter (at 9-cm depth). Compute the meter setting.

8-3. A patient is 22 cm thick in the anterior–posterior direction and is 32 cm thick in the lateral direction. 10- × 10-cm fields are used. An SSD technique (SSD = 100 cm) using 6-MV photons will be used to deliver treatment through a four-field "box" treatment plan, consisting of beams from the anterior, posterior, right lateral, and left lateral directions. A total dose of 200 cGy is to be delivered to the point at the intersection of the beam axes. Equal doses are to be given at the target point. What "given doses" will be required?

8-4. If equal given doses are to be delivered in problem 8-3, what dose at the target point would be delivered from each field?

8-5. An obliquely incident beam of 6-MV x rays is used to treat a patient. An 8- × 13-cm field at 80-cm SSD is used. The dose rate at d_m in this field size is 1.006 cGy/MU. The target point is off-axis at 8-cm depth, as measured along the central axis. However, the SSD above the target point is 84 cm. Use (a) the effective SSD method and (b) the ratio of TARs method to determine the corrected dose rate.

8-6. A patient is to be treated to a point lying behind bone of $\rho_e = 1.40$. 6 MV photons will be used, with a field size of 6 × 6 cm at 100-cm SSD. The bone is 2 cm thick and lies beneath 3 cm of soft tissue. The target point is 4 cm below the bone, in soft tissue: Use (a) the ratio of TARs method and (b) the power-law TAR method to determine the corrected percent depth dose.

8-7. An electron beam will be used to treat a tumor lying immediately behind a rib. The bone is 2 cm thick and is covered by 2 cm of tissue. What is the effective depth of the point?

8-8. Two high-energy photon beams are abutted to treat a spinal-axis field at 100-cm SSD. The superior field is 30 cm long, while the inferior field is 26 cm long. The fields are to abut at 6-cm depth. How large a gap at the skin should exist between the fields?

REFERENCES

1. Task Group 51, Radiation Therapy Committee, American Association of Physicists in Medicine. Protocol for clinical reference dosimetry of high-energy photon and electron beams. *Med. Phys.* 1999; **26**:1847–1870.
2. Khan, F. M. *Radiation Therapy Physics*, 3rd edition. Baltimore, Williams & Wilkins, 2003.
3. International Commission on Radiation Units and Measurements, Report 50: *Prescribing, Recording and Reporting Photon Beam Therapy,* 1993.
4. International Electrotechnical Commission, Report 60976, 1st edition, Geneva, October 1989.
5. Sear, R. A theoretical approach to the radiation dose-rate distribution from combined x- and gamma-ray beams: With special reference to wedge-filtered beams. *Phys. Med. Biol.* 1959; **4**:10.
6. Cohen, M. Physical aspects of roentgen therapy using wedge filters. *Acta Radiol.* 1959; **52**:65/158. *Acta Radiol.* 1960; **53**:153.
7. Sonntag, A., Jordanow, D., and Bunde, E. Wedge filters in cobalt-60 teletherapy. *Electromedica* 1968; **3**:65.
8. Van Roosenbeck, B., and Grimm, J. Wedge filters: Their construction and use with a 22 meV betatron. *AJR* 1961; **85**:926.
9. Leavitt, D., Martin, M., Moeller, J. H., and Lee, W. L.. Dynamic wedge field techniques through computer-controlled collimator motion and dose delivery. *Med. Phys.* 1990; **17**:87–91.
10. Clarkson, J. A note on depth doses in fields of irregular shape. *Br. J. Radiol.* 1941; **14**:265.
11. Cundiff, J., Cunningham, J. R., Golden, R., Holt, G., Lanzl, L. H., Meurk, M. L., Ovadia, J., Page, V., Pope, R. A., Sampiere, V. A., Saylor, W. L., Shalek, R. S., and Suntharalingam, N. The calculation of dose in the radiation treatment of Hodgkin's disease. In *Proceedings of the Hodgkin's Disease Dosimetry Workshop.* Houston: Radiological Physics Center, 1970.
12. Hallberg, J. R., Ibbott, G. S., Carson, P. L., Hendee, W. R., and Aymar, M. A. Computational analysis and dosimetric evaluation of a commercial irregular fields computer program. *Med. Phys.* 1977; **4**:528.
13. Archambeau, J. O., Forell, B., Doria, R., Findley, D. O., Jurisch, R., and Jackson, R. Use of variable thickness bolus to control electron beam penetration in chest wall irradiation. *Int. J. Radiat. Oncol., Biol. Phys.* 1981; **7**:835–846.
14. Bewley D. K., Brodshaw, A. L., Greene, D., Haybittle, J. L., and Secretan, L. F. Central axis depth dose data for use in radiotherapy. *Br. J. Radiol.* 1983;**17**:1–147.
15. Boge, R. J., Edland, R. W., Matthes, D. C. Tissue compensators for megavoltage radiotherapy fabricated from hollowed styrofoam filled with wax. *Radiology* 1974; **111**:193–198.
16. Ellis, F., Hall, E., and Oliver, R. A compensator for variations in tissue thickness for high energy beam. *Br. J. Radiol.* 1959; **32**:421.
17. Arora, V. R., and Weeks, K. J. Characterization of gypsum attenuators for radiotherapy dose modification. *Med. Phys.* 1994; **21**:77–81.
18. Ibbott, G., and Hendee, W. Beam-shaping platforms and the skin-sparing advantage of ^{60}Co radiation. *Am. J. Roentgenol.* 1970; **108**:193.
19. Hendee, W., and Garciga, C. Tissue compensating filters for ^{60}Co teletherapy. *Am. J. Roentenol.* 1967; **99**:939.
20. Willis, R., and Casebow, M. Tissue compensation with lead for ^{60}Co therapy. *Br. J. Radiol.* 1969; **42**:452.
21. International Commission on Radiation Units and Measurements. *Determination of Absorbed Dose in a Patient Irradiated by Beams of x- or γ-Rays in Radiotherapy Procedures.* ICRU Report No. 24, 1976.
22. Almond, P. R., Wright, A. E., and Boone, M. L. N. High-energy electron dose perturbations in regions of tissue heterogeneity. *Radiology* 1967; **88**:1146.

23. Dutreix, J. Dosimetry. In Gayarre, G., et al., (eds.). *Symposium on High-Energy Electrons.* Madrid: General Directorate of Health, 1970.

24. Pohlit, W., and Manegold, K. H. Electron-beam dose distribution in inhomogeneous media. In Kramer, S., Suntharalingam, N., and Zinninger, G. F. *High Energy Photons and Electrons.* New York: 1976. Wiley & Sons, 1976.

25. Massey, I. Dose distribution problems in megavoltage therapy. *Br. J. Radiol.* 1962; **35**:736.

26. Spring, E., and Anttila, P. Empirical formulas for tissue correction factors in cobalt teletherapy. *Acta Radiol. Ther.* 1968; **7**:230.

27. Hazuka, M. B., Stroud, D., Adams, J., Ibbott, G. S., and Kinzie, J. J. Prostatic thermoluminescent dosimeter analysis in a patient treated with 18 MV X-rays through a prosthetic hip. *Int. J. Radiat. Oncol., Biol. Phys.* 1993; **25**:339–343.

28. International Commission on Radiation Units and Measurements, Estimation of Integral Absorbed Dose. *Clinical Dosimetry.* Recommendations of the ICRU, Report l0d: National Bureau of Standards Handbook 87, Appendix III, 1963.

29. Grein, E. E., Lee, R., and Luchka, K. An investigation of a new amorphous silicon electronic portal imaging device for transit dosimetry. *Med. Phys.* 2002; **29**:2262–2268.

30. Batho, H. F. Lung corrections in ^{60}Co beam therapy. *J. Can. Assoc. Radiol.* 1964; **15**:79.

31. Young, M. E. J., and Gaylord, J. D. Experimental tests of corrections for tissue inhomogeneities in radiotherapy. *Br. J. Radiol.* 1970; **43**:349.

32. Sontag, M. R., and Cunningham, J. R. Corrections to absorbed dose calculations for tissue inhomogeneities. *Med. Phys.* 1977; **4**:431.

33. Sontag, M. R., Cunningham, J. R. The equivalent tissue/air ratio method for making absorbed dose calculations in a heterogeneous medium. *Radiology* 1978; **129**:787.

34. Sundblom, I. Dose planning for irradiation of thorax with cobalt in fixed beam therapy. *Acta Radiol.* 1965; **3**:342.

35. Werner, B. L., Das, I. J., Khan, F. M., and Meigooni, A. S. Dose perturbation at interfaces in photon beams. *Med. Phys.* 1987; **14**:585–595.

36. Kornelson, R. O., and Young, M. E. J. Changes in the dose-profile of a 10 MV x-ray beam within and beyond low density material. *Med. Phys.* 1982; **9**:114.

37. Holt, J. G., et al. Memorial electron beam AET treatment planning system. In Orton, C. G., and Bagne, F. (eds.). *Practical Aspects of Electron Beam Treatment Planning.* New York, American Institute of Physics, 1978.

38. Laughlin, J. S. High energy electron treatment planning for inhomogeneities. *Br. J. Radiol.* 1965, **38**:143.

39. Laughlin, J. S., et al. Electron-beam treatment planning in inhomogeneous tissue. *Radiology* 1965; **85**:524.

40. Almond, P. R. Radiation physics of electron beams. In Tapley, N. D. (eds.). *Clinical Applications of the Electron Beam.* New York, Wiley & Sons, 1976.

41. Mayneord, W. Energy absorption: III. The mathematical theory of integral dose and its application in practice. *Br. J. Radiol.* 1944; **17**:359.

42. Meredith, W., and Massey, I. *Fundamental Physics of Radiology.* Baltimore, Williams & Wilkins, 1968.

43. International Commission on Radiation Units and Measurements. *Prescribing, Recording and Reporting Photon Beam Therapy.* Report 62 (Supplement to ICRU Report 50), 1999.

CHAPTER

9

DIAGNOSTIC IMAGING AND APPLICATIONS TO RADIATION THERAPY

OBJECTIVES   188

INTRODUCTION   188

RADIOGRAPHY   189

X-Ray Film   189
Intensifying Screens   191
Radiographic Grids   193
Digital Radiography   194
Digital X-Ray Detectors   195

FLUOROSCOPY   196

Image Intensification   196
Television Display of Fluoroscopic Images   198

TREATMENT SIMULATORS   199

COMPUTED TOMOGRAPHY   200

History   200
Principles of Computed Tomography   201

Reconstruction Algorithms   202

ULTRASONOGRAPHY   203

NUCLEAR MEDICINE   206

Properties of Radioactive Pharmaceuticals   206
Nuclear Medicine Imaging   207

EMISSION COMPUTED TOMOGRAPHY   209

Single-Photon Emission Computed Tomography   210
Positron Emission Tomography   210

MAGNETIC RESONANCE IMAGING   211

FUNCTIONAL MAGNETIC RESONANCE IMAGING   213

SUMMARY   214

PROBLEMS   216

REFERENCES   216

Radiation Therapy Physics, Third Edition, by William R. Hendee, Geoffrey S. Ibbott, and Eric G. Hendee
ISBN 0-471-39493-9 Copyright © 2005 John Wiley & Sons, Inc.

■ OBJECTIVES

After studying this chapter, the reader should be able to:

- Explain the equipment and procedures for acquiring radiographic images, as well as explain the characteristics of both analog and digital radiographs.
- Identify the features and purposes of x-ray film, intensifying screens, radiographic grids, and digital x-ray detectors.
- Outline the process of fluoroscopy, the features of image intensifiers, and the television display of fluoroscopic images.
- Discuss the mechanism and value of x-ray and CT treatment simulation in radiation therapy.
- Delineate the features of transmission CT images and the process of acquiring these images.
- Provide an in-depth explanation of the acquisition and features of ultrasound images.
- Discuss how nuclear medicine images (including SPECT and PET images) are acquired, and the attributes and limitations of these images.
- Explain magnetic resonance imaging (including fMRI) and how it contributes to treatment planning in radiation therapy.

■ INTRODUCTION

For several decades after the discovery of x rays, medical radiology evolved as the application of ionizing radiation to the diagnosis and treatment of human disease and injury. Over this period, radiologic specialists were trained in both diagnostic applications (diagnostic radiology) and therapeutic procedures (therapeutic radiology). In the early years, many radiologists practiced as both diagnosticians and therapists. After World War II, however, both diagnostic and therapeutic radiology grew in complexity. For example, radiation therapy became immensely more sophisticated with the advent of ^{60}Co and its requirements for more sophisticated treatment planning and monitoring to replace the visual landmarks (e.g., skin reddening and blistering) used with superficial and orthovoltage therapy. In the early 1970s, diagnostic and therapeutic radiology were finally recognized as separate specialties, with separate training programs, accreditation committees for residencies, and certification procedures for specialists. Radiation therapists became known as radiation oncologists, and the term "radiation therapist" was transferred to the technologists who deliver treatments under the supervision of radiation oncologists. Most academic institutions established departments of radiation oncology independent of (diagnostic) radiology, and physicists increasingly focused their expertise onto technical challenges in a single discipline such as radiology, radiation oncology, or nuclear medicine. Residency programs in radiology included almost no training in radiation oncology, and educational programs in radiation oncology contained only a token exposure, if any, to diagnostic imaging.

Over the past two decades, treatment planning and monitoring in radiation therapy have become increasingly complex. High-energy accelerators for x-ray and electron-beam treatments, computers, mathematical algorithms, sophisticated software programs, the heightened presence of physicists and computer specialists, an increased regulatory burden, and a growing demand for quality control all contribute to this complexity. Also enhancing the complexity is expanding use of imaging techniques, especially fluoroscopy, radiography, computed tomography (CT), and magnetic resonance imaging (MRI) for treatment simulation, treatment planning, and three-dimensional visualization of tumors and surrounding anatomic structures. The acceptance of imaging techniques as an essential part of radiation therapy demands that radiation oncologists acquire a fundamental understanding of these techniques,

In 1946 three ^{59}Co disks were activated in nuclear reactors to produce the first ^{60}Co sources to be used for radiation therapy. Two were activated by the Atomic Energy of Canada Ltd. (AECL) at Chalk River, Canada, and one was activated at the Oak Ridge National Laboratory in Tennessee.

The three ^{60}Co sources were installed in 1951 in teletherapy units in Saskatoon, Saskatchewan; Toronto, Ontario; and Houston, Texas.

their strengths and limitations, and their applications to treatment planning and monitoring in radiation therapy. The acquisition of this understanding is the purpose of this chapter.

■ RADIOGRAPHY

Radiography is the process by which information carried to a film by an x-ray beam is recorded, displayed, and interpreted to yield a diagnosis or reveal the location and extent of patient disease or injury.

X-Ray Film

X-ray film is an emulsion on one or both sides of a transparent film base. The emulsion contains granules of a silver halide, usually silver bromide, suspended as a crystal lattice in a gelatin matrix and covered with a protective coating. The emulsion is sensitive to visible light and ultraviolet light and to ionizing radiation.

When light photons or x rays interact with a film emulsion, electrons are released from the silver halide granules and trapped in *sensitivity centers* in the crystal lattice of the granules. The trapped electrons attract and neutralize mobile silver ions (Ag^+) in the lattice, leading to deposition of metallic silver across the film in response to the intensity of radiation incident on each region of film. This deposition of metallic silver is termed a *latent image* because it is not visible in the emulsion.

When an exposed film is placed in a developing solution, the silver atoms present at sensitivity centers serve to catalyze the deposition of additional silver atoms from the solution onto the film base. Unaffected granules of silver halide are then removed from the film base by placing the film in a fixing solution containing sodium or ammonium thiosulfate. Finally the film is washed and dried to yield an image in which the degree of blackening reflects the concentration of metallic silver, and therefore the amount of light or x radiation, interacting in the emulsion at each location. As described in Chapter 5, the blackening affects the transmission of visible light through the film, expressed as the *optical density* (OD), where OD = log (1/T), and T is the fractional transmission of light through the film.

Example 9-1

A small area on a radiograph transmits 10% ($T = 0.1$) of the incident light. What is the optical density of the area?

$$OD = \log(1/T) = \log(1/0.1) = \log(10) = 1$$

A second film with a uniform OD of 1 is placed over the radiograph. What is the OD of the combination of the uniform film and small area on the radiograph?

$$T = (0.1) \cdot (0.1) = 0.01$$

$$OD = \log(1/T) = \log(1/0.01) = \log 100 = 2$$

The relationship of OD and radiation exposure is described by the *characteristic curve* for the film (Figure 9-1). The region below the *straight-line* portion of the curve is the *toe*, and the region above the straight line portion is the *shoulder*. The range of exposures over which useful optical densities are achieved is termed the *exposure latitude*, and the difference in optical density between two exposures (i.e. the steepness of the straight-line portion of the curve) is described as the *film contrast*. The contrast can be described by the *average gradient* of the film, where

$$\text{Average gradient} = [D_2 - D_1]/[\log X_2 - \log X_1]$$

and X_1 and X_2 are the exposures required to produce optical densities D_1 and D_2.

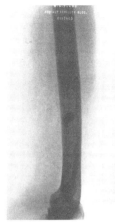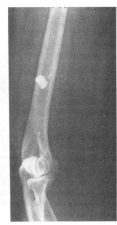

MARGIN FIGURE 9-1
Comparison of early and "modern" radiographs. An unusual historical item showing an early radiograph and "follow-up" made 35 years later. The patient was a girl who had been shot by a rifle bullet in 1897. The radiographic examination was made in the laboratory of Wolfram C. Fuchs in Chicago. After the examination, gold-toned contact prints were made from the *original glass plate*. One was sent to her physician; another was given to the patient and is reproduced on the left. The patient was reexamined in 1932 with "modern" x-ray film right, and the bullet may still be seen in its original position.[1]

For a few years following the discovery of x rays, radiography was thought of as a special area of photography, and photographers established "Röntgen studios" for photographic sittings using x rays.

The first radiographs were made with glass plates coated with a photographic emulsion. Occasionally radiographs are still referred to as "x-ray plates."

The first commercial x-ray film with a plastic film base was introduced in 1913 when the supply of glass from Belgium was impeded by World War I. The film base was cellulose nitrate, a highly flammable material. Cellulose nitrate was largely replaced with cellulose acetate following a disastrous fire at Cleveland Hospital in 1929. Cellulose acetate was replaced by a polyester film base in the early 1960s.

Optical density is a useful concept because it varies logarithmically with the transmission or brightness of the image. The human eye also responds logarithmically to image brightness.

A film that transmits 50% of the incident light has an optical density of 0.3 [$\log(1/0.5) = \log(2) = 0.3$].

Characteristic curves for film are also known as sensitometric or Hurter-Driffield [H–D] curves, with the latter expression named after the two photographers who developed the characteristic curve method.

Exposure latitude and film contrast are reciprocal concepts; increasing one decreases the other.

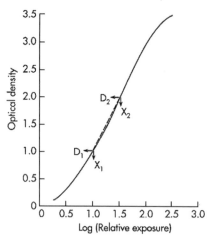

FIGURE 9-1
Characteristic curve for an x-ray film.[2]

Example 9-2

An x-ray film yields an OD of 2 for an exposure of 100 mR (10^{-1}R) and an OD of 1 for an exposure of 10 mR (10^{-2}R). What is the average gradient of the film?

$$\text{Average gradient} = [D_2 - D_1]/[\log X_2 - \log X_1]$$
$$= [2 - 1]/[\log 10^{-1} - \log 10^{-2}]$$
$$= 1/[-1 - (-2)]$$
$$= 1$$

The *film gamma* is the maximum gradient or slope of the characteristic curve, defined at the approximate center (the inflection point) of the characteristic curve.

The length of the toe of the characteristic curve, and therefore the position of the curve along the exposure axis, is described by the *film speed or film sensitivity*:

The inflection point of a characteristic curve is the point where the slope is constant (neither increasing nor decreasing).

Film speed = 1/[Exposure (R) to produce an OD of 1.0 above base density]

The toe is short for high-speed (fast) film and longer for lower-speed (slow) film. The speed of a film depends primarily on the size of the silver halide granules, with larger granules yielding a faster film. A fast film requires fewer x-ray or light interactions to form an image. Hence, a fast film furnishes a "noisier" image, in which fine detail may be less visible.

A fast film provides images at shorter exposures; however, the images tend to reveal less detail because they are "noisy."

Example 9-3

What is the speed of an x-ray film that requires 10 mR to provide an optical density of 1.0 above base density?

Film speed = 1/[Exposure (R) to produce an OD of 1.0 above base density]
$$= 1/0.01$$
$$= 100$$

Areas where x-ray film is stored must be very well protected from ambient radiation; an exposure of just a few MR can cause a significant increase in film fog.

A film processed without exposure to radiation has a small optical density resulting principally from absorption of light in the film base, which may be tinted slightly to yield a pleasing visual background. This intrinsic optical density is termed the *base density* of the film. Most x-ray film has a base density in the range of 0.07. When film is exposed to background radiation, chemical vapors, elevated temperatures, or physical pressure (e.g., by stacking film so that some sheets bear the weight of other sheets higher in the stack), metallic silver may be deposited in the emulsion without purposeful exposure to x rays. This deposition is referred to as *film fog*. A film density greater than about 0.2 contributed by the base density plus fog is considered unacceptable.

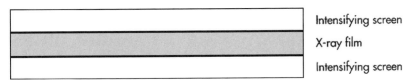

FIGURE 9-2
Intensifying screens and double-emulsion x-ray film.

The processing of x-ray film is one of the critical elements in producing high-quality images. Development time and temperature must be carefully controlled to yield images with satisfactory contrast and detail and without artifacts that can interfere with the visibility of important structures in the image. Quality control of the processing operation is achieved by the technique of *film sensitometry*, in which an image of a test object (step wedge) with graded thicknesses of absorbing material is obtained. Measurements of optical density at locations in the processed film corresponding to different thicknesses of absorber are compared with those for a standard image to ensure that processing conditions have not changed from the time when the standard image was obtained.

Intensifying Screens

Only a small percentage of the energy in a diagnostic x-ray beam is absorbed when a film is exposed directly to x-rays. Direct exposure to x rays is an inefficient process and is used only when images with fine detail (e.g., when looking for hairline fractures in the extremities) are required and relatively long exposure times are tolerable. For most x-ray examinations, the x-ray film is sandwiched between *intensifying screens* that furnish a light image in response to variations in exposure to the screens (Figure 9-2). The light image is then recorded by film that is sensitive to the wavelengths of light emitted by the screen.

Until the early 1970s, most intensifying screens contained crystalline calcium tungstate as a fluor that emitted light in the blue (420 nm) region. Calcium tungstate [$CaWO_4$] screens absorb 20% to 50% of the incident x rays depending on the screen thickness. A thicker screen (referred to as a "fast" screen) absorbs more x radiation but yields less detail in the image because the light diffuses from its origin in the screen on its way to the film emulsion. Thinner screens (termed *detail screens*) are less efficient but provide images with greater detail because less diffusion occurs over the shorter distance from screen to film. Screens of intermediate speed are termed *par-speed screens* and represent a compromise between speed and detail. These screens are widely used in radiography.

The K-absorption edge of tungsten (69.5 keV), the principal absorbing element in calcium tungstate screens, is above the energy of most photons in a diagnostic x-ray beam. X-ray absorption could be increased by replacing tungsten with an element of reduced Z so that the K-absorption edge occurs in the range of 30–50 keV and is thereby matched more appropriately to the average energy of x rays in the beam. Candidates for improved x-ray absorption include the rare-earth elements gadolinium, lanthanum, and yttrium. These elements, complexed in oxysulfide or oxybromide crystals and embedded in a plastic matrix, form the active component of *rare-earth intensifying screens* that have largely replaced calcium tungstate screens for conventional radiography. Rare-earth screens yield not only increased x-ray absorption, but also increased light output compared with calcium tungstate screens. The latter property is referred to as a greater *conversion efficiency* of x-ray energy to light. The two properties provide shorter exposure times and several other advantages for rare-earth screens compared with calcium tungstate screens.[1]

Example 9-4

Compare the number of visible light photons emitted by a calcium tungstate screen with the number emitted by a gadolinium oxysulfide screen. Assume that 100 x rays, each having an energy of 30 keV, strike the screen. The following data are given:

Film processing is a frequent cause of degraded image quality and image artifacts.

The first $CaWO_4$ x-ray intensifying screens were designed by Thomas Edison in 1896. Intensifying screens were first used at Columbia University in the same year.

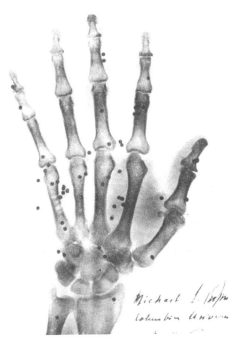

MARGIN FIGURE 9-2
First screen-film radiograph obtained by M. Pupin of Columbia University in February 1896. The radiograph demonstrates a shotgun wound to the hand.[1]

Rare-earth screens evolved in the early 1970s from research on new phosphors for television screens and instrument panels for aircraft and manned space flights.

Rare-earth phosphors used in intensifying screens include gadolinium oxysulfide, lanthanum oxybromide, yttrium oxysulfide, and barium fluorochloride.

	Calcium Tungstate	Gadolinium Oxysulfide
Absorption (%)	40	60
Conversion (%)	5	20
Spectral emission peak (nm)	420	555

The energy per visible photon emitted (with the simplifying assumption that all photons are emitted at the spectral peak energy) is

$$\text{keV} = \frac{1.24}{\lambda \, (\text{nm})}$$

$$= \frac{1.24}{420}$$

$$= 2.95 \times 10^{-3} \, \text{keV} \cong 3 \, \text{eV for calcium tungstate}$$

$$= \frac{1.24}{550}$$

$$= 2.25 \times 10^{-3} \, \text{keV} \cong 2 \, \text{eV for gadolinium oxysulfide}$$

The energy converted to visible light photons emitted from each screen is

$$\text{Energy emitted} = (100)(30 \times 10^3 \, \text{eV})(0.40)(0.05)$$

$$= 6 \times 10^4 \, \text{eV for calcium tungstate}$$

$$= (100)(30 \times 10^3 \, \text{eV})(0.60)(0.20)$$

$$= 36 \times 10^4 \, \text{eV for gadolinium oxysulfide}$$

The number of visible photons emitted from each screen is

$$\text{No. of photons emitted} = \frac{6 \times 10^4 \, \text{eV}}{3 \, \text{eV/photon}}$$

$$= 2 \times 10^4 \, \text{photons for calcium tungstate}$$

$$= \frac{36 \times 10^4 \, \text{eV}}{2 \, \text{eV/photon}}$$

$$= 18 \times 10^4 \, \text{photons for gadolinium oxysulfide}$$

Thus the lower energy per visible photon and the higher absorption and conversion efficiencies all act to produce more visible photons per incident photon for the gadolinium oxysulfide screen versus the calcium tungstate screen.

Source: Reference 2, with permission.

Radiographs (*port films*) obtained with high-energy photon beams used in radiation therapy are used to document the position of treatment fields and to confirm that the region to be treated is enclosed within the fields. These radiographs can be produced by direct exposure of the film to radiation. However, intensifying screens may be useful to shorten exposure times and to reduce the effects of scattered radiation on image detail and contrast. Because intensifying screens used in diagnostic radiology are not efficient absorbers of high-energy photons, lead sheets are often used to sandwich the x-ray film. The incident photons interact in the lead sheets, releasing photoelectrons and Compton electrons that impinge on the x-ray film to cause silver deposition. Compared with diagnostic x-ray images, port films provide lower image contrast because higher-energy photons interact in tissue principally by Compton interactions. These interactions yield images that mainly depict differences in physical density rather than atomic number in the patient (see Chapter 3).

Port films are widely used in radiation therapy to ensure the adequacy of a treatment plan, verify beam alignment, and evaluate the degree of shrinkage of a

Over the years, various techniques have been devised to improve the verification of alignment of treatment fields with the anatomic region to be treated. Today these techniques are approaching real-time verification of alignment during treatment.

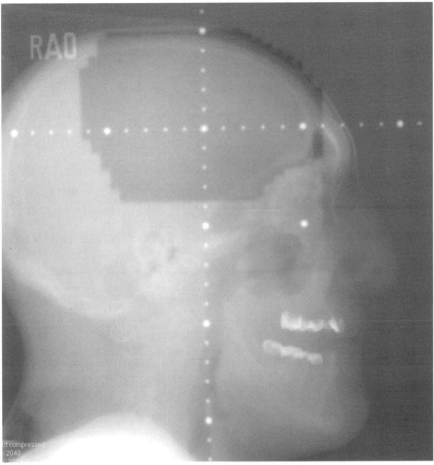

FIGURE 9-3
Port film demonstrating blocked treatment field (dark region) for a patient with a high grade glioma. (Courtesy of Waukesha Memorial Hospital.)

tumor during a course of treatment. The double-exposed port film for a 6-MV x-ray beam in Figure 9-3 shows the treatment field (the inner dark rectangle) superimposed on a larger exposed area that reveals the surrounding anatomy. On occasion, a slow film is left under the patient during the entire treatment to produce a treatment verification film.

Radiographic Grids

Information is conveyed to a film by primary x radiation transmitted through the patient. Radiation scattered from the patient and striking the film conceals patient information by producing a general photographic fog on the film. The amount of scattered radiation increases with the volume of irradiated tissue and can be reduced by confining the area of the x-ray beam to just the region of interest in the patient. Hence, proper collimation of the x-ray beam improves the x-ray image and reduces the radiation dose to the patient.

In addition to limiting the x-ray beam to the smallest cross-sectional area that encompasses the region of interest in the patient, further limitation of scattered photons usually is needed. Two solutions are possible because a scattered photon differs from a primary photon in two ways: It has less energy and it has a different direction. The first possible solution is not applicable to an x-ray beam, however, because the primary photons in the beam encompass a broad range of energies. Scattered photons fall within this energy range and cannot be distinguished from primary photons based

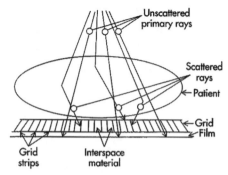

FIGURE 9-4

A radiographic grid is used to remove scattered radiation emerging from the patient. Most primary x rays are transmitted through the grid without attenuation.[2]

The first radiographic grid was described by Gustav Bucky in 1913. His grid removed scattered radiation relatively well, but created distracting lines in the images. Three radiologists, Bucky, Eugene Caldwell, and Hollis Potter, almost simultaneously conceived of the idea of moving the grid during exposure to blur the images of the grid lines. The moving grid today is referred to as a "Bucky" or a "Bucky–Potter mechanism." Caldwell has been lost in anonymity.

The Bucky moving grid was marketed in 1921 by General Electric. Bucky was a German citizen, and his patent on the moving grid concept was confiscated by the U.S. government at the end of World War I. He never received any royalties for his invention.

The grid ratio GR is

$$GR = \frac{\text{Grid strip height}}{\text{Grid strip separation}}$$

The contrast improvement factor CIF is

$$CIF = \frac{\text{Image contrast with grid}}{\text{Image contrast without grid}}$$

on energy. The second possible solution is applicable to an x-ray beam, because all of the primary x rays emanate from a common source (the focal spot of the x-ray tube) and follow predictable straight-line paths through the patient. Photons scattered in the patient deviate significantly from these straight-line paths and can be removed by a mechanical device (*a radiographic grid*) placed between the patient and the x-ray film or screen-film combination.

A radiographic grid (Figure 9-4) contains thin strips of a dense, high-Z material, such as lead or tungsten, separated by a material such as fiber, aluminum, or plastic that is relatively transparent to x rays. The thin (0.01 to 0.1 mm) strips are aligned parallel to the primary x rays so that they are not intercepted during their transit through the grid. The scattered x rays impinge on the grid in directions different from the primary x rays and must cross one or more lead strips before reaching the film. In all likelihood, the scattered photons will interact in a lead strip before reaching the film. In this manner, the radiographic grid uses the different direction of scattered x rays compared with primary x rays to remove the scattered photons from the x-ray beam. Hence, the grid helps to preserve the information in the image.

The efficiency of removal of scattered radiation by a grid is described by the *grid ratio*, defined as the height of the grid strips divided by the distance of separation of one strip from the next. Although grids with ratios as high as 16 are available commercially, grid ratios of 8–12 are used most often. Higher ratios provide little additional removal of scattered x rays and must be aligned carefully with the primary x-ray beam to prevent interception of primary x rays, resulting in *grid cut-off* (non-uniform exposure of the x-ray film). The *contrast improvement factor* of a grid is the ratio of image contrast with the grid compared with that without the grid in place. The number of grid strips per inch (lines per inch) is also important in describing the ability of a grid to remove scattered radiation, referred to colloquially as "grid cleanup." Grids with as many as 100 lines per inch are available. As a grid removes scattered x rays, more primary radiation is required to expose the film to yield the desired optical density. The *Bucky factor* is the exposure to the film without the grid divided by the exposure to the film with the grid in place, so that the desired OD is obtained for a wide x-ray field and relatively thick patient.

Although grid strips are thin, they still intercept the few primary x rays that impinge directly on them. Hence, the strips project a pattern of closely spaced fine lines in the image. This image is usually tolerable, especially for grids with thin strips and many lines per inch. The image of the grid strips can be removed by moving the grid laterally over a short distance during exposure. By moving the grid, the image of the grid strips is blurred across the film and is rendered invisible in the image. The capacity of the grid to remove scattered x rays is unaffected by the motion of the grid.

Digital Radiography

Recording of x-ray images on film is considered an analog method of information acquisition because the spatial and contrast information is captured in a continuous (i.e., nonsegmented) manner. In a digital image, the spatial information is presented as a matrix of small cells (picture elements or *pixels*), with each pixel presented as a gray level interpreted from a number for the particular pixel stored in the memory of a computer. The number is a "density value" for the tissue represented in the pixel. Several techniques are available to acquire radiographic information digitally or to convert analog images into digital format. These techniques are gradually gaining acceptance in radiology as interest grows in manipulating images by computer-based image processing programs. A second impetus for digital radiography is the desire to transmit images across *local area networks* (*LANs*) from their site of production to a location in the same institution where they are interpreted and used in patient care. A further incentive for digital radiology is to use *teleradiology* methods to transmit images across large distances for diagnostic interpretation and consultation. Local area networks are particularly useful for transmitting digital images in the hospital from the radiology department to the radiation oncology service, where they are used in treatment planning. Such networks are often called *miniPACS*, in which PACS is an acronym for *p*icture *a*rchiving and *c*ommunications *s*ystems.[3]

Some digital radiography systems employ a bank of radiation detectors, such as scintillation probes, photodiodes, or semiconductor devices, that scan across the patient in synchrony with a scanning fan-shaped x-ray beam. This *slit-scanning technique* yields an image with little scattered radiation.[4] The electrical signals from the detectors are converted to digital format, in which the magnitude of the signal is interpreted as a number ranging from perhaps 1 to 256 (2^0 to 2^8) and presented in the image as segmental gray levels displayed across a matrix of 512×512, 1024×1024, or 2048×2048 pixels. Another approach to digital radiography involves the digital conversion of the electrical signal from a television camera that views the output screen of a large image intensifier (image intensifier and television cameras are discussed in the following section on fluoroscopy).[5]

Storage phosphor technology is one approach to digital radiography that has been deployed in many clinical settings. In this technique, the x-ray image is projected and stored on a plate containing a photostimulable phosphor, such as barium fluorobromide. When the plate is scanned some time later with an intense focused laser, visible light is emitted from the phosphor in proportion to the energy absorbed earlier from the x-ray beam. The light output from the plate is detected with a photomultiplier tube (pmt) or other light-sensing detector, and it is digitized to produce a signal that can be viewed as an image on a high-resolution television monitor or photographic film. Digital radiography using storage phosphor technology sometimes is referred to as *computed radiography*.

Digital X-Ray Detectors

Over the next few years, digital x-ray detectors are likely to become available as replacements for more traditional methods of x-ray detection such as image intensifiers and intensifying screens and film. The most promising approach to digital x-ray detection is the use of "charge-coupled" devices (CCDs) produced by the technique of photolithography. A CCD is an integrated circuit formed by depositing an insulating oxide layer on a semiconductor wafer (usually silicon), followed by a series of electrodes called "gates." The product is an array of metal-oxide-semiconductor (MOS) capacitors (termed "storage wells") that can store electrical charge produced by the radiation or incident light. The stored charge is read out by transferring it from its storage location to a single readout preamplifier by synchronous operation of the gates above the storage wells. To date, only small two-dimensional CCD arrays of several square centimeters in area have been produced. However, work is progressing rapidly on making arrays large enough for clinical x-ray imaging.[7]

Radiographic images can be digitized by scanning them with a laser beam, with a light detector on the opposite side of the film used to measure the intensity of transmitted light. The signal from the detector is converted into digital form for transmission to remote locations, where it modulates the intensity of a light beam

Several academic medical centers have established teleradiology links with community hospitals to provide expert consultation on radiologic interpretation. In some cases these links have been extended to hospitals in remote locations, including foreign countries.

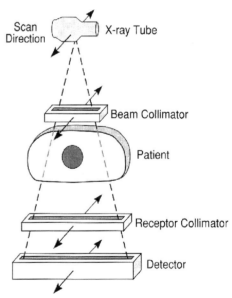

MARGIN FIGURE 9-3
Scanning slit radiography as a means of reducing contrast degradation by scatter. This is one of several ways in which a radiographic image can be entered directly into a computer without going through the intermediate step of forming an image on film or on a photostimulable phosphor plate.[6]

scanned across an x-ray film to reconstruct the original image. This technique is used in teleradiology to send images to other locations in the same institution or community or across much greater distances. Once the film image is digitized, it can be transmitted to remote locations over a telephone wire (twisted pair) or fiber-optic cable, or by a microwave or satellite link.

Example 9-5

What is the spatial resolution when an 8- × 10-in. radiograph is scanned into a 1024 × 1024 digital matrix?

Resolution element (pixel size) dimensions:

$$\text{Horizontal } (8 \text{ in.})(25.4 \text{ mm/in.})/1024 = 0.20 \text{ mm}$$

$$\text{Vertical } (10 \text{ in.})(25.4 \text{ mm/in.})/1024 = 0.25 \text{ mm}$$

Line pairs per millimeter: $1/2(1/r)$, where r = pixel dimension:

$$\text{Horizontal } 1/2(1/0.20 \text{ mm}) = 2.5 \text{ line pairs per mm}$$

$$\text{Vertical } 1/2(1/0.25 \text{ mm}) = 2.0 \text{ line pairs per mm}$$

The spatial resolution of the digitized image is significantly less than the 6–10 line pairs per millimeter available in the original radiograph.

Example 9-6

What is the computer storage required for the digital image in Example 9-5 if each pixel has a capacity of 256 (2^8 or 8 bits or 1 byte) of gray-scale information?

$$\text{Storage} = 1024 \times 1024 \times 8 = 8.4 \times 10^6 \text{ bits (more than one megabyte)}$$

Edison believed that fluoroscopy, rather than radiography, was the future of x-ray imaging. He designed the first fluoroscopic screen, which he initially called a "vitascope" and later a "fluoroscope."

■ FLUOROSCOPY

Radiography furnishes images that reveal the anatomy of the patient at a particular moment in time. The production of a continuous stream of images that depicts instantaneous changes in patient anatomy is referred to as *fluoroscopy*. In earlier years, fluoroscopy was performed by allowing x rays emerging from the patient to impinge directly on a fluorescent screen. The light image produced on the screen was viewed directly by the radiologist. In the early 1950s, the image intensifier was developed to provide a much brighter fluoroscopic image that does not require dark adaptation for viewing fluoroscopic images in a completely darkened room. Today the fluoroscopic image is usually viewed by capturing the image from the image intensifier with a television camera and using a television monitor to display the captured image.

Image Intensification

An *image intensifier* is diagrammed in Figure 9-5. X-rays from the patient impinge on a fluorescent input screen that is 5–12 in. in diameter. The fluorescent emulsion is a thin coating of CsI that emits a pattern of visible light in direct proportion to the x-ray intensity incident across the input screen. The light, in turn, falls on a contiguous photocathode surface from which electrons are ejected in response to the incident light. The electrons are focused and accelerated toward an anode that is maintained at a positive potential of 25–35 kV with respect to the photocathode. The electrons pass through the anode and impinge on the output screen, where a minified light image is produced of much greater intensity than the image on the input screen. The entire process occurs inside an evacuated glass envelope contained inside a metal-alloy housing that shields the intensifier from stray magnetic fields. The image-intensification process is accompanied by several transformations of the

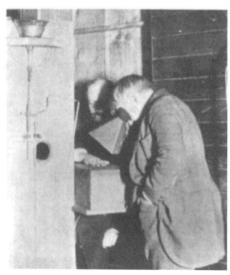

MARGIN FIGURE 9-4
Thomas Edison using the "vitascope" to view the hand of his assistant, Clarence Dally. Dally subsequently died of radiation-induced cancer and is considered the first casualty of x-irradiation.

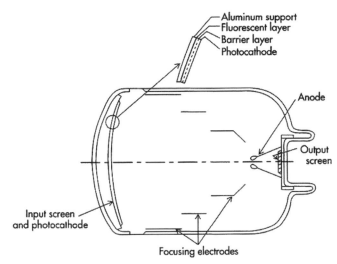

FIGURE 9-5
Cross section of an x-ray image intensifier.

carrier of patient information. The information is transferred from x rays to visible light, from visible light to electrons, and finally from electrons back to visible light emerging from the output screen as an intense but minified visible image.

The *brightness gain* of an image intensifier is described as the brightness of the image on the output screen of the intensifier compared with the brightness of the image produced by the same x-ray beam impinging directly on a fluorescent screen. The brightness gain is the product of two factors: the *minification gain* caused by the increased brightness resulting from minification of the image on the output screen and the *electronic gain* achieved by accelerating the electrons from the photocathode through several thousand volts on their way toward the anode. The minification gain is simply the ratio of the (diameter)^2 of the input screen divided by the (diameter)^2 of the output screen. The electronic gain is not easily calculable but is typically on the order of 40 or 50.

Example 9-7

What is the brightness gain of an image intensifier with a 9 in. diameter input screen, 1 in. diameter output screen, and electronic gain of 50?

$$\text{Minification gain} = [(\text{diameter input screen})/(\text{diameter output screen})]^2$$

$$= (9 \text{ in.}/1 \text{ in.})^2$$

$$= 81$$

$$\text{Electronic gain} = 50$$

$$\text{Brightness gain} = (\text{minification gain})(\text{electronic gain})$$

$$= (81)(50)$$

$$= 4050$$

By changing the voltage on the focusing electrodes, many image intensifiers can select the region of the input screen that is projected onto the output screen. This flexibility permits the intensifier to project a near life-size image (normal viewing mode) or a magnified image (magnified viewing mode). If one stage of magnification is provided, the intensifier is termed a *dual-field image intensifier*. An intensifier that furnishes two stages of magnification is called a *triple-field image intensifier*. To

Early image intensifiers employed CdZnS as the fluorescent screen. CsI was introduced in the early 1970s as a replacement for CdZnS.

The image intensifier was introduced into radiology in 1952, and it became accepted in the early 1960s as a replacement for the stand-alone fluoroscopic screen. The image intensifier yields a much brighter image compared with a simple fluorescent screen, and radiologists no longer had to "dark adapt" for several minutes to be able to see the fluoroscopic image.

The brightness gain of a stand-alone fluoroscopic screen is unity. Comparison of this value with the brightness gain computed in Example 9-7 illustrates the improvement in image brightness achieved with the image intensifier.

compensate for the loss in minification gain that accompanies viewing in magnified mode, the exposure rate is increased when magnification of the image is selected.

Example 9-8

What exposure rate increase is required to maintain the brightness of the output screen when a dual-field image intensifier is changed from normal (9-in. diameter) to magnified (6-in. diameter) viewing mode?

$$\text{Minification gain} = [(\text{diameter input screen})/(\text{diameter output screen})]^2$$

$$9 \text{ in.:} \quad \text{gain} = (9/1 \text{ in.})^2 = 81$$
$$6 \text{ in.:} \quad \text{gain} = (6/1 \text{ in.})^2 = 36$$

$$\text{Reduction in minification gain} = 81/36 = 2.25$$

The exposure rate must be raised by a factor of 2.25 in switching from normal to magnified viewing mode.

Television Display of Fluoroscopic Images

A television system for viewing fluoroscopic images consists of five components:

- Television camera
- Transmission channel
- Television monitor
- Camera control unit
- Image storage device

A television monitor for viewing fluoroscopic images is similar in principle to a home television set. However, it displays black and white rather than color images, and does not need a tuning circuit to intercept different broadcast frequencies.

In television viewing of fluoroscopic images, a camera control unit is required to ensure that the electron scanning beams in the camera and the monitor are exactly synchronized.

Digital detectors such as charge-coupled devices provide a direct readout of electrical charge, obviating the need for a scanning electron beam from a television camera. As these radiation detectors are deployed in the future, television cameras will become unnecessary.

Today, most image-intensified fluoroscopic images are viewed on a television monitor. The televised image is produced by coupling a television camera optically to the output screen of the image intensifier. The television camera, usually of the plumbicon or vidicon type, scans the light image on the output screen and produces an electrical signal with an amplitude that varies instantaneously with the light intensity at each point on the output screen. This signal is transmitted by cable to a television monitor, a technique referred to as *closed-circuit television*. In the monitor, the electrical signal is used to modulate the intensity of an electron beam that scans across a fluorescent screen in synchrony with the scanning electron beam in the television camera. In this manner, a light image is created on the fluorescent screen of the television monitor that replicates the image on the output screen of the image intensifier.

The spatial resolution in the vertical direction of a television image varies with the number of horizontal sweeps of the electron beam in the television camera and therefore the number of corresponding horizontal sweeps of the electron beam used to create the image on the television monitor. Images with a large number (e.g., 875 or 1024) of horizontal sweeps (scan lines) in a television monitor yield a greater vertical resolution compared with that in images with a lower number (e.g., 525 or 625) of horizontal scan lines.

To prevent brightness flicker in the image, the electron beam in the television camera first scans along even-numbered sweeps (2,4,6,...). The resulting set of horizontal scan lines constitutes a single *field* of the television image. This image is followed immediately by sweeps of the electron beam along odd-numbered lines (1,3,5,...) to produce a second television field. The two fields are interlaced to form a single *frame* of the television image. With voltage alternating at a frequency of 60 Hz, each field is completed in 1/60 second, and a television frame is presented every 1/30 second.

The spatial resolution in the horizontal direction of a television image depends on the number of resolution elements available along a single horizontal scan line in the image. The number of horizontal resolution elements depends in turn on the bandwidth (sometimes called the frequency bandpass) of the television system. The bandwidth is the highest frequency at which the electrical signal can be modulated without distortion in response to varying light intensity on the output screen of the intensifier. Bandwidths for closed-circuit television typically range from about 3.5 MHz (3.5 million cycles per second) to 12 MHz. Bandwidths up to 20 MHz are available in high-resolution (high-definition) television [HDTV]) systems, but such systems are too expensive at present for routine use in diagnostic imaging.

In the computation of the vertical and horizontal resolutions of a television image, additional factors must be considered. For the vertical resolution, the following examples may be used[8]:

$$\text{Vertical resolution} = (\text{Horizontal sweeps/frame})(\text{Kell factor})$$

where the Kell factor is the fraction of horizontal sweeps of the electron beam that are actually effective in preserving detail in the image. The Kell factor is about 0.7 for most television systems. The horizontal resolution can be computed with the expression[9]

$$\text{Horizontal resolution} = \frac{2(\text{bandwidth})(\text{horizontal function})(\text{aspect ratio})}{(\text{frames/sec})(\text{lines/frame})}$$

In this expression, (1) the bandwidth is expressed in hertz, (2) the horizontal fraction is the quotient of the time required to complete on horizontal sweep divided by the time required for the horizontal sweep plus the time required to return the electron beam (the retrace) to a position for the next horizontal sweep, (3) the number of frames/sec is usually 30, (4) the lines/frame is the number of horizontal scan lines per frame, (5) the aspect ratio is the ratio of the width of a television frame to its height, and (6) the expression is multiplied by 2 because resolution is described in terms of the total number of resolution elements, both light and dark, that are visible in the television image. Most television images provide about equal resolution in the horizontal and vertical directions.

Example 9-9

What approximate bandwidth is required for a 60-Hz interlaced 525-line television system to provide equal spatial resolution in the horizontal and vertical dimensions? Assume a horizontal fraction of 0.83 and an aspect ratio of 1:

$$\text{Vertical resolution} = (\text{Number of active sweeps/frame})(\text{Kell factor})$$

$$= (525)(0.7)$$

$$= 370 \text{ lines/frame}$$

The horizontal resolution is therefore also 370 lines/frame:

$$\text{Horizontal resolution} = \frac{2(\text{bandwidth})(\text{horizontal fraction})(\text{aspect ratio})}{(\text{frames/sec})(\text{lines/frame})}$$

$$370 \text{ lines/frame} = \frac{2(\text{bandwidth})(0.83)(1)}{(30)(525)}$$

$$\text{Bandwidth} = \frac{(370)(30)(525)}{2(0.83)(1)}$$

$$= 3.5 \times 10^6 \text{ sec}^{-1}$$

$$= 3.5 \text{ MHz}$$

■ TREATMENT SIMULATORS

A treatment simulator is an x-ray imaging device that simulates the geometry of a radiation treatment unit. Most simulators provide both fluoroscopic imaging and radiography for production of permanent hard-copy images. A simulator is used to present diagnostic images of a tumor and surrounding tissues in the exact configuration encountered during radiation therapy. With a simulator, the proper configuration of treatment fields can be confirmed, and the correct alignment of shielding blocks and surface landmarks can be verified.

Compared with conventional radiography, features of early x-ray computed tomography included:

a. spatial resolution that was poorer by a factor of at least 10×;
b. imaging times that were 100–1000× longer
c. cost that was 10× greater

These disadvantages were more than compensated by x-ray CT's ability to provide cross-sectional images with greatly improved contrast resolution.

The term "tomography" is derived from the Greek word *tomos*, meaning "section."

William Oldendorf was a neuroscientist interested in improving the differentiation of brain tissue. In particular, he was searching for a better imaging method than pneumoencephalography for studying the brain. In this search, Oldendorf developed a rudimentary CT scanner in the early 1960s. Many scientists believe he should have shared in the 1970 Nobel Prize in Medicine.

Hounsfield termed his technique "computerized transverse axial tomography." This expression was later abbreviated to "computerized axial tomography" and was referred to as "CAT scanning." After sufficient ridicule had been directed toward this acronym, the expression *computed tomography* (CT scanning) was adopted by major journals in Medical imaging.

In the early 1960s the physicist Allen Cormack explored the generation of cross-sectional displays of attenuation coefficients for use in treatment planning for radiation therapy. He published his results in the *Journal of Applied Physics*. He received only one reprint request. It was from members of the Swiss Avalanche Research Center, who were interested in possible use of his method to predict snow depths.

Simulators offer many advantages for treatment planning and monitoring in radiation therapy. Because they employ x-ray beams of diagnostic quality, they provide more definitive images with improved contrast compared with port films obtained with the treatment unit. Because they duplicate the geometry of the treatment unit, they furnish more accurate displays of tissue configuration and radiation beam alignment compared with images obtained with conventional diagnostic x-ray equipment. They are located outside the treatment room, so the time-consuming process of patient setup can be conducted without impeding the use of the treatment unit for other patients. Simulators permit measurements of patient contours, tissue thicknesses, and tumor margins for construction of bolus, tissue-compensating filters, and shielding blocks.

A relatively recent addition to treatment simulation is the use of CT-based simulators (CT-Sim). This topic is explored in Chapter 11.

■ COMPUTED TOMOGRAPHY

In conventional radiography, subtle differences of a few percent in x-ray transmission through the body are not visible in the image because (1) the projection of three-dimensional anatomic information onto a two-dimensional image receptor obscures subtle differences in x-ray transmission through different structures in the body; (2) conventional image receptors (film, screens, and image intensifiers) are unable to resolve differences smaller than a few percent in the intensity of incident radiation; and (3) large-area x-ray beams used in conventional radiography produce significant amounts of scattered radiation that interfere with the visualization of subtle differences in x-ray transmission.

Each of these limitations in conventional radiography is significantly reduced in *CT*, and differences in x-ray transmission (subject contrast) of a few tenths of a percent are revealed in the image. Although the spatial resolution of a millimeter or so provided by CT is notably poorer than that provided by conventional radiography (~0.1 mm), the superior visualization of subject contrast and the display of anatomy across planes (e.g., cross-sectional [sometimes called transaxial], coronal, and sagittal sections), which are not available with conventional radiography, make CT exceptionally useful for visualizing anatomy in many regions of the body.

History

The revolutionary imaging technology of CT was introduced to clinical medicine in 1972 with announcement of the EMI Ltd head scanner developed by Hounsfield.[10] The technique of image reconstruction from projections employed in the EMI scanner had been used in other fields, such as radioastronomy,[11] electron microscopy,[12,13] and optics,[14,15] and was based on a mathematical algorithm developed by Radon in 1917.[16] The advantages of CT in clinical medicine quickly became apparent, and many companies joined the race in the mid-1970s to produce a better scanner.[17] By the end of the decade, four "generations" of CT scanners had appeared, and several of the companies had become financial casualties or had decided to redirect their attention to other ventures. Today, CT units are marketed principally by the major instrument companies servicing the medical marketplace. More than 4000 CT units are installed today in U.S. hospitals alone, at a cost of a million dollars or more per unit.[1]

Computed tomography has been a major influence on the evolution of imaging technologies in medicine over the past two decades. Some once-popular imaging techniques, such as brain scans in nuclear medicine and pneumoencephalography in radiology, have virtually disappeared, whereas others, such as cerebral angiography and myelography in radiology, have been impacted significantly. Imaging methods such as single-photon emission computed tomography (SPECT), positron emission tomography (PET), and MRI employ image reconstruction techniques similar to those developed for CT. Others, such as real-time and gray-scale ultrasonography, functional studies in nuclear medicine, and digital radiography, employ computer-based digital methods for data acquisition and processing that were introduced originally by CT. Treatment planning in radiation therapy has been assisted greatly by CT. Medical imaging has experienced major changes over the past two decades that were initiated with the recognition of the clinical advantages of CT in the early 1970s.

Principles of Computed Tomography

In early versions of a CT scanner, a narrow beam of x rays is scanned across the patient in synchrony with a radiation detector on the opposite side of the patient. The x-ray detector may be a pressurized ionization chamber, a scintillation detector, or a semiconductor diode. The transmission I of x rays through a patient of thickness x is $I = I_0 e^{-\mu x}$ with the patient assumed to have a uniform composition with linear attenuation coefficient μ. For a patient with many ("n") regions, each with a different thickness and attenuation coefficient, the x-ray transmission is $I = I_0 e^{-\sum \mu_i x_i}$, where $-\sum \mu_i x_i = -(\mu_1 x_1 + \mu_2 x_2 + \cdots + \mu_n x_n)$ and the fractional transmission $I/I_0 = e^{-\sum \mu_i x_i}$. With a single transmission measurement, the separate attenuation coefficients cannot be determined because too many unknown values of μ_i exist in the equation for fractional transmission. However, multiple measurements of x-ray transmission obtained at different orientations of the x-ray source and detector permit computation of the separate coefficients. This computation yields a cross-sectional matrix of attenuation values corresponding to a slice of tissue through the patient. Each of the attenuation values can be expressed as a *CT number* calculated as

$$\text{CT number} = 1000 \left[\frac{\mu_i - \mu_w}{\mu_w} \right]$$

where μ_i is the attenuation value of a particular volume element of tissue (voxel) and μ_w is the linear attenuation coefficient of water for the average energy of x rays in the CT beam. Each of the CT numbers can be assigned a particular shade of gray, and the matrix of CT numbers can be presented as a cross-sectional (transaxial) gray-scale display. This gray-scale display constitutes the CT image. Successive CT sets of transmission measurements displaced slightly from each other through the patient yield a series of cross-sectional images representing contiguous "slices" through the body. Each slice possesses a *slice thickness* that can be varied from about 1 mm to 1 cm. Furthermore, corresponding voxels in successive slices can be combined mathematically to yield coronal and sagittal images that complement the transaxial images provided routinely by the CT scanner.

In first-generation CT scanners, the x-ray source provided a pencil-like x-ray beam that was scanned in translational motion across the patient at several (e.g., 180) orientations that differed slightly in direction (e.g., 1 degree) from the preceding and succeeding scan. This translate–rotate scanning geometry required several minutes to accumulate x-ray transmission data for a single image, and patient motion interfered with image quality. The time-consuming procedure for data acquisition prevented application of the technique to areas of the body other than the head because patient motion is too severe in those areas. Succeeding generations of CT scanners have principally reflected efforts to reduce scanning times to a few seconds or less and to improve spatial resolution by introducing intrinsic methods of quality control. Second-generation scanners replaced the pencil-like x-ray beam with a fan-shaped beam that employs translate–rotate motion at angular increments of several degrees to reduce scanning times to 20 seconds or so. Third-generation scanners use a fan-shaped x-ray beam and a bank of multiple detectors that undergo purely rotational motion to reduce scan times to as short as 1 to 2 seconds. Fourth-generation scanners use a stationary circular array of detectors and a fan-shaped x-ray beam to provide scan times comparable to those with a third-generation scanner. Fifth-generation scanners employ a novel approach to x-ray production to reduce scan times to several

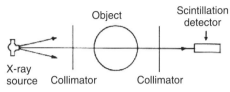

MARGIN FIGURE 9-5
In a first-generation computed tomographic scanner, x-ray transmission measurements are accumulated while an x-ray source and detector are translated and rotated in synchrony on opposite sides of the patient.

X-ray CT images are often described as "density distributions" because they provide a gray-scale display of linear attenuation coefficients that are closely related to the physical density of tissues.

Spiral CT scanners today employ multiple detector rings to scan several slices through the body during each gantry rotation. These scanners are referred to as multi-slice CT scanners.

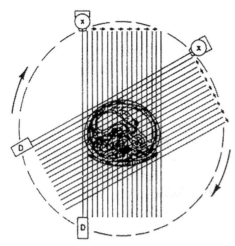

MARGIN FIGURE 9-6

First-generation scanner using a pencil x-ray beam and a combination of translational and rotational motion.

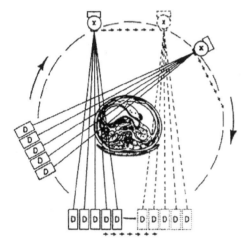

MARGIN FIGURE 9-7

Second-generation scanner with a fan x-ray beam, multiple detectors, and a combination of translational and rotational motion.

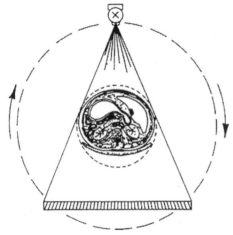

MARGIN FIGURE 9-8

Third-generation scanner with rotational motion of the x-ray tube and detector array.

milliseconds. These scanners yield images that are restricted by image noise caused by limitations in the number of x rays used to determine the attenuation coefficients of different voxels. Most CT scanners in use today employ third-generation or fourth-generation geometry.[17] The scanning geometries characteristic of different generations of CT scanners are depicted in the margin.

Reconstruction Algorithms

The foundation of CT is the construction of images from projections by use of a mathematical *algorithm*. Various algorithms have been used, including simple backprojection, integral equations (the *convolution method*), Fourier transformation, and series expansion.[18] Image reconstruction can be illustrated by the technique of simple backprojection applied to translate–rotate geometry.

In *simple backprojection*, each path of x-ray transmission through the body is divided into multiple equally spaced elements, and each element is assumed to contribute equally to the total attenuation of x rays along the transmission path. In Figure 9-6, transmission path A is divided into 10 equally spaced volume elements (voxels), and each element is assumed to contribute 1% attenuation to the total 10% attenuation along the path. Path B of x-ray transmission measured at a different orientation intersects path A at one of the voxels. The total attenuation along path B is 20%, and each of the 10 voxels along the path is assumed to contribute 2% to the attenuation. The two attenuations at the intersecting voxel are added to yield a summed attenuation of 3%. A third transmission path C also intersects the common voxel and adds an additional 3% to the summed attenuation value. For a translate–rotate geometry with 180 angular orientations, the total attenuation of the common voxel is the sum of 180 separate values, with each value measured for an x-ray path obtained at a particular angular orientation of the x-ray source and detector. Every voxel in the anatomic cross section is intersected by 180 paths of x-ray transmission, and the attenuation for each is the sum of 180 individual measurements. As a result, the cross-sectional gray-scale display of attenuation values presents picture elements (pixels) corresponding to the volume elements (voxels) of tissue in the patient, with grayness in the pixel corresponding to the attenuation in the voxel. This display constitutes the CT image compiled by the method of simple backprojection.

Simple backprojection has one major limitation: It produces images with serious blurring artifacts in regions where adjacent voxels differ significantly in their attenuation values. Suppression of these artifacts requires a modification of the simple backprojection technique in which a deblurring function is combined (convolved) with the transmission data before the transmission data are backprojected. The most common deblurring function is a *frequency ramp filter* that increases signal amplification linearly with frequency up to a cutoff frequency, where the amplification drops to zero. Because a ramp filter also amplifies the noise, an *ad* hoc filter such as a Hamming or Hann filter is introduced to reduce or "roll off" the amplification of the ramp filter at higher frequencies.

The technique of convolving the transmission data with a deblurring function is referred to as the *convolution method* of image reconstruction. This method is the most popular reconstruction algorithm used today in CT. One of its advantages is that the image can be compiled while x-ray transmission data are being collected.

Computed tomography is a useful imaging technique for delineating surface contours, tumor volumes, and the position of surrounding normal structures in treatment planning for radiation therapy.[19−21] It also provides attenuation values helpful in determining corrections for tissue heterogeneity during the delivery of radiation treatments.[22,23] Most commercial CT units offer software packages for extension to treatment planning applications. Many of the packages permit direct transfer of images from the CT unit to the treatment planning computer, in which isodose distributions can be superimposed to delineate satisfactory treatment plans for the patient. In treatment planning computers without direct linkage to a CT unit, the CT contours can be entered manually for use in treatment planning. An example of an isodose distribution superimposed on a cross-sectional CT image is shown in Figure 9-7.

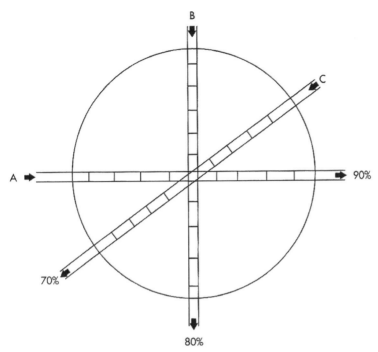

FIGURE 9-6
Principle of simple back construction method of image reconstruction from projections. See text for explanation.

■ ULTRASONOGRAPHY

Ultrasound imaging (*sonography*) is a useful technique for delineating surface contours and internal structures important to identification of satisfactory treatment plans in radiation therapy. In this imaging method, a piezoelectric crystal at the face of an ultrasound transducer is used to generate a mechanical disturbance (pressure wave) that is propagated through tissue directly in front of the transducer. The wave is

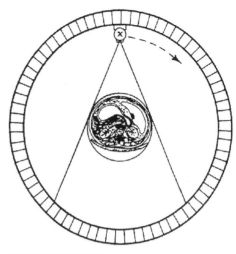

MARGIN FIGURE 9-9
Fourth-generation scanner with rotational motion of the x-ray tube and a stationary array of several hundred detectors.

Filtered backprojection removes the star-like blurring seen in simple backprojection. It is the principal reconstruction algorithm used in CT scanners.

The scanning technique employed by first-generation CT scanners is referred to as "rectilinear pencil-beam scanning."

The first five clinical CT units marketed by EMI Ltd. were installed by early 1973 in London, Manchester, Glasgow, Rochester (MN), and Boston.

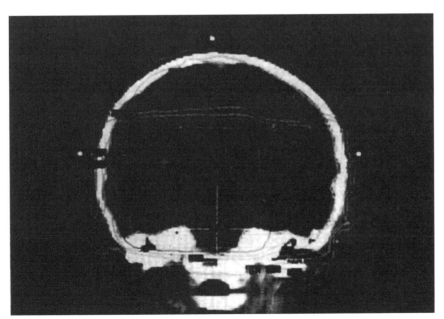

FIGURE 9-7
Complex isodose distribution superimposed on a cross-sectional computed tomographic image. (Courtesy of George T. Y. Chen, University of Chicago, now at Massachusetts General Hospital.)

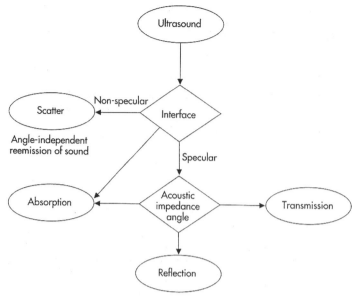

FIGURE 9-8
Ultrasound reflection and refraction at an interface between tissues in the body.

initiated by applying a momentary electrical shock to the piezoelectric crystal that sets the crystal into vibration. This vibration introduces the pressure wave into the medium. The frequency (1–10 MHz) of the pressure wave is in the ultrasound range well above the frequency range to which the human ear is responsive (20 Hz to 20 kHz).

As an ultrasound wave moves through the body, it encounters various interfaces between tissues that reflect and refract (change the direction of) the ultrasound energy (Figure 9-8). At any interface, the amount of energy reflected back toward the transducer depends on the difference in acoustic impedance across the interface. The acoustic impedance Z of a tissue is the product of the physical density ρ of the tissue and the speed v of ultrasound through the tissue ($Z = \rho v$).

Piezo is Greek for "pressure"

A *transducer* is any device that converts (transduces) energy from one form to another.

Piezoelectricity was discovered by Jacques and Pierre (husband of Marie) Curie in the 1880s.

During World War I, Langevin and others developed the use of pulse-echo sound to detect submarines, map the ocean floor, and detect underwater obstacles. The latter application was stimulated by the Titanic disaster of 1912. During World War II, the pulse-echo method evolved into the sophisticated technique of Sound Navigation and Ranging (SONAR).

Example 9-10

The fraction of ultrasound reflected at an interface is described by the ultrasound reflection coefficient

$$\alpha_R = \left[\frac{Z_2 - Z_1}{Z_2 + Z_1} \right]^2$$

and Z_1 and Z_2 are the acoustic impedances of tissues on each side of the interface. What is the fraction of ultrasound energy reflected at the interface between the chest wall and lung if the ultrasound velocity is assumed to be the same in both tissues and the physical densities are assumed to be approximately 1 g/cm^3 in the chest wall and 0.001 g/cm^3 in lung?

$$\alpha_R = \left[\frac{Z_2 - Z_1}{Z_2 + Z_1} \right]^2$$

$$= \left[\frac{1 - 0.001}{1 + 0.001} \right]^2 = 0.996$$

That is, 99.6% of the ultrasound energy is reflected, and only 0.4% is transmitted at the interface.

When the difference in acoustic impedance is great across an interface, most of the energy is reflected, and little is transmitted across the interface into the second medium. For this reason, ultrasonography is not useful in examining the thorax because the great difference in physical density between the chest wall and the lung prevents the ultrasound from penetrating across the interface. Ultrasonography is useful for measuring the thickness of the chest wall in treatment planning because reflected ultrasound yields a clear delineation of the surface contour and the inner boundary of the chest wall. Ultrasonography also presents problems in examining structures in the shadow of bone because much of the ultrasound energy is reflected at the soft tissue–bone interface, and that which is transmitted is strongly absorbed in bone.

Ultrasonography is particularly useful for delineating tissues that differ only slightly in their acoustic impedances, provided that enough energy is reflected at the interface between the tissues to furnish a measurable signal as reflected ultrasound returning to the transducer. For example, ultrasonography is used to distinguish cysts from solid lesions in the breast following their identification as suspicious regions in mammography because enough ultrasound energy is reflected to outline the boundaries of the lesion. Furthermore a solid lesion produces additional reflections in the lesion's interior, whereas the inner region of a cyst is anechoic (i.e., it does not produce internal reflections [*echoes*] of ultrasound energy).

Ultrasound energy reflected from an interface between tissues in the body returns as a pressure wave of reduced amplitude to the transducer. As it is absorbed by the piezoelectric crystal in the transducer, it generates a small electrical signal that is captured and processed. The angular orientation of the ultrasound transducer as the signal is received defines the direction of the returning pressure wave and therefore the position of the interface that produced it. The time t between transmission of the ultrasound energy and receipt of the returning signal defines the depth of the interface according to the expression

$$\text{Depth} = (v \cdot t)/2$$

where v is the velocity of ultrasound. Division by 2 is required in this expression because the time t includes both the time to reach the interface and the time for the echo to return to the transducer. The velocity v of ultrasound varies slightly among different soft tissues, but a value of 1540 m/sec often is assumed in computations of the depth of reflecting interfaces.

> Echocardiography is possible because soft-tissue pathways into the mediastinum are accessible.

Example 9-11

An echo is detected 130 μsec after an ultrasound pulse is transmitted into tissue. What is the depth of the interface that produced the echo?

$$\text{Depth} = (v \cdot t)/2$$
$$= (154,000\,\text{cm/sec})(130 \times 10^{-6}\,\text{sec})/2$$
$$= 10\,\text{cm}$$

Reflected ultrasound energy is returned to the transducer most efficiently when the interface is at right angles to the ultrasound beam. However, tissue interfaces in the body can be at any angle with respect to the surface contour of the patient. To obtain images of these interfaces, the ultrasound transducer usually is rocked as it is moved across the patient's surface so that the ultrasound beam intersects interfaces at close to a right angle at least part of the time during a scan. This two-phase motion with the transducer coupled to the skin with a thin layer of gel is referred to as *compound contact scanning*.

In the early years of ultrasound imaging, a single transducer was moved manually across the body surface to obtain an ultrasound image. This process was relatively slow and required a highly-skilled operator to acquire an acceptable image. Recent scanners provide *multitransducer arrays* that permit more rapid imaging and the acquisition of real-time images in which artifacts caused by patient motion are subdued

> The first compound contact scanner was built in 1962 by Thompson, Holmes and colleagues at the University of Colorado.

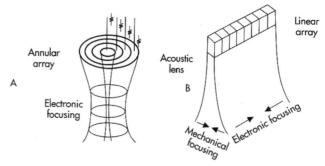

FIGURE 9-9
Multitransducer arrays for real-time ultrasound imaging.[2]

(Figure 9-9). More complete explanations of the technology and applications of ultrasound imaging are available in standard texts on the physics of medical imaging.[2,24]

In addition to determinations of chest wall thickness, ultrasound imaging is useful for localizing a variety of normal and abnormal structures in the head and neck, breast, upper abdomen, lower pelvis, and retroperitoneum. These applications of ultrasonography to treatment planning and delivery in radiation therapy are described in the literature.[25−27]

■ NUCLEAR MEDICINE

Nuclear medicine is a form of functional imaging in which physiology, metabolism, and biochemistry, rather than anatomic structure, are the principal features portrayed in images. In this discipline, a radioactive nuclide (*radionuclide*) is administered to a patient, usually tagged to a specific gamma-emitting radioactive pharmaceutical selected for its tendency to concentrate in a specific organ or tissue of interest in the patient. Gamma rays emitted by the nuclide escape from the body and are measured with an external detector. The measurement process yields a "map" of the accumulation, distribution, and excretion of the pharmaceutical in the organ or tissue of interest.

The use of radioactively tagged compounds as biochemical tracers has been of great importance in biology since the discovery of radioactivity. Radioactive tracers have contributed in a major way to the many advances in biology and the basic sciences underlying medicine (e.g., biochemistry, physiology, pharmacology, and cellular and molecular biology) that have occurred over this century. However, the routine use of radioactively tagged pharmaceuticals (*radiopharmaceuticals*) in clinical medicine awaited three major advances that occurred in the middle of the twentieth century. These advances were: (1) the availability of nuclear reactors as sources of artificially produced radioisotopes that followed World War II and was facilitated by the Atoms for Peace program of the Atomic Energy Commission; (2) the development of the scintillation camera by Anger in the late 1950s[28]; and (3) the evolution of the radionuclide generator, specifically the ^{99}Mo^{99m}Tc radionuclide generator, at about the same time. Today, close to half of all hospitalized patients in the United States experience at least one nuclear medicine procedure, and most potential candidates for radiation therapy undergo one or more nuclear medicine procedures for purposes such as staging cancer and determining the likelihood and extent of its dissemination.

Properties of Radioactive Pharmaceuticals

Radionuclides are selected for diagnostic nuclear medicine based on properties that make them desirable for medical imaging. Among these desirable properties are:

- A relatively short physical half-life so that the radionuclide can be administered to the patient in sufficient activities to yield enough gamma rays to produce an

---

Nuclear diagnostic studies can be categorized into four general groups:

- Localization
- Dilution
- Flow or diffusion
- Biochemical and metabolic properties

Many of these properties were first demonstrated in the 1920s by George Hevesy, a Hungarian physicist working in Denmark. One of his more well-known experiments was use of a radioactive tracer to prove that the hash served at his boarding house contained meat he had left on his plate the evening before.

In accepting the Nobel Prize for Chemistry in 1943, de Hevesy stated: "The most remarkable result obtained in the study of the application of isotope indicators is perhaps the discovery of the dynamic state of the body constituents. The molecules building up the plant or animal organism are incessantly renewed."

Scintillation cameras are sometimes referred to as gamma cameras or Anger cameras.

The first commercial scintillation camera was installed at Ohio State University in 1962.

acceptable image, yet with little residual activity so that problems of disposing residual materials and patient wastes are reduced

- A relatively short biologic half-life so that residual activity in the patient does not produce unacceptable radiation doses
- The emission of little particulate radiation (e.g., beta particles and conversion and Auger electrons) because these radiations do not contribute to the examination but increase the radiation dose to the patient
- The emission of gamma rays of an energy well matched to the detection efficiency of the measurement apparatus (e.g., the scintillation camera)
- The availability of a specific gamma-ray energy that is well separated from gamma rays of lower energy so that scattered photons can be rejected based on their lower energy
- High specific activity so that the radionuclide can be tagged with high efficiency into the selected pharmaceutical
- Ease of labeling of the radionuclide into the pharmaceutical

One radionuclide that satisfies these requirements reasonably well is ^{99m}Tc, and 85% or so of all nuclear medicine procedures are performed with this material. ^{99m}Tc is produced in a radionuclide generator in which the condition of transient equilibrium (see Chapter 1) is achieved between the parent ^{99}Mo and the progeny ^{99m}Tc.

Pharmaceuticals also have specific properties that make them desirable as imaging agents in nuclear medicine. Among these properties are:

- Their availability in a specific chemical form without competing chemical isomers that exhibit different physiologic behaviors
- Chemical stability *in vitro* so that the pharmaceutical can be stored before use, and *in vivo* so that the radionuclide does not dissociate from the pharmaceutical once it is inside the body
- Predictable and reproducible behavior in the body
- A high target/nontarget ratio in the body so that the radiopharmaceutical will deposit in the region of interest without delivering excessive radiation doses to other organs and tissues
- Traceable kinetics that permit determination of quantitative parameters important to the assessment of physiologic function
- A biologic half-life that is long enough to accommodate the nuclear medicine study, yet short enough to permit rapid elimination of the tagged pharmaceutical after the study has been completed

The development of *receptor-specific radiopharmaceuticals* is one of the more promising areas of nuclear medicine today. Some of these pharmaceuticals, including radioactively tagged monoclonal antibodies, may soon permit identification of the presence of specific types of cancer cells at much lower concentrations than those measurable by current imaging techniques. Although much work remains to improve the sensitivity and specificity of receptor-specific radiopharmaceuticals, their appeal as a promising approach to cancer detection and staging is unmistakable.[29]

Nuclear Medicine Imaging

In nuclear medicine, gamma rays emitted by a radionuclide tagged to a specific pharmaceutical localized in a particular organ or tissue of the patient are measured by a radiation detector positioned outside the patient. To obtain an image of the distribution of the radionuclide in the patient, the site of interaction of gamma rays in the detector must be correlated with the origin of the gamma rays inside the patient. To provide this correlation, a collimator is placed between the detector and the patient. Different collimators are available, including pinhole, converging, and diverging collimators. The most common collimator is the parallel multihole collimator depicted in Figure 9-10. With this collimator, the origin of a gamma ray interacting in the

The element technetium has no stable isotopes, and consequently does not occur in nature. It was first discovered in 1937 by the Italian physicist E. Segrè in molybdenum heat shields and deflectors discarded from E. O. Lawrence's first cyclotron at Berkeley. Segrè was awarded the 1959 Nobel Prize in Physics for the discovery of the antiproton.

Advantages of ^{99m}Tc for nuclear medicine studies include:

- Short high life (6 hr)
- Ideal γ-ray energy (140 keV)
- Little particulate radiation
- Ease of labeling
- Administration of relatively high activities

The first applications of radioactive tracers to experimental medicine were studies by Blumgart, Weiss, and Yens in 1926 that used a decay product of radium to measure the circulation time of blood.

To be effective, receptor-specific pharmaceuticals must satisfy several criteria, including:

- Demonstration of reasonable pharmacokinetics
- Ability to overcome biological barriers to targeted delivery
- Development of strategies for signal amplification
- Improvement in the speed and sensitivity of imaging methods

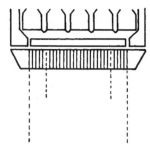

MARGIN FIGURE 9-10
Parallel multihole collimator

Other collimators used for specific applications include the pinhole collimator and the converging collimator.

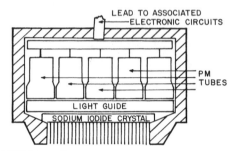

MARGIN FIGURE 9-11
Detector assembly of a scintillation camera.

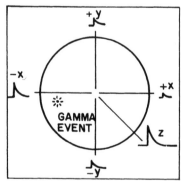

MARGIN FIGURE 9-12
In the position-encoding matrix for each PM tube, the PM signal is separated into four signals of relative sizes that reflect the position of the particular PM tube within the PM tube array.

A lower limit of 70 keV, together with an upper limit of 600 keV, defines the range of useful γ-ray energies for nuclear imaging.

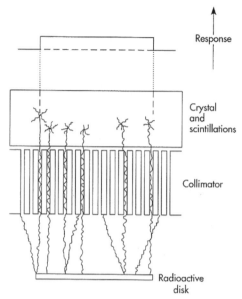

FIGURE 9-10
Parallel multihole collimator for nuclear medicine imaging.

detector is confined to a small region of the patient directly below the detector. Primary gamma rays from other regions of the patient cannot reach the interaction site because they are intercepted and absorbed by the high-Z (lead or tungsten) septa in the collimator. In this manner, the collimator imposes a spatial relationship between the interaction sites in the detector and the origin of gamma rays in the patient. Use of a collimator greatly restricts the efficiency of gamma-ray detection in nuclear medicine because fewer than 1/100 of the gamma rays emitted from the patient are transmitted by the collimator and reach the detector. Without a collimator, however, the sites of interaction of gamma rays in the detector could not be used as a map of the distribution of radioactivity in the patient, and the acquisition of useful nuclear medicine images would be impossible.

In most applications, the radiation detector in nuclear medicine is a large (up to 50-cm diameter), relatively thin (0.6 to 1.2 cm) NaI(T 1) scintillation crystal. Mounted above the crystal are many photomultiplier tubes (pmts). When an interaction occurs in the crystal, light is released and detected by the pmts. The amount of light reaching each pmt, and therefore the size of the electrical signal from it, depends on the lateral distance between the pmt and the interaction site of the gamma ray in the crystal. By electronically analyzing the relative size of the signals from the pmts, the location of the interaction site, and therefore the origin of the gamma ray in the patient, can be identified. This analysis results in the formation of four electrical signals ($+x$, $-x$, $+y$, $-y$) that reveal the position of the interaction site in the crystal.

The gamma-ray origin identified by this technique may be one of two types. It could represent the site of release of a primary gamma ray from a molecule of the radiopharmaceutical deposited at the site. However, it could also represent the location where a primary photon originating elsewhere in the body is scattered toward the scintillation detector. Both the primary and scattered gamma rays originating at the site could traverse the collimator and interact in the crystal. They can be distinguished, however, because a scattered photon is less energetic than a primary photon and therefore stimulates less light emission when it interacts in the crystal. To accomplish this distinction, the electrical signals from all the pmts are added, and the sum (the Z pulse) is compared in *a pulse height analyzer* to the size of a signal expected when a primary gamma ray interacts in the crystal. If the signal is smaller than expected for a primary gamma ray, interaction of a scattered photon is assumed and the pulse is rejected.

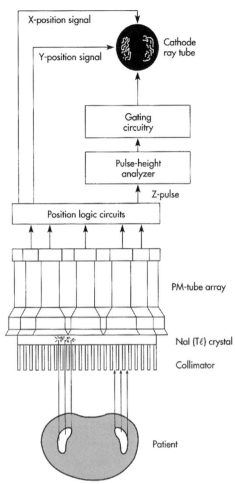

FIGURE 9-11
Schematic of a scintillation camera. (From J. A. Sorensen and M. E. Phelps,[30] used with permission.)

Electrical signals (Z pulses) representing interaction of primary gamma rays in the NaI(Tl) crystal are transmitted to the display device in the scintillation camera. Each signal activates a short burst of electrons from a filament. The electrons are directed toward a fluorescent screen in a cathode-ray tube (CRT). The four position signals ($+x$, $-x$, $+y$, $-y$) for the interaction are applied to deflection electrodes surrounding the electrons so that they strike the fluorescent screen at the location corresponding to the interaction site of the gamma ray in the crystal. In this manner, an image of brief light flashes is compiled on the screen that can be photographed to reveal the distribution of sites of gamma-ray interactions in the crystal and hence the distribution of radioactivity in the patient. A diagram of a scintillation camera is shown in Figure 9-11. A more complete explanation of the scintillation camera and principles of nuclear imaging in general are available in standard texts on the physics of medical imaging.[2,24]

■ EMISSION COMPUTED TOMOGRAPHY

Tomography is the process of collecting data about an object from multiple views (projections) and then using these data to construct an image of a "slice" through the object. This approach to imaging can be applied to nuclear medicine by detecting γ grays emitted from a radiopharmaceutical distributed within the body. The term emission computed tomography (ECT) refers to this procedure. Tomographic images

Scintillation cameras that digitize the signals after pulse-height and positioning analysis are called *hybrid analog–digital cameras*. Scintillation cameras that digitize the signals before pulse-height and positioning analysis are called *all-digital cameras*. Virtually all scintillation cameras marketed today are all-digital cameras. These cameras furnish more precise pulse-height and positioning analysis, and they yield images with superior spatial resolution.

acquired by detecting annihilation photons released during positron decay are referred to as positron emission tomography (PET). Tomographic images computed from the registration of interactions of individual γ rays are known as single-photon emission computed tomography (SPECT).

Single-Photon Emission Computed Tomography

This nuclear imaging technique has several features in common with x-ray transmission CT. Multiple views are acquired to produce an image in one or more transverse slices through the patient. In fourth-generation x-ray CT, the x-ray tube rotates and the detectors are stationary. Most SPECT systems employ a rotating detector (a scintillation camera) and a stationary source of γ rays (the patient). One, two, or three scintillation cameras are mounted on a rotating gantry. Each scintillation "head" encompasses enough anatomy in the axial direction to permit acquisition of multiple image "slices" in a single scan.

One major difference between SPECT and x-ray CT is that a SPECT image represents the distribution of radioactivity across a slice through the patient, whereas an x-ray CT image reflects the attenuation of x rays across a slice of tissue. In SPECT, photon attenuation interferes with the imaging process because fewer photons are recorded from voxels at greater depths in the patient. A correction must be made for this attenuation. Methods for attenuation correction usually involve estimating the body contour, sampling the patient from both sides (i.e., 360° rather than 180° rotation), and constructing a correction matrix to adjust scan data for attenuation.

SPECT has many clinical applications, including cardiac imaging, liver/spleen studies, and chest–thorax procedures.[1] It is also important for imaging receptor-specific pharmaceuticals such as monoclonal antibodies, because it provides improved detection and localization of small sites of radioactivity along the axial dimension.

Positron Emission Tomography

The principle of SPECT is applicable to positron emission tomography (PET). In PET, however, the radiation detected is annihilation radiation released as positrons interact with electrons. The directionality of the annihilation photons (511-keV photons emitted in opposite directions) provides a way to localize the origin of the photons and hence the radioactive decay process that resulted in their emission.

In a typical PET system (Figure 9-12), the patient is surrounded by a ring of detectors. When detectors on opposite sides of the patient register annihilation photons simultaneously (i.e., within a nanosecond), the positron decay process that created the photons is assumed to have occurred along a line between the detectors. The PET image reveals the number of decays (counts) occurring in each of the volume elements (voxels) represented by picture elements (pixels) in the image.

Radionuclides suitable for PET imaging include ^{11}C, ^{13}N, ^{15}O, ^{18}F, ^{62}Cu, ^{68}Ga, and ^{82}Rb. Many of these nuclides have very short lives, and a cyclotron for their instantaneous production must be close to the PET imager. To date, however, all clinical PET applications have employed ^{18}F-labeled fluorodeoxyglucose (^{18}FDG). The 1.7-hour half-life of this nuclide permits it to be obtained from a nearby supplier.

It is more challenging to obtain multiple image slices in PET than in SPECT. Most PET scanners use several detector rings for this purpose. Attenuation corrections are intrinsically more accurate in PET than in SPECT because the pair of annihilation photons defines a line through the patient such that the sum of the path lengths is constant irrespective of where the photons originate along the line.

PET imaging with ^{18}F-FDG is very useful in radiation oncology for assessing the spread of a primary cancer, detecting metastases, and monitoring the patient during and after treatment. Particularly useful for this purpose are scanners that combine PET and CT imaging in the same unit so that the PET images can be overlaid on x-ray CT images. PET imaging is rapidly becoming recognized as an essential imaging tool for radiation oncology.

In earlier SPECT units, the detectors rotated in a circular orbit around the body. In newer units, the detectors follow an elliptical path so that they remain close to the skin surface during the entire scan.

Transverse-section SPECT units can also provide coronal and sagittal images by interpolation of data across multiple transverse planes.

For 360° SPECT imaging, a single-head unit must rotate 360°; a dual-head unit must rotate 180°; and a triple-head unit must rotate 120°. Hence, data acquisition is three times faster with a triple-head unit compared with a single-head unit.

In transverse SPECT, data acquisition can either be continuous (i.e., the detector(s) move continuously) or discontinuous (i.e., the detector(s) stop rotating during data acquisition). The latter method is referred to as "step and shoot."

Since the directionality of annihilation photons provides information about the origin of the photons, collimators are not needed in PET imaging. This approach, referred to as *electronic collimation*, greatly increases the detection efficiency of PET imaging.

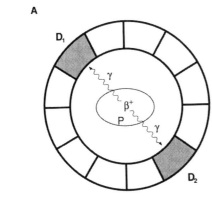

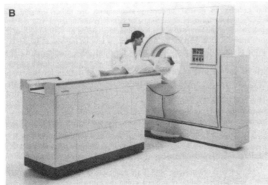

FIGURE 9-12
A: In positron emission tomography (PET), two detectors D_1 and D_2 record the interaction of 0.511-MeV photons in coincidence, indicating that a positron decay event has taken place somewhere along a line connecting the two detectors within the patient P. **B:** PET scanner (Siemens ECAT953B brain scanner) at the MRC cyclotron Unit, London. (Part B courtesy of Siemens Medical Systems, Inc.)

MAGNETIC RESONANCE IMAGING

Magnetic resonance is arguably the most important development in medical imaging since the discovery of x rays in 1895. The technology is based on the delineation of the magnetic properties of the proton by Frisch and Stern in 1933[33] and demonstration of the principle of magnetic resonance by Rabi in 1939.[34] The detection in 1945 by Bloch[35] and Purcell[36] of radio signals from nuclei placed in a magnetic field led to development of the technique of nuclear magnetic resonance, which has contributed in many ways to analytical chemistry and biochemistry. In 1971, Damadian[37] employed nuclear magnetic resonance to observe differences in magnetic properties between normal and cancerous tissues in rats. Two years later, Lauterbur[38] published the first magnetic resonance image. Since that time, magnetic resonance imaging (MRI) has assumed a position of growing importance in medical imaging. Today, MRI and angiography, along with functional neuroimaging with magnetic resonance techniques, hold great promise for revealing characteristics of the human body in health, disease, and injury that heretofore have been inaccessible and incompletely understood at best.

Both the proton and the neutron behave like tiny magnets as a result of their spin about their own axis. Nuclei with even numbers of protons and neutrons do not exhibit magnetic properties, however, because the magnetic properties of the constituent nucleons tend to cancel one another. In nuclei with an odd number of protons or neutrons, complete cancellation of the magnetic properties of the nucleons is not possible. Hence, these nuclei have a residual magnetic moment (i.e., they behave as a small atomic magnet). Ordinary hydrogen ^{1}H has the strongest magnetic moment because it contains only one nucleon, a proton, and no additional proton or neutron

The PET scanner was developed in the early 1950s by Brownell, Sweet, and Aronow at Massachusetts General Hospital.[31,32]

The first multicrystal PET unit was developed in the mid-1970s by TerPogossian, Phelps, and Hoffman of Washington University in St. Louis.

PET Radionuclides

Nuclide	$T^1/_2$ (minutes)
^{11}C	20.4
^{13}N	10
^{15}O	2
^{18}F	110
^{62}Cu	9.8
^{68}Ga	68
^{82}Rb	1.25

Otto Stern received the 1943 Nobel Prize in Physics. Isador Rabi was awarded the Nobel Prize in Physics in 1944. Felix Bloch and Edward Purcell shared the 1952 Nobel Prize in Physics.

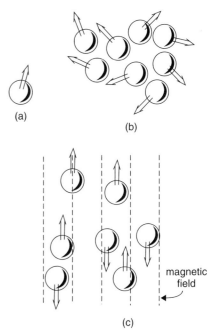

MARGIN FIGURE 9-13
A: Proton magnetic moment direction is indicated by arrow. **B:** In a typical material, magnetic moments are oriented randomly. **C:** If a magnetic field is applied, magnetic moments align themselves along the direction of the field. Note that some are parallel, others are antiparallel.

The rotational frequency ω is also known as the frequency of precession or Larmor frequency.

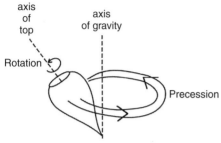

MARGIN FIGURE 9-14
Motions of a spinning top. Rotation or spin of the top about its own axis is first-order motion. Precession of the top about the vertical axis (axis of gravity) is second-order motion.

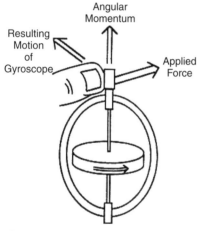

MARGIN FIGURE 9-15
A spinning object demonstrates a property known as angular momentum, shown as an arrow along the axis of the spinning object. When force is applied to an object having angular momentum, the resulting motion is at right angles to the force.

is available to counteract its magnetic moment. Other nuclei with an odd number of nucleons, including ^{13}C, ^{19}F, ^{23}Na, and ^{31}P, exhibit a smaller magnetic moment.

Although each nucleus in a sample of hydrogen (or other material that contains nuclei with a magnetic moment) acts like a small magnet, the sample itself exhibits no net magnetism because the magnetic moments of the individual nuclei are oriented randomly and cancel out. If such a sample is placed in an intense magnetic field, however, the nuclei tend to align themselves either with or against the applied magnetic field. In this orientation, the magnetic moments of the individual nuclei rotate (wobble or "precess") around the direction of the applied field in much the way a spinning top tends to wobble around the direction of the earth's gravitational field. This rotational frequency is

$$[\omega = gB]$$

where g is the gyromagnetic ratio of the particular nuclei and B is the strength of the magnetic field, usually described in tesla. The orientation and wobbling actions produce a component vector of the magnetic moments of the nuclei in the direction of the applied field and a smaller component at right angles to the applied field. Because the magnetic moments of the sample nuclei wobble out-of-phase with one another, the components of the nuclear magnetic moments in a direction perpendicular to the applied field tend to cancel one another. Hence, no net magnetic moment in a direction perpendicular to the applied magnetic field is measurable for the sample.

As described previously, the rotational frequency ω of the nuclei in a magnetic field is characteristic of the type of nuclei and the strength of the applied field. This frequency is in the radiofrequency (rf) range. If a brief pulse of rf energy is applied to the sample while the nuclei are precessing, two things happen: (1) The alignment of the nuclei is altered so that their magnetic component in a direction perpendicular to the applied magnetic field is changed, and (2) their rotation is affected so that they precess about the applied magnetic field in phase. The result of these effects is that the sample assumes a net magnetic moment in some direction other than parallel to the applied magnetic field.

Example 9-12

Find the resonance frequency ω for protons ($g = 42.58 \, \text{MHz/T}$) in a 1.5-tesla MRI unit.

$$\omega = gB$$
$$= (42.58 \, \text{MHz/T})(1.5 \, \text{T})$$
$$= 63.9 \, \text{MHz}$$

Immediately after application of an rf energy pulse to a sample, the nuclei begin to resume the status that they occupied before the rf was applied. In the process, the energy that was delivered to the sample by the rf pulse is released, and it can be measured with an rf antenna (a signal coil) coupled closely to the sample. The rf signal detected by the signal coil decreases (decays) over several milliseconds according to two time constants $T1$ and $T2$. The time constant $T1$, known as the *spin-lattice* or *longitudinal relaxation time*, describes the rate of return of the magnetic moment of the sample to its original orientation before the rf pulse was applied. The time constant $T2$, known as the *spin–spin* or *transverse relaxation time*, describes the rate at which the rotating nuclei dephase to the out-of-phase condition they displayed before the rf pulse was applied. Three characteristics of the signal of radiated rf energy can be measured and used to characterize the rf signal from the sample. These characteristics are the intensity of the signal (representative of the *spin density* related to the concentration of rotating nuclei in the sample), the spin–lattice relaxation time $T1$, and the spin–spin relaxation time $T2$. These three characteristics of the sample form the basic parameters used to produce a magnetic resonance image.

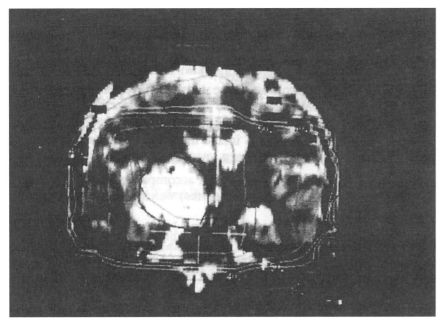

FIGURE 9-13
Complex isodose distribution superimposed on a cross-sectional magnetic resonance image. (Courtesy of George T. Y. Chen, University of Chicago).

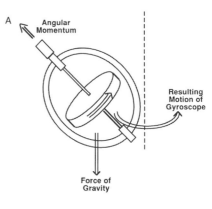

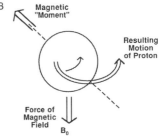

MARGIN FIGURE 9-16
Diagram of forces acting to cause precession. Angular momentum and gravity interact to cause precession of a gyroscope. Magnetic moment and a magnetic field interact to cause precession of a proton.

A variety of methods have been developed to apply the rf energy to a sample and to collect and measure the rf signal radiated from a sample. These methods are known as pulse sequences and are described in detail in texts on magnetic resonance and the physics of medical imaging.[1,40,41] Pulse sequences yield images with exquisite spatial and contrast information about anatomic structure and function in the patient. Included in this information are data important to delineating various features of biologic tissue, such as the presence and extent of tumors, the shape of normal structures in the immediate vicinity of a tumor, and the distinction between recurrent tumor and radiation necrosis. An isodose distribution superimposed on a magnetic resonance image is illustrated in Figure 9-13. Magnetic resonance imaging is gaining recognition as a useful adjunct to treatment planning and quality control in radiation therapy and is sure to grow in importance in the future as additional applications are identified and developed.[42]

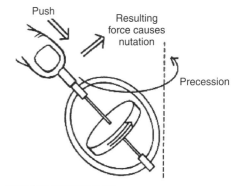

MARGIN FIGURE 9-17
Attempting to push a gyroscope in the direction of precession causes the gyroscope to change its angle of precession. Change in the angle of rotation is referred to as nutation.

■ FUNCTIONAL MAGNETIC RESONANCE IMAGING

Most biological tissues exert a weak repulsive force to counteract an applied magnetic field. This effect is termed *diamagnetism*, and the tissues are said to be diamagnetic. Oxygenated blood (oxyhemoglobin) is diamagnetic. In tissue containing deoxygenated blood, the deoxyhemoglobin in the blood has unpaired electrons that create a highly localized region in which T_2 is shortened. This effect is termed *paramagnetism*, and the region exhibiting the effect is typically two to three times the radius of the blood vessel nourishing the region.

Neuronal activity in a region of the brain stimulates a localized increase in blood flow, cerebral blood volume, and oxygen delivery in the region. The increased blood flow "drives out" the deoxyhemoglobin and replaces it with oxygenated blood. This process removes the T_2-shortening effect of deoxyhemoglobin, and the change can be seen in MR images weighted to reveal T_2 differences. The changes in T_2 signal can be seen within seconds after initiation of neuronal stimulation, which supports the theory that the change in MR signal is related to the movement of oxygenated blood through the capillary bed and into venuoles. That is, the oxyhemoglobin is serving as a naturally occurring contrast agent that yields MR signals corresponding

It is recommended that all patients undergo screening prior to admittance into the magnetic resonance scanner. The screening should check for the presence of foreign materials within the patient that may produce an adverse effect in the presence of static or changing magnetic fields. In addition, the FDA recommends particular caution with regard to the following conditions[42]:

a. Patients with greater than normal potential for cardiac arrest.
b. Patients who are likely to develop seizures or claustrophobic reactions.
c. Decompensated cardiac patients, febrile patients, and patients with impaired ability to perspire.
d. Patients who are unconscious, heavily sedated, or confused, and with whom no reliable communication can be maintained.
e. Examinations which are carried out at a room temperature above 24°C or relative humidity above 60%.

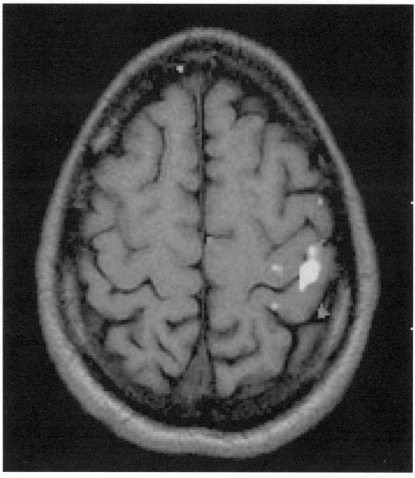

FIGURE 9-14
fMRI image of brain activation (light areas on right side of figure) in the sensory-motor cortex related to finger tapping (Courtesy of John Ulmer, M.D., Medical College of Wisconsin.)

to the spatial and temporal pattern of neuronal activation in the brain. Display of this pattern yields a functional map of neuronal activity in the brain. Acquisition of these maps is referred to as functional magnetic resonance imaging (fMRI).

Functional MRI is revolutionizing the study of brain function. Before fMRI, brain function was studied principally by analyzing neurological and behavioral abnormalities in individuals who had suffered losses in brain function through birth defects and accidents. The technique of fMRI is proving to be very useful in mapping functional areas of the brain before tumor resection (Figure 9-14), and it is helpful in the evaluation of patients following strokes and other neurovascular events (Figure 9-15). It also is adding greatly to the knowledge base of structure and function in the cognitive sciences.

■ SUMMARY

- The characteristic curve of an x-ray film is a plot of optical density as a function of the logarithm of the exposure.
- The characteristic curve reveals information about the density, latitude, contrast, base density and sensitivity of an x-ray film.
- Intensifying screens (usually $CaWO_4$ or rare-earth) are used to increase the sensitivity of the film-based image receptor to impinging x rays.
- Port films are used in radiation therapy to document the position of treatment fields and to confirm that the treated region is enclosed within the fields.

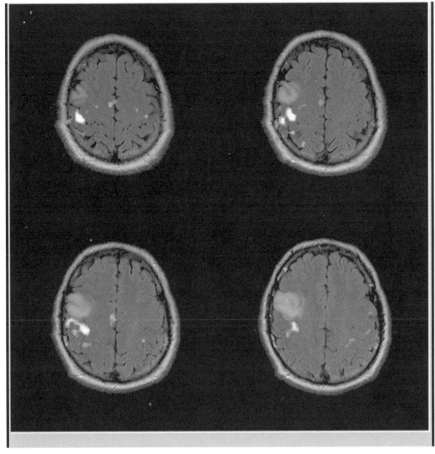

FIGURE 9-15
fMRI T_2-weighted image that reveals a tumor (gray area) anterior to the sensory-motor cortex (yellow-orange area). (Courtesy of John Ulmer, M.D., Medical College of Wisconsin.)

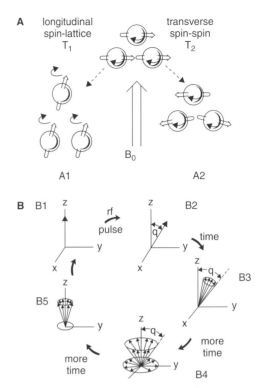

MARGIN FIGURE 9-18
A: Two relaxation processes in a sample of nuclear spins. There are several terms for each process. **A1:** Longitudinal relaxation occurs as the spins return to alignment with the static magnetic field, B_0. **A2:** Transverse relaxation occurs as the spins precess "out of phase." **B:** Spin-spin relaxation diagrammed in the rotating frame of reference. **B1:** Magnetic moment of the sample is aligned with the magnetic field. **B2:** Immediately after an RF pulse, the magnetic moment of the sample can be represented by a single vector. **B3:** As the magnetization vector begins to break up or diphase as a result of localized nonuniformities in the applied field, components of the vector begin to fan out in the xy plane. **B4:** When there are an equal number of components in all directions in the xy plane, the components cancel one another and the MR signal disappears. **B5:** As time passes, the cone representing the precessing but dephased magnetic moment continues to narrow because of spin-lattice relaxation. **B1:** Finally the magnetic moment once again is realigned with the applied field.[39]

- Radiographic grids are used to reduce the scattered radiation that otherwise would reach the image receptor and degrade image quality.
- Digital x-ray detectors, including storage phosphors and charge-coupled devices, are being used with increasing frequency in radiography.
- Image-intensification fluoroscopy provides a continuous x-ray image that reveals patient anatomy in "real time."
- Most x-ray fluoroscopic images are displayed on television monitors with interlaced frames.
- A treatment simulator is an x-ray or CT imaging device that simulates the geometry of a radiation treatment unit.
- X-ray transmission computed tomography provides planar and three-dimensional anatomical information with exquisite contrast resolution.
- Ultrasonography reveals interfaces between tissues that differ slightly in acoustic impedance Z [$Z =$ (velocity of ultrasound)(density of medium)].
- Nuclear medicine employs pharmaceuticals labeled with a radioactive nuclide to reveal information about the physiology, metabolism, and biochemistry, as well as the anatomy, of tissues.
- SPECT and PET employ single-photon and positron-emitting radioactive nuclides to produce two- and three-dimensional images from projections acquired with scintillation detector-based cameras.
- Magnetic resonance imaging techniques provide images with excellent contrast resolution based on subtle differences in tissue magnetization over time.
- Functional magnetic resonance imaging (fMRI) reveals areas of the brain involved in sensing and responding to a variety of external and internal stimuli.

PROBLEMS

9-1. Two areas of a radiograph have optical densities of 1 and 2. What is the ratio of light transmission through the two areas?

9-2. A film with an average gradient of 1 yields of difference of 0.3 in optical density for two exposures X_2 and X_1. What is the ratio of the exposures?

9-3. A high-speed screen-film combination yields an optical density of 1.0 above the base and fog density for an exposure of 1 mR. What is the speed of the film-screen combination?

9-4. Twice the exposure is required to produce a given optical density with a grid in place. What is the Bucky factor of the grid?

9-5. How many bytes of computer memory are used to store a 2048 × 2048 digital image that presents 256 shades of gray?

9-6. What is the spatial resolution in 1p/mm of a 4-in.^{2} x-ray image stored in a 512 × 512 digital matrix?

9-7. What is the brightness gain of an image intensifier with a 6-in.-diameter input screen, 0.5-in.-diameter output screen image, and electronic gain of 40?

9-8. Determine the exposure rate increase that accompanies a switch from normal (6-in. diameter) to magnified (4.5-in. diameter) viewing mode in an image intensifier.

9-9. Determine the CT numbers for air ($\mu \approx 0$) and compact bone ($\mu \approx 2\mu_w$).

9-10. A fluid-filled cyst has an acoustic impedance of 1.50, and the liver has an acoustic impedance of 1.65. (Note the units of acoustic impedance of kg-m^{-2}-sec^{-1} × 10^{-4} appropriate for these values can be neglected in the computation.) Determine the percent of ultrasound reflected at the liver–cyst interface.

9-11. How much time is required for an ultrasound pulse to return to the transducer following reflection from an interface 12 cm below the surface?

9-12. What is the rotational frequency of protons in a 1.5 MRI unit?

REFERENCES

1. Fuchs, A. W. Evolution of roentgen film. *AJR* 1956; **75**:30–48.
2. Hendee, W. R., and Ritenour, E. R. *Medical Imaging Physics*, 4th edition. New York, John Wiley & Sons, 2001.
3. Mun, S. K., et al. (eds.). *The First International Conference on Image Management and Communication in Patient Care: Implementation and Impact.* Washington, DC, IEEE Computer Society Press, Institute of Electrical and Electronics Engineers, 1989.
4. Barnes, G., Ceare, H., and Brezovich, I. Reduction of scatter in diagnostic radiology by means of a scanning multiple slit assembly. *Radiology* 1976; **120**: 691–694.
5. Smathers, R. L., and Brody, W. R. Digital radiology: Current and future trends. *Br. J. Radiol.* 1985; **58**:285–307.
6. Wolbarst, A. B. *Physics of Radiology.* Norwalk, CT, Appleton & Lange, 1993.
7. Rowlands, J. A. X-ray imaging: Radiography, fluoroscopy, computed tomography. In *Biomedical Uses of Radiation: Part A—Diagnostic Applications,* W. Hendee (ed.). Weinheim, Germany, Wiley-VCH, 1999, pp. 97–174.
8. Kell, R., Bedford A., and Fredenhall, G. A. determination of optimum number of lines in a television system. *RCA Rev.* 1940; **5**:8.
9. Templeton, A. W., Dwyer, S. J., Jansen, C., Garrotto, L., Rathke, J. E., and Tolan, J. H. Standard and high-scan line television systems. An experimental and clinical evaluation. *Radiology* 1968; **91**:725–730.
10. Hounsfield, G. Computerized transverse axial scanning (tomography). Part I: Description of system. *Br. J. Radiol.* 1973; **46**:1016–1022.
11. Bracewell, R. Strip integration in radio astronomy. *Aust. J. Phys.* 1956; **9**:198–217.
12. DeRosier, D., and Klug, A. Reconstruction of three dimensional structures from electron micrographs. *Nature* 1968; **217**:130–134.
13. Gordon, R., Bender, R., and Herman, T. Algebraic reconstruction techniques (ART) for three-dimensional electron microscopy and x-ray photography. *J. Theor. Biol.* 1970; **29**:471–481.
14. Berry, M., and Gibbs, D. The interpretation of optical projections. *Proc. R. Soc [A]* 1970; **314**:143–152.
15. Rowley, P. Quantitative interpretation of three-dimensional weakly refractive phase objects using holographic interferometry. *J. Opt. Soc. Am.* 1969; **59**:1496–1498.
16. Radon, J. Über die Bestimmung von Funktionen durch irhe integralwerte laengs gewisser Mannigfaltigkeiten (on the determination of functions from their integrals along certain manifolds). *Ber. Saechsische Akad. Wiss. (Leipzig) Math.-Phys. Klasse* 1917; **69**:262.
17. Hendee, W. R. *Physical Principles of Computed Tomography.* Boston, Little, Brown & Co., 1983.
18. Swindell, W., and Webb, S. X-ray transmission computed tomography. In *The Physics of Medical Imaging*, S. Webb (ed.). Philadelphia: Adam Hilger, 1988.
19. Dobbs, H. J., and Parker, R. P. The respective roles of the simulator and computed tomography in radiotherapy planning: A review. *Clin. Radiol.* 1984; **35**:433–439.
20. Dobbs, J. H., and Webb, S. Clinical applications of x-ray computed tomography in radiotherapy planning. In S. Webb (ed.) *The Physics of Medical Imaging.* Philadelphia: Adam Hilger, 1988.
21. Harrison, R. M., and Farmer, F. T. The determination of anatomical cross-sections using a radiotherapy simulator. *Br. J. Radiol.* 1978; **51**:448–453.
22. Ragan, D. P., and Perez, C. A. Efficacy of CT assisted two-dimensional treatment planning in analysis of 45 patients. *AJR* 1978; **131**:75–79.
23. Silver, M. D., Nishiki, M., Tochimura, K., Arita, M., Drawert, B. M., Judd, T. C. CT imaging with an image intensifier: Using a radiation therapy simulator as a CT scanner. In *Image Physics: Proceedings of the Society of Photo-Optical Instrumentation Engineers.* 1991; **1443**:250–260.
24. Curry, T. S., Dowdey, J. E., and Murry, R. C. *Christensen's Physics of Diagnostic Radiology*, 4th edition. Philadelphia, Lea & Febiger, 1990.
25. Carson, P. L., et al. Ultrasound imaging as an aid to cancer therapy—part I. *Int. J. Radiat. Oncol. Biol. Phys.* 1975; **1**:119–132.
26. Carson, P. L., et al. Ultrasound imaging as an aid to cancer therapy—part II. *Int. J. Radiat. Oncol. Biol. Phys.* 1976; **2**:335.
27. Fessenden, P., and Hand, J. W. Hyperthermia therapy physics. In *Radiation Therapy Physics,* A. R. Smith (ed.). Berlin, Springer-Verlag, 1995, pp. 315–363.
28. Anger, H. Scintillation camera. *Rev. Sci. Instrum.* 1958; **29**:27–33.
29. Srivastava, S. C., and Mausner, L. F. (ed.). Radiolabelled monoclonal antibodies: Chemical, diagnostic and therapeutic investigations. *Nucl. Med. Biol.* 1987; 13.
30. Sorensen, J. A., and Phelps, M. E. *Physics in Nuclear Medicine.* Orlando, Grune and Stratton, 1987.
31. Brownell, G., and Sweet, W. Localization of brain tumors. *Nucleonics* 1953; **11**:40–45.
32. Aronow, S., Brownell, G., Lova, S., and Sweet, W. Statistical analysis of eight

years' experience in positron scanning for brain tumor localization. *J. Nucl. Med.* 19562; **3**:198.

33. Frisch, R., and Stern, O. Über die magnetische ablenkung von Wasserstoff-Molekulen und das magnetische moment das protons I. *Z. Physik* 1933, **85**:4–16.

34. Rabi, I. I., Millman, S., Kusch, P., Zacharias, J. R. Molecular beam resonance method for measuring nuclear magnetic moments. *Phys. Rev.* 1939; **55**:526–535.

35. Bloch, R. The principle of nuclear induction. In *Nobel Lectures in Physics, 1946–1962.* New York, Elsevier Science Publishing, 1964.

36. Purcell, E. M. Research in nuclear magnetism. In *Nobel Lectures in Physics, 1946–1962.* New York, Elsevier Science Publishing, 1964.

37. Damadian, R. Tumor detection by nuclear magnetic resonance. *Science* 1971; **171**:1151–1153.

38. Lauterbur, P. C. Image formation by induced local interactions: Examples employing nuclear magnetic resonance. *Nature* 1973; **242**:190–191.

39. Morgan, C. J., and Hendee, W. R. *Introduction to Magnetic Resinance Imaging.* Denver, Multi-Media Publishers, 1984.

40. Stark, D. D., and Bradley, W. G. (eds). *Magnetic Resonance Imaging.* St. Louis, Mosby–Year Book, 1988.

41. Thomas, S. R., and Dixon, R. L. (eds.). *NMR in Medicine: Instrumentation and Clinical Applications: Medical Physics Monograph No. 14.* New York, American Institute of Physics, 1986.

42. Guidance for the submission of premarket notifications for Magnetic Resonance Diagnostic Devices, Food and Drug administration, Center for Devices and Radiologic Health, Computed Imaging Devices Branch, Office of Device Evaluation, FDA, Rockville, MD, www.fda.gov/chrh/ode/mri340.pdf, November 14, 1998.

10

COMPUTER SYSTEMS

OBJECTIVES   220

HISTORY OF COMPUTERS   220

TERMINOLOGY AND DATA REPRESENTATION   221

Number Systems   221

CONVERSION FROM ONE SYSTEM TO ANOTHER   223

BITS, BYTES, AND WORDS   223

REPRESENTATION OF DATA   224

Indication of States   224
Numeric Data   225
Alphanumeric Data   225
Analog-to-Digital and Digital-to-Analog Conversion   225
Representation of Graphic Data   227

COMPUTER ARCHITECTURE   230

Memory   230
Central Processing Unit   231
Input/Output Devices   232

Mass Storage Devices   232

COMPUTER SOFTWARE   234

PROGRAMMING LANGUAGES   234

Computer Languages   234
Low-Level Languages   235
High-Level Languages   235

NETWORKING   237

Network Components and Structure   238
Interfaces   238
Transmission Media   239
Data Compression   239
Display Stations and Standards   240

COMPUTER REQUIREMENTS FOR TREATMENT PLANNING   241

SUMMARY   241

PROBLEMS   242

REFERENCES   242

Radiation Therapy Physics, Third Edition, by William R. Hendee, Geoffrey S. Ibbott, and Eric G. Hendee
ISBN 0-471-39493-9 Copyright © 2005 John Wiley & Sons, Inc.

■ OBJECTIVES

After studying this chapter, the reader should be able to:

- Provide a historical perspective on the development of computers and computer networking.
- Express quantities in different number systems and convert expressions from one system to another.
- Delineate the processes and uncertainties in converting analog to digital data and vice versa.
- Demonstrate the features, advantages and limitations of digital images.
- Discuss the characteristics and contributions of computer components, including memory, CPU, and I/O and mass storage devices.
- Explain the differences in various levels of software languages.
- Describe the structure and components of computer networks and their functions, including interfaces, transmission media, data compression, display stations, and network standards.

■ HISTORY OF COMPUTERS

Computers were introduced into radiology departments in the early 1970s. Because of their usefulness for storing, manipulating, and displaying large amounts of data, computers quickly were incorporated into clinical nuclear medicine. They were also quickly adopted in radiation therapy, primarily for calculating and displaying composite isodose distributions for multifield treatments.

A computer is any device that records and manipulates numbers or symbols. Early examples of computers include the sticks and clam shells used by primitive man to record transactions. Electrical circuits and analog computers have been constructed to perform calculations but are generally restricted to one or a few specific tasks. Digital computers, which use a large number of electrical switches to record values, offer great flexibility and are easily adapted to multiple purposes.

An early calculating device was the abacus, usually constructed with beads that slide on wooden or metal rods. Some documentation suggests that primitive forms of the abacus were in use by the Babylonians as early as 3000 BCE.[2] The abacus is still routinely used in many cultures.

The first calculating machine was probably the invention of Wilhelm Schickard in 1623.[3] This device could add and subtract automatically, and multiply and divide semiautomatically. Constructed of toothed wheels fitted with pins that engaged adjacent wheels, this device was modeled after clocks developed in China and the Middle East during the first millenium A.D. A mechanical calculating device was invented by Pascal.[4,5] It was an adding machine that operated on the same principle as the modern mechanical automobile odometer. Pascal's machine could also convert sums of money from one currency to another.

In 1833, a device called the analytical engine was invented by the English mathematician Babbage.[7] Its purpose was to produce navigational tables for use in commercial shipping. It was noteworthy because it used decks of punched paper cards to program different functions. Although the analytical engine was not actually put into practice, its design led to Hollerith's invention of a mechanical calculating machine for the U.S. Census Bureau.[8] In addition to programming, punched paper cards were used to enter data into the calculating machine. The data could be stored, sorted, and organized into an early type of "database."

The first true electronic digital computer was built in 1939 at Iowa State University by Atanasoff and Berry.[9] This device was designed to help solve large arrays of linear equations in quantum mechanics.

A turning point in computer technology was reached with use of the vacuum tube in computational circuits. This development allowed construction of the Electronic

Some say that the human brain is simply a computer; others argue vehemently against this notion.

In the 1930s the word "computer" meant a person, usually female, whose job was performing computations.[1]

Babbage once remarked that his analytical engine "could do everything but compose country dances."[6]

Numeric Integrator and Calculator (ENIAC) by Mauchly and Eckert at the University of Pennsylvania in 1945.[10] This computer was built to prepare ballistics tables for artillery in World War II. In contrast to the compact dimensions of modern computers, the ENIAC filled several large rooms.

The ENIAC was quickly found to be inadequate because it had no way of storing results or, more importantly, programs. A means for creating a "memory" had to be developed. One early design used a delay device by which up to 500 numbers circulated through a "storage tank." The numbers were actually represented by ultrasonic pulses traveling through a tank of mercury. A memory device of this type was built in 1947 and incorporated into the Electron Delay Storage Automatic Calculator (EDSAC), which became operational in 1949.[12]

In the early 1940s, Alan Turing and several other mathematicians were sequestered in Betchley, England to penetrate the ENIGMA code used by German U-boats to sink Allied ships. The result of this effort was the COLOSSUS computer, which contributed significantly to the ultimate Allied victory in World War II.

The development of the transistor shortly after World War II brought about a revolution in the design of computers. Transistors control the flow of electricity in much the same way as vacuum tubes, but they are much smaller and use considerably less power. By the 1960s, techniques had been developed to manufacture small silicon wafers called integrated circuits (ICs, also known as microchips). These devices contain many transistors connected in complex circuits. IBM used the capability of ICs to develop a new line of computers, called the 360 series. Other companies soon followed, including AT&T, Exxon, and Digital Equipment Corporation (DEC). Many of the early manufacturers of computers ultimately dropped out as competition became fierce and aggressive marketing strategies created giants such as IBM and DEC.

As the technology for making ICs advanced, computers could be made much more powerful. The computer industry developed large computers called mainframes, as well as minicomputers such as DEC's PDP-8 that was first marketed in 1965. The PDP-8 was one of the first in a long line of minicomputers marketed at a modest price. In the late 1960s, DEC modified the PDP-8 computer to market one of the first dedicated treatment planning computers, the "RAD-8."

Further reductions in size of computer components have led to the development of tremendously powerful computers assembled into packages that fit on a desktop or even a laptop. In 1971, Intel Corporation introduced the first processor built entirely on a single silicon chip. The chip contained 2300 transistors. Because of its small size, the 4004 chip, called a microprocessor, could be manufactured inexpensively in bulk. Since that time, the manufacturing process has improved so much that Intel's "P6" microprocessor contains 5.5 million transistors. With this smaller size has come increased speed. The P6 microprocessor can perform 133 million operations per second, and clever instruction-handling techniques increase this speed even more. Computers built around such processors are 100,000 times more powerful than the computer behemoths of the 1950s. At today's rate, microprocessor performance is doubling every 18 months. Additional uses for microprocessors continue to be developed. Today they are found in numerous scientific instruments and in consumer items ranging from automobiles to kitchen appliances and toys.

The Atanasoff and Berry computer was the first to use vacuum tube circuits for computation.

Mauchly and Eckert were awarded a patent for the ENIAC, but it was later ruled invalid because of prior public release of information by their competitors von Neumann and Goldstine. Consequently, Mauchly and Eckert never profited from their invention.[11]

The ENIAC contained 17,468 vacuum tubes, weighed 60,000 pounds, occupied 16,200 cubic feet, and used 174 kilowatts of power. In 1995 its function was duplicated on a 7.44×5.79 mm^2 chip.

Alan Turing was a genius, but also a tragic figure. He committed suicide by cyanide poisoning in 1954. The play Breaking the Code depicts Turing's adult life.

Alan Turing was included along with his fellow mathematician Kurt Gödel, in Time Magazine's March 29, 1999 list of the greatest scientists and thinkers of the twentieth century.

The observation that microprocessor performance doubles every 18 months is known as Moore's Law.

In February 1996, the chess-playing computer Deep Blue defeated world chess champion Gary Kasparov. The significance of this victory has been vigorously debated in the artificial intelligence community.

■ TERMINOLOGY AND DATA REPRESENTATION

Number Systems

Base 10

Humans count and calculate using a base-10 number system, probably because we have 10 fingers. The term "base 10" indicates that the number system has 10 digits (0 to 9). A power of 10 is denoted by the position of a digit within a number.

The base 10 number system is also referred to as the decimal system.

TABLE 10-1 A Sequence of Numbers Represented in Decimal and Binary Form

Decimal	Binary	Decimal	Binary
1	1	11	1011
2	10	12	1100
3	11	13	1101
4	100	14	1110
5	101	15	1111
6	110	16	10000
7	111	17	10001
8	1000	18	10010
9	1001	19	10011
10	1010	20	10100

Development of the binary notation of numbers is often attributed to the German mathematician Gottfried Leibniz (1646–1716).

In binary notation, positive numbers less than unity are represented as infinite strings of 1s and 0s. For example,

$$\tfrac{1}{4} = .01000000\ldots$$

$$\tfrac{1}{3} = .01010101\ldots$$

$$1/\pi = .0101000101\ldots$$

where the denominators are successive powers of two. That is, $1/3 = 1/4 + 1/16 + 1/64 + \cdots$

Numbers are represented by listing appropriate digits in a meaningful sequence. For example, the number 1983 actually represents $1 \times 10^3 + 9 \times 10^2 + 8 \times 10^1 + 3 \times 10^0$, where 10^0 equals 1. Multiplication or division by 10 is a simple process; it requires only that the digits in the number be shifted by one to the left of the decimal to multiply by 10, or to the right of the decimal by one digit to divide by 10. For example, $198.30 \times 10 = 1983.0$, and $198.30 \div 10 = 19.830$.

Base 2

A counting system involving only two digits (0 and 1) is used by computers because the two digits can be expressed easily by electronic means. For example, a switch in the off position can indicate 0, and a switch in the on position can indicate 1. Because this counting system has two digits, it is called base 2 or the binary system. As in the decimal system, numbers in the binary system are formed by placing digits in a sequence, where the position of a digit indicates its value. The binary number 1011 actually represents $1 \times 2^3 + 0 \times 2^2 + 1 \times 2^1 + 1 \times 2^0$, where $2^3 = 8$, $2^2 = 4$, $2^1 = 2$, and $2^0 = 1$. That is, the binary number 1011 is identical in value to the decimal number 11.

Counting in the binary system is performed just as counting in the decimal system; to increment a number by 1, the digit 1 is added to the least significant (farthest to the right) digit of the number. If the least significant digit is already 1, when adding another 1, it is replaced by 0, and 1 is "carried" to the next more significant digit. The digit 0 is sometimes called a place holder because its function is to assist in correctly identifying the value of other digits in the number.

Multiplying by 2 in the binary system is analogous to multiplying by 10 in the decimal system; the digits in the number simply are shifted by one to the left to multiply by 2, and by one to the right when dividing by 2. (Example 10-1). A sequence of numbers in binary and decimal form is shown in Table 10-1.

Example 10-1

Multiply the binary number 101 by 2 twice (the equivalent of multiplying by the decimal number 4).

$101 \times 2 = 1010$ (the digits are shifted to the left one place and a zero is inserted in the least significant position)

$1010 \times 2 = 10100$ (the process is repeated)

Compare the results with the values listed in Table 10-1.

In converting a quantity from one base numbering system to another, the quantity itself does not change. That is, the quantity "Twenty Things" does not change irrespective of whether it is expressed as 20 (decimal), 10100 (binary), 24 (octal), or F5 (hexadecimal).

	Decimal (Base 10)		Binary (Base 2)					Octal (Base 8)		Hexadecimal (Base 16)	
Place	Tens	Ones	Sixteens	Eights	Fours	Twos	Ones	Eights	Ones	Sixteens	Ones
Power of base	10^1	10^0	2^4	2^3	2^2	2^1	2^0	8^1	8^0	16^1	16^0
		0					0		0		0
		1					1		1		1
		2				1	0		2		2
		3				1	1		3		3
		4			1	0	0		4		4
		5			1	0	1		5		5
		6			1	1	0		6		6
		7			1	1	1		7		7
		8		1	0	0	0	1	0		8
		9		1	0	0	1	1	1		9
	1	0		1	0	1	0	1	2		A
	1	1		1	0	1	1	1	3		B
	1	2		1	1	0	0	1	4		C
	1	3		1	1	0	1	1	5		D
	1	4		1	1	1	0	1	6		E
	1	5		1	1	1	1	1	7		F
	1	6	1	0	0	0	0	2	0	1	0
	1	7	1	0	0	0	1	2	1	1	1
	1	8	1	0	0	1	0	2	2	1	2
	1	9	1	0	0	1	1	2	3	1	3
	2	0_{10}	1	0	1	0	0_2	2	4_8	1	4_{16}

FIGURE 10-1
Representation of the decimal numbers 0_{10} and 20_{10} in other bases.

Other Numbering Systems

Other numbering systems are used when it is convenient. For example, base 8 (also called octal) is useful when the digits 0 to 7 can be used, which is the case when three binary digits are available. Base 16 (or hexadecimal) is used when digits representing the decimal numbers 0 to 15 are required or practical. Such numbers can be expressed with four binary digits, and the symbols 0, 1, . . . , 9, A, B, C, D, E, and F are used to indicate the 15 digits. The representation of a series of decimal numbers in other numbering systems is shown in Figure 10-1.

■ CONVERSION FROM ONE SYSTEM TO ANOTHER

Conversion from the decimal system to another base requires division of the original number by powers of the new base. For example, to convert the decimal number 419 into binary form, 419 is first divided by 2^8 (or 256), then the remainder is divided by 2^7 (or 128), and so on. This process is illustrated in the margin. Conversion into decimal from any other base requires multiplication of successive powers of the base.

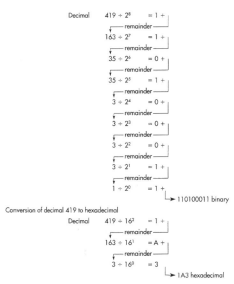

MARGIN FIGURE 10-1
Conversion of a decimal number into binary and hexadecimal.

■ BITS, BYTES, AND WORDS

The fundamental unit of data in a computer is called a bit (for *binary digit*). As a binary number, a bit can be used to represent either of two states, such as on or off. In modern computer memories, each bit is represented by a transistor, and so can indicate whether a voltage is present or absent at the transistor terminal. In magnetic storage media such as disks and tape, a bit represents a small area on the storage media that can be magnetized or not to indicate its state.

Bits are grouped into numbers called bytes, each generally consisting of eight bits. Bytes, therefore, can be conveniently used to indicate numbers between 0 and $2^8 - 1$,

In computer jargon, a zero or a one is a single "bit" of information.

or 255. As will be seen later, a byte is a convenient unit of storage, because it may be used to represent many types of data. Computer memory is generally described in terms of the number of available bytes. Because this number is frequently very large, the terms kilobytes, megabytes, gigabytes and terabytes are used (Margin Figure 10-2). The prefixes kilo, mega, and giga are actually approximations; as is shown in Margin Figure 10-2, the actual number of memory locations is only approximately a multiple of 10^3.

1 kilobyte = 2^{10} bytes = 1,024 bytes
1 megabyte = 2^{20} bytes = 1,048,576 bytes
1 gigabyte = 2^{30} bytes = 1,073,741,824 bytes
1 terabyte = 2^{40} bytes = 1,099,511,627,776 bytes

MARGIN FIGURE 10-2
Units used to describe computer storage capacity.

Example 10-2

Convert the binary number 10111 into decimal form.
Answer:

$$(1 \times 2^4) + (0 \times 2^3) + (1 \times 2^2) + (1 \times 2^1) + (1 \times 2^0) = 16 + 0 + 4 + 2 + 1 = 23$$

Example 10-3

Convert the hexadecimal number F7A into decimal.

The hexadecimal digit F has the decimal value 15, whereas A has the value 10. Therefore

$$F7A = (15 \times 16^2) + (7 \times 16^1) + (10 \times 16^0)$$
$$= (15 \times 256) + (7 \times 16) + (10)$$
$$= 3840 + 112 + 10$$
$$= 3962$$

Bits are also grouped into larger units called words. Words are typically 16 bits (corresponding to 2 bytes), 32 bits (corresponding to 4 bytes), or 64 bits (corresponding to eight bytes). The grouping of bits into words facilitates the expression of larger integers. For example, a 32-bit word can be used to express integers between 0 and $2^{32} - 1 = 4,294,967,295$. The size of the word determines the amount of computer memory that can be accessed. A computer with 16-bit words can directly access only 65,535 memory locations ($2^{16} - 1$). Because each memory location typically stores one byte of data, this amount of memory is also known as 64 kilobytes. Today, many computer applications require access to much larger amounts of memory, and even home computers are frequently equipped with 100 or more megabytes of memory. Access to these large volumes of memory requires 32-bit and even 64-bit words.

The number of instructions that a computer can execute per second is a measure of the speed of the computer. The speed is usually expressed in units of millions of instructions per second or MIPS. Today's PCs can perform up to 100 MIPS. Special-purpose computers have been built with speeds up to 10^{12} (prefix "tera") instructions per second (TIPS).

■ REPRESENTATION OF DATA

Indication of States

Modern computers are designed to solve a variety of problems and to assist humans working in a variety of circumstances. For example, a contemporary desktop computer may be used to run a word-processing program, perform complex mathematical computations, and display images. This multitasking performance requires the computer to store and process many different types of data in digital form. The word-processing program requires the computer to present and operate on alphanumeric data (text). Programs that perform calculations require the computer to store numerical values in digital form. Earlier, it was shown how computers store integers of values ranging from 0 to a maximum dictated by the number of bits in the computer word. Computers often are required to manipulate negative numbers, fractions, and very large or very small numbers.

Numeric Data

The storage of positive integers in a computer's memory has already been described. It was shown that an 8-bit binary number can easily represent numbers from 0 to 255 ($2^8 - 1$). However, it is often necessary to represent negative numbers in computer memory. To do so, the computer may reserve one bit to indicate the sign of the number, and use the remaining bits (in this case, 7) to indicate the value of the number up to 127 (2^7 or $128 - 1$). Many computers today use an alternate method called "two's complement notation" to represent signed integers. An 8-bit binary number can therefore be used to repressent numbers between -127 and $+127$. The binary number 00000001 represents the decimal number 1, whereas 01111111 represents positive 127. The binary number 10000000 represents -127, whereas 11111111 represents the decimal number -1. Although this notation may seem slightly awkward, it simplifies the addition of numbers in the computer's memory.

Very large and very small numbers are often required for scientific calculations. Avogadro's number (6.023×10^{23} molecules per gram-mole) and the charge on an electron (1.6×10^{-19} coulombs) are examples. Numbers such as these may be represented in "floating point" form. Floating point is similar to exponential notation, in which a number is expressed as a decimal quantity multiplied by 10 raised to a power. Similarly, a number can be written as a binary quantity multiplied by 2 raised to a power. Typically, four 8-bit bytes are used to store floating point numbers, with one bit used to identify the sign (0 = plus, 1 = minus), 8 bits for the exponent, and 23 bits for the mantissa. For example, Avogadro's number could be stored as: 0000 0001 1111 1110, 0100 0110, where the first binary number represents a sign bit (in this case, 0, indicating a positive number) followed by a 23-bit mantissa (000 0001 1111 1110$_2$ = 510$_{10}$). The second binary number represents an exponent of the base 2 ($2_2^{0100\ 0110} = 2^{70} \approx 1.181 \times 10^{21}$). The product of these two numbers is 510 $\times$ $1.181 \times 10^{21} = 6.023 \times 10^{23}$. The actual method used for storing the mantissa and exponent varies among computer systems.

Alphanumeric Data

The storage of text, in the form of alphanumeric symbols, requires a conversion table between binary integers and alphanumeric symbols. The output of a computer, such as the text of a word-processor document, requires the conversion of binary integers into the shapes humans recognize as letters and symbols. The 26 letters of the alphabet, the digits 0 to 9, and a number of special symbols (such as $, !, =, etc.) are referred to collectively as the alphanumeric character set. With the inclusion of upper- and lowercase letters and additional symbols, the alphanumeric character set may consist of as many as 128 elements. Table 10-2 shows the American National Standard Code for Information Exchange (ASCII). This is one of the most widely used schemes for encoding alphanumeric information.

Analog-to-Digital and Digital-to-Analog Conversion

Measurable quantities may be displayed in one of two forms: analog and digital. The use of an analog display indicates that the quantity being measured may vary in continuous fashion. For example, a voltage may be displayed on a meter whose needle moves from zero to some maximum value. The quantity displayed may have any value within the range. Our ability to measure the quantity depends only on our ability to read the meter. A watch or clock with continuously moving hands is an example of an analog display of time. Our ability to measure time is limited only by our ability to read the position of the hands on the clock. On the other hand, a quantity may be represented digitally. Digital quantities are discrete and can assume only specific values separated by intervals. A digital voltmeter may display only integer numbers of volts (0, 1, 2, etc.), and a digital watch may display only integer numbers of minutes (e.g, 10:23).

Large-size words permit computations with greater precision and reduced rounding errors.

Instructions for floating-point computations are more time-consuming than for fixed-point (integer) computations.

One million floating-point operations per second is abbreviated as IMFLOPS. Parallel-processing supercomputers can attain floating-point processing speeds of >300 MFLOPS, and so-called "massively parallel systems" with several hundred microprocessors achieve giga-FLOP speeds.

Quantum Computers. In the quest for greater computing power, one area of research involves using some of the properties of objects, such as small numbers of photons, electrons, or nuclei, whose behavior is dominated by quantum mechanical effects.

Once such phenomenon is "quantum teleportation" in which a state that could represent one bit of information (such as the direction of electromagnetic fields in a light beam) may be changed instantaneously over large distances. The implications for high-speed communications are obvious.

Another potentially useful property of a quantum mechanical system is that it exists in all possible combinations of states up to the moment of measurement. This property suggests that the various states could represent ones and zeros in computations and that, until the moment of measurement, the "quantum computer" could explore all possible combinations of solutions to a problem. One way to construct such a system of quantum mechanical spins involves the same nuclear magnetic resonance phenomenon in liquid samples that is used in magnetic resonance imaging of the human body.[12]

TABLE 10-2 American National Standard Code for Information Interchange (ASCII)

Character	Binary Code	Character	Binary Code
A	100 0001	0	011 0000
B	100 0010	1	011 0001
C	100 0011	2	011 0010
D	100 0100	3	011 0011
E	100 0101	4	011 0100
F	100 0110	5	011 0101
G	100 0111	6	011 0110
H	100 1000	7	011 0111
I	100 1001	8	011 1000
J	100 1010	9	011 1001
K	100 1011		
L	100 1100		
M	100 1101	Blank	010 0000
N	100 1110	.	010 1110
O	100 1111	(	010 1000
P	101 0000	+	010 1011
Q	101 0001	$	010 0100
R	101 0010	*	010 1010
S	101 0011	)	010 1101
T	101 0100	–	010 1101
U	101 0101	/	010 1111
V	101 0110	,	010 1100
W	101 0111	=	011 1101
Y	101 1001		
Z	101 1010		

When digitizing an analog signal, the maximum digitization error err_{max} is

$$err_{max} = R_a/N = R_a/2^n$$

and the average digitization error err_{avg} is

$$err_{avg} = err_{max}/2 = R_a/2^{n+1}$$

In these expressions, R_a is the range (minimum to maximum measured analog value), and N is the number of distinct digitization increments.[12]

Computers described in this chapter are digital computers. They operate only with digital quantities. However, much of the information collected in science, as well as in medicine, is presented in analog form. Therefore, conversion from analog to digital form, and back again, is often necessary. For example, the electrical signals from radiation detectors such as ionization chambers are in analog form. To represent the signal of an ionization chamber in a computer requires conversion of the analog signal to digital form. Conversely, the use of a computer to control a piece of equipment (even a simple device such as a motor) may require conversion of the computer output to an analog signal. An example of an analog output from a computer is the musical sounds produced by contemporary computer systems. The representation of an analog quantity by a digital number requires that the representation be limited to a finite number of alternatives. For example, it may be desirable to represent the signal from an ionization chamber as a 3-bit binary number. This binary number can provide at most eight different values. The output of the ionization chamber may vary between 0 and 10 volts. The eight available binary values can be used to display voltages between 0 and 10 volts if each binary value corresponds to 1.25 volts (Figure 10-2). An analog voltage between 0 and 1.25 volts might be recorded as 0, whereas a value between 1.25 and 2.50 might be recorded as 1.25 volts, and so on. The error associated with this digitizing process may be as large as 1.25 volts, the difference between adjacent binary values. However, the average digitization error (assuming that the analog values were uniformly distributed between 0 and 10 volts) is half the digitization increment, or 0.625 volts.

Such a crude digitizer may be acceptable in some circumstances, but in most scientific applications, greater resolution is required. A 16-bit digitizer would be able to display voltages in the range of 0–10 volts with a resolution of $10V/2^{16} = 0.00015$ volts. The maximum error is equal to the resolution, and the average error (for analog values that are uniformly distributed between 0 and 10 volts) is half of the resolution, 0.000075 volts.

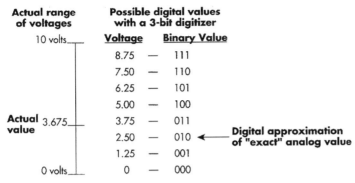

FIGURE 10-2
A 3-bit digitizer is used to record voltage signals over the range of 0–10 V. Because only eight digital values are possible for a 3-bit digitizer, one scheme, illustrated here, would assign all voltages between 0 and 1.25 V to the value 0 V (binary 000), all voltages between 1.25 and 2.50 V to the value 1.25 V (binary 001), and so on.

Example 10-4

Determine the maximum and average digitization error (in cm) of the position-sensing circuit of an isodose plotter. The detector axis is 50 cm long, and a potentiometer provides a position-dependent voltage ranging from 0 to 15 V. The voltage is monitored by a 12-bit analog-to-digital converter (ADC).

The digitizer resolution is

$$\frac{15\,\text{V}}{2^{12}} = 0.0037\,\text{V}$$

The maximum digitization error is therefore

$$\frac{0.0037\,\text{V}}{15\,\text{V}}(50\,\text{cm}) = 0.012\,\text{cm}$$

The average error is 0.00185 V, corresponding to 0.006 cm. The problem can also be solved by noting that a 12-bit ADC is capable of 4096 values and therefore has a precision of one part in 4096. The maximum digitizing error is therefore

$$\frac{50\,\text{cm}}{4096} = 0.012\,\text{cm}$$

Representation of Graphic Data

To store images in a computer, the image must be divided into small sections called picture elements, or pixels (Figure 10-3). Each pixel is assigned a single numeric value that denotes the color, if a color image is stored, or the shade of gray (referred to as the gray level), if a black and white image is stored. A digital image therefore consists of a list of binary numbers corresponding to individual pixels in the image (Figure 10-4). The number of bits used for each binary value (corresponding to each pixel) determines the number of different colors or shades of gray available. For example, a digital image in which each pixel is represented by a 3-bit binary number can have only 2^3 or eight different colors or shades of gray (Figure 10-5). Clearly, the faithfulness of the computer-rendered image to the original photograph is improved as the "bit depth" (the number of bits in the binary number used to describe the color or gray level) is increased.

Computers may generate images directly in digital form. For example, computed tomography (CT), magnetic resonance (MR), and computed radiography (CR) images are produced directly by digital computers. The number of pixels used to create an image has a profound influence on the quality of the image. The use of only a small number of pixels results in a coarse, perhaps even an unidentifiable, image. As the number of pixels used increases, the quality of the image improves, to the point that

The set of pixels comprising an image is referred to as the *image matrix*. Matrix sizes are powers of two (e.g., 64 × 64, 512 × 512, 2048 × 2048, etc.)

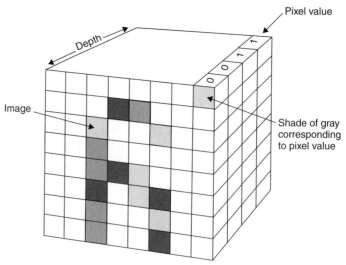

FIGURE 10-3
A digital image may be thought of as a three-dimensional object composed of a number of small cubes, each of which contains a binary digit (bit). The image appears on the front surface of the block. The "depth" of the block is the number of bits required to describe the color or gray level for each pixel. The total number of cubes that make up the large block is the number of bits required to store the image.

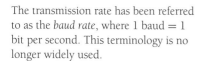

The transmission rate has been referred to as the *baud rate*, where 1 baud = 1 bit per second. This terminology is no longer widely used.

it may be indistinguishable to the eye from the original (Figure 10-6). Likewise, a digital image produced by a computer (such as a CT image) with a large number of pixels is said to be a "high-resolution" image. The observer may not even be able to detect the individual pixels. The use of large numbers of pixels to produce images has the benefits of improved quality and better resolution, but has the disadvantage of requiring larger computer capacity to store the image. Image matrix sizes are generally powers of two, reflecting the binary nature of computer storage. For example, CT images are typically 256 × 256 ($2^8 \times 2^8$) pixels, or 512 × 512 ($2^9 \times 2^9$) pixels. If the bit depth of these images is 8 bits, the image formats would require 524,288 or 2,097,152 bits of information each, respectively. Typically, the images would be stored in bytes of 8 bits each, requiring $2^{16} = 65,536$ or $2^{18} = 262,144$ bytes, respectively.

An additional disadvantage of large image matrices is the time required to transmit an image from one computer to another. Transfer of data in serial form requires transmission of the bits of information one at a time along the connection between the two computer systems. The *transmission rate* is the number of bits of information

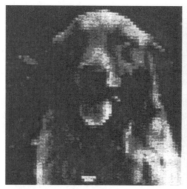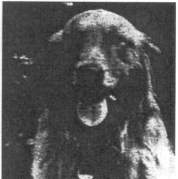

FIGURE 10-4
The photograph on the **left** has been digitized for the purpose of manipulation and storage in a computer. (From Hendee, W. R., and Ritenour, E. R., *Medical Imaging Physics.*[12])

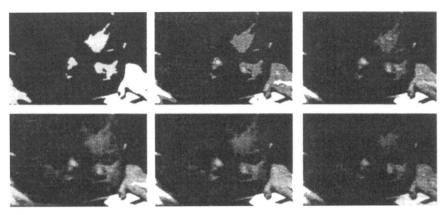

FIGURE 10-5
As the bit depth of a digital image is increased, the number of shades of gray that are stored for each pixel is increased. The images shown here are, from **top left**, 1 bit (2 shades), 2 bit (4 shades), 3 bit (8 shades), 4 bit (16 shades), 6 bit (64 shades), 8 bit (256 shades). Each image has a matrix size of 768 × 512 pixels. (From Hendee, W. R., and Ritenour, E. R., *Medical Imaging Physics.*[12])

that can be transmitted per second. Transmission rates range from a few megabits per second (Mbps) for "twisted cable" (telephone wire) to several terabits per second (Tbps) for fiber-optic cable. Clearly, larger image matrices take longer to transmit from one computer to another.

Example 10-5

The connection between two computers permits images to be transferred at a transmission rate of 9600 bits per second. Calculate the length of time required to transfer a 128 × 128 matrix of pixels, each consisting of 8-bit binary numbers.

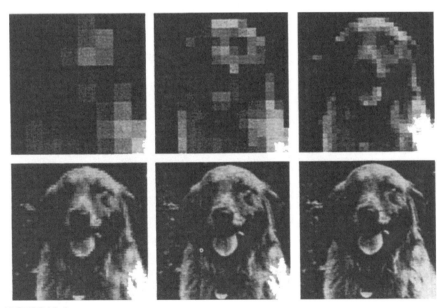

FIGURE 10-6
As the matrix size of a digital image is increased, the relative size of each pixel decreases and the image appears more like the original (lower right). The images shown here, beginning at **top left**, consist of 8^2, 16^2, 64^2, 128^2, and 256^2 pixels. Each image has a bit depth of 8, corresponding to 256 shades of gray. (From Hendee, W. R., and Ritenour, E. R., *Medical Imaging Physics.*[12])

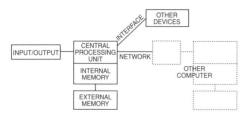

MARGIN FIGURE 10-3
Computer system hardware.

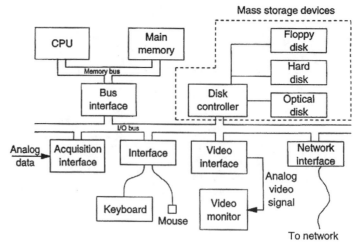

FIGURE 10-7
A block diagram of a modern computer. (From Bushberg, J. T., et al. *The Essential Physics of Medical Imaging.*[13] Used with permission.)

The total number of bits making up such an image is $128 \times 128 \times 8 = 131,072$. At 9600 bits per second, the time required to transmit the image is $131,072/9600 = 13.65$ seconds.

COMPUTER ARCHITECTURE

Reference has been made earlier in this chapter to computer memory. Computers actually consist of a number of components, including memory, which are linked together by pathways called data buses (Figure 10-7). The main memory of the computer stores the program (as a sequence of instructions) that is being executed, as well as the data being processed. A central processing unit (CPU) executes the instructions in the program to process the data. Input/output (I/O) devices are required to enable the operator to enter information into and retrieve information from the computer. Typical I/O devices include a keyboard, mouse or other pointing device, video monitor, mass storage device, and printer or plotter. A data bus is a group of wires or fibers used to transfer data in parallel. This method is more efficient than the process of serial data transfer described earlier, in which data are transferred one bit at a time along a single connection. With parallel data transfer, bits may be transferred simultaneously along each of several connections. A data bus consisting of eight connections can transfer an 8-bit byte in the same time required for a serial interface to transfer a single bit.

Memory

Computer memory provides temporary storage for the computer program (a sequence of instructions to the computer) as well as for the data currently being processed by the computer. The memory consists of a large number of data storage locations, each typically consisting of one byte. Each storage location is uniquely identified with an address. Memory addresses usually start at zero and increase sequentially. A computer having "1 megabyte" of memory actually has 1,048,576 memory locations, identified by addresses ranging from 0 to 1,048,575. Most contemporary computers have a certain amount of random access memory (RAM). RAM refers to memory into which the computer can both write and read data. A disadvantage of most modern RAM is that it is volatile, meaning that data stored in it are lost when the electrical power is switched off. To write to the memory, a computer must first send the address of the

Computer hardware is any physical component of a computer. Computer software is any set of instructions used to operate the computer or perform mathematical operations.

Device	Input	Output
Keyboard	X	
Light pen	X	
Joystick	X	
Mouse	X	
Modem	X	X
Hard copy		X
Display screen		X
Printer		X
X/Y plotter		X
Touchscreen	X	X
Disk/tape drive	X	X
Digitizer	X	
Network interface	X	X
Equipment interface	X	X

location in memory into which a datum is to be written, and then send the datum. To read from memory, the computer sends the address from which a datum is to be read and, in return, is sent the datum at that location. To be able to access a full 1 megabyte of memory, a computer must be able to send addresses as large a 1,048,575, or $2^{20} - 1$. This requires a word length of at least 20 bits; typically 24 or even 32 bits are used.

Another type of memory is read-only memory (ROM). A computer can only read data from ROM; it cannot write or alter data. The primary advantage of ROM is that data stored in it are not lost when the computer's electrical power is switched off. ROM is used to store frequently used programs provided by the manufacturer for performing important functions such as preparing the computer for operation when power is turned on.

To provide greater flexibility and make upgrading simpler, some standardized software is provided on programmable read-only memory chips (PROMs). These chips are intended to be removed and replaced by the user as different software capabilities are required. Under some circumstances, PROMs can be reprogrammed by the manufacturer, often through a modem connection.

The amount of memory required for a computer depends on its intended applications. For example, a computer used for word processing requires sufficient memory to store the word-processing program, together with the document being written. A typical word-processing program may require as much as 2 megabytes of memory, while word-processing documents are rarely longer than 100 kilobytes. A computer with less available RAM may still be able to run a word-processing program, but only a portion of the program can be loaded into RAM at one time. Hence, only a subset of the available commands and functions are available at one time. Making another function available requires that another portion of the program be loaded into memory (replacing the portion previously loaded). This process delays execution of the program. Manipulation of large amounts of data, such as medical images, requires large amounts of memory to be available for the data. Modern computer workstations designed for handling medical images frequently have as much as 96 megabytes of RAM, or even more.

The term *memory* to denote the storage capacity of the computer was suggested by John von Neumann in 1945. The first all-purpose computers marketed by IBM were called "johniacs." This acknowledgment reflects von Neumann's many contributions to computer design, including the concept of a program code to direct computer operations.

Computer memory can be thought of as (a) "internal memory" that is directly accessible during an instruction cycle and (b) "external memory" such as a magnetic tape, magnetic disk, or optical storage device.

Modem is an acronym for "*mo*dulate, *dem*odulate."

Central Processing Unit

The central processing unit (CPU) is the central control mechanism of the computer. It is a collection of electronic circuits that can execute a small number of rather simple functions. For example, the CPU fetches and executes the instructions of a computer program in sequence. Typically, instructions tell the CPU to perform one of four tasks:

- Transfer a unit of data (typically a byte or a word) from one memory location, storage register, or I/O device to another.
- Perform a mathematical operation between two numbers.
- Compare the value of two numbers or other pieces of data.
- Change the address of the next instruction in the program to be executed.

For example, a program instruction may instruct the CPU to add two numbers. This operation requires the following steps.

1. Locate the first number from an I/O device or RAM.
2. Store this number in a temporary location and record the address of that location.
3. Locate the second number from an I/O device or RAM.
4. Identify the temporary storage location where the result is to be placed.
5. Perform the addition function and store the result in the identified temporary storage location.

6. Report the result of the operation back to the main program and look for the next instruction.

Most currently available computers function by using a technique called serial processing. This approach requires that one task is completed before another is begun. In many applications, the result of one task is the input for the next, and serial processing is necessary. In some applications, however, the completion of one task is independent of at least some other tasks. In these cases, it may be possible for one computer processor to work on one task while a separate processor works on another. This capability is known as multitasking. If a program is written to perform the same operation on numerous elements of data, then two processors could simultaneously operate on two pieces of data, executing the task twice as quickly. These tasks are said to be performed "in parallel." A computer that can perform tasks in parallel is termed a parallel processor.

One type of parallel processor is the "array" processor. An array processor uses a single instruction to perform the same computation on all elements of a large matrix of data. Tremendous savings in computer time may be achieved by using an array processor to manipulate digital images. Such processors are routinely used in CT and MR imaging units, and they are becoming standard on all types of digital imaging systems.

Another special processor that is used routinely in radiology is the "arithmetic processor." Many mathematical functions such as exponential quantities, square roots, and trigonometric functions can be calculated in clever but time-consuming fashion by repeated application of procedures such as addition. A faster and usually more accurate alternative involves the use of an arithmetic processor, a device that executes fewer steps in performing discrete mathematical operations. The arithmetic processor is optimized to perform mathematical functions only. It is called on by the CPU to provide these functions and return the results to memory.

> Supercomputers with parallel-processing capability can attain data-processing speeds of >300 million "floating-point" operations per second (MFLOPS). So-called "massively parallel" systems with several hundred microprocessors achieve giga-FLOP and tera-FLOP speeds.[14]

> An array processor is essentially a small-scale parallel processor.

Input/Output Devices

Input and output (I/O) devices form the operator interface of a computer. Components such as a keyboard, mouse, video monitor, and printer fall into this category. These devices can send or receive data serially (using a single data line) or in parallel.

A keyboard, for example, converts each alphanumeric symbol into a digital code representing the symbol. When the letter A is struck, the keyboard transmits a sequence of voltage pulses of high (e.g., 5 volts) and low (e.g., 0 volts) levels. These pulses are interpreted as ones and zeroes, making up the ASCII character representation $0100\ 0001_2$ (see Table 10-2).

Similarly, a printer receives a sequence of pulses, representing the ones and zeroes making up the binary code for an ASCII character. The printer interprets the code and correspondingly rotates a character wheel, squirts tiny droplets of ink, or fires a laser to deposit black powder on paper, causing the appropriate character to be printed on paper.

Another component used for data transfer is a *modem*. This device connects a computer to, and transmits data across, a telephone line. A modem must convert (modulate) a digital signal into an audible one, and then convert (demodulate) audible signals back to digital ones. Many modems incorporate proprietary data compression algorithms and error-checking capabilities that enable them to transfer data accurately at speeds equivalent to 100,000 bits per second or more.

Mass Storage Devices

The programs and data used by computers are stored permanently on devices incorporating magnetic or optical encoding. The memory, or RAM, of a computer is used only to store a copy of the program being executed and the data being manipulated.

As mentioned earlier, the stored information is lost if power to the RAM is interrupted. In addition, when the memory is required to run a different program or to manipulate new data, the previous information stored in the memory may be overwritten. Before they are lost, new data created by the program should be written to a mass storage device.

Common mass storage devices include magnetic disks, optical disks, and magnetic tape. Magnetic disks and tape store data by magnetizing small regions called domains. When the domains are oriented together by a magnetic field, their combined magnetic fields become detectable. The local magnetic field produced by the write head of a magnetic disk drive can magnetize groups of domains in small regions of the disk. The same head, when operating in its "read" mode, can detect the pattern of magnetization. The pattern of magnetization is not lost when power is removed, so the magnetic storage devices are said to be "nonvolatile."

Magnetic tape devices, like those used for recording music, store data sequentially. For example, a 2400-foot reel of tape can store more than 150 megabytes of data, at a density of 6400 bytes per inch. A modern digital audio tape (DAT) cassette can hold as much as 8 gigabytes. Tape is most useful for making backups of other media, or for transferring large volumes of data such as digitized medical images. Data stored on tape cannot be edited; it is only possible to write additional data after records are already written (provided there is room). Tape is relatively slow, because data must be written and read sequentially. However, tape is relatively inexpensive.

Magnetic disks have been manufactured in a variety of formats. Flexible (or "floppy") diskettes are inexpensive but hold comparatively little information, typically 1.4 megabytes. They are also somewhat unreliable and are most useful for backups or short-term storage of data. Hard disks are available in both fixed and removable formats, with capacities from a few megabytes to many gigabytes.

Both floppy and hard disks are coated with magnetizable material. The information embedded in the disk is read with a read/write head that hovers a small distance above the disk. Data are stored along concentric *tracks*, which themselves are divided into *sectors*. The head moves radially across the disk to access different tracks. Frequently, two opposing heads are provided, and data are stored on both sides of the disk.

Data are generally written in *blocks*, and a directory stored on the disk identifies the usage of each block. A large program or data file may require a number of blocks, but, depending on the capabilities of the drive, the blocks may not have to be contiguous. Instead, the final record of each block is a *pointer* to the next block in the series used for the file. While it is potentially possible to change a single bit on a hard disk, an edited file is generally rewritten to a new location on the disk, and the previous locations are made available for new data.

The time required to move the read/write head to a desired location on the disk is called the *access time*. Typical access times range from a few milliseconds to a few hundred milliseconds. The *data transfer rate* describes the speed with which data can be written to or read from the disk. Typical rates range from a few hundred kilobytes to 10 megabytes or more per second.

Hard disk drives can be permanently damaged if the head physically contacts the disk. Usually, before a disk drive is moved (such as the disk drive in a portable computer), a mechanism is activated to "park" the head in a secure location. Disk drives must be enclosed to protect them from dust or dirt. Because the head travels only a few micrometers above the disk, a hair or speck of dust can scratch the disk or damage the head (Figure 10-8).

Optical disks (such as compact disks, or "CDs") are removable glass or plastic disks with a thin coating of metal. To write data to the disk, a laser burns a pattern of holes in the metal coating. This pattern can be read by a laser to retrieve the data. Some optical disks allow data to be written only permanently. These units are called "worm" drives (for "write once, read many" times). Other devices have been developed that allow rewriting of optical disks.

The term "jukebox" is used for a mechanical device that stores and selects multiple storage disks (CD ROMs, DVDs, etc.). These devices resemble the jukeboxes that select and play vinyl records. The expression "juke" is from Gullah, a language spoken by descendants of West African slaves living on islands off the Georgia and South Carolina coasts. In Gullah, juke means "bad" or "disorderly." Roadside drinking establishments in the southeastern United States became known as "juke joints," and the record-playing devices in juke joints became known as jukeboxes.

12 cm diameter optical disks, known as CD ROMs, have become standard for musical recording and routine PC use. Higher-capacity disks are known as digital video disks (DVDs).

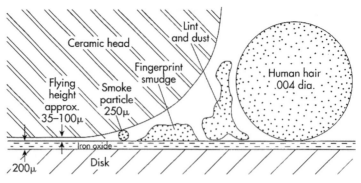

FIGURE 10-8
The read/write head of a hard disk drive travels only a small distance above the disk. Dirt or a hair can cause catastrophic damage.[15]

■ COMPUTER SOFTWARE

The instructions that cause computers to perform their intended functions are organized into *programs* that are collectively referred to as *software*. Software includes simple programs to add two numbers together, as well as word-processing programs, and programs to perform complex calculations with large amounts of data. Programs also exist to simplify development of other programs.

All modern computers run a program called an *operating system*. For example, Microsoft Windows is an operating system. Many computer workstations (a generation of desktop computers with fast processors and large amounts of memory) run a version of an operating system called Unix. The operating system monitors the various pieces of hardware and handles the transfer of data from one to another. It continually monitors input devices such as a keyboard or mouse, and it interprets the instructions received from these devices. The instructions may tell the operating system to read a copy of a file into the memory, then send the file to the printer.

Applications are programs developed for specific purposes such as word processing. In response to a command from the mouse or keyboard, the operating system may read an application from a disk, store it in memory, and begin executing it. Control of the computer then passes to the application.

Running the operating system is termed "booting" the computer, taken from the phrase "to pull oneself up by the bootstraps"—that is, to be a self-starter.

■ PROGRAMMING LANGUAGES

Computer Languages

Instructions to a computer that enable it to perform a desired function are contained in programs. Programs required to make a computer function are referred to as *software* (in contrast to the hardware that makes up the computer itself). A program consists of a series of instructions, arranged in a logical sequence, which when executed cause the computer to perform a set of operations. The program may be simple (e.g., instructing the computer to display a word or sentence on a monitor) or complex (e.g., word-processing and spreadsheet programs). Complicated programs often are broken up into smaller sections called *subroutines*, in which a single function or operation is handled.

The instructions that comprise a program must be written in a manner that is intelligible to the computer. Instructions that are easily interpreted by a computer are not directly translatable by humans. Consequently, several different levels of language have been developed to convert programs from the languages understood by humans to the languages understood by computers.

Since software refers to one or more computer programs, the expression *software program* is redundant.

The expression "bug" for a computer malfunction was coined in 1951 by Grace Hopper, Ph.D., a U.S. Navy admiral, after she found an actual bug in an electronic relay of a malfunctioning computer.

```
10 PRINT "CALCULATE POWERS of 2"
20 FOR I = 1 TO 10
   30 LET A = 2**I
   40 REM The double asterisk indicates an exponent
   50 PRINT "The";I;" Exponent of 2 is "; A
60 NEXT I
70 END
```

FIGURE 10-9
A simple BASIC language program.

Low-Level Languages

Low-level languages are those that are understood by a computer without translation. These languages are referred to as *object code*, or *machine language*. When printed, an object code appears to be a meaningless list of numbers and letters. The digits and letters may be hexadecimal numbers, each representing a single instruction. For example, a particular hexadecimal code may be an instruction to the CPU to retrieve a value from memory, with the address of the value to be read given by the next instruction.

Object code is difficult for humans to interpret, even those skilled at writing programs in this language. A slightly more intelligible code is *assembly language*. This code substitutes mnemonics for each of the instructions contained in object code. These instructions, although cryptic, are at least recognizable, and they make writing programs in low-level languages a little easier. Mnemonic codes correspond one-to-one with object code instructions.

High-Level Languages

To facilitate the development of programs, high-level languages have been developed. These languages use commands that resemble the English language. An example of a high-level language is the BASIC program portrayed in Figure 10-9. This figure illustrates several common elements of computer programs. Instructions to the computer are listed in a logical sequence, and the sequence is defined by *line numbers*. Some instructions are intended to be repeated a selected number of times, or until some criterion is met. These instructions are placed in a *loop*. In Figure 10-9, the loop is defined by the "For" and "Next" statements (the intervening commands have been indented for clarity, a common practice by programmers). Instructions must be included to deliver the results to the person operating the program. In this example, the "Print" statements cause the text within quotes and the numeric values represented by the symbols *I* and *A* to be printed on an output device connected to the computer.

When high-level programming language is used, the computer must be equipped with a program to *interpret* or *compile* programs written in the high-level language. The distinction between the two is easily made: An *interpreter* is a program that decodes the user's program (such as the BASIC program in Figure 10-9) one line at a time, acts on the instructions contained in that line, and then goes on to the next line. Each time a line is encountered, even if it falls within a loop, it must be interpreted anew. A *compiler* creates a new program in assembly language from the user's program. The assembly language program may be modified further and combined with other subroutines to finally produce a program in object code. This final version requires no interpretation and can be executed at maximum speed by the computer. However, it is almost impossible to be understood by humans, or to change. Instead, changes must be made in the original high-level program, which must then be compiled and linked once more before it is executed. The advantage is that once a program reaches its final form, the computer can execute it rapidly and as often as necessary.

An example of a section of a C program, and the corresponding assembly language code generated by the compiler, are shown in Figure 10-10. The program is very

Basic is one of many high-level programming languages. Other high-level programming languages in common use include FORTRAN, PASCAL, Visual BASIC, C, C++ and SQL.

A computer is much faster than an interpreter in converting a high-level language program into object code. However, instructions in the program are almost impossible to change once the compiler has completed the translation.

c program language:

```
#include <stdio.h>

main ()
    {
    float a;
    float b;
    float c;

    /*
    * Display a prompt.
    */

    printf("Enter values A, B: ");

    /*
    * Read values A and B from standard input. */

    scanf("%f,%f",&a,&b);

    /*
    * Put product of A and B in C.
    */

    c=a*b;

    /*
    * Print product on screen.
    */

    printf("The product of A and B is: %f",c);

}
```

Assembly code generated by the compiler:

```
.SPACE     $TEXT$,SORT=8
.SUBSPA    $CODE$,QUAD=0,ALIGN=4,ACCESS=0x2c,CODE_ONLY,SORT=24
main
.PROC
.CALLINFO          CALLER,FRAME=16,SAVE_RP
.ENTRY
STW        %r2,-20(%r30)    ;offset 0x0
LDO        64(%r30),%r30    ;offset 0x4
ADDIL      LR'M$2-$global$,%r27          ;offset 0x8
LDO        RR'M$2-$global$(%r1),%r26     ;offset 0xc
LDIL       L'printf,%r31    ;offset 0x10
.CALL      ARGW0=GR,RTNVAL=GR            ;in=26;out=28;
BLE        R'printf(%sr4,%r31)           ;offset 0x14
COPY       %r31,%r2         ;offset 0x18
ADDIL      LR'M$2-$global$+20,%r27       ;offset 0x1c
LDO        RR'M$2-$global$+20(%r1),%r26  ;offset 0x20
LDO        -64(%r30),%r25   ;offset 0x24
LDO        -60(%r30),%r24   ;offset 0x28
LDIL       L'scanf,%r31     ;offset 0x2c
.CALL      ARGW0=GR,ARGW1=GR,ARGW2=GR,RTNVAL=GR    ;in=24,25,26;out=28;
BLE        R'scanf(%sr4,%r31)            ;offset 0x30
COPY       %r31,%r2         ;offset 0x34
LDO        -48(%r30),%r1    ;offset 0x38
FLDWS      -16(%r1),%fr4L   ;offset 0x3c
FCNVFF,SGL,DBL         %fr4L,%fr4  ;offset 0x40
LDO        -48(%r30),%r31   ;offset 0x44
FLDWS      -12(%r31),%fr5L  ;offset 0x48
FCNVFF,SGL,DBL         %fr5L,%fr5  ;offset 0x4c
FMPY,DBL %fr4,%fr5,%fr6     ;offset 0x50
FCNVFF,DBL,SGL         %fr6,%fr5R  ;offset 0x54
LDO        -48(%r30),%r19   ;offset 0x58
FSTWS      %fr5R,-8(%r19)   ;offset 0x5c
ADDIL      LR'M$2-$global$+28,%r27       ;offset 0x60
LDO        RR'M$2-$global$+28(%r1),%r26  ;offset 0x64
LDO        -48(%r30),%r20   ;offset 0x68
FLDWS      -8(%r20),%fr6L   ;offset 0x6c
```

FIGURE 10-10

A short section of a C language program is converted into a number of assembly language statements by the compiler. (Courtesy of Yeong-Yeong Liu of Computerized Medical Systems, St. Louis, MO.)

```
         FCNVFF,SGL,DBL                  %fr6L,%fr7   ;offset 0x70
         LDIL       L'printf,%r31        ;offset 0x74
         .CALL      ARGW0=GR,ARGW2=FR,ARGW3=FU,RTNVAL=GR        ;in=26;out=28;fpin=107;
         BLE        R'printf(%sr4,%r31)          ;offset 0x78
         COPY       %r31,%r2             ;offset 0x7c
         LDW        -84(%r30),%r2        ;offset 0x80
         BV         %r0(%r2)             ;offset 0x84
         .EXIT
         LDO        -64(%r30),%r30       ;offset 0x88
         .PROCEND  ;out=28;


         .SPACE     $TEXT$
         .SUBSPA    $CODE$
         .SPACE     $PRIVATE$,SORT=16
         .SUBSPA    $DATA$,QUAD=1,ALIGN=8,ACCESS=0x1f,SORT=16
     M$2
         .ALIGN     8
         .STRINGZ "Enter values A, B: \x00%f,%f"
         .BLOCKZ    2
         .STRINGZ "The product of A and B is: %f"
         .IMPORT    $global$,DATA
         .SPACE     $TEXT$
         .SUBSPA    $CODE$
         .EXPORT    main,ENTRY,PRIV_LEV=3,RTNVAL=GR
         .IMPORT    printf,CODE
         .IMPORT    scanf,CODE
         .END
```

FIGURE 10-10
(*Continued*)

simple; it prompts the operator to enter two numbers, the numbers are multiplied together, and the result is displayed. The operational part of the program is contained between the brackets, and the portions offset by "/*" are comments that are ignored by the computer.

The corresponding assembly code is much more lengthy. Text that follows a semicolon on each line is a comment. Clearly, C code is much more compact and readable than the resulting assembly language.

In recent years, very high level programming languages have been developed that enable the programmer to use statements that are even closer to English. Examples of such software include MATHCAD (Mathematics Computer-Aided Design) and MATLAB (Mathematics Laboratory).

MATHCAD is a registered trademark of MathSoft, Inc., 201 Broadway, Cambridge, MA 02139. MATLAB is a registered trademark of The MathWorks, Inc., 24 Prime Park Way, Natick, MA 01760.

◼ NETWORKING*

The increased use of computers in all areas of medicine, including diagnostic imaging, creates the desire to link the computers together, thereby making information present in one computer available to all computers in an institution or community. This linking of computers, called "networking," is a topic of current interest.[16–19]

In the late 1960s, the US Department of Defense wanted to develop a computer network that would survive a nuclear attack. The network would continue to deliver streams of digital data, even if a number of its components or linkages were destroyed. The solution was "packet switching," a system in which data streams are broken into smaller pieces, called cells or frames. Each cell contains not only a piece of the data, but also information such as the place of the cell in the original sequence, the priority of this stream of data compared with other data streams, and so forth. One key feature of packet switching is that each cell also contains the address of the component to which it is being sent. Another key feature of packet switching is that the network consists of interconnected routers. Each router is a computer whose purpose is to maintain information about the addresses of surrounding routers. When a packet arrives at a router, it is automatically sent on to another router that is "closer" to its destination. Thus, if part of the network is disabled, the routers update their

*This section on networking is taken from Hendee, W. R., and Ritenour, E. R. *Medical Imaging Physics*, 4th edition New York, John Wiley & sons, 2001.

History of the Internet. The World Wide Web was created in March 1989, at CERN, a high-energy particle physics laboratory on the Franco–Swiss border. Tim Berners-Lee, a physicist at CERN, proposed the idea of using a hypertext system that would link data from diverse information sources and different computer platforms.

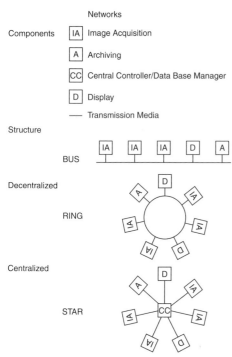

MARGIN FIGURE 10-4
Components and structures commonly used in image networks.

information and simply send cells via different routes. This earliest wide-area network was known as Arpanet, after the Department of Defense's Advanced Research Projects Administration.

When electronic mail (e-mail) was developed, the usefulness of Arpanet became apparent to a wider community of users in academics and in government, and the number of network users continued to grow. Arpanet was officially decommissioned in 1989. By that time, a wide community of users required that the network be continued. The administration of the network was turned over to the National Science Foundation. The network of routers, file servers, and other devices that have become the foundation of modern communications has been known as the Internet since 1989.

In 1989, the World Wide Web (WWW) was first proposed at CERN, a high-energy physics laboratory on the border between France and Switzerland. This proposal embodied all of the modern components of the WWW, including file servers that maintain "pages" of data in standard format with "hypertext" links to other sources of data or other servers. In 1991 there were only 10 file servers on the WWW, at various physics laboratories. Today, the number of servers is well into the millions.

Network Components and Structure

Computer networks for medical imaging are known by many names, such as information management, archiving, and communications systems (IMACS), picture archiving and communications systems (PACS), digital imaging networks (DIN), and local area networks (LAN). These networks face some fundamental problems including (1) how to transmit images quickly, (2) how to avoid bottlenecks or "data collision" when the network is experiencing heavy use, (3) how to organize and maintain the data base or "log" that records the existence of images and their locations on the system, and (4) how to retain as many images as possible on the network for as long as necessary.

The main components of a computer network and its typical organization are shown in Margin Figure 10-4. Components include image acquisition (CT, ultrasound, etc.), archiving (tape, disk, etc.), central controller, data base manager, and display station. Components that allow the network to communicate with the outside world through display and archiving techniques are referred to as "nodes." All components are not necessarily nodes. For example, several ultrasound units might be connected to a single formatting device that translates the digital images into a standard format recognizable by the network. The formatting device communicates directly with the network and is the node for the ultrasound units.

Networks can be divided into two categories on the basis of their overall structure. Centralized networks use a single computer (a central controller) to monitor and control access to information for all parts of the network. A distributed network contains components that are connected together with no central controller. Tasks are handled as requested until a conflict arises such as more demands being placed on a component than it can handle. While it may appear chaotic, a distributed network has the advantage that other components are not affected by slowdown or stoppage of one or more components of the system. In particular, there is no central controller that would shut the whole system down if it malfunctions.

Interfaces

The interface of an imaging device such as a CT scanner with a computer network is usually a more complex matter than simply connecting a few wires. Transfer of images and other data requires that the network must be ready to receive, transmit, and store information from the device. These operations could interfere with other activities taking place on the network. Therefore, the imaging device may have to send an "interrupt" signal that indicates that a transmission is ready. The data may have to be transmitted in blocks of specified size (e.g., 256-kbyte transmission packets) that are recognizable to the network as part of a larger file of information.

The above-mentioned problems require both hardware and software solutions. Programs that control transmission of data to and from various components are called "device drivers." The physical connectors must also be compatible with (i.e., can be attached and transmit signals to) other network components. Both hardware and software are implied in the term "interface." Connecting a component to a computer or computer network in such a way that information may be transmitted is described as interfacing the component. There have been a number of attempts to standardize interfaces for imaging devices, including the American College of Radiology/National Electronics Manufacturers Association (ACR/NEMA) standards.[20]

Transmission Media

Components of a network may be physically separated by distances varying from a few feet to several hundred miles or more. The transmission of digital information requires a transmission medium that is appropriate to the demands of the particular network. Once of the most important factors to consider is the rate at which data are transmitted, measured in bits per second (bps).

Example 10-6

A network is capable of transmitting data at a rate of 1 megabit per second (Mbps). If each pixel has a bit depth of 8 bits, how long will it take to transmit 50 512 × 512 images?

Since each pixel consists of 8 bits, the total number of bits is

$$50 [8 \text{ bits/pixel} \times (512 \times 512 \text{ pixel})] = 50(2^3 \times 2^9 \times 2^9) \text{ bits}$$
$$= 50(2^{21}) \text{ bits}$$
$$= (50)(2 \text{ Mbits}) = 100 \text{ Mbits}$$

The transmission time is then

$$\frac{100 \text{ Mbits}}{1 \text{ Mbps}} = 100 \text{ seconds}$$

One of the least expensive transmission media is telephone wire (sometimes called "twisted pairs"). It is inexpensive and easy to install and maintain. However, the transmission rate does not usually exceed a few Mbps. Higher rates up to hundreds of Mbps are achievable with coaxial cable. However, coaxial cable is more expensive, needs inline amplifiers, and is subject to electric interference problems in some installations. The highest transmission rates are achievable with fiber-optic cable. This transmission medium consists of glass fibers that transmit light pulses, thereby eliminating electrical interference problems. Transmission rates for fiber-optic cables are currently just below a terabit per second (Tbps).

Data Compression

Images are transmitted faster and require less storage space if they are composed of fewer bits. Decreasing the number of pixels reduces spatial resolution, however, and decreasing the bit depth decreases contrast sensitivity. It is possible, however, to "compress" image data in such a way that fewer bits of information are needed without significant loss of spatial or contrast resolution.

Digital Communications Options

Copper Wire:
Modulator/Demodulator (modem): 56 kbps
Integrated Services Digital Network (ISDN): 64 or 128 kbps
Digital Subscriber Line (DSL)
  Several versions up to 4 Mbps
Asynchronous DSL 3–4 Mbps to the home
  <1 Mbps from the home

Hybrid-Fiber/Coax:
Cable Modem
  40 MBps to the home, *but* multiple
    users slow it down
<10 MBps from cable box to your computer

Wireless (high-frequency GHz radio waves):
Local Multi-Point Distributed Services (LMDS)
  Data rates of up to 155 Mbps
  Problems: "rain fade," trees, etc.
Cellular Telephone
  Now: 10–50 kbps
  Future: 1 Mbps
Satellites
  Data rates of up to 210 Mbps
  Problems: price

Direct Fiber:
Fiber-to-the-Home
  Now: <10-Mbps Ethernet for most PCs
    <100-Mbps FDDI for some devices
    10's of Gbps Asynchronous Transfer Mode
  Future: Tbps

One way to reduce the number of bits is to encode pixel values in some sequence (e.g., row by row) to indicate the value of each pixel and the number of succeeding pixels with the same value. This decreases the total number of bits needed to describe the image, because most images have several contiguous pixels with identical values (e.g., the black border surrounding a typical CT image). Other techniques for data compression include analysis of the probability of occurrence of each pixel value, and assignment of a code to translate each pixel value to its corresponding probability. Such a "probability mapping" uses fewer bits for the more probable pixel values.[21]

In the examples above, the full information content of the image is preserved. When the image is expanded, it is exactly the same as it was before compression. These approaches to data compression are known as lossless (bit-preserving, or nondestructive) techniques. They may yield a reduction in the number of required bits by a factor of 3 or 4. When a greater reduction is needed, methods of data compression may be used that do not preserve the exact bit structure of an image, but still maintain acceptable diagnostic quality for the particular application. These techniques, known as irreversible (non-bit-preserving or destructive) data compression methods, can reduce the number of bits by an arbitrarily high factor.

An example of an irreversible data compression method involves the use of the Fourier transform to describe blocks of pixel values in the image. Some of the high- or low-frequency components of the image are then eliminated to reduce the number of bits required to store the image. When an inverse transform is used to restore the image, the loss of high or low spatial frequencies may not significantly detract form the diagnostic usefulness of the image.

Display Stations and Standards

The part of a computer network that is most accessible to the observer is the digital display or monitor, usually referred to as the image workstation. Some display stations are capable of displaying more data than are presented on the screen at one time. They may, initially, show images at reduced resolution (e.g., 1024 × 1024) while preserving the full "high-resolution" data set (e.g., 2048 × 2048) in memory. The stored data can be recalled in sections through user-selectable windows. Alternatively, only part of the image may be presented, but the part that is presented may be "panned" or moved around the full image.

Recalling stored digital imaging data in sections at higher resolution is analogous to viewing an analog image with a magnifying lens.

Standards for digital matrix size and remote display of medical images that are acceptable for primary diagnosis from computer monitors have been established by the American College of Radiology (ACR).[22] These standards will continue to evolve as equipment performance (particularly display monitors) continues to improve. Current versions of the standards are available on the ACR web site (www.acr.org). Currently, two classes of images are recognized; small matrix systems and large matrix systems. Small matrix systems (CT, MRI, ultrasound, nuclear medicine, and digital fluoroscopy) must have a format of at least 5k × 5k × 8 bits. The display must be capable of displaying at least 5k × 0.48k × 8 bits. Large matrix systems (digitized radiographs, computed radiography) are held to a standard based upon required spatial and contrast resolution. For these imaging methods, the digital data must provide a resolution of at least 2.5 line pairs per millimeter and a 10-bit gray scale. The display must be capable of resolving 2.5 line pairs per millimeter with a minimum of 8-bit gray scale.

The development of the DICOM standard was initiated by the American College of Radiology (ACR) and the National Electrical Manufacturer's Association (NEMA) in 1985, and it continues to evolve as equipment capabilities change.

The industry-standard format for transferring images between components of a network is the Digital Imaging and Communications in Medicine or DICOM standard. The standard consists of specifications for various data "fields" that must occur in the image header. These fields describe attributes such as the matrix size of the image, whether it is part of a series (e.g., one slice of a multi-slice CT series), and patient demographic data.

Although the capabilities of "high-end" workstations are far from being standardized, some general features have been. A monitor should be able to display enough written information concerning the patient to obviate the need for transport of paper documents. The display station should be able to run image-processing software as well as provide simple display functions such as variable window level, window width, and magnification. Dimensional reconstruction and tissue segmentation (display of bones only or vessels only) are becoming more common.

COMPUTER REQUIREMENTS FOR TREATMENT PLANNING

No special or unusual requirements are imposed on computer systems for radiation therapy treatment planning. Today, treatment planning computers are assembled from components available "off the shelf" from a variety of manufacturers. Over the years, treatment planning software has been developed to run on standard desktop computers such as those made by Apple and IBM. As the capabilities of desktop computers have increased, these system have become more powerful and suitable for treatment planning applications. Comprehensive treatment planning systems have been developed for high-end workstations such as those marketed by Silicon Graphics, Hewlett-Packard, and Sun. These systems have superb graphics capabilities as well as fast processors, and they are able to handle large amounts of data. For example, a number of CT or MRI images can be stored. Modern 3D treatment planning computers also require large amounts of memory to store the calculated dose matrix.

Computers for treatment planning require several methods of data entry. Most systems are equipped with a *digitizer* for entering patient contours, field shapes, and, in some cases, beam data. These systems require a mouse or some other pointing tool, as well as a keyboard. To enter CT or other images, a tape drive, optical disk drive, or Ethernet connection may be used. A high-quality video monitor is needed, because the developing treatment plan frequently must be viewed by several people simultaneously. Finally, an output device is required, most often a multi-pen plotter capable of drawing the patient outline, treatment fields, and isodose curves. When CT or other images are used for treatment planning, a color graphics printer may be needed.

SUMMARY

- Although computers in various forms have been available for centuries, it was the development of the transistor that ushered in the modern era of computers and information networking.
- Quantities can be expressed in many number systems; the most common systems are base 10 (decimal), base 2 (binary), base 8 (octal) and base 16 (hexadecimal).
- A single unit of information is a bit (**bi**nary digi**t**); multiples of bits make up bytes (8 bits) and words (16 or 32 bits).
- Many signal detectors and display systems are analog devices; analog-to-digital (ADCs) and digital-to-analog (DAC) converters function as interfaces between these devices and computer systems.
- Digital images are two-dimensional matrices of pixels, with each pixel providing a bit depth for display of gray-scale information.
- Computer memory contains operational programs for the computer, and provides temporary storage for data being processed by the computer.
- The central processing unit (CPU) is the central control mechanism for the computer.
- Many input/output (I/O) devices are available, and several can serve both purposes.

- Mass data storage devices include magnetic tape, magnetic disks and optical disks (CD-ROMS and DVDs).
- Computer languages exist at several levels, with high-level languages resembling the English language.
- Computer networks for medical imaging are frequently referred to by the acronyms IMACS, PACS, DIN, and LAN.
- Networks can be separated into two categories: centralized networks and distributed networks.
- Transmission media for information networks range from telephone lines to fiber-optic cable.
- In the transmission of digital images, data compression is usually required to reduce the data conversion and transmission time.
- Standards for transmitting images between components in a LAN are known as DICOM standards.
- Standards for image transmission from remote locations (teleradiology) have been established by the American College of Radiology.
- No special requirements are imposed on computer systems used for radiation therapy treatment planning.

PROBLEMS

10-1. Show that multiplying a binary number by a power of 2 is performed by moving the decimal point a number of times equal to the power.

10-2. Convert the binary number 1110 0110 1001 1101 into octal, decimal, and hexadecimal.

10-3. Convert the decimal number 1995 into binary, octal and hexadecimal.

10-4. In two's-complement notation and an 8-bit register, the binary number 1111 0100 represents the decimal value −12. Show that the addition of 0001 1010 (decimal 26) yields 0000 1110 (decimal 14).

10-5. The digitizer tablet of a treatment planning computer is stated to have a resolution of 0.25 mm. The tablet is 50 cm wide. How many bits long must the binary word representing position be? If the digitizer produces an analog voltage ranging from −15 V to +15 V, what increment of voltage corresponds to each increment in the binary value?

10-6. A CT image consists of 256 × 256 pixels. A compression algorithm is used to reduce the "depth" of each pixel to 6 bits. How long will it take to transmit this image over a network operating at 28.8 kb (thousand bits per second)?

10-7. Modern modems operate at speeds of 28.8 kb. How long might it take to transfer this chapter at 28.8 kb? The chapter consists of approximately 12,000 characters, each represented by one 8-bit word.

10-8. How many CT scans could be stored on magnetic tape, at a storage density of 6,400 8-bit bytes per inch? Each scan is 512 × 512 pixels, and each pixel is 8 bits deep. The tape is 2400 feet long.

REFERENCES

1. Davis, M. *The University Computer: The Road from Leibniz to Turing.* New York, W. H. Norton, 2001.
2. Considine, D. M. (ed.). *Von Nostrand's Scientific Encyclopedia*, 5th edition. New York, Van Nostrand Reinhold, 1976.
3. Moreau, R. *The Computer Comes of Age.* Cambridge, MA, MIT Press, 1984. (Translated by J. Howlett.)
4. Kuni, C. C. *Introduction to Computers and Digital Processing in Medical Imaging.* St. Louis, Mosby–Year Book, 1988.
5. Spencer, D. D. *Introduction to Information Processing*, 3rd edition. Columbus, OH, Charles E. Merrill, 1981.
6. Huskey, V. R., and Huskey, V. D. Lady Lovelace and Charles Babbage. *Ann. Hist. Comput.* 1980; **2**:299–329.
7. Ritenour, E. R. *Computer Applications in Diagnostic Radiology, Instructor's Manual.* St. Louis, Mosby–Year Book, 1983.
8. Stubbe, J. W. *Computers and Information Systems.* New York, McGraw-Hill, 1984.
9. Mackintosh, A. R. The first electronic computer. *Phys. Today* 1987; **March**:25–32.
10. Mauchly, K. R. *IEEE Annals in the History of Computing,* Vol. 6. Piscataway, NJ, IEEE Computer Society, 1984, p. 116.
11. Stern, N. *From ENIAC to UNIVAC: An Appraisal of the Eckert–Mauchly Machines.* Bedford, MA, Digital Press, 1981.
12. Hendee, W. R., and Ritenour, E. R. *Medical Imaging Physics*, 4th edition. New York, John Wiley & Sons, 2001.
13. Bushberg, J. T., Seiberta, J. A., Leidholdt, E. M. and Boone, J. M. et al., *The Essential Physics of Medical Imaging.* Baltimore, Williams & Wilkins, 1994.
14. Glantz, J. Microprocessors deliver teraflops. *Science* 1996; **271**:598.

15. Hendee, W. R. *The Selection and Performance of Radiological Equipment*. Baltimore, Williams & Wilkins, 1985.

16. Johnson, N. D., Garofolo, G., and Geers, W. Demystifying the hospital information system/radiology information system integration process. *J. Digital Imaging* 2000 **13**(2 Suppl. 1):175–179.

17. Langer, SG: Architecture of an image capable, Web-based, electronic medical record. *J. Digit. Imaging* 2000, **13**(2):82–89.

18. Abbing, H. R. Medical confidentiality and electronic patient files. *Med. Law* 2000; **19**(1):107–112.

19. Staggers, N. The vision for the Department of Defense's computer-based patient record. *Military Med.* 2000, **165**(3):180–185.

20. Wang, Y., Best, D. E., Hoffman, J. G., Bushberg, J. T., Seibert, J. A., Leidholdt, E. M., Boone, J. M. ACR/NEMA digital imaging and communications standards: Minimum requirements. *Radiology* 1988; **166**:529–532.

21. Huang, H. K. *PACS: Basic Principles and Applications*. New York, John Wiley & Sons, 1999, Chapter 6.

22. American College of Radiology. *Handbook of Teleradiology Applications*. Reston, VA, ACR, 1997.

COMPUTER-BASED TREATMENT PLANNING

OBJECTIVES   246

INTRODUCTION   246

BEAM DATA ENTRY   247

PATIENT DATA ENTRY   248

VIRTUAL SIMULATION TECHNIQUES   252

IMMOBILIZATION AND LOCALIZATION   253

PHOTON BEAM COMPUTATIONAL ALGORITHMS   258

THE ANALYTICAL METHOD   258

MATRIX TECHNIQUES   258

SEMIEMPIRICAL METHODS   259

Clarkson Method   259
Differential Scatter–Air Ratio Calculation   262
Heterogeneity Corrections   262
Three-Dimensional Integration Methods   263

ELECTRON BEAM COMPUTATIONAL ALGORITHMS   265

SELECTION OF IDEAL TREATMENT PLAN   265

BIOLOGICAL MODELING   267

FORWARD PLANNING   267

INVERSE PLANNING   270

INTENSITY-MODULATED RADIATION THERAPY   270

Treatment Planning Techniques   270
Setting the Objective Function   272
Optimization   274
Conversion to Deliverable Treatment   274

DYNAMIC DELIVERY TECHNIQUES   277

TOMOTHERAPY   278

Serial Tomotherapy   278
Helical Tomotherapy   278

TREATMENT PLANNING CHALLENGES   280

Treatment Field Geometry   280
Lateral Disequilibrium in High-Energy Beams   280
Interface Effects   280

SUMMARY   280

PROBLEMS   281

REFERENCES   282

Radiation Therapy Physics, Third Edition, by William R. Hendee, Geoffrey S. Ibbott, and Eric G. Hendee
ISBN 0-471-39493-9 Copyright © 2005 John Wiley & Sons, Inc.

In speaking of relativity, Albert Einstein said "For a believing physicist, the distinction between the past, the present, and the future is only an illusion."

"Monitor units" refers to a number that is set on the treatment machine to deliver the intended treatment. It is typically related through machine calibration to the radiation dose administered to a simulated patient. For example, 1 monitor unit for a 6-MV x-ray beam may be set to equal 1 cGy for a 10-cm × 10-cm field at the point of maximum dose along the central beam axis in a water phantom set up at either 98.5-cm source-to-surface distance ("SAD calibration") or 100-cm source-to-surface distance ("SSD calibration"). The monitor unit came into use with modern linear accelerators to replace timer settings used with cesium and cobalt machines.

The ICRU is an international group of volunteer experts that publishes reports and guidances on a wide variety of topics related to ionizing radiation.

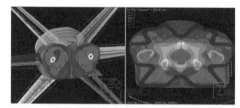

MARGIN FIGURE 11-1
CT image obtained through the pelvis of a patient undergoing radiation therapy. The prostate, rectum, and bladder are outlined, and a planning target volume is drawn around the prostate to include a margin. Conformal shaped beams are placed to deliver a uniform dose to the target.

■ OBJECTIVES

By studying this chapter, the reader should be able to:

- Describe the role of virtual simulation in radiation therapy planning.
- Differentiate between immobilization and localization, and describe current techniques used.
- Discuss various dose calculation algorithms.
- Understand methods of heterogeneity correction in treatment planning.
- Give examples of situations favorable to forward planning and inverse planning.
- Define intensity modulated radiation therapy and methods of delivery.
- Differentiate between serial tomotherapy and helical tomotherapy.

■ INTRODUCTION

Broadly speaking, the term *treatment planning* refers to all processes and decisions that lead to a plan of action for treating a patient with radiation. Processes include a physician's analysis and interpretation of diagnostic procedures, consultations with other specialists, decisions supporting treatment with external radiation, simulation of proposed treatment fields, and estimates and calculations of intended dose distributions. This chapter, which focuses on the last of these topics, uses a narrower interpretation of *treatment planning* to describe the procedures and calculations, both manual and automated, that yield dose distributions in patients receiving radiation therapy.

Manual techniques for treatment planning were described in Chapter 8. Manual calculations of dose to selected points in a patient are performed routinely, generally to determine the treatment time or monitor unit setting. Estimation of complete dose distributions by manual methods is rarely done today, because the availability of computers, even in departments of modest size, makes such laborious work unnecessary. Manual methods must be learned, however, to provide the insight and understanding necessary to correctly interpret computer-generated results and to determine their validity. On rare occasions when a treatment planning computer is not available, manual methods may prove valuable in constructing dose distributions for actual patients.

The treatment planning process can be described in the following manner:

1. A physician determines the target volume to be irradiated, on the basis of physical examination, surgery, and imaging studies. Computed tomography (CT) is one of the most commonly used imaging techniques for treatment planning, although magnetic resonance imaging (MRI), radiography, angiography, radionuclide imaging, and other techniques also are used. The physician then identifies the dose to be delivered to the target volume. This "dose prescription" is generally based on the physician's experience and on published reports and recommendations. In some cases the dose prescription is dictated by the requirements of a clinical trial. The clarity of the prescription, and the ease with which it is communicated, may be improved through use of the terminology recommended by the International Commission on Radiation Units and Measurements (ICRU).[1] These recommendations are described in detail in Chapter 8.

2. The physician often will also identify sensitive normal tissues, so-called *organs at risk*, and specify an upper limit of dose for these tissues. These limiting doses are based on the physician's experience, as well as on the determination of *tolerance doses* for the organs, above which an unacceptable frequency of complications might be expected.

3. Through consultation with a medical physicist and a dosimetrist, the physician selects a treatment beam and energy to be used. In some circumstances, the choice of beam energy may be guided by the location of the target organ.[2] The choice of electron beam energy generally is dictated by the maximum depth of the target tissue.

In more complicated cases, the beam modality and energy are chosen by comparing alternate treatment plans generated as described in Step 4.

    4. Finally, a treatment plan is generated and optimized. The procedure is guided by a number of goals[3]:

- The dose gradient throughout the tumor should be minimal.
- The tumor dose should be significantly greater than the dose anywhere else in the irradiated volume.
- The *integral dose* (see Chapter 8) should be kept as low as possible.
- The shape of the high-dose volume should conform to the planning target volume (PTV).
- The dose to sensitive normal structures (organs at risk) should be kept below levels that have a significant probability of causing damage.
- The dose distribution should consider regions of possible tumor extension or lymphatic spread (these should be included in the PTV).

Early treatment-planning computers simply reproduced manual methods already in use. As more powerful computers have become available, increasingly complex techniques have become practical. For example, Monte Carlo simulations are now used for benchmarking treatment-planning software, as well as for calculating certain beam characteristics employed in some commercial software.

    During the 1980s and early 1990s, a transition occurred from two-dimensional planning to systems that began to encompass the three-dimensional nature of the patient and certain aspects of treatment planning. The term *three-dimensional treatment planning* is used to describe two somewhat different aspects of this transition. Some systems permit the entry of image data, such as from a CT scanner, that is then manipulated and displayed in other orientations to demonstrate the three-dimensional nature of the patient's anatomy. Other systems perform a true three-dimensional calculation of the absorbed radiation dose. This is accomplished by considering radiation interactions and the scattering of radiation throughout the patient volume, including the effects of heterogeneities on both primary and scattered radiation. Some treatment planning systems provide one of these capabilities but not the other, while other systems provide both. Although considerably more complex and demanding of computer resources, three-dimensional treatment planning is both cost-effective and practical in modern radiation oncology departments.[5]

    The increased capabilities of modern computer systems have improved the quality and accuracy of treatment planning calculations. With this increased accuracy has come increased confidence in the ability to deliver curative radiation doses to target organs while sparing sensitive normal structures. Techniques of shaping radiation dose distributions geometrically to the target volume are referred to as *conformal therapy*[6] (see Chapter 16). The increased use of conformal therapy permits the delivery of higher doses to the target volume while maintaining acceptable doses to adjacent normal tissues. This capability improves the probability of tumor control without a corresponding increase in treatment complications.[5]

▥ BEAM DATA ENTRY

All treatment planning systems require the entry of data that describe the radiation beam. The amount of data required depends on the computational algorithm, varying from almost none to thousands of measurements that completely map the radiation beam for a variety of field sizes. Systems that require the entry of almost no measured beam data rely upon a detailed description of the design of the accelerator head, collimator, and accessories. Dependence of a system on a large amount of measured data is thought by some to be a disadvantage, because substantial effort is required to accumulate the large amount of data. The accuracy of any treatment planning system is ultimately determined by comparison with measured data. Complete validation of a treatment planning system requires comparison between calculations and

The treatment planning process:

- Identify target volume.
- Identify organs at risk.
- Select treatment beam and energy.
- Generate optimal treatment plan.

From the beginning, a fundamental rule of radiation therapy has been "Immature cells and cells in an active stage of division are more sensitive to radiation than are cells which have already acquired their adult morphological and physiologic character." This rule is known as the Law of Bergonie and Tribondeau (Bergonie, J., and Tribondeau, L., Interpretation of some results of radiotherapy. *Compt. Rend. Acad. Sci.* **143**:983–985, 1906).

Monte Carlo simulation is a computational technique in which statistical methods are used to simulate a large number of radiation interactions.[4]

Three-dimensional treatment planning allows physicians to impose x-ray beams directly on the image, replacing previous methods of looking at a transverse image and manually transferring image information to planar x-ray films obtained by simulation. This advance has increased accuracy in treatment field design while saving physicians significant time.

The term "conformal radiotherapy" was coined in 1961 by Takahashi of Japan to connote techniques to match the high dose region of treatment to the irregular three-dimensional shape of the treatment volume.

"Conformal avoidance radiotherapy" refers to the technique of designing a radiation field to exclude a three-dimensional organ(s) at risk. This approach is useful for tumors that are not easily defined by a boundary, and with regional treatment areas that surround or are close to critical structures.

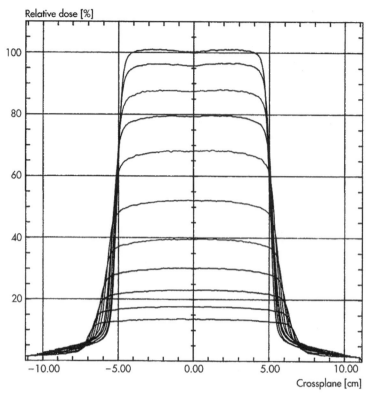

FIGURE 11-1
Graphic representation of several measured beam profiles of the type entered into a treatment planning computer. The illustration shows a number of profiles made along lines perpendicular to the central axis at several depths in a phantom.

Measured data required for treatment planning systems typically include cross-beam profiles, depth dose curves, and relative output factors.

X-ray beam data can be entered into a treatment-planning computer by use of

- A keyboard
- A graphics digitizer tablet
- A direct pathway from the beam-scanning system

Niels Bohr once commented, "Never express yourself more clearly than you think."

measurements over a wide variety of treatment conditions, necessitating a large volume of measured data.[7] Hence, it is unrealistic to expect that the choice of algorithm or commercial treatment planning computer can eliminate or even have significant impact on the amount of measured data that is required.

The entry of beam data is managed by one of three methods. In situations in which a large amount of measured data is not required, it may be practical to enter measured values through a keyboard. Larger amounts of data may be entered more easily by digitizing plots of data with a graphics digitizer tablet. An example of measured beam profiles of the type entered into many treatment planning systems is shown in Figure 11-1.

When very large volumes of measured data are required, it may be more convenient to transfer the data electronically from a beam scanning system directly into the treatment planning computer. This capability is available from a number of manufacturers of treatment planning and beam scanning systems.

■ PATIENT DATA ENTRY

When a treatment plan is to be generated, certain information specific to the individual patient is required. At minimum, for anything other than simple point-dose calculations, a transverse contour of the patient in the plane of the beam central-axis is required. Several methods for obtaining contour information are available, including the simple use of solder wire and plaster bandages. Caution must be exercised when using these methods, because it is easy to distort the wire or plaster when removing it from the patient and transferring the contour information to paper. Several devices have been described for obtaining patient contours.[8–12] One device is shown in Figure 11-2.

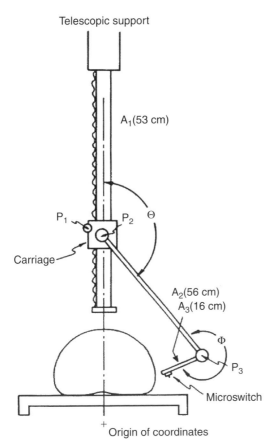

FIGURE 11-2
Device for obtaining the external contour of a patient. (From Doolittle, A. M. Jr., Berman, L. B., Vogel, G., Agostinelli, A. G., Skomro, C., and Schulz, R. J. An electronic patient-contouring device. *Br. J. Radiol.* 1977; **50**:135–138. Used with permission.)

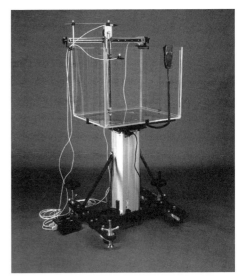

MARGIN FIGURE 11-2
Representative beam scanning system. The system consists of a water tank, computer-controlled positioning system, and radiation detectors. The software driving the computer also displays measurement results and can analyze data with a variety of protocols. Data can often be saved in a format for direct input into the treatment planning system.

In most cases, the use of only a single external contour of the patient provides insufficient information for treatment planning. Although such a contour enables the calculation of percent depth doses and permits corrections for oblique entry of the beam, it does not demonstrate the relationship between the dose distribution and the patient's anatomy. Without additional information, the superposition of calculated doses over the target volume and other anatomical structures cannot be determined accurately. Corrections for inhomogeneous tissues cannot be made unless the location and composition of such tissues are known. To resolve these difficulties, alternative systems for obtaining patient anatomical information have been investigated. Primary among these systems is the use of CT images.[13] CT images are attractive for treatment planning because they clearly demonstrate the anatomy in the patient's transverse plane. An image plane can be chosen that is coincident with the plane of rotation of the gantry of a treatment unit.

The use of CT images for radiation therapy treatment planning has become widely accepted, and for some types of treatment it is considered the standard of care. An example of a CT image obtained for treatment planning is shown in Figure 11-3.

Several important issues must be considered when using CT images for treatment planning. For diagnostic imaging, patients are generally positioned on a curved table top, quite unlike the flat treatment couches used in radiation therapy. The choice of couch shape can significantly alter not only the quality of the image, but also the relationship of external landmarks to internal anatomy[14] (Figure 11-3). Patient motion during imaging must be avoided, because it can cause artifacts and reduce image quality. Consequently, it is advisable to instruct the patient to create an intermediate physiologic condition, for example, by taking a shallow breath prior to the scan.

With the widespread availability of images from computed tomography and magnetic resonance imaging that can be read directly into the treatment planning system, the use of manually defined external patient contours is becoming less common.

For increased reproducibility of patient setup for radiation therapy, a flat table top is often used.

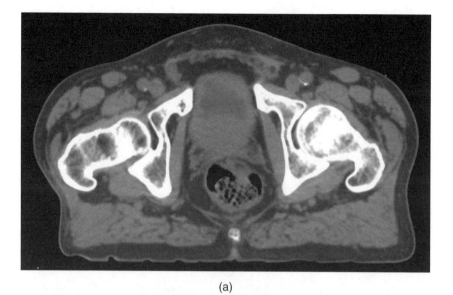

(a)

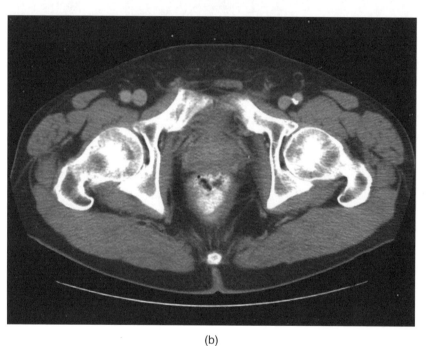

(b)

FIGURE 11-3
Comparison of patient CT images taken with (**A**) a flat table top and (**B**) a curved table top. (From Hobday, P., Hodson, N. J., Husband, J., Parker, R. P., and Macdonald, J. S. Computed tomography applied to radiotherapy treatment planning: Techniques and results. *Radiology* 1979; **133**:477–482. Used with permission.)

Homogeneous dose calculations assume that all tissues within patients have a uniform density equal to that of water. Heterogeneous dose calculations utilize tissue densities determined by a CT scan. While it may be argued that including heterogeneities yields more accurate dose distributions, much of the historical data for determining effectiveness in radiation oncology are based on homogeneous dose calculations.

Computed tomography also provides information about the physical density of anatomical tissues. Computed tomographic images are composed of varying shades of gray, where the brightness of each pixel is related to the linear attenuation coefficient of the x rays used for imaging. However, the interaction of photons in a radiation therapy beam is not governed by the attenuation coefficients obtained at diagnostic x-ray energies. Instead, because the most common interaction is Compton scattering, the frequency of photon interaction is dependent on the electron density (electrons per cubic centimeter) of the medium. Therefore, the relationship between CT number and relative electron density must be determined for each CT scanner, and this relationship

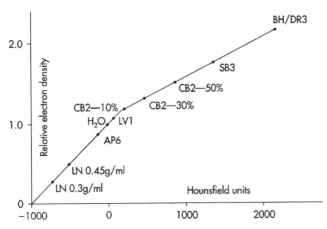

FIGURE 11-4

Relationship between CT number and electron density. The relationship is not necessarily a smooth function, and it may be different from one CT scanner to another. (From Constantinou, C., Harrington, J. C., and DeWerd, L. A. An electron density calibration phantom for CT-based treatment planning computers. *Med. Phys.* 1992; **19**:325–327. Used with permission.)

must be used to convert CT images into images of relative electron density.[15] Many treatment planning systems include software to perform this translation. Once images of relative electron density are prepared, the computer can perform a *heterogeneity correction* with one of the methods outlined later in this chapter.

The use of attenuation coefficients determined at diagnostic energies can lead to inaccurate corrections for heterogeneities. A representative graph of CT number versus electron density is shown in Figure 11-4. Not all treatment planning systems are capable of using patient density information in a pixel-by-pixel format. In these cases, it is necessary to outline individual organs and assign an average (or "bulk") relative electron density to the entire organ.

Magnetic resonance (MR) images are also used for treatment planning, but caution must be exercised in using them. MR images are subject to various artifacts, some of which may cause distortions in patient anatomy.[16] In addition, the brightness of an MR image (pixel value) is not related to tissue density but, instead, to one or more MR variables such as the proton density, as well as to the relaxation constants T1 or T2. The relationship between tissue density and pixel value is much more complex in MR than it is in CT imaging. On the other hand, MR images portray soft tissue differences much better than do CT images, and they are often considered preferable for locating tumors within tissues. Positron emission tomography (PET) imaging also is being used increasingly in treatment planning. Some investigators have described ways to correlate MR images and PET scans with CT images.[17]

A large amount of treatment planning information is obtained from images produced by a radiation therapy simulator. These images rarely show a tumor target volume directly, although its location can be inferred from the position of other anatomical landmarks such as bony structures. The simulator shows the relationship of the proposed treatment field to these landmarks. Several efforts have been made to combine the planar imaging capability of a simulator with the cross-sectional imaging capability of a CT scanner. In such devices, the gantry of the simulator is rotated around the patient, while the x-ray tube is operated continuously. The fluoroscopic image intensifier—or, alternatively, a separate set of detectors—monitors the transmission of radiation through the patient as the gantry is rotated. From these transmission measurements, a "fan-beam CT" image is generated. While the quality of images produced in this fashion does not compete with conventional CT scanners, some argue that the quality is adequate for radiation therapy treatment planning.[18] In all other aspects, the images may be used exactly as those obtained with a conventional CT scanner.

Otto Stern (1888–1969), with his colleague Walter Gerlach, attempted to discern the magnetic properties of silver atoms by observing where they struck a glass plate after passing through a region with a magnetic field that was turned on and off. No displacement could be seen on the glass plate at first, but a displacement gradually became visible as the silver turned to black silver sulfide in reaction with sulfur on Stern's breath resulting from his indulgence in cheap cigars. This experiment, known as the Stern–Gerlach experiment, was pivotal to the development of nuclear magnetic resonance and magnetic resonance imaging. (From Otto Frisch. *What Little I Remember.* New York, Cambridge University Press, 1979).

Because of their ability to distinguish soft tissue contrast, magnetic resonance images are commonly used in radiation therapy to define treatment targets as well as critical structures. Examples include pre-surgical definition of brain tumors to show regions of tumor and edema, display of the prostate/rectal interface in patients treated for prostate cancer, and depiction of metastatic lesions particularly of the spine and brain.

Functional images from PET scans and anatomical information from CT scans complement each other. This complementarity has led to development of an imaging system that combines both modalities. The PET/CT unit has a single patient couch with PET and CT scanners enclosed in the housing. A PET/CT unit is able to fuse the information from the two imaging techniques to provide valuable information on the anatomic location of metabolic activity.

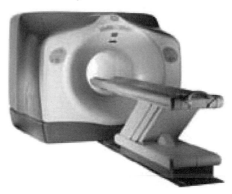

MARGIN FIGURE 11-3

PET/CT unit, the General Electric Discovery LS.

The "simulator" is a device that mimics the geometry of the treatment unit. It is used to position the patient for treatment and to determine the location of the central beam axis (isocenter). Generally, the patient is positioned under fluoroscopic guidance, and planar x-ray films are taken to define the treatment field.

To obtain the resolution typical of a conventional simulation x-ray film, virtual simulation studies may require images every few millimeters. Also, to provide sufficient patient anatomy superior and inferior to the target, the length of the patient scanned may extend well above and below the target. A 30-cm length scanned in 2-mm increments yields 150 CT images that must be fed into the planning computer.

■ VIRTUAL SIMULATION TECHNIQUES

In the preceding paragraph, it was shown how a radiation therapy simulator can be used to create computed tomographic images. In the process of *virtual simulation*, a conventional CT scanner is used to (a) produce images comparable to those generated by a radiation therapy simulator and (b) to duplicate the patient-alignment functions of a simulator.[19–22] Virtual simulation consists of first obtaining many (often 100 or more) parallel transverse CT images. The images must be thin (i.e., small slice thickness) and contiguous for best results. In the computer workstation, the image information is reformatted and reconstructed to yield three-dimensional representations of the patient.

A full set of parallel CT images contains an enormous amount of data, the presentation of which can be complicated and confusing. To address this difficulty, different methods of displaying three-dimensional information have been developed.[23] They include the use of selective *volume rendering* techniques,[24–26] in which only tissues corresponding to a selected range of densities are displayed, and the use of semitransparent structures so that other structures can be seen through them (see Figure 11-5).

To enable the visualization of patient anatomy with respect to the proposed treatment beam, a technique known as *beam's eye view* (BEV) has been developed. In this approach, patient anatomy is displayed as if it were being viewed from the source of radiation. The central axis of the beam appears as a dot in the center of the image, and the edges of the field are shown as a rectangle at the location of the isocenter of the treatment unit. Through the use of real-time three-dimensional

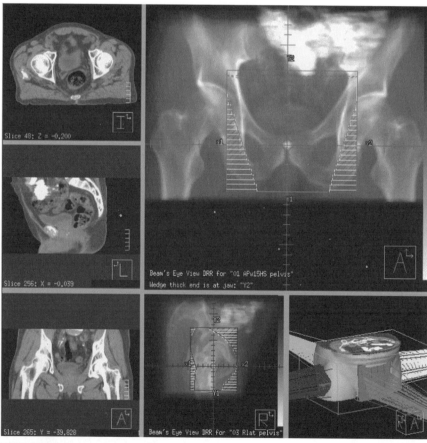

FIGURE 11-5
Reconstruction of CT images can present patient information in a variety of ways.
Counterclockwise from top left: Transverse, sagittal, coronal, lateral DRR, 3D reconstruction, and anterior DRR.

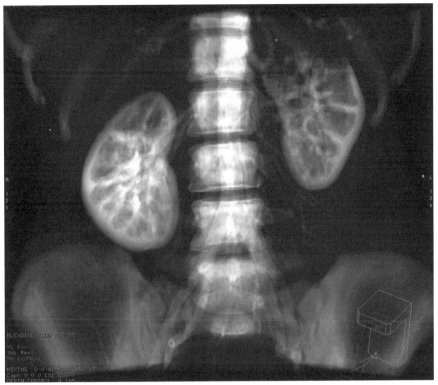

FIGURE 11-6
Digitally reconstructed radiograph. Features available with many systems allow visualization of soft tissue structures as well as bony anatomy without the use of contrast. Thin slices provide detail similar to that of conventional simulation films.

display techniques, patient anatomy can be rotated and translated to simulate gantry rotation and couch motion, and the rectangle representing the radiation beam can be rotated to simulate collimator rotation. Finally, beam-shaping blocks, or the leaves of a multileaf collimator, can be drawn in some systems to indicate the shape of a customized field.

As a final step in the virtual simulation procedure, a *digitally reconstructed radiograph* (DRR) can be generated (Figure 11-6).[27,28] A DRR is a map of average attenuation coefficients computed along each of a large number of rays drawn from the source of radiation to the location of a "virtual film." The result is an image comparable to a simulator film, and many systems include additional features to enhance the DRR image. The CT images contain soft tissue and bony information in a matrix format, and the computer can reconstruct this information in ways to provide the physician with valuable information. For example, structures such as the kidneys can be visualized without injecting a contrast agent into the patient (Figure 11-6).

Many systems also permit multi-modality image fusion, such as superimposing magnetic resonance images (MRIs) on CT images. In this way the physician can use the increased tissue contrast provided by MRI to aid in design of the treatment fields. Image fusion, once tedious and time-consuming, is increasingly an automated process utilizing techniques such as *mutual information*. The physician or physicist can then fine tune the fusion based on experience.

The "beams-eye view" replaces the conventional simulation image. By moving the CT data set relative to the beam and updating the beams-eye view in real time, "virtual fluoroscopy" is performed that allows the physician to accurately position the isocenter in the virtual patient.

The Russian emigrant physicist George Gamow said of Niels Bohr, "Probably Bohr's most characteristic property was the slowness of his thinking and comprehension."

Although CT and MRI images may display pixel values using different lookup tables, the similarities in anatomy are characterized as mutual information. The process of correlating and aligning the anatomy yields an accurate image fusion.

■ IMMOBILIZATION AND LOCALIZATION

Inclusion of a laser alignment system may make it possible to substitute a CT scanner-based virtual simulator (Figure 11-7) for a conventional radiation therapy simulator.[15] In fact, many centers have abandoned their conventional simulator and are using the

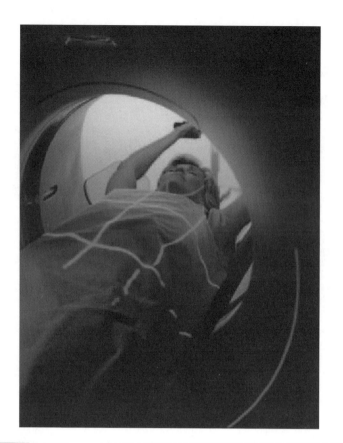

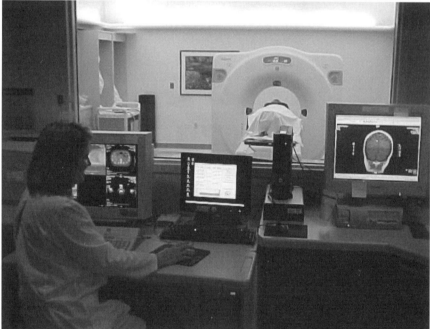

FIGURE 11-7
CT simulation, showing patient setup to fit easily through the bore of the scanner, and lasers used to mark setup points. The console area has the CT control console, laser positioning system, and PACs viewing workstation.

space to house a virtual simulator. When making such a transition, a few issues must be considered:

1. Differences in Geometry Between the Virtual Simulator and the Treatment Machine. The principal limitation here is the physical bore size of the CT scanner, on the order of 70 cm, compared with the relatively unobstructed treatment setup on the linear accelerator. This is particularly a problem for breast treatments where the arm is raised above the patient's head and may not be very mobile after surgery. For large patients, the field of view of the scanner may not be great enough to provide the patient's external contour. Larger-bore scanners exist to solve these problems (e.g., 85 cm), but budget constraints for many departments limit their availability, particularly if the scanner is shared with the radiology department.

2. Inability of the Couch to Move Laterally, and Vertical Limits of Couch Movement. Most scanners have an internal laser system, but it often does not perform at the exacting levels required for radiation therapy because the lasers are mounted on the moving gantry. Fixed wall lasers have to be shifted out of the "isocenter" of the CT scanner, since that point is within the bore of the scanner. In addition, the bore limits couch movement compared with conventional simulation, with no lateral movement or rotation and limited vertical movement. To solve these problems, movable lasers are available which are shifted a known distance out of the bore. These lasers can be programmed directly from the virtual simulation software to indicate isocenter position.

3. Philosophy of Technique. There are two schools of thought with regard to virtual simulation. The first is to use the simulator to create a three-dimensional model of the patient, with the actual simulation performed as a post-processing procedure that does not require the patient to stay on the table. In this way, the time of the simulation (and one of the patient's first experiences in treatment) is kept to a minimum. This approach requires the patient to be marked with reference points prior to leaving, and any shift in the actual treatment isocenter must take place at a later time. The second school of thought is to follow the traditional simulation technique, which requires the patient to be present until the simulation is complete. In this case, the isocenter can be marked directly on the patient, avoiding any future shift. With the additional contouring on the CT images, however, this process can often take much longer than a traditional simulation, thereby causing discomfort to the patient. Some centers accept a compromise where the physician sets the isocenter, but all contouring and beam placement take place after the patient has left.

Defining the target and other structures precisely on the CT images with the patient in treatment position allows the beam portals to be precisely aligned. This provides many options such as reduced margins and dose escalation to increase the patient's chance of cure. Consistency is critical in patient setup between time of virtual simulation and treatment, as well as in localization of the target. Immobilization and localization devices to achieve this goal come in two principal varieties: (a) external fixation and localization devices and (b) internal image-based localization.

Common external fixation and localization devices include molds and masks shaped to the patient's external surface to provide a reproducible setup from treatment to treatment (Figure 11-8). Fine tolerances on couch position for these systems can be achieved by using devices that are locked to the treatment couch in positions to match the virtual simulation. Video subtraction of the patient's external surface may be used to position the patient (Figure 11-9). In this case, room cameras compare the difference image at the time of treatment to a reference image.

A similar concept is to use a camera system with external fiducials such as small reflective balls to position the patient. If the balls are referenced to a fixed part of patient anatomy (e.g., the hard palette by mounting them on a custom dental bite block), setup accuracy required for stereotactic radiotherapy can be achieved. The fiducials monitor patient position during treatment to ensure that the patient does not move.

Patient motion during treatment, particularly respiratory motion, is an area of great concern. For example, a lung tumor exhibits a complex cyclic motion, requiring

Werner Heisenberg (1901–1976), developer of matrix mechanics and the Uncertainty Principle, led the German project to develop an atomic bomb during World War II. In 1944 the professional baseball player Moe Berg, who knew some physics, was sent by the US OSS (forerunner of the US CIA) to attend a lecture by Heisenberg in Zurich. He was to determine from Heisenberg's lecture whether the German project was progressing. If progress was being made, Berg was to assassinate Heisenberg with a pistol he had smuggled into the lecture. Heisenberg did not mention the German atomic bomb project, and Berg did not draw his pistol.

When transferring from conventional to virtual simulation, three principal issues are:

1. Differences in geometry between the treatment unit and CT scanner gantries, particularly CT bore size limitations.
2. Limitations in CT couch movement in positioning the patient.
3. Philosophy of technique; whether to create a three-dimensional model of the patient and perform the simulation with the patient absent, or to adhere to the conventional simulation process and keep the patient on the table.

Two key concepts in creating reproducible patient setups are immobilization and localization. Immobilization devices are created at the time of simulation to position the patient and restrict motion. Localization techniques are typically applied at the time of treatment, and they use information obtained at the time of simulation to accurately position the isocenter.

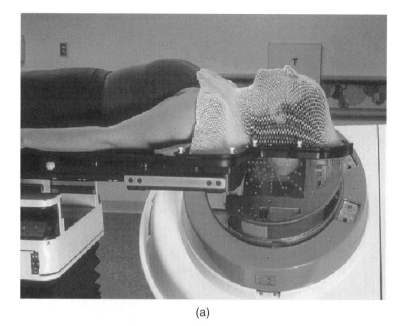

(a)

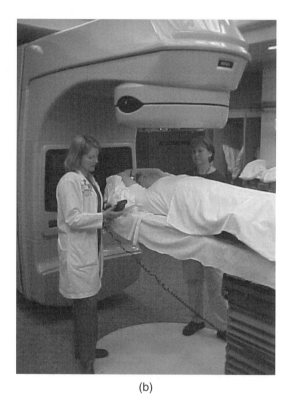

(b)

FIGURE 11-8
A: Immobilization of patient for head and neck treatment. This system incorporates shoulder immobilization and extends off the end of the treatment couch. **B:** Immobilization for breast treatment with both arms extended above the patients head and use of a custom molded device for repositioning.

expanded margins to account for movement during treatment. The technique of respiratory gating addresses this issue, whereby the patient's breathing cycle is characterized at the time of simulation.[29–31] As the patient breathes, the motion is tracked using external fiducials and displayed graphically. Acceptable limits for treatment are determined by the clinical staff and used to control when the treatment beam will

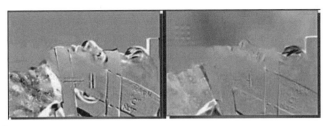

FIGURE 11-9
Video subtraction technique. The image on the left shows slight misalignment that has been corrected in the image on the right.

be on, as shown in Figure 11-10. With this technique in place, the clinician is better able to localize the moving target during treatment and thus reduce margins. It also reduces the effect of organ motion on complex treatment fields such as IMRT (discussed later in this chapter).

Internal or image-based localization is used to reduce setup error between treatments, based on image information available at the time of treatment. Ultrasound

External fiducials commonly employ markers such as reflective balls, with a camera system used to monitor their position. This information can be used to position the patient and accurately localize the target. In addition, the fiducial locations can be used to trigger the beam on and off in response to patient motion such as breathing.

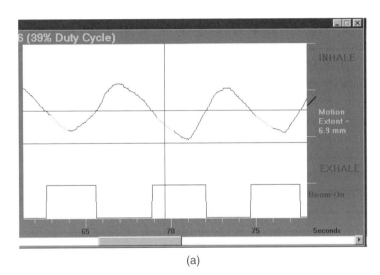

(a)

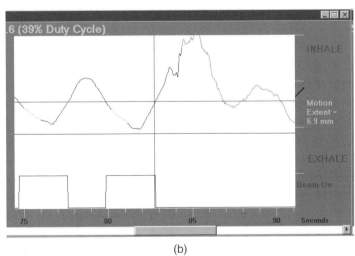

(b)

FIGURE 11-10
Respiratory gating. Breathing cycle (top curve in each figure) has thresholds set to control when the beam is turned on and off (bottom curve). **A:** Normal breathing. **B:** Patient coughs or moves causing the beam to turn off until normal breathing resumes.

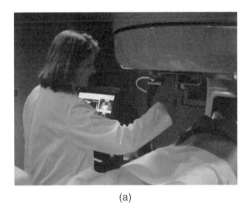

(a)

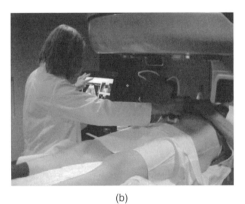

(b)

MARGIN FIGURE 11-4
Ultrasound imaging at the time of treatment can be used to localize the prostate and other tissues that are subject to movement between treatments. **A:** The scanner is referenced to the treatment unit by placing the probe in a rigid mount attached to the head of the linac. **B:** Ultrasound images of the prostate are compared with the expected position derived from the planning system in order to align the patient for treatment.

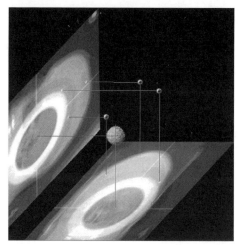

MARGIN FIGURE 11-5

X-ray localization utilizing implanted fiducials. Two orthogonal films are taken, and the gold fiducials (three small spheres) are digitized from each image. By triangulation and with known positions of the markers relative to the target (larger sphere), the target can be accurately positioned for treatment.

Photon beam computational methods may be classified as

- Analytical
- Matrix
- Semiempirical
- Three-dimensional integration

The increased speed of modern computers has largely eliminated limitations of slower algorithms, and is making highly computer-intensive processes like Monte Carlo a reality in treatment planning.

The analytical method:

- uses one equation for depth dose and one for the cross-beam profile
- computes the dose at a point by multiplying these two equations.

images of the prostate and x-ray images of bony anatomy are common methods currently in practice.[32–37] To be effective, these methods must be quick and provide information to accurately position the patient (e.g., couch shifts). Real-time systems provide rapid feedback and include ultrasound, x-ray fluoroscopy, and electronic portal imaging detectors (EPID). Internal fiducials are also commonly used, either (a) implanted in the skull for stereotactic radiosurgery and radiotherapy or (b) implanted in the target itself (e.g., prostate). Axial imaging techniques at the time of treatment are also used to provide a cross-sectional view of the patient (see the section on Tomotherapy).

Quite often, the patient setup for virtual simulation and subsequent treatment involves a combination of external and image-based localization. The external positioning device provides a reproducible setup, and the image based localization system accurately positions the target. The data provided by the virtual simulation process are transferred to the treatment planning computer for dose computation, usually via the hospital network using a Dicom protocol.

PHOTON BEAM COMPUTATIONAL ALGORITHMS

The ICRU has divided photon beam calculation methods into four classifications.[38] Listed in approximate chronological order of their development, they are the *analytical* method, the *matrix* method, the *semiempirical* method, and the *three-dimensional integration* method.

The analytical and matrix methods were developed when computers in radiation therapy were not very powerful. These methods permit computation of the dose distribution in a single plane in a reasonable amount of time, and development of multiple alternative plans is possible. As more complex and accurate computational algorithms became available, they were implemented on available computer hardware. The calculation times increased, and it was common for computers to be provided with both a rapid but less accurate algorithm and a slow but more accurate algorithm. The slower algorithm could be reserved for generation of a final treatment plan only after an acceptable beam arrangement had been determined using the faster technique. As computer speeds have increased and advances have been made in treatment planning programs, this limitation has been largely eliminated, allowing both fast and accurate dose calculation.

THE ANALYTICAL METHOD

One of the earliest analytical techniques for radiation therapy treatment planning was developed in the 1960s by Sterling et al.[39] The method is based on two equations: One equation models the central axis percent depth dose, and the other models the beam profile as a function of depth and off-axis distance. The dose at any point in the irradiated volume is the product of the result of these two calculations. The analytical method has been extended and improved, and a current implementation considers the effects of field blocking and wedge attenuation.[40]

MATRIX TECHNIQUES

In the early 1970s, several treatment planning computer systems were developed to perform calculations based on measurements of large amounts of beam data. These measurements were stored in matrix form and aligned with rays diverging from the radiation source. A diverging matrix is illustrated in Figure 11-11.[41] The matrix itself is formed by first drawing diverging *fan lines* that radiate from the source. In a water phantom, these fan lines intersect *depth lines* located at selected depths below the surface and drawn perpendicular to the central axis. Measurements are made along

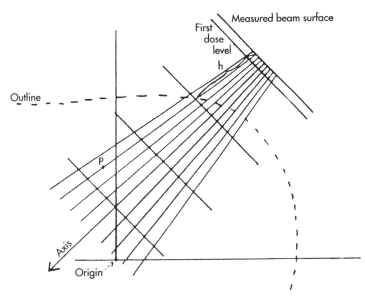

FIGURE 11-11

A fan-line/depth-line diverging array for representing measurements of beam characteristics. The beam array is shown superimposed upon a patient contour. (From Milan, J., and Bentley, R. E. The storage and manipulation of radiation dose data in a small digital computer. *Br. J. Radiol.* 1974; **47**:115–121. Used with permission.)

the central axis and at intersections between the depth lines and fan lines. The data are stored in two tables: a table of percent depth dose values and a table of off-axis ratios. The off-axis ratios are normalized to the central axis value along each depth line. Both tables are compiled for representative field sizes spanning the clinical range of interest.

A treatment plan is generated by retrieving, for each beam in the treatment plan, the appropriate central axis depth dose table and appropriate set of beam profiles. The beam profiles are taken from the table that corresponds to the width of the beam being planned (the dimension of the field shown on the plane of the treatment plan; see Figure 11-11). The central axis depth dose table is taken from the field size corresponding to the equivalent square of the treatment field. In both cases, interpolation may be used when the field dimensions fall between dimensions for which data have been compiled.

This computational technique has the advantage of speed, because data can be retrieved quickly from a mass storage device (hard disk) for each beam in the treatment plan. The method has the perceived disadvantage that a large amount of measured data must be stored before treatment planning can be performed. As mentioned earlier, however, the data required for treatment planning are generally no more than that required for the normal commissioning of a treatment unit.

◼ SEMIEMPIRICAL METHODS

Clarkson Method

It has long been recognized that the dose at a point in a patient is the sum of the dose from two contributions: primary radiation and scattered radiation. In the mid-1970s, efforts were directed to modeling the primary and scattered radiation independently to provide more accurate estimates of the dose at a point resulting from changes in field characteristics at a distance from the point. Probably the most well known of these methods is the *Clarkson scatter integration* technique.[42] The technique is described in detail in Chapter 8.[43] A computer implementation of the Clarkson scatter integration technique incorporates several improvements over the manual calculation method.

Dmitri Mendeleyev (1834–1907) constructed the periodic table of the elements after a dream in which all of the elements fell into place. Years later he gave the Faraday Lecture of the Chemical Society of Great Britain in the Royal Institute of London. The honorarium for the lecture was provided in a silk purse in the Russian national colors. Mendeleyev kept the purse but emptied the gold sovereigns on a table, declaring that nothing would induce him to accept money from a society that had paid him the high compliment of inviting him to do honor to the memory of Michael Faraday in a place made sacred by his labors. (Obituary of Dmitri Mendeleyev by Sir Edward Thorpe from W. Gratzer, *Eurekas and Euphoria,* New York, Oxford University Press, 2002.

Matrix techniques:

- use two-dimensional tables for various field sizes to determine the dose from a beam
- generate beam profiles from (a) the width of the beam on a CT image and (b) depth dose from the equivalent square field size
- are very fast in displaying the dose on a given axial image.

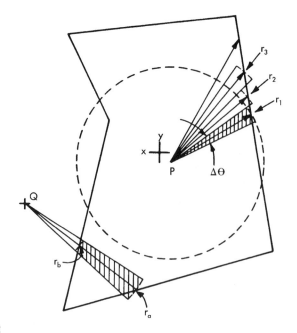

FIGURE 11-12

The Clarkson scatter integration procedure. When implemented by computer, the field is generally divided into sectors that span no more than 10°. (From Cunningham, J. R. Keynote address: Development of computer algorithms for radiation treatment planning. *Int. J. Radiat. Oncol. Biol. Phys.* 1989; **16**:1367–1376. Used with permission.)

Shown in Equation (8-3) is the expression for calculating the dose in an irregularly shaped field using the Clarkson scatter integration technique.

$$D_T = D_C \cdot S_C \cdot F \cdot \frac{1}{TAR_C} \cdot \left(\frac{SCD}{SSD + g + d} \right)^2 (P \cdot TAR_{0.d} + SAR_{\text{avg}}) \quad \textbf{(8-3)}$$

The scatter integration is performed by the computer in exactly the same fashion as if it were performed manually (refer to Chapter 8), although the field may be divided into more sectors than might be used for manual calculations (Figure 11-12).

The *primary off-axis factor, P,* can be calculated with a model that considers the primary radiation to be affected by three components: penumbra, block or collimator transmission, and flattening filter effects.

The *penumbra correction* models the variation in primary dose rate in the penumbra region created by the shadow of the collimator jaws and by field blocking. In some implementations of the algorithm, the penumbra correction is based on the *Wilkinson extended source model* shown in Figure 11-13.[44] This model originally described a ^{60}Co source as a broadened distribution of activity. The source activity was depicted as being greatest on the axis of the source, and decreased at distances away from the axis. The presence of scattered radiation high in the collimator caused the effective source to appear wider ("extended") than the actual source. The model has been applied to accelerators to describe the apparent source of radiation. A simple exponential expression is used, assuming radial symmetry:

$$l_r = \frac{\beta^2}{2\pi} \cdot e^{-\beta r}$$

where r is the distance from the center of the source, and $\beta^2/2\pi$ is required for normalization. β is calculated as follows:

$$\beta = \frac{\alpha}{PEN}$$

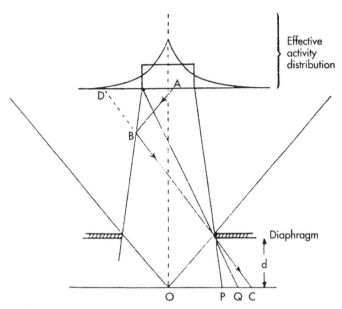

FIGURE 11-13
The geometry for the Wilkinson extended source model. Radiation reaching points at locations represented by P, Q, and C may appear to come from different parts of an "extended" source. (From Wilkinson, J. M., Rawlinson, J. A., and Cunningham, J. R. *An extended source model for the calculation of the primary component of a cobalt-60-radiation beam in penumbral regions.* Presented at American Association of Physicists in Medicine Workshop, Chicago, II, 1970. Used with permission.)

where

$$PEN = SD \frac{(SSD + d - SDD)}{SDD}$$

Therefore

$$\beta = \frac{\alpha \cdot SSD}{SD(SSD + d - SDD)}$$

where SD is the source diameter, d is the depth below the surface at the point of calculation, SSD is the source-to-surface distance, and SDD is the source-to-diaphragm distance, or the distance from the source to the final field-defining aperture. PEN therefore is the width of the geometric penumbra at the depth of interest. The penumbra correction is calculated by integrating the function over the area of the extended source as observed from the calculation point. In practice, the integration is performed analytically, in a manner similar to the summation of the scatter function. The presence of blocking is taken into account by computing β from a unique value of α entered for each block:

$$W = \sum_i \frac{\delta}{2\pi} \left[1 - (1 + \beta r_i) e^{-\beta r_i} \right]$$

The block or collimator transmission factor is included in the primary off-axis factor, to yield a more accurate estimate of the dose under the blocks or collimator. The transmission term is equal to the block transmission factor at calculation points that fall under the block. The expression reflects the penumbra that exists below the block edges; it falls to zero outside blocked regions.

$$Bl = \left(\frac{tran}{2} \right) \left\{ 1 - G \left[1 - (1 + \beta r) e^{-\beta r} \right] \right\}$$

where $G = \pm 1$ to indicate that the point is inside or outside the block, and *r is the*

James Chadwick, discoverer of the neutron, was interned for 5 years in a German prison camp during World War I. During this time he investigated radioactivity by studying a thorium-containing toothpaste marketed by the Auer Company. The toothpaste also contained a substance that fluoresced as the α particles from thorium were absorbed. The toothpaste was advertised as providing an "iridescent smile." (W. Gratzer, *Eurekas and Euphorias,* New York, Oxford University Press, 2002.

distance from the point to the nearest block edge. β has the same form as before, but α and *tran* may be defined uniquely for each block.

A *flattening filter correction* is employed when calculations are performed for linear accelerators. The original implementation of the Clarkson scatter integration technique was developed for cobalt units, for which the primary dose rate was quite constant from the central axis to a point near the edge of the field, where it began to decrease. In an accelerator x-ray beam, the primary dose rate may actually increase at distances away from the central axis, an effect manifested as "horns" in the isodose distributions from many linear accelerators. A flattening filter correction is required to model this increase in dose rate away from the central axis. The flattening filter correction *FF* is

$$FF = 1 + Ar + Br^2 + Crd$$

where r and d are as defined above. A, B, and C are determined empirically by the user to correctly model the shape of the dose distribution.

Finally, the *primary off-axis correction factor* is computed by combining these three terms:

$$P = (W + Bl) \cdot FF$$

Differential Scatter–Air Ratio Calculation

A significant shortcoming of the Clarkson scatter summation technique is its assumption that scattered radiation is generated with uniform intensity throughout the field, with the exception of regions shielded by the collimator or blocks. Factors that alter the primary photon fluence at depth, such as the presence of partially transmitting filters (wedges) or nonuniform surface contours, are ignored. The differential scatter–air ratio (dSAR) technique accounts for variations in the amount of scattered radiation at different locations in the patient[45] (Figure 11-14).

The dSAR method can be combined with the conventional Clarkson scatter integration technique, so that the scattered radiation reaching a point of interest from each of the numerous field sectors drawn around the point is integrated along each sector. The resulting dSAR is similar to a point spread function that defines the scattered radiation from a pencil beam of photons.

Heterogeneity Corrections

The three calculation methods described above rely on data measured in homogeneous water phantoms, with the assumption that the patient also is homogeneous. Several techniques have been described for correcting for the presence of heterogeneities. These methods, described in Chapter 8, include the *ratio of tissue–air ratios* method, the *power law tissue–air ratio* method,[46,47] and the *equivalent TAR* method.[48] The computerized implementation of each of these methods of heterogeneity correction is essentially identical to the manual technique. Once the dose at a point has been calculated using either an analytical, matrix, or semiempirical method, a heterogeneity correction is applied to compensate for the presence of inhomogeneous tissue within the field. Both the ratio of TARs method and the power law TAR method are "one-dimensional" techniques, in that they consider only the effect of heterogeneities that fall on a line from the source to the point of calculation. Heterogeneities that lie away from this line are not considered, nor are the lateral extent of heterogeneities. The equivalent TAR technique does consider the effect of heterogeneities that fall away from the line connecting the source and the point of interest. Although this technique does not explicitly account for the dose attributed to secondary electrons, it is inherently three-dimensional. However, most of the existing planning systems that have implemented this algorithm collapse the three-dimensional patient volume into a two-dimensional slice through the isocenter, in order to reduce calculation time. This approach makes the technique essentially a "2 1/2-dimensional" calculation.

For semiempirical methods, the primary radiation is considered to be affected by three components:

1. penumbra
2. block or collimator transmission
3. flattening filter effects

These are combined into the primary off-axis factor, P, used in a Clarkson integration to compute dose.

The *Differential Scatter–Air Ratio Method* allows variations in the amount of scattered radiation to be considered, based on the distance from a reference point and the presence of beam modifiers such as wedges.

Louis de Broglie created the equation linking a particle's momentum to its wavelength while serving during World War I as a meteorological observer stationed in an aerie in the Eiffel tower in Paris.

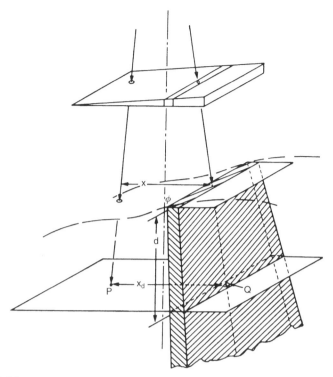

FIGURE 11-14

Diagram depicting differential scatter–air ratios. The crosshatched region represents a volume element of an irradiated phantom. Radiation is scattered from it to points such as P, which is at a distance x from the volume element. (From Cunningham, J. R. Keynote address: Development of computer algorithms for radiation treatment planning. *Int. J. Radiat. Oncol. Biol. Phys.* 1989; **16**:1367–1376. Used with permission.)

Three-Dimensional Integration Methods

Several investigators have developed proposals for three-dimensional calculation of dose distributions. Many of these techniques rely on *Monte Carlo* calculations.[28,49–53] The Monte Carlo technique is described briefly earlier in this chapter. The technique can be used in a limited fashion to develop a description of the distribution of dose following a limited number of photon interactions within a patient. For example, the Monte Carlo method has been used to generate dose distributions for monoenergetic pencil beams of photons that are forced to intersect at the center of a large volume of water.[54,55] This three-dimensional dose distribution represents the transport of photons and electrons away from the primary interaction site. It is commonly referred to as a *dose spread array, point spread function,* or simply a *kernel.* The dose in a treatment volume then is computed by superimposing the dose kernel throughout the three-dimensional irradiated volume, weighted by the total energy released per unit mass at each point. The change in dose distribution near the field boundaries is considered by modeling the change in primary photon fluence at these boundaries. The effects of heterogeneities are included by (a) determining the change in primary photon fluence as a result of passage through the heterogeneity and (b) scaling the dimensions of the dose kernel according to the density of the patient.

A number of investigators have used different Monte Carlo codes to compute dose kernels.[56,49,4,57] One method by which a primary dose spread array is computed using the EGS3 Monte Carlo code is shown in Figure 11-15.[57] The resulting dose spread array in an isodose format is shown in Figure 11-16. In this illustration, only the dose distribution resulting from *first-scattered* radiation from the site of the primary interaction is shown. Because radiation is frequently scattered two or more times, the dose at any point in a patient results not only from primary interactions and from radiation that has been scattered once, but also from radiation that has been scattered two or more times.

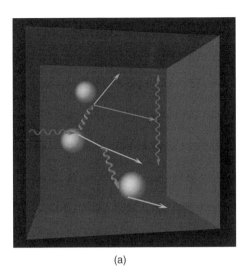

(a)

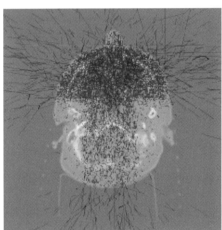

(b)

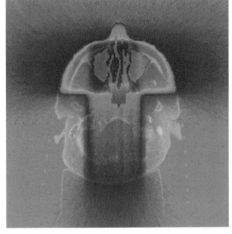

(c)

MARGIN FIGURE 11-6

Monte Carlo example. **A:** Single photon interaction. **B:** 1.7×10^5 particles. **C:** 6.8×10^7 particles. (From Nomos, Peregrine treatment planning system.)

The "dose spread array," "point spread function," or "kernel" refers to a method of characterizing dose deposition in tissue for a particular energy spectrum in the beam.

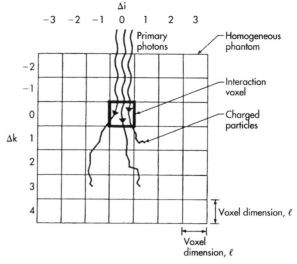

FIGURE 11-15
Schematic representation of the generation of a primary dose spread array. (From Mackie, T. P., Scrimger, J. W., and Battista, J. J. A convolution method of calculating dose for 15-MV x rays. *Med. Phys.* 1985; **12**:188–196. Used with permission.)

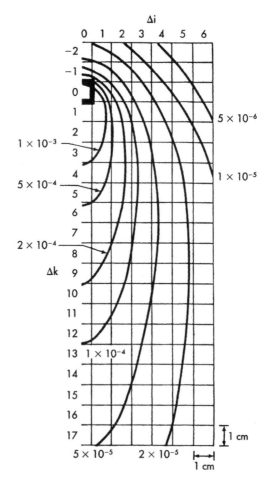

FIGURE 11-16
Truncated first scatter (TFS) dose spread array in isodose format. (From Mackie, T. R., Scrimger, J. W., and Battista, J. J. A convolution method of calculating dose for 15-MV x rays. *Med. Phys.* 1985; **12**:188–196. Used with permission.)

The availability of advanced computer technologies has prompted the development of treatment planning software that uses *convolution* techniques.[4,28,54–58] Typically, a number of kernels computed for different photon energies are summed together according to the spectrum of the clinical photon beam. These kernels are then *convolved* with the spectrum of the primary photon fluence, to compute the dose distribution throughout a three-dimensional volume. These calculations are complex and time-consuming, but as computer power and speed have increased, they have become more practical for clinical treatment planning systems.

ELECTRON BEAM COMPUTATIONAL ALGORITHMS

A number of computational algorithms similar to those used for photon beams have been applied to electron beams. The matrix methods are directly applicable to electron beams, provided that the location of fan lines and depth lines are adjusted to be consistent with the shape of the dose distribution for each electron beam energy. However, matrix techniques do not exactly model the unique ways in which electron beams interact with inhomogeneous tissues. For more accurate modeling, several analytical techniques have been pursued, including the use of the age-diffusion equation.[59,60] The central axis depth dose distribution for electron beams has also been modeled using an equation in the form of the Fermi–Dirac distribution function.[61]

The *pencil beam* method is the calculation technique that has enjoyed the greatest popularity, and that has demonstrated the greatest potential for accurate electron beam dose distribution calculations.[62–65] The technique is analogous to the method described earlier for photon beams. In a high-energy electron beam, however, the spatial distribution of absorbed energy is dictated by multiple scattering of electrons. The dose spread array covers a smaller area, because of the decreased range of electrons. The dose distribution in a broad beam can be generated by superposition of many electron pencil-beam distributions. Extension of the pencil-beam method to three dimensions has been accomplished,[65] and efforts have been made to incorporate heterogeneity corrections.[66–69]

SELECTION OF IDEAL TREATMENT PLAN

Development of the ideal treatment plan requires a process for altering treatment planning parameters (either manually or automatically) to yield a uniform dose throughout the planning target volume (PTV), while keeping the dose low to organs at risk (OAR).[70] For conventional treatment planning, this is conducted by trial and error and is influenced by the combined experience of the planner and the physician. Alternative treatment plans are generated sequentially, and the improvement or deterioration of the plan is noted, until an ideal plan is reached.

To improve the process of optimizing a treatment plan, several computational techniques are available that yield useful statistical information about the plan. *Dose–volume histograms* (DVH) are graphic representations that relate the dose received by the patient and the volume of tissue receiving the dose.[71–73] Figure 11-17 illustrates the procedure for developing a dose–volume histogram. Figure 11-17A shows a simple treatment plan using three fields encompassing a square target volume. Figure 11–17B shows the calculated dose distribution, mapped onto a square array. The dose received at the center is indicated within each square. The doses are indicated in Gy. Figure 11-17C illustrates a "direct" or "differential" DVH. The direct DVH is a histogram of dose bins, and the frequency with which each dose occurs. For example, every array location in Figure 11-17B at which the dose falls between 0 and 0.9 Gy has been summed into a bin identified as "0 Gy"; those at which the dose falls between 1.0 and 1.9 Gy have been summed into a bin identified as "1 Gy," and so on up to

In convolution techniques, dose is determined by integrating the product of the mass attenuation coefficient, the incident energy fluence, and the dose deposition kernel.

$$\frac{D(\vec{r})}{MU} = \frac{\Psi_0}{MU} \int \frac{\mu}{\rho}(\vec{r}') \frac{\Psi(\vec{r}')}{\Psi_0} K(\vec{r} - \vec{r}') \, d^3\vec{r}'$$

The Pauli Exclusion Principle states that no two electrons in an atomic system can possess the same four quantum numbers. Pauli's colleagues liked to quote the "second" Pauli Exclusion Principle. It stated that Pauli should be excluded from any and all physics laboratories, because his presence spelled destruction to any mechanical device or scientific apparatus.

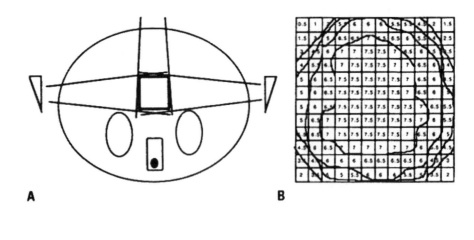

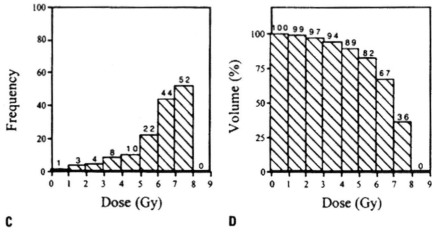

FIGURE 11-17

A: A simple hypothetical three field treatment plan. **B:** The resulting dose matrix for the plan shown in Part A. Dose values are in Gy, and isodose lines are in 1-Gy dose increments. **C:** A direct DVH. **D:** A cumulative DVH for the dose grid shown in part B. The dose bin size is 1 Gy. (From Ten Haken, R. K., Kessler, M. L., Martel, M. K., Lawrence, T. S. Use of dose–volume histograms and tumor control and normal-tissue complication probabilities for clinical planning. *In Syllabus: A categorical course in physics: Three-dimensional radiation therapy treatment planning.* Presented at the 80th Scientific Assembly and Annual Meeting of the RSNA, Oak Brook, II., 1994. Used with permission.)

9 Gy. Only one location recorded a dose between 0 and 0.9 Gy, while 52 locations recorded a dose between 7.0 and 7.9 Gy.

Direct DVHs of the type shown in Figure 11-17C are not often used. Instead, cumulative DVHs are considered more valuable in radiation therapy. A cumulative DVH is determined in a similar fashion as the direct DVH. A representative cumulative DVH is shown in Figure 11-17D. It exhibits two differences from the direct DVH. The vertical axis is labeled as the percent of total tissue volume that receives a dose equal to or greater than a particular dose. The horizontal axis is labeled in units of cumulative dose; in other words, the first bin records the volume of tissue at which the dose is *at least* 0 Gy, for which the value is obviously 100%. The second bin indicates the volume of tissue for which the dose is *at least* 1 Gy. Here, 99% of the volume of irradiated tissue has received at least 1 Gy. Only 36% of the irradiated volume has received a dose of at least 7 Gy, and 0% of the tissue has received a dose greater than 8 Gy.

Cumulative dose–volume histograms may be used to compare competing treatment plans. Figure 11-18 shows the DVHs for normal tissue for two alternative

Niels Bohr said "We shall never understand anything until we have found some contradictions."

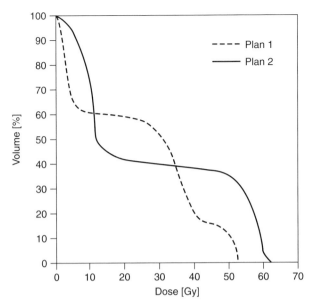

FIGURE 11-18
Cumulative normal tissue DVHs for two competing treatment plans.

treatment plans. Both treatment plans indicate relatively high doses to normal tissues, but the curve labeled "plan 2" clearly demonstrates that larger volumes of tissue receive a higher dose than with "plan 1." Comparison of DVHs can be used to select an optimum plan.[74]

The use of statistical decision theory has been proposed as one approach to selecting an ideal treatment plan.[75] The method involves the development of an objective function based on a statistical model of the biological response to radiation. This objective function is calculated from the dose distribution, and a score is determined. The plan exhibiting the "best" score is presumably the optimum treatment plan. The statistical method has been largely abandoned recently in favor of biological modeling techniques.

■ BIOLOGICAL MODELING

It has long been recognized that the distribution of absorbed dose is not the only criterion that might be used to select a superior treatment plan from several alternatives. Because biological response is probably not a linear function of dose, factors such as variable sensitivities of different tissues, effects of fractionation, and the possible use of biological modifiers must be considered. Some of these factors have been addressed through the development of models for *tumor control probability (TCP)* and *normal tissue complication probability (NTCP)*.[76–80] Representative graphs of TCP and NTCP are shown in Figure 11-19.[81] As of this date, only limited efforts have been made to correlate these biological models with clinical outcome data. However, the product of TCP and (1-NTCP) yields the probability of *uncomplicated tumor control.* A representative graph is shown in Figure 11-20.]

■ FORWARD PLANNING

The concept of *forward planning* (Figure 11-21) involves the modification of beam parameters based on observed isodose distributions or patient geometry.[82] Commonly, forward planning begins by setting up a common beam arrangement for the site being treated. Then the dose is computed, and "hot spots" are detected in the dose

The technique of "biological modeling" in radiation therapy involves maximizing the tumor control probability and minimizing the normal tissue complication probability. Both are sigmoidal functions of dose.

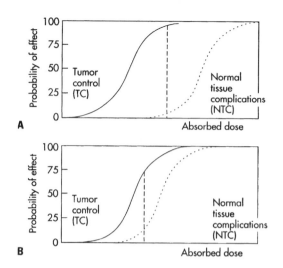

FIGURE 11-19
A schematic showing the tumor control probability and normal tissue complication probability as a function of dose. **A:** A favorable situation in which a high tumor-control probability can result with a small complication probability. **B:** A less favorable situation where a high tumor-control probability would result in a larger complication probability. (From Wambersie, A., Hanks, G., and Van Dam, J. Quality assurance and accuracy required in radiation therapy: Biological and medical considerations. In *Selected Topics in Physics of Radiotherapy and Imaging,* U. Madhvanath, K. S. Parthasarathy, and T. V. Venkateswaran (eds.). New Delhi, McGraw-Hill, 1988. Used with permission.)

Forward planning techniques may be utilized to achieve a more uniform dose to the target volume. It requires an initial calculation of dose with subsequent beams to block various dose levels.

distribution. Next, a set of sub-beams (also known as segments or control points) are generated to block the hot spots. Finally, the weighting of the beams is adjusted to provide a uniform dose across the treated region, either manually or automatically.

Most treatment planning systems can accommodate some form of forward planning. Several advantages are achieved by using a forward planning technique. First, the resulting beams are rather intuitive since they are based on observed dosimetry. Second, there are relatively few control points when compared with intensity modulation techniques. Third, quality assurance can often be accommodated by using the current clinical techniques in use. Finally, this approach can often save time in treatment planning and delivery, by eliminating trial and error approaches such as multiple wedge angles and/or orientations. In the case of breast tangents, for example, the dosimetrist may have to try a number of wedges and wedge orientations to get the best treatment plan. The forward planning technique can use a standard wedge in one field, and the segments on the other field effectively "clean up" the dose distribution. With this approach, the radiation therapists do not have multiple wedges and wedge orientations to contend with during treatment, thereby shortening the overall treatment time.

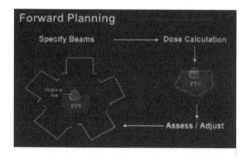

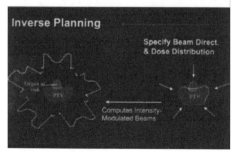

MARGIN FIGURE 11-7
In forward planning, a dose distribution is computed for external beams of specified size, direction, and weighting. In inverse planning, the size, direction, intensity modulation, and weighting of external beams are computed to deliver a predetermined dose distribution.

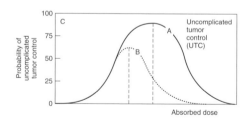

FIGURE 11-20
The "mantelpiece clock" overlap curve of TCP and (l-NTCP). Curves A and B correspond with use of the curves from Figure 11-19. This shows the probability of uncomplicated tumor control (P_{UTC}). (From Wambersie, A., Hanks, G., and Van Dam, J. Quality assurance and accuracy required in radiation therapy: Biological and medical considerations. In *Selected Topics in Physics of Radiotherapy and Imaging,* U. Madhvanath, K. S. Parthasarathy, and T. V. Venkateswaran (eds.). New Delhi, McGraw-Hill, 1988. Used with permission.)

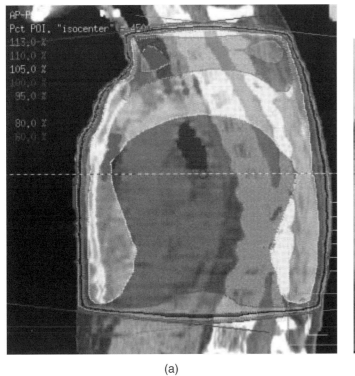

(a)

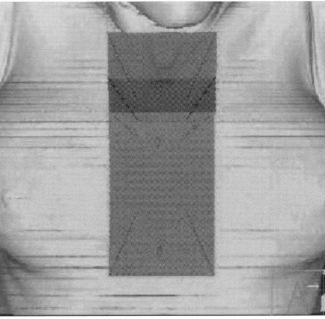

(b)

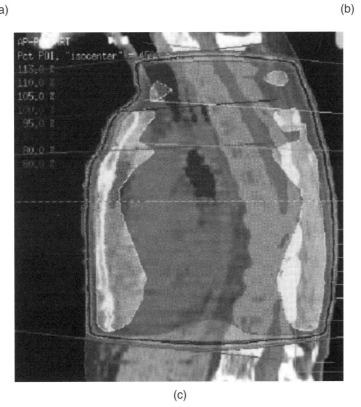

(c)

FIGURE 11-21

Forward planning example for AP/PA treatment of the mediatinum. **A:** Sagittal view of AP/PA treatment plan with open fields and no wedges. **B:** Anterior surface rendering showing the original field and two smaller fields ("subfields" or "segments") with the superior jaw position reduced to block higher dose levels in thinner parts of the patient. **C:** By adjusting the weights of the segments, a uniform dose throughout the entire region is obtained.

■ INVERSE PLANNING

Inverse planning is the name given to a prescribed technique of treatment optimization by automated methods.[83,84] For radiation therapy, it involves development of a treatment plan whereby the planning computer is given a set of objectives and beam parameters to adjust in iterative fashion to arrive at a satisfactory dose distribution. For example, the treatment planning computer could iteratively adjust the weights of the beams to provide the most uniform dose to the target. In this case, the objective is uniform dose to the target, and the adjustable beam parameter is the weight of each beam. Iterative problem-solving techniques in inverse planning, particularly with complex objective functions, is an ideal application for fast treatment planning computers.

■ INTENSITY-MODULATED RADIATION THERAPY

Individual beams can be divided into small beamlets (e.g., 5 mm × 5 mm), and the weight of each beamlet can be adjusted to provide a uniform dose to the target, while at the same time limiting the dose to normal tissues. This technique is known as *intensity-modulated radiation therapy* (IMRT).[85–88] In the case of a seven-beam arrangement of 10- × 10-cm fields broken into 5- × 5-mm beamlets, the result is 400 beamlets for each beam, or a total of 2800 adjustable parameters! It appears that beam direction is of great importance and cannot easily be modeled by the computer.[89,90] Therefore, the beam direction may be set by the operator; or, in some cases, a large number of beams may be positioned at predetermined angles. The computer then adjusts the beam weights to find the optimum solution (Figure 11-22). [91,92]

Treatment Planning Techniques

IMRT requires the clinician to accurately define the treatment objectives. This task can be quite involved, because choices must be made not only about what occurs within the target, but also what happens anywhere the beams intersect. Routinely, more beams are required in IMRT than with other techniques such as conformal three-dimensional (3-D) treatment planning, and these beams may be penetrating tissues that previously were outside the fields. For example, head and neck portals typically utilize lateral fields, but with IMRT it is common to use seven or nine beams around the circumference of the patient, causing irradiation of tissues such as the anterior portion of the mouth and the cerebellum that were previously blocked.[93] While it is true that the dose to these structures is significantly less than the target dose, they must be evaluated by the physician and monitored during treatment to quickly detect unanticipated side effects.

There are three general classifications of anatomical structures in radiation therapy:

1. Target Volumes. In transitioning from 3-D conformal treatment planning to IMRT, the definition of target volume has to be carefully reviewed. In head and neck cases, for example, it may be desirable for the physician to draw the volume on lateral DRRs as has traditionally been done. The target is then defined as everything in that field, except for the parotids and spinal cord. This "everything but" approach is known as *conformal avoidance radiotherapy*.[94–96] Planning computers commonly have sophisticated tools for defining regions to include or exclude structures. In the case of transferring a 3-D CRT volume to IMRT, one cannot assume that the margins for the PTV are the same in IMRT as they are in 3-D CRT. This discrepancy exists because the objectives in IMRT are dose-based or dose–volume-based, instead of geometrically based as in 3-D CRT. If the objective is to maintain similar dose margins for target coverage, then those margins must be correctly transferred to an objective for use in IMRT. For example, one can define the PTV by measuring the distance of the 97% isodose line to the target in a typical 3-D prostate plan, and transferring those

In inverse planning techniques, the computer iteratively weights the various beams segments and/or beamlets to achieve the dose distribution goal set by the operator.

The Uncertainty Principle, posited by Werner Heisenberg in 1927, states that the more you know about a particle's velocity (or momentum), the less you know about the particle's position (or time) when it possessed the particular velocity (momentum).

The Complementarity Principle, developed by Niels Bohr in 1928, states that matter (e.g., an electron) can behave as either a particle or a wave, but not both simultaneously.

The Copenhagen Interpretation, a fusion of Uncertainty and Complementarity, established that the position of an electron can be expressed only as a probability. This interpretation established probability as a fundamental feature of the atomic realm.

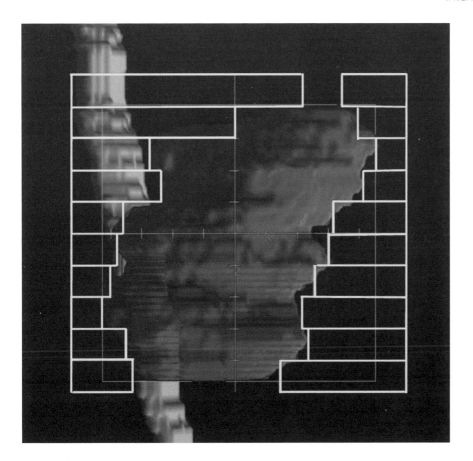

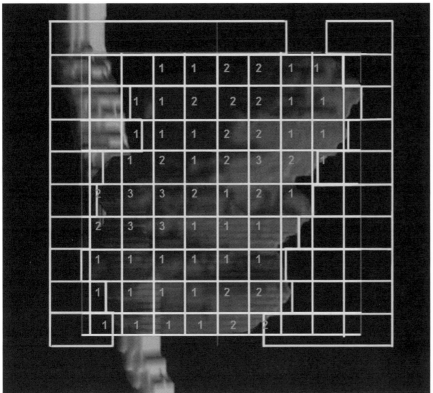

FIGURE 11-22
Initialization of optimization by defining field limits (first image), and creating beamlets with adjustable weights (second image).

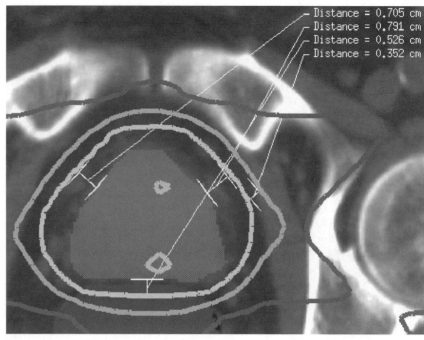

FIGURE 11-23
Defining dose volume based objectives from a conformal treatment plan to maintain similar dose margins in IMRT. The distances to the 95% and 80% line are measured and defined as minimum and maximum dose volume objectives. This ensures adequate target coverage while keeping dose compact within the region.

margins to a volume in an IMRT plan by expanding the prostate by the measured amount. Then, defining an objective to ensure that this PTV gets at least 97% of the prescription dose effectively transfers similar coverage between the 3-D plan and IMRT to maintain consistency in treatment margins as the new technology is adopted (Figure 11-23).

2. Critical Structures or Objects at Risk (OARs). With IMRT, defining critical structures becomes very important, because the beams are likely to be converging from many directions, and more OARs will be within the field. Also, if the computer does not know that a structure is present, it will not be able to avoid it. Since it is possible to obtain steep dose gradients with IMRT, adequate margins must be defined around critical structures such as the spinal cord to account for patient setup error and motion.[97,98]

3. Dose Shaping Structures. To obtain the desired dose distribution and beam characteristics, it may be advantageous to utilize structures that control the geometry of the dose distribution. These structures may or may not relate to actual patient anatomy. A rather simple example is to define normal tissue as everything that is not included in the target(s) and critical structures.

Structures considered in IMRT include:

1. Target volumes
2. Critical structures
3. Dose-shaping structures

Setting the Objective Function

Objective functions can be either dose-based or dose–volume-based.[99–102] For example, "give a minimum dose of 5000 cGy to the target" is an example of a dose-based objective. Likewise, "keep the dose below 2000 cGy to half of the parotids" is an example of a dose–volume-based objective, because it includes information on how much of the volume can receive a given dose. The objectives are entered into the planning system by defining the name of the structure, dose level to achieve or avoid, fraction or percent of volume, and importance relative to other clinical objectives (Figure 11-24). The values are often displayed on a dose–volume histogram to yield a graphical representation of the objectives.

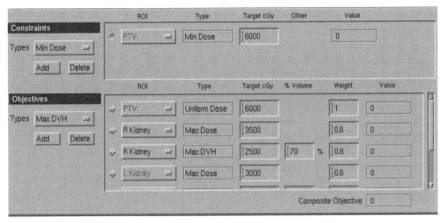

FIGURE 11-24

Objectives can be entered in a table such as the one above. The clinician must identify the region of interest, the type of objective, the dose level, volume (if dose–volume–based), and a weighting or importance value.

In developing objectives to be used clinically, physicians can refer to previous experience by looking at DVHs from similar cases and making improvements. One of the primary goals of IMRT for prostate cancer, for example, is to lower rectal dose. Previous DVHs for prostate patients provide a good baseline for how to set objectives to achieve that goal (Figure 11-25).

Alternatively, clinicians may set objectives by utilizing published data or experience from other institutions with IMRT capability (Figure 11-26).

Regarding dose-shaping objectives, trial and error may be used to obtain desirable dose distributions that satisfy physicians and physics staff. For example, if it is desired to keep overall beam weights similar for all fields, a ring structure at a large distance from the target can be utilized. The DVH for this structure is computed using uniform open fields of equal weight. This DVH is then used to create dose–volume objectives for that structure (Figure 11-27).

Objective functions used in IMRT can be determined from published clinical data, experience from other institutions, and from current planning techniques.

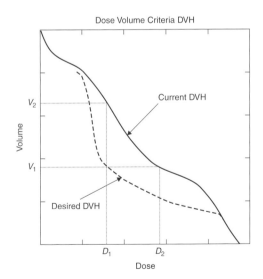

FIGURE 11-25

Dose–volume-based objective to make an improvement on the existing DVH. Generally, this technique is useful to lower the dose to a critical structure. (From Wu, Q., and Mohan, R. algorithms and functionality of an intensity modulated radiotherapy optimization system. *Med. Phys.* 2000; **27**(4): 701–711.)

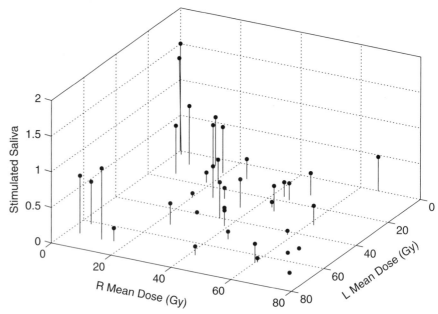

FIGURE 11-26
Stimulated saliva as a function of parotid dose. Either sparing one parotid or keeping the mean parotid dose less than 25 Gy should reduce the amount of xerostomia in patients. (From Chao, K. S., Deasy J. O., Markman, J., Haynie, J., Perez, C. A, Purdy, J. A., Low, D. A. A prospective study of salivary function sparing in patients with head-and-neck cancers receiving intensity-modulated or three-dimensional radiation therapy: Initial results. *Int. J. Radiol. Oncol. Biol. Phys.* 2001; **49**(4):907–916.

Optimization

The objectives are combined to define an *objective function or cost function,* a measure of the disagreement between the desired dose distribution and the calculated distribution. The objective function may be focused on achieving a uniformly homogeneous dose in the planning target volume, and minimizing the integral dose to organs at risk. This function is iteratively solved using one of several techniques, depending upon the planning system in use. One of the techniques commonly employed is the *simulated annealing* method (Figure 11-28). This algorithm searches for a treatment planning solution that corresponds to a minimum in the cost function.[103]

The end result of the optimization process is a *fluence map* for each beam. A fluence map (or intensity map) is a two-dimensional matrix of beamlet intensity for each beam. These matrices are commonly displayed as a two-dimensional gray scale image, or a three-dimensional map, as shown in Figure 11-29.

Although fluence maps appear to be complex, persons with experience can see common trends to assist in evaluating a treatment plan. These trends may include (a) a noticeable decrease in intensity in areas intersecting critical structures, (b) an increase in intensity outside a critical structure in the plane of gantry rotation to compensate for other beams with reduced intensity to avoid critical structures, and (c) an increase in intensity for projections that have the best "view" of the target. (Figure 11-30).

Conversion to Deliverable Treatment

The solution to the objective function obtained by optimization presents the ideal fluence to treat the patient. However, physical restrictions of the treatment unit usually require conversion of the ideal fluence map to something that can actually be delivered. The closest match to the ideal fluence map is achieved using x-ray beam compensators, because they can be machined to tight tolerances. More often, multileaf collimators are used to deliver the treatment. In this approach, the conversion

A cost function is a way to mathematically describe the desired result and to assign "penalties" for not achieving the desired result.

A "fluence map" is a two dimensional matrix of beam intensity for a given treatment beam. It has been given other names, such as "intensity map," "fluence matrix," and "opening density matrix."

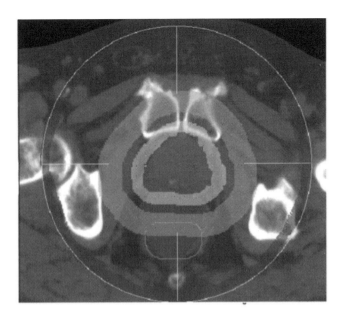

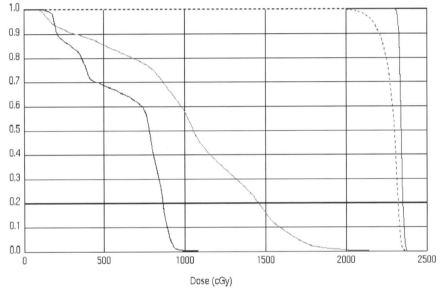

FIGURE 11-27
Dose-shaping structures and corresponding dose–volume histogram for a 3-D conformal treatment to be used in designing dose–volume–based objectives for IMRT. Each ring has a corresponding DVH, with the outermost ring having the lowest dose and progressing inwards.

process involves dividing the beam into a number of MLC patterns or *segments* to approximate the fluence map. As with the optimization process, there are a number of routines for accomplishing this task. Two common methods are IMFAST™ (Siemens) and K-means clustering.[104,105] In either case the result is segments that approximate the fluence map according to parameters such as minimum number of monitor units per segment, segment size, number of segments, and so on. When these segments are delivered by the treatment unit, a segment shape will be set, the beam will be turned on for the appropriate number of monitor units, and the beam will then step to the next segment. Since the beam is off while the MLC leaves are moving, the method is commonly known as "step and shoot" or "static" IMRT. Once the segments have been converted, the delivered dose distribution should be evaluated, together with the final dose–volume histogram, to ensure that all treatment objectives are met. In addition, the dose in areas outside the target volume should be examined closely to make sure that the dose in those areas is acceptable.

MLC conversion refers to the process of transferring the ideal fluence map into deliverable MLC segments. Two common routines are IMFAST^{TM} and K-means clustering.

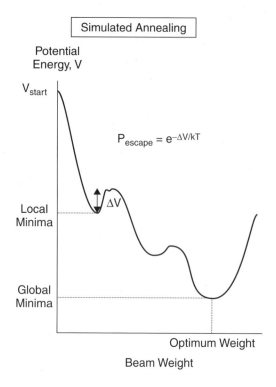

FIGURE 11-28
Optimization technique to prevent settling on a local minima solution. The optimizer has enough "velocity" to escape small local traps to find a global solution.

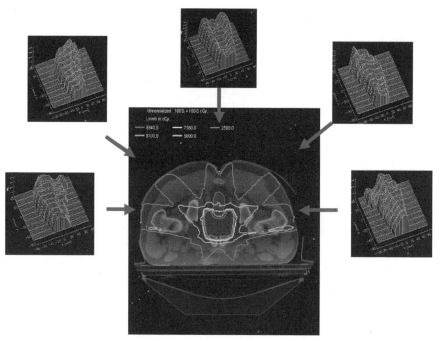

FIGURE 11-29
Five-field prostate IMRT showing three-dimensional fluence maps for each field and the corresponding dose distribution in the patient.

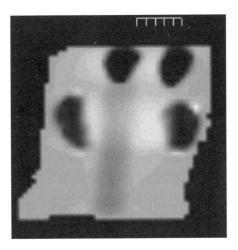

FIGURE 11-30
Fluence map for nasopharynx patient. The positions of the eyes and parotids are easily seen. The spinal cord is the slightly darkened region running vertically in the center of the image. Note the brighter area between the cord and parotids to make up for these areas being blocked from other beam directions.

■ DYNAMIC DELIVERY TECHNIQUES

The "sliding window" approach to treatment delivery involves moving the MLC leaves while the x-ray beam is on. This approach is more complex than step and shoot for the following reasons: (a) The "window" is often very narrow, resulting in narrow beam geometry; and (b) the MLC quality assurance protocol for dynamic delivery is more stringent, requiring leaf speed characterization. With the sliding window method, very complex distributions can be achieved as illustrated in Figure 11-31.

Allowing the gantry to arc while the leaves are moving is a technique known as *intensity-modulated arc therapy* (IMAT) or *dynamic arc therapy*.[106–108] This approach

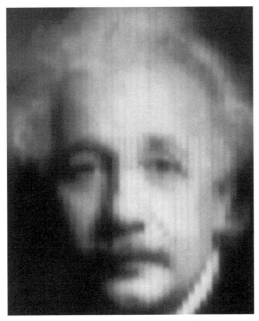

FIGURE 11-31
Complex intensity map illustrating the ability of IMRT to produce highly complex fields. The width of the leaves, oriented vertically, is the primary resolution limitation. (Courtesy of Varian.)

Clinical use of serial tomotherapy began in 1994. Since that time, thousands of patients have been treated with this technique, providing much of the clinical data for IMRT.

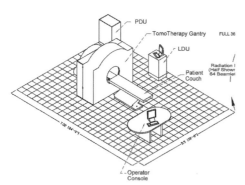

MARGIN FIGURE 11-8
Tomotherapy room layout.

Tomotherapy, Inc. was founded with a platform helical tomotherapy technology developed by Rock Mackie, Ph.D., a medical physicist at the University of Wisconsin.

Megavoltage CT uses the treatment linac and a bank of modified CT detectors to generate CT images. These images are comparable to conventional CT images, but are not subject to artifacts from high-density objects such as dental fillings or hip prostheses.

may require a few arc passes to completely deliver the treatment, because a given gantry angle can have only one MLC shape per arc. This method allows very complex dose distributions, but is challenging to plan and verify.

■ TOMOTHERAPY

Serial Tomotherapy

Serial tomotherapy, literally "slice therapy," has been in clinical use since 1994. The commercial system, Peacock™, combines a narrow MLC attachment to the linac (Mimic collimator) with precise couch increments to deliver a slice-by-slice treatment.[109,110] The MLC operates in binary mode, with the leaves either fully open or fully closed. Thousands of patients have been treated with this system, most of whom are patients with brain or head and neck cancers. The Peacock system has paved the way for other planning and delivery systems that are now available, because it provided much of the early clinical data demonstrating the benefits of IMRT.

Helical Tomotherapy

In the same manner that CT scanners have moved from axial to helical delivery, Tomotherapy Inc. has adopted a helical delivery system (Table 11-1).[111–115] The treatment unit looks much like a CT scanner, with a compact 6-MV linear accelerator replacing the x-ray tube. With this design, many of the components in a standard linear accelerator are not needed. For example, (a) the compact size eliminates the long cantilevered gantry and the bending magnet; (b) there are no electron energies and the target is fixed, so there is no carousel; and (c) since the beam is modulated by the MLC, there is no need for a flattening filter. The absence of a flattening filter provides a higher beam output compared with a conventional linac. A binary MLC is used, similar to the Mimic collimator previously mentioned.

A primary advantage of the tomotherapy system is that it fully integrates real-time patient imaging with the delivery of radiation treatments. The clinical success of conformal (and conformal avoidance) radiotherapy relies upon the ability to accurately localize the beam on a day-to-day basis. On-board axial image information is obtained using the megavoltage beam and a bank of CT detectors. So-called megavoltage CT (MVCT)[116] provides surprisingly good image quality and is not subject to artifact generation in high-density objects (e.g., dental fillings) (Figure 11-32). Also, an electron density conversion is not required because the imaging beam and treatment beam are one and the same. The imaging capabilities of this device offer a distinct advantage for comparison with virtual simulation.

In helical tomotherapy, the exit fluence at the detectors is used to reconstruct the dose delivered during the actual treatment. This information is fed back to the

TABLE 11-1   Helical Tomotherapy Specifications

- Patented helical slice delivery MLC with 360° continuous rotation and CT-like geometry.
- On-board megavoltage computed tomographic imaging; dose per CT is approximately 1.5–2.5 cGy
- Small, low-energy footprint (approximately 20′ × 20′)
- Max field size = 5 cm × 40 cm
- Max clinical dose rate at isocenter = 800–1100 cGy
- Energy = 6-MeV x rays
- 32 processor CPU with Convolution Dose Algorithm
- One planning console and one delivery console (multiple planning consoles available in future releases)

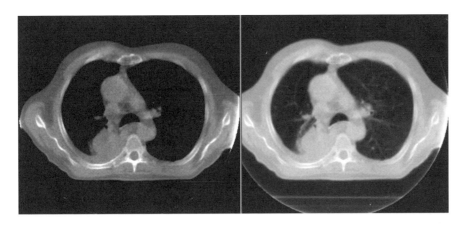

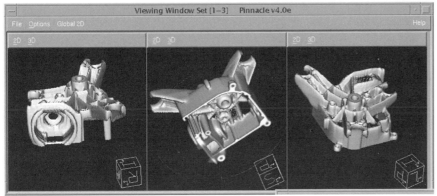

FIGURE 11-32
Megavoltage CT images. The top images show good contrast and resolution, and the bottom image shows a 3-D reconstruction of a carburetor, an object that would have been impossible to image accurately with conventional CT because of density artifacts.

planning system to monitor the dose delivered over the patient's course of therapy. This method of providing information from the actual treatment back to the planning computer is known as *adaptive radiotherapy* (Figure 11-33).[117] Changes to the treatment to achieve the intended goals can be made as the treatment progresses.

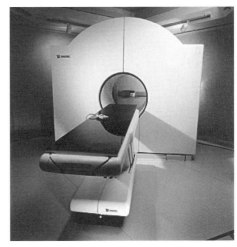

MARGIN FIGURE 11-9
The world's first helical tomotherapy treatment unit at the University of Wisconsin.

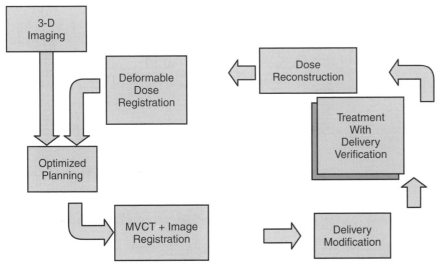

FIGURE 11-33
Adaptive radiotherapy. Information from the treatment itself, in the form of the exit dose received at the detectors, is used to determine how much dose was given and where it was given. This is fed back to the treatment planning module to update treatment progression and make necessary adjustments.

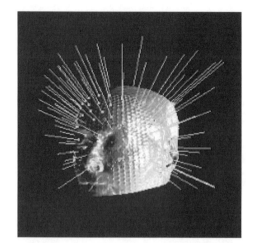

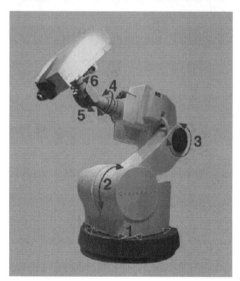

MARGIN FIGURE 11-10
Accuray's Cyberknife robot controlled linear accelerator for stereotactic radiosurgery and IMRT. The six degrees of freedom are indicated in the image. This treatment device merges state-of-the-art technology from the manufacturing industry (robotics) with advanced radiation delivery in the form of a compact linear accelerator.

■ TREATMENT PLANNING CHALLENGES

Treatment Field Geometry

Modern radiotherapy equipment is provided with capabilities far more sophisticated than the equipment commonly used for radiation therapy in the 1960s and 1970s, when much of the development work in treatment planning was performed. For example, the use of asymmetric collimators requires that computational techniques consider the variation of dose with off-axis distance.[118–120] Recent incorporation of multileaf collimators has created a demand for development of special calculation methods,[121] particularly with static and dynamic IMRT to fully account for the dosimetric influence of the MLC. Also, the use of very small diameter radiation fields, as used in stereotactic radiosurgery, requires special considerations.[122] In particular, dose calculations must be carried out at high resolution in order to accurately mimic the steep dose gradients encountered during radiosurgery. The acquisition of beam data for treatment planning with radiosurgery beams is similarly demanding, requiring measurements of very high precision.[123]

Lateral Disequilibrium in High-Energy Beams

A phenomenon described as *lateral electronic disequilibrium*[124–126] occurs as high-energy photons interact with tissue to yield high-energy Compton electrons that may travel several centimeters through tissue. Some of these electrons deposit dose outside of the photon beam. As a result, the dose within the field is reduced, the penumbra is broadened, and the dose deposition outside the field edges is increased. This effect is more pronounced in low-density tissue such as lung, where the Compton electrons can travel correspondingly larger distances. Only some of the most advanced computational techniques, such as the convolution algorithm and the differential pencil-beam method, can model the behavior of electrons under these conditions. Lateral disequilibrium also exists in very small fields (e.g., stereotactic radiosurgery) due to outscatter of electrons.

Interface Effects

The deposition of dose in the region of tissue interfaces is similarly complex. The sudden change in the probability of interaction of photons with the medium, combined with the transport of high-energy Compton electrons across the boundary, yields complex changes to the dose distribution. This effect may present a significant problem in the vicinity of air cavities such as the nasal sinuses. Most conventional computational algorithms cannot address the transport of electrons, although some of the newest three-dimensional techniques are able to address this problem quite acceptably. Monte Carlo methods are also able to effectively compute the dose across an interface.

■ SUMMARY

- Three-dimensional treatment planning includes two general aspects: (1) image data, such as from a CT scanner, that is then manipulated and displayed in other orientations to demonstrate the three-dimensional nature of the patient's anatomy and (2) performing a true three-dimensional calculation of the absorbed radiation dose.
- Conformal radiation therapy involves techniques of shaping radiation dose distributions geometrically to the target volume, usually based on transaxial CT images.
- With the availability of tissue density information from CT, the ability to perform heterogeneity corrections has gained increasing use in clinical treatment planning. Although much of the historical data is based on homogeneous calculations, the complexity of three-dimensional and IMRT planning techniques

often requires heterogeneity corrections, particularly when used to modify observed isodose distributions.

- The process of virtual simulation involves creating a three-dimensional model of the patient, usually from a contiguous CT scan data set. Isocenter placement, beam arrangement, and dose calculation can then take place on the "virtual placement."
- The concept of immobilization involves techniques to minimize patient motion during treatment in order to ensure accurate and reproducible setup for each treatment.
- Increased attention is being directed at target localization to improve accuracy and limit uncertainty in mobile structures such as the prostate. Techniques include real-time imaging with ultrasound and tomotherapy. Positioning may be relative to anatomical structures or fiducials, either implanted or external.
- The ICRU has divided photon beam calculation methods into four classifications:

  1. analytical
  2. matrix
  3. semiempirical
  4. three-dimensional integration

- Dose computation algorithms for treatment planning systems utilize a balance between speed and accuracy. More accurate algorithms, such as convolution/superposition and Monte Carlo, are becoming commonplace with modern computing systems.
- Dose volume histograms are graphical depictions of radiation dose to various structures of interest for the treatment plan.
- Heterogeneity corrections have utilized corrections based on the effective depth (e.g., Batho method), dose deposition kernal "stretching" (convolution/superposition), and large samples of simulated interactions (Monte Carlo).
- The biological response of tumors and critical structures has been addressed through the development of models for tumor control probability (TCP) and normal tissue complication probability (NTCP).
- The process of intensity modulated radiation therapy (IMRT) involves three general steps:

  1. Setting dose or dose–volume objectives, based on accurate and detailed structure definition.
  2. Iterative optimization using any of a number of available mathematical techniques to accomplish the objectives.
  3. Conversion to a deliverable treatment, such as step-and-shoot MLC segments or dynamic sliding window.

- Serial tomotherapy involves incremental slice-by-slice treatments (e.g., Peacock system from Nomos), and helical tomotherapy involves overlapping helical treatments on a device that looks much like a conventional CT scanner.

PROBLEMS

11-1. A three-dimensional treatment planning system utilizes a 20-cm × 20-cm × 15-cm dose calculation matrix. The dose grid resolution is 4 mm. If the matrix size is changed to 10 cm × 10 cm × 15 cm, and the resolution is changed to 5 mm, how many times faster will the calculation be?

11-2. For a head and neck treatment plan, the field size is 15 cm ×

15 cm. If there are nine fields and the pencil-beam algorithm uses 5-mm beamlets, how many adjustable intensity parameters are there?

11-3. On your planning system:
   a. A standard procedure for evaluating the accuracy of a calculation algorithm is to compare isodose curves calculated by the

computer with those measured in the treatment beam. Perform a treatment plan of a single photon beam incident perpendicularly on a rectangular phantom, and compare the calculated isodose curves with the measured data. Do the calculated data meet the customary standards for acceptability? (See Chapter 15.) The calculated dose should agree with the measured dose to within 2% in regions of shallow gradient or within 2-mm in regions of steep dose gradient.

b. For an intact breast patient, prepare a homogeneous treatment plan to give uniform dose. Then recalculate the plan with heterogeneity corrections. Note the differences between these techniques, particularly in the number of monitor units and the effect of wedges. These results will be more dramatic for lung treatments and mastectomy patients.

c. It is expected that with smaller electron beam cutout sizes, the point of maximum dose for the depth dose curve will shift toward the surface. How well does your planning system predict electron beam depth dose curves for small cutout sizes?

11-4. If IMRT treatment volumes are expected to be 30% of the patient volume on a typical linear accelerator (e.g., 30 patients/day), and the number of monitor units triples for these patients to deliver step and shoot segmented MLC shapes, how will this affect shielding calculations regarding head leakage? If the original design had an additional tenth value layer of shielding built in as a safety margin and only 6-MeV x rays are used for IMRT, do you think this will this still be enough?

REFERENCES

1. International Commission on Radiation Units and Measurements, Report No. 50: Prescribing, Recording and Reporting Photon Beam Therapy, Washington, DC, International Commission on Radiation Units and Measurements, 1993.
2. Laughlin, J. S., Mohan, R., and Kutcher, G. J. Choice of optimum megavoltage for accelerators for photon beam treatment, *Int. J. Radiat. Oncol. Biol. Phys.* 1986; **12**(9):1551–1557.
3. Hope, C. S., et al. Optimization of x-ray treatment planning by computer judgment, *Phys. Med. Biol.* 1967; **12**:531–542.
4. Mackie. T. R., et al. Generation of photon energy deposition kernels using EGS Monte Carlo code, *Phys Med Biol* 1988; **33**:1–20.
5. Perez, C. A., et al. Three-dimensional treatment planning and conformal radiation therapy: Preliminary evaluation, *Radiother. Oncol.* 1995; **36**:32–43.
6. Purdy, J. A., and Starkschall, G. (eds.). *A Practical Guide to 3-D Planning and Conformal Radiation Therapy.* Madison, WI, Advanced Medical Publishing, 1999.
7. Kutcher, G. J., et al. Comprehensive QA for radiation oncology: Report of AAPM Radiation Therapy Committee Task Group 40, *Med. Phys.*1994; **21**(4):581–618.
8. Andrew, J. W., et al. A video-based patient contour acquisition system for the design of radiotherapy compensators, *Med. Phys.* 1989; **16**:425–430.
9. Doolittle, A. M., et al. An electronic patient-contouring device, *Br. J. Radiol.* 1977; **50**:135–138.
10. Hills, J. F., Ibbott, G. S., and Hendee, W. R. Patient contours utilizing an ultrasound scanner interfaced to a minicomputer, *Med. Phys.*1979; **6**:309–311.
11. Kuisk, H. "Contour Maker" eliminating body casting in radiotherapy planning, *Radiology* 1971; **101**:203–204.
12. Rosenow, U. Various methods of determining the body contours of the patient, *Radiology* 1973; **38**:558–564.
13. Stewart, J. R., et al. Computed tomography in radiation therapy, *Int. J. Radiat. Oncol. Biol. Phys.* 1978; **4**:313–324.
14. Hobday, P., et al. Computed tomography applied to radiotherapy treatment planning: Techniques and results, *Radiology* 1979; **133**:477–482.
15. Constantinou, C., Harrington, J. C., and DeWerd, L. A., An electron density calibration phantom for CT-based treatment planning computers, *Med. Phys.* 1992; **19**:325–327.
16. Hendee, W. R., and Ritenour, E. R. *Medical Imaging Physics,* 4th edition.New York, John Wiley & Sons, 2002.
17. Pelizzari, C. A., et al. Accurate three-dimensional registration of CT, PET, and/or MR images of the brain, *J Comput. Assist. Tomogr.* 1989; **13**:20–26.
18. Jani, S. K. (ed.). *CT Simulation for Radiotherapy,* Madison, WI, Medical Physics Publishing, 1993.
19. Sherouse, G. W., and Chaney, E. L. The portable virtual simulator, *Int. J. Radiat. Oncol. Biol. Phys.* 1991; **21**:475–482.
20. Sherouse, G. W., et al. Virtual simulation in the clinical setting: Some practical considerations, *Int. J. Radiat. Oncol. Biol. Phys.* 1990; **19**:1059–1065.
21. Jani, S. *CT Simulation for Radiotherapy*. Madison, WI, Medical Physics Publishing, 1993.
22. Coia, L., Shultheiss, T., and Hanks, G. *A Practical Guide to CT-Simulation.* Madison, WI, Advanced Medical Publishing, 1995.
23. Rosenman, J., et al. Three-dimensional display techniques in radiation therapy treatment planning, *Int. J. Radiat. Oncol. Biol. Phys.* 1989; **16**:263–269.
24. Lee, J. S., et al. Volumetric visualization of head and neck CT data for treatment planning. *Int. J. Radiat. Oncol. Biol. Phys.* 1999; **44**(3):693–703.
25. Gehring, M., et al. A three-dimensional volume visualization package applied to stereotactic radiosurgery treatment planning. *Int. J. Radiat. Oncol. Biol. Phys.* 1991; **21**(2):491–500.
26. Reynolds, R. A., Sontag, M. R., and Chen, L. S. An algorithm for three-dimensional visualization of radiation therapy beams. *Med. Phys.* 1988; **15**(1):24–8.
27. Sherouse, G. W., Novins, K., and Chaney. E. L. Computations of digitally reconstructed radiographs for use in radiotherapy treatment design, *Int. J. Radiat. Oncol. Biol. Phys.* 1990; **18**:651–658.
28. Webb, S. *The Physics of Three-Dimensional Radiation Therapy: Conformal Radiotherapy, Radiosurgery and Treatment Planning,* Bristol, Institute of Physics Publishing, Ltd., 1993.
29. Ford, E. C., et al. Evaluation of respiratory movement during gated radiotherapy using film and electronic portal imaging. *Int. J. Radiat. Oncol. Biol. Phys.* 2002; **52**(2):522–531.
30. Vedam, S. S., et al. Determining parameters for respiration-gated radiotherapy. *Med. Phys.* 2001; **28**(10):2139–2146.
31. Ramsey, C. R., et al. Clinical efficacy of respiratory gated conformal radiation therapy. *Med. Dosim.* 1999; **24**(2):115–119.
32. Serago, C. F., et al. Initial experience with ultrasound localization for positioning prostate cancer patients for external beam radiotherapy. *Int. J. Radiat. Oncol. Biol. Phys.* 2002; **53**(5):1130–1138.
33. Morr, J., et al. Implementation and utility of a daily ultrasound-based localization system with intensity-modulated radiotherapy for prostate cancer. *Int. J. Radiat. Oncol. Biol. Phys.* 2002; **53**(5):1124–1129.
34. Lattanzi, J., et al. Ultrasound-based stereotactic guidance of precision conformal external beam radiation therapy in clinically localized prostate cancer. *Urology* 2000; **55**(1):73–78.
35. Lattanzi, J., et al. A comparison of daily CT localization to a daily ultrasound-based system in prostate cancer. *Int. J. Radiat. Oncol. Biol. Phys.* 1999; **43**(4):705–706.
36. Shimizu, S., et al. Use of an implanted marker and real-time tracking of the marker for the positioning of prostate and bladder cancers. *Int. J. Radiat. Oncol. Biol. Phys.* 2000; **48**(5):1591–1597.
37. Adler, J. R., Jr., et al. The Cyberknife: A frameless robotic system for radiosurgery. *Stereotact. Funct. Neurosurg.* 1997; **69**(1–4 Pt 2):124–128.
38. International Commission on Radiation Units and Measurements, Report No. 42: *Use of Computers in External Beam Radiotherapy Procedures with*

High-Energy Photons and Electrons, Washington, DC, International Commission on Radiation Units and Measurements, 1987.

39. Sterling, T. D., Perry, H., and Katz, L. Automation of radiation treatment planning, *Br. J. Radiol.* 1964; **37**:544–550.

40. Van de Geijn J, et al. *A unified 3-D model for external beam dose distributions.* Computers in Radiation Therapy. Proceedings of the 7th International Conference on the Use of Computers in Radiotherapy, Tokyo, 1980.

41. Milan, J., and Bentley, R. E. The storage and manipulation of radiation dose data in a small digital computer. *Br. J. Radiol.* 1974; **47**:115–121.

42. Clarkson, J. A note on depth doses in fields of irregular shape. *Br. J. Radiol.* 1941; **14**:265.

43. Cundiff, J. H., et al. A method for the calculation of dose in the radiation treatment of Hodgkin's disease. *Am. J. Roentgenol. Radium Ther. Nucl. Med.* 1973; **117**(l):30–44.

44. Wilkinson, J. M., Rawlinson, J. A., and Cunningham, J. R. *An extended source model for the calculation of the primary component of a cobalt-60 radiation beam in penumbral regions.* Presented at American Association of Physicists in Medicine Workshop, Chicago, September 17, 1970.

45. Cunningham, J. R. Keynote Address: Development of computer algorithms for radiation treatment planning, *Int. J. Radiat. Oncol. Biol. Phys.* 1989; **16**:1367–1376.

46. Cassell, K. J., Hobday, P. A., and Parker, R. P. The implementation of a generalized Batho inhomogeneity correction for radiotherapy planning with direct use of CT numbers. *Phys. Med. Biol.* 1981; **26**(5):825–833.

47. Wong, J. W., and Henkelman, R. M. Reconsideration of the power-law (Batho) equation for inhomogeneity corrections. *Med. Phys.* 1992; **9**:521–530.

48. Sontag, M. R., and Cunningham, J. R. The equivalent tissue–air ratio method for making absorbed dose calculations in a heterogeneous medium. *Radiology* 1978; **129**:791–794.

49. Boyer, A. L., and Mok, E. C. A photon dose distribution model employing convolution calculations. *Med. Phys.* 1985; **12**:169–177.

50. Ma, C. M., et al. A Monte Carlo dose calculation tool for radiotherapy treatment planning. *Phys. Med. Biol.* 2002; **47**(10):1671–1689.

51. Demarco, J. J., Chetty, I. J., and Solberg, T. D. A Monte Carlo tutorial and the application for radiotherapy treatment planning. *Med. Dosim.* 2002; **27**(1):43–50.

52. DeMarco, J. J., Solberg, T. D., and Chetty, I. Monte Carlo methods for dose calculation and treatment planning: A revolution for radiotherapy. *Adm. Radiol. J.* 1999; **18**(8):24–27.

53. Miften, M., et al. Comparison of RTP dose distributions in heterogeneous phantoms with the BEAM Monte Carlo simulation system. *J. Appl. Clin. Med. Phys.* 2001; **2**(1):21–31.

54. Mohan, R., Chui, C., and Lidofsky, L. Differential pencil beam dose computation model for photons. *Med. Phys.* 1986; **13**:64–73.

55. Pijpelink, J., Van den Temple, Y., and Hamers, R. *A pencil beam algorithm for photon beam calculations.* Nucletron-Oldelft Activity,Report No. 6, 21–32, 1995.

56. Ahnesjö, A. Collapsed cone convolution of radiant energy for photon dose calculation in heterogeneous media. *Med. Phys.* 1989; **16**:577–592.

57. Mackie, T. R., Scrimger, J. W., and Battista, J. J. A convolution method of calculating dose for 15-MV x rays. *Med. Phys.* 1985; **12**:188–196.

58. Boyer, A. L., et al. Fast Fourier transform convolution calculations of x-ray isodose distributions in homogeneous media. *Med. Phys.* 1989; **16**:248–253.

59. Ayyangar, K., Leonard, C., and Suntharalingam, J. Computerization of electron beams for treatment planning. *Med. Phys.* 1980; **7**:440.

60. Kawachi, K. Calculation of electron dose distribution for radiotherapy treatment planning. *Phys. Med. Biol.* 1975; **20**:571–577.

61. Shabason, L., and Hendee, W. R. An analytic expression for central axis electron depth dose distributions. *Int. J. Radiat. Oncol. Biol. Phys.* 1979; **5**:263–267.

62. Hogstrom, K. R., Mills, M. D., and Almond, P. R. Electron beam dose calculations. *Phys. Med. Biol.* 1981; **26**:445–459.

63. Lillicrap, S. C., Wilson, P., and Boag, J. W. Dose distributions in high energy electron beams: Production of broad beam distributions from narrow beam data. *Phys. Med. Biol.* 1975; **20**:30–38.

64. Mah, E., et al. Experimental evaluation of a 2D and 3D electron pencil beam algorithm. *Phys. Med. Biol.* 1989; **34**:1179–1194.

65. Shiu, A. S. *Three-dimensional electron beam dose calculations.* Doctoral dissertation, Houston, Texas, University of Texas Graduate School of Biomedical Sciences. 1988.

66. Almond, P. R., Wright, A. E., and Boone, M. L. N. High-energy electron dose perturbations in regions of tissue heterogeneity. II. Physical models of tissue heterogeneities. *Radiology.* 1967; **88**:1146–1153.

67. Holt, J. G., et al. Memorial electron beam AET treatment planning system. In *Practical Aspects of Electron Beam Treatment Planning*, C. G. Orton, and F. Bagne (eds.). New York, American Institute of Physics, 1978.

68. Laughlin, J. S., et al. Electron-beam treatment planning in inhomogeneous tissue. *Radiology* 1965; **85**(3):524–531.

69. Laughlin, J. S. High energy electron treatment planning for inhomogeneities. *Br. J. Radiol.* 1965, **38**:143–147.

70. McDonald, S. C., and Rubin, P. Optimization of external beam radiation therapy. *Int. J. Radiat. Oncol. Biol. Phys.* 1977; **2**:307–317.

71. Drzymala, R. E., et al. Dose–volume histograms. *Int. J. Radiat. Oncol. Biol. Phys.* 1991; **21**:71–78.

72. Drzymala, R. E., et al. Integrated software tools for the evaluation of radiotherapy treatment plans. *Int. J. Radiat. Oncol. Biol. Phys.* 1994; **30**:909–919.

73. Lawrence, T. S., Tesser, R. J., and Ten Haken, R. K. Application of dose volume histograms to treatment of intrahepatic malignancies with radiation therapy. *Int. J. Radiat. Oncol. Biol. Phys.* 1990; **19**:1041–1047.

74. Schell, M. C., et al. Evaluation of radiosurgery techniques with cumulative dose volume histograms in linac-based stereotactic external beam irradiation. *Int. J. Radiat. Oncol. Biol. Phys.* 1991; **20**:1325–1330.

75. Schultheiss, T. E., and Orton, C. G. Models in radiotherapy: Definition of decision criteria. *Med. Phys.* 1985; **12**:183–187.

76. Kutcher, G. J., and Burman, C. Calculation of complication probability factors for non-uniform normal tissue irradiation: The effective volume method. *Int. J. Radiat. Oncol. Biol. Phys.* 1989; **16**:1623–1630.

77. Lyman, J. T. Complication probability as assessed from dose volume histograms. *Radiat. Res.* 1985; **104**:S13–S19.

78. Martel, M. K., et al. Analysis of tumor dose-volume histograms in relationship to local progression free survival for lung cancer patients. *Int. J. Radiat. Oncol. Biol. Phys.* 1993; **27**(suppl 1):238.

79. Niemierko, A., and Goitein, M. Implementation of a model for estimating tumor control probability for an inhomogeneously irradiated tumor. *Radiother. Oncol.* 1993; **29**:140–147.

80. Niemierko, A., and Goitein, M. Optimization of 3D radiation therapy with both physical and biological end points and constraints. *Int. J. Radiat. Oncol. Biol. Phys.* 1992; **23**:99–108.

81. Wambersie, A., Hanks, G., and Van Dam, J. Quality assurance and accuracy required in radiation therapy: Biological and medical considerations. In *Selected Topics in Physics of Radiotherapy and Imaging*, U. Madhvanath, K. S. Parthasarathy, and T. V. Venkateswaran (eds.): New Delhi, McGraw-Hill, 1988.

82. Xiao, Y., et al. An optimized forward-planning technique for intensity modulated radiation therapy. *Med. Phys.* 2000; **27**(9):2093–2099.

83. Hristov, D., et al. On the implementation of dose-volume objectives in gradient algorithms for inverse treatment planning. *Med. Phys.* 2002; **29**(5):848–856.

84. Chui, C. S., and Spirou, S. V. Inverse planning algorithms for external beam radiation therapy. *Med. Dosim.* 2001; **26**(2):189–197.

85. IMRT collaborative working group, Intensity modulated radiotherapy: Current status and issues of interest. *Int. J. Radiat. Oncol. Biol. Phys.* 2001; **51**(4):880–914.

86. Webb, S. *The Physics of Conformal Radiotherapy.* Bristol, UK, Institute of Physics Publishing Ltd., 1997.

87. Purdy, J., et al eds. *3D Conformal and Intensity Modulated Radiation Therapy: Physics and Clinical Applications.* Madison, WI, Advanced Medical Publishing, 2001.

88. Brokaw, M. *Intensity Modulated Radiation Therapy. Optimizing Clinical Quality and Financial Performance.* Oncology Roundtable, The Advisory Board Company, 2002.

89. Brahme, A. Optimization of radiation therapy. *Int. J. Radiat. Oncol. Biol. Phys.* 1994; **28**:785–787.

90. Soderstrom, S., and Brahme, A. Selection of suitable beam orientations in radiation therapy using entropy and Fourier transform measures. *Phys. Med. Biol.* 1992; **37**:911–924.

91. Oldham, M., and Webb, S. The optimization and inherent limitations of 3D conformal radiotherapy treatment plans of the prostate. *Br. J. Radiol.* 1995; **68**:882–893.

92. Starkschall, G., and Eifel, P. J. An interactive beam-weight optimization tool for three-dimensional radiotherapy treatment planning. *Med. Phys.* 1992; **19**:155–163.

93. Eisbruch, A., et al. Dose, volume and function relationships in parotid salivary glands following conformal and intensity modulated irradiation of head and neck cancer. *Int. J. Radiat. Oncol. Biol. Phys.* 1999; **45**(3):577–587.

94. Lamdau, D., et al. Cardiac avoidance in breast radiotherapy: A comparison of simple shielding techniques with intensity-modulated radiotherapy. *Radiother. Oncol.* 2001; **60**(3):247–255.

95. Mackie, T. R., et al. Tomotherapy. *Semin. Radiat. Oncol.* 1999; **9**(1):108–117.

96. Purdy, J. A. Advances in three-dimensional treatment planning and conformal dose delivery. *Semin. Oncol.* 1997; **24**(6):655–671.

97. McKenzie, A., van Herk, M., and Mijnheer, B. Margins for geometric uncertainty around organs at risk in radiotherapy. *Radiother. Oncol.* 2002; **62**(3):299–307.

98. Oiuwen, W., et al. The potential for sparing of parotids and escalation of biologically effective dose with intensity-modulated radiation treatments of head and neck cancers: A treatment design study. *Int. J. Radiat. Oncol. Biol. Phys.* 2000; **46**(1):195–205.

99. Chao, K. S., et al. *Intensity Modulated Radiation Therapy for Head and Neck Cancers*. Philadelphia, Lippincott, Williams and Wilkins 2002.

100. Zelefsky, M., et al. Clinical experience with intensity modulated radiation therapy (IMRT) in prostate cancer. *Radiother. Oncol.* 2000; **55**:241–249.

101. Sternick, S. (ed.). *Theory & Practice of Intensity Modulated Radiation Therapy*. Madison, WI, Advanced Medical Publishing, 1997.

102. Wu, Q., and Mohan, R. Algorithms and functionality of an intensity modulated radiotherapy optimization system. *Med. Phys.* 2000; **27**(4):701–711.

103. Mageras, G. S., and Mohan, R. Application of fast simulated annealing to optimization of conformal radiation treatments. *Med. Phys.* 1992; **20**:639–647.

104. Potter, L. D., et al. A quality and efficiency analysis of the IMFAST segmentation algorithm in head and neck "step & shoot" IMRT treatments. *Med. Phys.* 2002; **29**(3):275–283.

105. Que, W. Comparison of algorithms for multileaf collimator field segmentation. *Med. Phys.* 1999; **26**(11):2390–2396.

106. Yu, C. X., et al. Clinical implementation of intensity-modulated arc therapy. *Int. J. Radiat. Oncol. Biol. Phys.* 2002; **53**(2):453–463.

107. Wong, E., Chen, J. Z., and Greenland, J. Intensity-modulated arc therapy simplified. *Int. J. Radiat. Oncol. Biol. Phys.* 2002; **53**(1):222–235.

108. Ma, L., et al. Optimized intensity-modulated arc therapy for prostate cancer treatment. *Int. J. Cancer.* 2001; **96**(6):379–384.

109. Salter, B. J. NOMOS Peacock IMRT utilizing the Beak post collimation device. *Med. Dosim.* 2001; **26**(1):37–45.

110. Low, D. A., and Mutic, S. A commercial IMRT treatment-planning dose-calculation algorithm. *Int. J. Radiat. Oncol. Biol. Phys.* 1998; **41**(4):933–937.

111. Mackie, T. R., et al. Tomotherapy: A new concept for the delivery of dynamic conformal radiotherapy. *Med. Phys.* 1993; **20**(6):1709–1719.

112. Olivera, G. H., et al. Tomotherapy. In *Modern Technology of Radiation Oncology*. J. Van Dyk (eds.). Madison, WI, Medical Physics Publishing, 1999.

113. Shepard, D. M., et al. Iterative approaches to dose optimization in tomotherapy. *Phys. Med. Biol.* 2000; **45**(1):69–90.

114. Kapatoes, J. M., et al. A feasible method for clinical delivery verification and dose reconstruction in tomotherapy. *Med. Phys.* 2001; **28**:528–542.

115. Lu, W., et al. *A generalization of adaptive radiotherapy and the registration of deformable dose distributions*. Proceedings of the 13th International Conference on Computers in Radiotherapy, Heidelberg, Germany, 2000.

116. Ruchala, K. J., et al. Megavoltage CT image reconstruction during tomotherapy treatments. *Phys. Med. Biol.* 2000; **45**(12):3545–3562.

117. Wu, C., et al. Re-optimization in adaptive radiotherapy. *Phys. Med. Biol.* 2002; **47**(17):3181–3195.

118. Khan, F. M., Gerbi, B. J., and Deibel, F. C. Dosimetry of asymmetric x-ray collimators. *Med. Phys.* 1986; **13**:936–941.

119. Kwa, W., et al. Dosimetry for asymmetric x-ray fields. *Med. Phys.* 1994; **21**:1599–1604.

120. Thomas, S. J., and Thomas, R. L. A beam generation algorithm for linear accelerators with independent collimators. *Phys. Med. Biol.* 1990; **35**:325–332.

121. Chui, C.-S., LoSasso, T., and Spirou, S. Dose calculation for photon beams with intensity modulation gener ated by dynamic jaw or multileaf collimations. *Med. Phys.* 1994; **21**:1237–1244.

122. Peters, T. M., et al. Stereotactic neurosurgery planning on a personal-computer-based work station. *J. Diagn. Imag.* 1989; **2**:75–81.

123. Bjarngard, B. E., Tsai, J.-S., and Rice, R. K. Doses on the central axes of narrow 6-MV x-ray beams. *Med. Phys.* 1990; **17**:794–799.

124. Haider, T. K., and el-Khatib, E. E. Differential scatter integration in regions of electronic non-equilibrium. *Phys. Med. Biol.* 1995; **40**(1):31–43.

125. Woo, M., Cunningham, J. R., and Jezioranski, J. J. Extending the concept of primary and scatter separation to the condition of electronic disequilibrium. *Med. Phys.* 1990; **17**:588–595.

126. Young, M. E., Kornelsen, R. O. Dose corrections for low-density tissue inhomogeneities and air channels for 10-MV x rays. *Med. Phys.* 1983; **10**(4):450–455.

CHAPTER

12

SOURCES FOR IMPLANT THERAPY

OBJECTIVES   286

RADIUM SOURCES   286

Construction of Radium Sources   287
Types of Radium Sources   287

SPECIFICATION OF BRACHYTHERAPY SOURCES   289

RADIUM SUBSTITUTES   290

Cesium   290
Cobalt   291
Tantalum and Iridium   291
Gold, Iodine, and Palladium   291
Americium-241 and Cesium-131   291

OPHTHALMIC IRRADIATORS   292

IMPLANTABLE NEUTRON SOURCES   292

RADIATION SAFETY OF BRACHYTHERAPY SOURCES   292

Storage   292
Test for Uniform Distribution of Activity   293
Evaluating the Safety of Brachytherapy Sources   293

SUMMARY   293

PROBLEMS   293

REFERENCES   294

Radiation Therapy Physics, Third Edition, by William R. Hendee, Geoffrey S. Ibbott, and Eric G. Hendee
ISBN 0-471-39493-9 Copyright © 2005 John Wiley & Sons, Inc.

Implant therapy is generally referred to as "brachytherapy" (short-distance therapy) and was once called "plesiotherapy" (from the Greek "plesios" meaning "close").

Radium molds were once used widely for treating superficial lesions but have been superseded to a large extent by treatment with superficial x rays and electrons.

Today, plaques are used frequently for the treatment of choroidal melanoma, a tumor that develops beneath the retina.

Interstitial implants are widely used for the treatment of intraoral and superficial lesions and for treatment of tumors in accessible organs such as the prostate.

Most intracavitary implants are used for the treatment of cancer of the cervix and uterus, with the sealed sources placed in the intrauterine cavity and around the cervix.

In recent years, intravascular brachytherapy has been used for treatment of recurrent coronary artery stenosis.

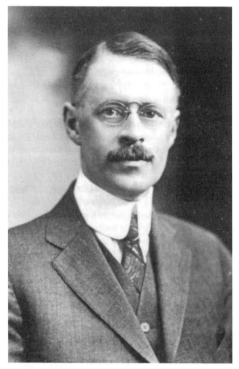

MARGIN FIGURE 12-1
William Duane, circa 1905. With permission from the American Institute of Physics.

■ OBJECTIVES

After reading this chapter, the student should:

- Understand the historical evolution of brachytherapy from the use of radium and radon sources to the present use of a variety of nuclides.
- Recognize the important and useful characteristics of the nuclides used for brachytherapy today.
- Be able to compute the equivalent mass of radium for a source of known activity.
- Understand the relationship between several terms for describing the strength of a brachytherapy source.
- Be able to explain the concept of radioactive equilibrium and calculate the activities as a function of time for two sources in equilibrium.

The implantation of sealed sources of radioactive material in or near a tumor is one of the oldest methods for treating cancer with ionizing radiation. In the past, the radioactive material employed most frequently for implant therapy was radium (^{226}Ra) in secular equilibrium with its decay products. Today, sources such as cesium (^{137}Cs), iridium (^{192}Ir), iodine (^{125}I), and palladium (^{103}Pd) are used as replacements for radium.

Techniques for implant therapy may be divided into four categories:

1. *Molds or plaques* are composed of radioactive sources that are displaced slightly above the skin in the region of a superficial lesion. The distance between the sources and the lesion seldom is greater than 1 or 2 cm. The intervening space is often filled with material such as wax or plastic.
2. *Interstitial implants* are composed of radioactive needles, wires, or small encapsulated sources called "seeds" that are inserted into a lesion or into tissue in the immediate vicinity of a lesion.
3. *Intracavitary implants* are composed of radioactive sources that are placed in a body cavity.
4. *Intraluminal implants* involve the introduction of radioactive sources into the lumen of a vessel, duct, or airway.

Radioactive implants may be *temporary or permanent*. Temporary implants usually require that the patient be hospitalized for the duration of treatment, which generally lasts no more than a few days. At the end of the treatment, the sources are removed. In many cases, the sources are stored for subsequent use. Permanent implants, practical only for interstitial treatments, require that the sources remain in the tissue indefinitely. Sources with relatively short half-lives are used, so that the majority of the dose is delivered within a few weeks or months.

The choice of activity and nuclide often yields a low dose rate at the patient's external surfaces, and the patient presents little or no risk of radiation exposure to others. These patients can be released from the hospital as soon as their medical condition permits.

■ RADIUM SOURCES

Radium was used in the treatment of cancer almost immediately after its discovery by Marie and Pierre Curie. Within the next two decades, the separation of radioactive radon gas from decaying radium was achieved, and the radon gas, encapsulated into glass tubes, also was used for treatment. During this time, encapsulation techniques were developed to filter the beta particles from the decaying radium and radon sources, to prevent tissue necrosis close to the radioactive sources.

In the decades from 1920 to 1950, much clinical experience with radium and radon was obtained. Most of the techniques used in modern brachytherapy were developed during this period. Although radium and radon are rarely used in medicine today, the techniques developed with these sources are of great importance to modern brachytherapy and are described here.

Radium sources used for implant therapy contain ^{226}Ra in secular equilibrium with its decay products. Secular equilibrium can be established for a radium source because the half-life for radioactive decay is much greater for ^{226}Ra (1,600 years) than for any of the decay products of this nuclide. About one month is required for a new source of radium to approach secular equilibrium. To establish secular equilibrium, the source must be sealed to prevent the escape of gaseous radon-222. The decay scheme from ^{226}Ra to stable lead (^{206}Pb) is shown in Margin Figure 12-2. This sequence of radioactive transformations is part of the uranium decay series, of which ^{226}Ra is the sixth member. Although the γ rays used for radiation therapy are released primarily during the decay of ^{214}Pb (RaB) and ^{214}Bi (RaC) (Margin Figure 12-3),[1] pure sources of these nuclides are not used for therapy because their half lives are too short. The γ rays of highest energy in the decay scheme are the 2.2-MeV and 2.4-MeV γ rays emitted by ^{214}Bi. The average energy is about 0.8 MeV for the γ rays emitted from a sealed source of radium[2,3] (Table 12-1). On the average, 2.22 γ rays are emitted by a sealed source of radium for each decay of ^{226}Ra.

Construction of Radium Sources

Diagrammed in Margin Figure 12-4 are radium needles used in the past for interstitial implants, along with radium tubes that were used primarily for molds and intracavitary treatments. The radium was supplied in the form of a salt (radium sulfate or radium chloride), which was mixed with an inert filler such as magnesium oxide or barium sulfate. The small crystals of radium salt and filler were contained within cylindrical cells about 1 cm long. The cells were made of gold foil 0.1 to 0.2 mm thick and were sealed to prevent the escape of radon gas. Each source of radium contained 1 to 3 cells surrounded usually by a wall of platinum, which was reinforced with iridium (10%). The thickness (usually 0.5 or 1 mm) of the platinum–iridium wall was sufficient to absorb alpha and beta radiation from the source. Gamma rays were attenuated only slightly by the wall.

The exposure rate is 8.25 roentgen per hour (R/hr) at a distance of 1 cm from a 1-mCi point source (or 0.825 R/hr at 1 m from a 1-Ci source) of ^{226}Ra that is in secular equilibrium with its decay products and that is enclosed within a 0.5-mm Pt–Ir wall.[2,4] The value of 8.25 R·cm^2/hr·mCi is referred to as the *exposure rate constant* Γ_∞ for ^{226}Ra in secular equilibrium with its decay products. The exposure rate constant for radium should be increased by 2% for each 0.1 mm of wall thickness less than 0.5 mm; it should be decreased by 2% for each 0.1 mm of wall thickness greater than 0.5 mm.

Types of Radium Sources

Illustrated in Margin Figure 12-5 are three types of radium needles that have been used in the past for interstitial implants. *Uniform linear-density needles* were manufactured using full-intensity (0.66 mg/cm), half-intensity (0.33 mg/cm), or quarter-intensity (0.165 mg/cm) loadings. Needles with linear densities of 0.5 mg/cm and 0.25 mg/cm also were found useful. *Indian club needles* had a greater activity at one end and were useful for implants with one uncrossed end. *Dumbbell needles* had a greater activity at each end and were used for implants with both ends uncrossed. Tubes for intracavitary and mold therapy usually were furnished in multiples of 5 mg of radium and usually were constructed with a platinum–iridium wall 1 mm thick.

Also available in the past have been nasopharyngeal applicators containing as much as 50–100 mg of radium in a thin capsule of 0.2–0.3 mm of metal alloy (monel metal). These sources are particularly hazardous and should be disposed of if present in an institution.

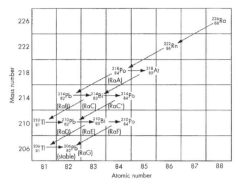

MARGIN FIGURE 12-2
Sequence of radioactive transformations for ^{226}Ra and its decay products. (From Hendee, W. R. *Medical Radiation Physics*, 1st edition. Chicago, Mosby–Year Book, 1970.)

A young physicist named William Duane worked with the Curies in 1907–1912 to separate radon gas from radium. Duane was the first professor of physics at the University of Colorado. Among other accomplishments, he is noted for having been one of the first in the United States to build an ionization chamber.

Radium sources are rarely found in clinical use in the United States today, having been replaced with safer alternatives. However, a few sources have been retained by clinics and the ADCLs for use as calibration standards.

The exposure rate constant Γ_∞ is related to the *specific gamma-ray constant* Γ but includes the x rays produced following internal conversion and photoelectric absorption events in the radium salt and in the encapsulation.

A supplier of radium sources was expected to specify:

1. The active length of each source (the distance between the ends of radioactive material in the core).
2. The actual length of each source.
3. The activity of each source (preferably including a standardization certificate).
4. The diameter and filtration of each source.

TABLE 12-1 Physical Properties of Radioactive Nuclides Used in Brachytherapy

Element	Isotope	Beta Particle Energy (MeV)[a]	Gamma Ray Energy (MeV)[b]	Exposure Rate Constant (R·cm²/hr·mCi)	Half-Life	HVL in Water (cm)[c]	HVL in Lead (mm)[c]	Clinical Uses	Source Form
Americium	^{241}Am	0.0039–0.0932	0.0139–0.0595	0.1216	432.2 yr	—	1.26	Intracavitary temporary implants	Tubes
Californium	^{252}Cf	2.13–2.15 neutrons	0.7–0.9	3.768[d]	2.645 yr	—	—	Temporary intracavitary implants	Tubes
Cesium	^{137}Cs	0.514–1.17	0.662	3.28	30 yr	8.2	6.5	Temporary intracavitary and interstitial implants	Tubes, needles
Cobalt	^{60}Co	0.313	1.17–1.33	13.07	5.26 yr	10.8	11	Temporary implants	Plaques, tubes, needles
Gold	^{198}Au	0.96	0.412–1.088	2.327	2.7 days	7.0	3.3	Permanent implants of prostate and other sites	Seeds
Iodine	^{125}I	None	0.0355	1.45[e]	59.6 days	2.0	0.02	Permanent interstitial implants of prostate, lung, and other sites, temporary implants of eye	Seeds
Iodine	^{131}I	0.25–0.61	0.08–0.637	2.2	8.06 days	5.8	3.0	"Cocktail" for thyroid therapy	Liquid, capsules
Iridium	^{192}Ir	0.24–0.67	0.136–1.062	4.62[f]	74.2 days	6.3	3.0	Temporary interstitial implants of Head, neck, breast, and other sites	Wires, Seeds
Palladium	^{103}Pd	—	0.020–0.0227	1.48	17 days	—	0.01	Permanent implants of prostate	Seeds
Phosphorus	^{32}P	1.71	None	—	14.3 days	0.1	0.1	Sodium phosphate injection, for bone and blood diseases; chromicphosphate pleural and intraperitoneal effusions	Liquid
Radium and decay products	^{226}Ra	0.017–3.26	0.047–2.44	8.25[g]	1622 yr	10.6	8.0	Temporary intracavitary and interstitial implants	Tubes, needles
Radon and decay products	^{222}Rn	0.017–3.26	0.047–2.44	8.25[g]	3.83 days	10.6	8.0	Permanent implants, many sites	Seeds
Ruthenium	^{106}Ru, ^{106}Rh	3.5 MeV max.	—	—	366 days	—	—	Temporary implants of eye	Plaques
Samarium	^{145}Sm	—	0.0382–0.0614	—	340 days	—	—	Medical uses currently under consideration	Seeds
Strontium	^{89}Sr	1.46	None	—	50 days	—	—	Injection for widespread bone metastases	Liquid
Strontium	^{90}Sr, ^{90}Y	0.54–2.27	None	—	28.9 yr 64 hr	0.15	0.14	Temporary application for shallow lesions (outpatient treatments)	Applicator
Tantalum	^{182}Ta	0.18–0.514	0.043–1.453	6.71	115 days	10.0	12	Temporary interstitial implants	Wires
Ytterbium	^{169}Yb	—	0.060–0.100	1.58[f]	32.0 days	—	—	Temporary and permanent implants	Seeds

[a] A dash separates the minimum and maximum energies of the β-particles in the spectra. All energies listed are the maximum energy of each particle.

[b] A dash separates the minimum and maximum energies of the γ rays in the spectra.

[c] Assumes narrow beam geometry, a condition usually not found in practical brachytherapy applications.

[d] For an encapsulated source with a wall thickness equivalent to 0.5 mm Pt-Ir alloy.[39] For radium and radon, the exposure rate constant is expressed in R · cm²/hr · mg.

[e] For an unfiltered point source with $\delta > 11.3$ keV.[40,41]

[f] Neutrons/fission.

[g] This value is reduced to 1.208 by the attenuation of the filtration incorporated into commercially available seeds, together with a correction for anisotropy.[42]

◼ SPECIFICATION OF BRACHYTHERAPY SOURCES

Sources for brachytherapy may be specified in one of several ways. As indicated earlier, radium sources have been specified in terms of the mass of radium in milligrams incorporated into the source. To facilitate their introduction into clinical use, sources composed of nuclides intended as substitutes for radium were originally, and in some cases still are, specified in terms of milligram equivalents of radium (mg-Ra-eq). This figure is the mass of radium required to produce the same exposure rate at 1 cm from the substitute source. For radium substitutes, the relationship between mCi and mg-equivalents is determined from the ratio of the exposure rate constants for the two nuclides (Example 12-3).

Example 12-1

What is the exposure rate at 5 cm from a 10-mg radium point source having a wall thickness of 1 mm?

The exposure rate constant for a radium source with a wall thickness of 0.5 mm is $8.25 \ R \cdot cm^2/hr \cdot mg$. It is

$$(8.25)(0.98)^5 = 7.46 \ R \cdot cm^2/hr \cdot mg$$

for a source with 1-mm-thick walls. The exposure rate is

$$(7.46)(10 \ mg)/(5 \ cm)^2 = 2.98 \ R/hr$$

at 5 cm from a 10-mg source.

Sources may also be specified in terms of their activity. The use of activity to specify a brachytherapy source is complicated by the influence of the source encapsulation on the exposure rate at some distance from the source. Sources with identical activities but with different encapsulation thicknesses may yield significantly different exposure rates at a distance. The *apparent activity* A_{app} of a source is determined from a measurement of the exposure rate at a distance; it describes the activity of that nuclide that would produce the same exposure rate when unencapsulated.

The National Council on Radiation Protection and Measurements Report No. 41 recommends specification of brachytherapy sources in terms of the exposure rate at 1 m from and perpendicular to the long axis of the source at its center.[3] More recently, the AAPM,[6] the British Commission on Radiation Units and Measurements,[7] and the Comite Français Measure des Rayonnements Ionisants[8] have recommended that brachytherapy sources be specified in terms of their air-kerma strength. The air-kerma strength (S_k) is the air-kerma rate measured at a specified distance, usually 1 m. Air-kerma strength is expressed in units of $\mu Gy \cdot m^2/hr$ or $cGy\text{-}cm^2/hr$. Air-kerma strength is related to the exposure rate X (R/hr) at a reference point in free space by the equation

$$S_k = X \cdot d^2 \cdot k \cdot \overline{W}/e \qquad (12\text{-}1)$$

where d is the distance along the perpendicular bisector of the source longitudinal axis to the point of measurement (usually 1 m), and the product $k \cdot \overline{W}/e$ has the value 0.876 cGy/R. In the United States, brachytherapy sources are calibrated by the AAPM-Accredited Dosimetry Calibration Laboratories (ADCLs), in terms of one or more of these units. Manufacturers likewise specify source calibrations in different ways, and users must apply caution when converting from an unfamiliar dose rate unit to a dose prescription unit.

Example 12-2

What is the air-kerma strength of a radium point source having an activity of 1 mg?

The exposure rate at 1 cm from a 1-mg radium point source is 8.25 R/hr. The air-kerma strength is determined from Equation (12-1) as

$$(8.25)(1 \ cm)^2(0.876) = 7.23 \ cGy \cdot cm^2/hr$$

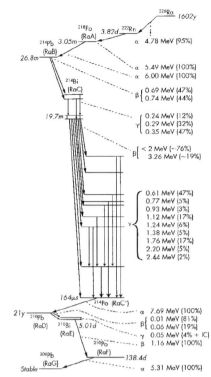

MARGIN FIGURE 12-3
A simplified decay scheme of ^{226}Ra and its decay products showing the radiations of greatest importance in brachytherapy. (Adapted from Lederer, C. M., Hollander, J. M., and Perlman, I. *Tables of Isotopes*, 6th edition. New York, John Wiley & Sons, 1967. Used with permission.)

Until recently, it was generally assumed that 1 mCi of radium has a mass of 1 mg. It is now known that 1 mg of radium actually has an activity of approximately 0.98 mCi.

The AAPM recommends against the use of *apparent activity* for clinical treatment planning.[5]

The international community uses the term *reference air-kerma rate* (RAKR), which is defined as the air-kerma rate at 1 m from the source in $\mu Gy/hr$.

S_K is expressed in units of $\mu Gy \cdot m^2/hr$ or, equivalently, $cGy \cdot cm^2/hr$.

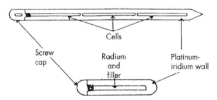

MARGIN FIGURE 12-4
A radium needle (**top**) and a radium tube (**bottom**). (From Hendee, W. R. *Medical Radiation Physics*, 1st edition. Chicago, Mosby–Year Book, 1970.)

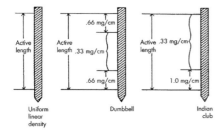

MARGIN FIGURE 12-5
Types of radium needles. (From Hendee, W. R. *Medical Radiation Physics*, 1st edition. Chicago, Mosby–Year Book, 1970.)

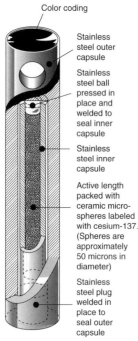

MARGIN FIGURE 12-6
A cut-away view of a model 6D6C ^{137}Cs source. (Courtesy of 3M Medical-Surgical Division, St. Paul, MN.)

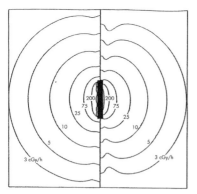

MARGIN FIGURE 12-7
Comparison between isodose curves from a ^{226}Ra (10.7 mg) source and a ^{137}Cs source (10 mg·Ra·eq) manufactured by Oris Corporation. Both sources have an air-kerma strength of 72 μGy·m^2/hr. (Courtesy of Jeffrey F. Williamson, Ph.D., Virginia Commonwealth University, Richmond, VA.)

■ RADIUM SUBSTITUTES

The use of radium sources is associated with several hazards. Seepage of radon (^{222}Rn) from a radium source is prevented by enclosing the source in a doubly sealed capsule. Nevertheless, "leaky" radium sources have occurred and have caused extensive radioactive contamination. Because of the buildup of radon gas, the pressure inside a new source of radium is slightly greater than atmospheric pressure. The internal pressure continues to increase over the years because:

1. Alpha particles emitted by ^{226}Ra and its decay products become gaseous atoms of helium after losing their kinetic energy.
2. The radiation-induced hydrolysis of water contained in the mixture of radium salt and filler produces gaseous O_2 and H_2. For this reason, care is taken to remove as much water as possible from the radium salt and filler.

Some believe that the increase in internal pressure, combined with the gradual loss of physical strength of the capsule, causes the probability of rupture of a radium source to increase with the age of the source. Radium sources should not be heated above 100°C because the pressure of a gas increases with temperature.[9]

Radium sources may be bent or broken by improper handling or, less frequently, by circumstances beyond the control of the user. The numerous hazards associated with the use of radium and radon have prompted the development of a number of substitute sources.

Cesium

The most common radium substitute is cesium-137. This source has largely replaced radium as an implant source. Sources of ^{137}Cs may be obtained as tubes or needles containing radioactive microspheres embedded in a ceramic matrix. A representative ^{137}Cs source is shown in Margin Figure 12-6. The tubes are typically 2.65 mm in external diameter with lengths of approximately 20 mm and active lengths of 14 mm. Larger and smaller sources are available. Generally, the activity of sources of ^{137}Cs is described in units of mg-equivalents of radium (mg-Ra-eq). Activities range between 5 and 40 mg-Ra-eq. These sources are safer than radium, because the radioactive material is a solid rather than a powder and because no gaseous radioactive products are produced during the decay of ^{137}Cs. The exposure rate constant for ^{137}Cs is 3.28 R·cm^2/hr·mCi. To determine the equivalent mass of radium, the activity in mCi is multiplied by the ratio of exposure rate constants for cesium and radium:

$$\text{Equivalent mass of radium} = \text{Activity in mCi} \cdot \frac{3.28\,\text{R}\cdot\text{cm}^2/\text{hr}\cdot\text{mCi}}{8.25\,\text{R}\cdot\text{cm}^2/\text{hr}\cdot\text{mg}}$$

Example 12-3

A new ^{137}Cs source is described by its manufacturer as containing 20 mg-equivalents of radium. How many mCi of cesium are contained in the source?

The activity is determined from Equation (12-2) as follows:

$$\text{mCi of } ^{137}\text{Cs} = 20\,\text{mg-Ra-eq} \cdot \frac{8.25\,\text{R}\cdot\text{cm}^2/\text{hr}\cdot\text{mg}}{3.28\,\text{R}\cdot\text{cm}^2/\text{hr}\cdot\text{mCi}}$$

$$\text{Activity} = 50.3\,\text{mCi}$$

^{137}Cs is a particularly well-suited substitute for radium, because it produces dose distributions in tissue that are virtually identical to those of radium (Margin Figure 12-7). Its 30-year half-life and single γ ray (0.662 MeV) help to make it a practical choice.

Cobalt

Sources of cobalt-60 were used in the past for interstitial and intracavitary implants. These sources were constructed as small wires of cobalt enclosed within a sheath of stainless steel or platinum–iridium. The short half-life of ^{60}Co (5.24 years) is an undesirable feature for a radium substitute, and these sources are rarely found in medical practice today.

Over a distance of at least 5 cm, the variation in dose rate is about equal for sources of radium, ^{137}Cs, and ^{60}Co. This relationship is depicted in Margin Figure 12-8.

Tantalum and Iridium

Sources of tantalum-182 were used as brachytherapy sources in the past, but have been replaced by sources with better characteristics. ^{182}Ta sources were provided as flexible wires about 0.2 mm in diameter encased in a platinum sheath with walls 0.1 mm thick. These sources could be inserted into locations that are not easily accessible to larger sources.[10–16] The 115-day half-life of ^{182}Ta is too long for this nuclide to be used as a permanent implant, and the maximum γ-ray energy of 1.45 MeV produces a less-than-desirable dose distribution. Tantalum-182 has largely been replaced by iridium-192, which has a 74-day half-life and emits γ rays with an average energy of 0.38 MeV. Iridium is available either as wire or as seeds. Iridium-192 wire is manufactured with a core of 25% iridium and 75% platinum either 0.1 or 0.3 mm in diameter made from 10% iridium and 90% platinum, which is encased in 0.1 mm of pure platinum to form seeds approximately 3 mm long.

The high specific activity of ^{192}Ir (more than 9000 Ci/g) makes it an attractive source for use when high dose rates are required. Sources with nominal activities of 10 Ci (3.7 × 10^{11} Bq, or $S_K = 4 × 10^4$ μGy · m^2/hr) are routinely used in high-dose rate (HDR) remote-afterloading equipment. These devices deliver dose rates as high as 700 cGy/min at 1 cm.[17,18] Consequently, HDR units must be operated in shielded rooms to avoid significant exposure to staff and other persons. A representative HDR source is shown in Margin Figure 12-9. A representative HDR remote afterloading brachytherapy unit is shown in Margin Figure 12-10.

Gold, Iodine, and Palladium

Radioactive gold-198 has a 2.7-day half-life and emits γ rays of 0.412 MeV. Seeds of ^{198}Au are still used on occasion as a radon seed substitute for permanent implants.[19] However, seeds of ^{125}I (half-life = 59.6 days) have essentially replaced ^{198}Au in medical use. Iodine-125 decays by electron capture and emits γ rays and x rays with energies in the range of 28–35 keV. With its low energies, ^{125}I is easily shielded with small thicknesses of lead (HVL = 0.02 mm of lead). Numerous designs of ^{125}I seeds are available, and several are shown in Margin Figure 12-11. The final panel of Margin Figure 12-11 shows a comparison of the angular dose distribution around several iodine seeds.[20–23]

Palladium-103 is also a reactor-produced nuclide with a half-life of approximately 17 days that undergoes decay by electron capture (Margin Figure 12-12). During decay, characteristic x rays in the range of 20 to 23 keV are emitted. The low photon energy and short half-life make ^{103}Pd an attractive isotope for permanent implants in organs such as the prostate.[24]

Americium-241 and Cesium-131

Americium-241 has been considered for specific brachytherapy applications. With its long half-life (432 years) and low photon energy (60 keV), ^{241}Am shows some promise as a substitute for radium in the treatment of gynecological disease. However, the low specific activity means that sources of ^{241}Am are quite large and unsuitable for other applications. The low γ energy makes practical the use of thin lead foils to protect sensitive organs.

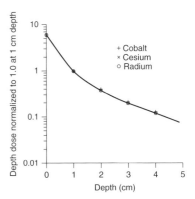

MARGIN FIGURE 12-8

Dose falloff as a function of distance in a tissue-equivalent phantom for sources of radium (10-mg, 0.5-mm Pt (Ir)), ^{137}Cs (17.1 mg·Ra·eq, 3M model 6D6C capsule), and ^{60}Co (15.0 mg·Ra·eq, Abbott model 6796 Actacel capsule). Each source is 3.1 mm in diameter and 20 mm long, with an active length of 14 mm. Measurements are normalized to 1.00 at 1 cm depth. (From Hendee, W. R. *Medical Radiation Physics*, 1st edition. Chicago, Mosby–Year Book, 1970. Courtesy of Lahr, T., and Grotenhuis, I. *An Evaluation of the Depth–Dose Relationship for Radium, Co-60 and Cs-137 Sources.* St. Paul, MN., 3M Company. Used with permission.)

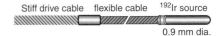

MARGIN FIGURE 12-9

A representative ^{192}Ir source for HDR remote afterloading brachytherapy. (Courtesy of Nucletron Corporation.)

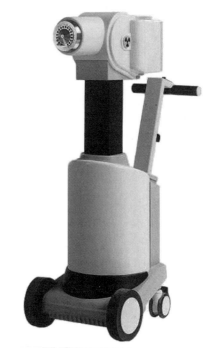

MARGIN FIGURE 12-10

An HDR remote afterloading brachytherapy unit. (Courtesy of Nucletron Corporation.)

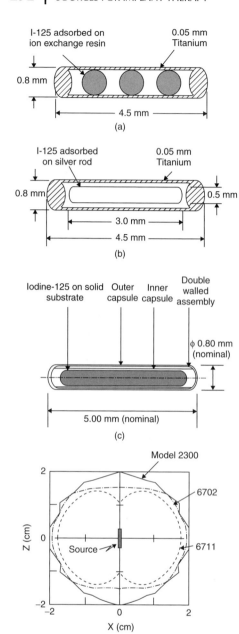

Three models of ^{125}I source. **A:** Mediphysics model 6702 seed, composed of ^{125}I adsorbed on spheres of ion exchange resin, separated by a gold sphere for radiographic localization. **B:** Mediphysics model 6711 seed containing ^{125}I adsorbed on a silver rod. **C:** Best Industries model 2300 seed containing ^{125}I adsorbed on a solid substrate. **D:** Comparison of the dose distribution around these three seeds. (From Weaver, K. A., Anderson, L. L., and Meli, J. A. Source characteristics. In *Interstitial Brachytherapy: Physical, Biological, and Clinical Considerations*, Anderson L. L., Nath, R., Weaver, K. A., et al. (eds.). New York, Raven Press, 1990 (for parts A, B, and C). From Nath, R., and Melillo, A. Dosimetric characteristics of a double wall ^{125}I source for interstitial brachytherapy. *Med. Phys.* 1993; 20:1475–1483. (for D). Used with permission).

Cesium-131 has a half-life of 9.7 days and photon energies in the range of 30 keV. Medical uses for this isotope are just now being considered.

OPHTHALMIC IRRADIATORS

Certain ophthalmologic conditions such as pterygium, vascularization, or ulceration of the cornea, as well as certain intraorbital malignancies such as melanomas, may be treated effectively with small radioactive applicators positioned on or near the sclera for a short period of time.[25,26] Applicators for the treatment of pterygium contain strontium-90 in secular equilibrium with yttrium-90. The low-energy beta particles from ^{90}Sr (0.54-MeV maximum) are absorbed by the encapsulation of the applicator, but the higher-energy betas from ^{90}Y (2.27-MeV maximum) penetrate the applicator and enter the sclera of the eye. The dose rate at the center of an applicator surface may be as high as 100 cGy/s.[27] The dose rate may vary greatly across the surface of an applicator. This dose rate may be made more uniform by constructing a compensating filter designed to fit over the end of the applicator.[28] The dose rate from a beta applicator decreases to about 5% of the surface dose rate at a depth of 4 mm, the depth of the lens below the cornea.[29]

Eye plaques are quite widely used to treat malignancies of the eye, such as choroidal melanoma.[30] These plaques may be loaded with γ-emitting sources such as ^{125}I or ^{103}Pd, or with beta emitters such as ruthenium-106 in equilibrium with rhodium-106 (see Chapter 13).

IMPLANTABLE NEUTRON SOURCES

Tubes containing radioactive californium (^{252}Cf) have been investigated as a replacement for radium.[31–33] Artificially produced ^{252}Cf (half-life = 2.65 years) fissions spontaneously with the release of 2.34×10^6 fast neutrons per second per microgram. Gamma rays also are emitted when ^{252}Cf fissions spontaneously. The range of neutrons released during fission is short compared with the penetration of γ rays. Californium-252 sources are constructed with platinum encapsulation to limit the γ-ray emission. Consequently, sources of ^{252}Cf deliver a high tumor dose with less radiation to surrounding normal structures. Also, hypoxic tumor cells may be destroyed more efficiently with ^{252}Cf because neutrons provide an oxygen enhancement ratio near unity. The small number and high cost of ^{252}Cf sources available limit their use to experimental therapy. Those sources are discussed in greater detail in Chapter 16.

RADIATION SAFETY OF BRACHYTHERAPY SOURCES

Storage

Because of their small size and the ease with which they may be misplaced, brachytherapy sources present a radiation safety hazard in radiation oncology facilities. Consequently, secure storage facilities and meticulous inventory techniques are required. Storage in an appropriately shielded container is essential, and the shielded container itself must be stored in a locked room, with access limited to persons directly involved in brachytherapy procedures. A lead safe is required for storage of radium and cesium sources, as well as for other sources of high-activity and energetic photon emissions. Sources emitting only low-energy photons are more easily shielded but also require secure storage.

Facilities required to handle and store brachytherapy sources in a safe manner vary with the amount of activity involved and the use of the sources. A few facilities have been described in the literature.[9,34–38] Radioactive sources for implant therapy always should be handled remotely or with forceps, and never directly with the hands. Whenever possible, sources should be viewed indirectly with mirrors rather than by direct vison.

Test for Uniform Distribution of Activity

An autoradiograph of a sealed radioactive source may be obtained by resting the source for a few seconds against an unexposed x-ray film. Simultaneously, the film may be exposed to low-energy x rays. Shown in Margin Figure 12-13 is an autoradiograph of a 1-mg radium needle exposed to x rays generated at 70 kVp. The increased optical density of certain regions of the image reflects the exposure of these regions to γ radiation from radium inside the needle. The image of the needle is visible under the blackened areas, permitting examination of the distribution of radioactive material along the core of the needle. The distribution is acceptable if it is relatively uniform along the entire length of the needle. It is advisable to examine new brachytherapy sources radiographically before they are accepted from the manufacturer. This is particularly advisable when radium sources are used, because the distribution of activity can become nonuniform. However, nonuniform distributions of activity have been observed with ^{125}I sources, and irregular spacing of ^{192}Ir seeds within catheters has occurred. Both situations are readily detected with autoradiography.

Evaluating the Safety of Brachytherapy Sources

Several methods have been developed for testing brachytherapy sources for leakage.[37] Three methods are described here:

1. The source may be swabbed with a moistened cotton swab. Any activity present on the surface of the source will be removed by the cotton swab, which is then placed into a scintillation counter. The removed activity is determined by first calibrating the spectrometer with a known source.
2. The leakage of radon gas from radium sources may be evaluated by placing a few needles or tubes in a test tube containing either cotton or activated charcoal. After a few hours, the sources are returned to the storage container and the cotton is monitored with a Geiger counter or scintillation detector. Radioactivity on the cotton or activated charcoal suggests that one of the sources is leaking. To identify the leaking source, the test must be repeated for each source individually.
3. A few needles or tubes are placed in a vial containing liquid scintillation "cocktail." After 1–2 hours, the sources are removed and residual activity is detected by analyzing the cocktail in a liquid scintillation counter. Residual activity in the vial indicates a leaking source. This method has been criticized because leaks in the source may be plugged temporarily by the liquid counting solution. Leaking sources should be sealed in a container and returned to the manufacturer.

■ SUMMARY

- Radium and radon seeds, the original brachytherapy sources, are no longer used; they have been replaced by sources of ^{137}Cs, ^{192}Ir, ^{182}Ta, ^{125}I and ^{103}Pd.
- Radioactive implants may be temporary (long-lived sources are used) or permanent (short-lived sources are used).
- Air-Kerma strength $\lfloor \mu Gy \cdot m^2/hr$ or $cGy \cdot cm^2/hr \rfloor$ is the current preferred expression to describe brachytherapy sources.

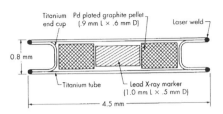

MARGIN FIGURE 12-12
Best Industries model 200 palladium-103 seed. The ^{103}Pd is plated on graphite pellets separated by a lead radiographic marker. (From Weaver, K. A., Anderson, L. L., and Meli, J. A. Source characteristics. In *Interstitial Brachytherapy: Physical, Biological and Considerations*, Anderson, L. L., Nath, R., Weaver, K. A., Nori, D., Phillips, T. L., Son, Y. H., Chiu-Tsao, S. T., Meigooni, A. S., Meli, J. A., and Smith, V. (eds.). New York, Raven Press, 1990. Used with permission.)

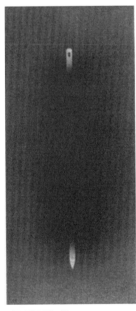

MARGIN FIGURE 12-13
Autoradiograph of a 1-mg radium needle exposed to x rays generated at 70 kVp. The activity is relatively uniform along each of the cells in the core of the needle. (From Hendee, W. R. *Medical Radiation Physics*, 1st edition. Chicago, Mosby–Year Book, 1970.)

PROBLEMS

12-1. For most radioactive sources, the rate of emission of γ rays decreases continuously. However, the rate of emission of γ rays from a sealed source of radium-226 (^{226}Ra) increases to a constant value over the first 30 days or so after the ^{226}Ra is placed in the sealed container. Why?

12-2. What is the activity in mCi of ^{226}Ra, radon-222 (^{222}Rn), ^{255}Po (polonium), and ^{214}Po in a 10-mg source of radium in secular equilibrium? What is the mass in grams of ^{222}Rn in the source?

12-3. What is the volume occupied by a "carrier-free" sample of radium sulfate (RaSO$_4$) that contains 1 mg of ^{226}Ra? The density of RaSO$_4$ is 5.42 g/cm^3. Does this volume of sample fill a 1-mg needle used for interstitial implants? If not, how is a nonuniform distribution of radioactive material avoided?

12-4. What is the activity of a 1-mg·Ra·eq ^{192}Ir source? A 1 mg·Ra·eq ^{60}Co source?

12-5. What is the air-kerma strength of a 1-mCi ^{125}I source?

12-6. What activity ^{125}I source will produce the same exposure rate at 10-cm distance in air as a 1-mCi ^{198}Au source?

REFERENCES

1. Lederer, C. M., Hollander, J. M., and Perlman, I. *Table of Isotopes*, 6th edition. New York, John Wiley & Sons, 1967.
2. Hendee, W. R. *Medical Radiation Physics*, 1st edition. Chicago, Mosby–Year Book, 1970.
3. National Council on Radiation Protection and Measurements. *Specification of gamma ray brachytherapy sources*, Report No. 41. Washington, DC, NCRP Publications, 1974.
4. Payne, W. H., and Waggener, R. G. A theoretical calculation of the exposure rate constant for radium-226, *Med. Phys.* 1974; **1**:210.
5. Williamson, J. F., Coursey, B. M., DeWerd, L. A., Hanson, W. F., Nath, R., and Ibbott, G. S. On the use of apparent activity (A_{app}) for treatment planning of ^{125}I and ^{103}Pd interstitial brachytherapy sources: Recommendations of the American Association of Physicists in Medicine Radiation Therapy Committee Subcommittee on Low-Energy Brachytherapy Source Dosimetry. *Med. Phys.* 1999; **26**(12):2529–2530.
6. AAPM Task Group No. 32. *Specification of brachytherapy source strength*, Report No. 21, June 1987.
7. British Committee on Radiation Units and Measurements. Specification of brachytherapy sources. *Br. J. Radiol.* 1984; **57**:941.
8. Comité Français Measure des Rayonnements Ionisants, *Recommendations pour la determination des doses absorhees en curietherapie*, CFMRI Report No. 1, 1983.
9. Meredith, W., and Massey, J. *Fundamental Physics of Radiology*. Baltimore, Williams & Wilkins, 1968.
10. Cohen, L. Protracted interstitial irradiation of tumors using ^{182}Ta. *Br. J. Radiol.* 1955; **28**:338.
11. Haybittle, J. Dosage distributions from "hairpins" of radioactive tantalum wire. *Br. J. Radiol.* 1957; **30**:49.
12. Sakhatshiev, A., and Moushmov, M. A new type of radioactive wire source. *Radiology* 1967; **89**:903.
13. Son, Y., and Ramsby, G. Percutaneous tantalum-182 wire implantation using guiding-needle technique for head and neck tumors. *Am. J. Radiol.* 1966; **96**:37.
14. Trott, N., and Whearley, B. Tantalum-182 wire gamma ray applicators for use in ophthalmology. *Br. J. Radiol.* 1956; **29**:13.
15. VanMiert, P., and Fowler, J. The use of tantalum-182 in the treatment of early bladder carcinoma. *Br. J. Radiol.* 1956; **29**:508.
16. Wallace, D., Stapleton, J., and Turner, R. Radioactive tantalum wire implantation as a method of treatment for early carcinoma of the bladder. *Br. J. Radiol.* 1952; **25**:421.
17. Meigooni, A. S., Kleiman, M. T., Johnson, J. L., Mazloomdoost, D., and Ibbott G. S. Dosimetric characteristics of a new high-intensity ^{192}Ir source for remote afterloading. *Med. Phys.* 1997; **24**(12):2008–2013.
18. Goetsch, S. J., Attix, F. H., Pearson, D. W., and Thomadsen, B. R., Calibration of ^{192}Ir high-dose-rate afterloading systems. *Med. Phys.* 1991; **18**(3):462–467.
19. Slanina, I., and Wannenmacher, M. Interstitial radiotherapy with ^{198}Au seeds in the primary management of carcinoma of the oral tongue. *Int. J. Radiol. Biol. Phys.* 1982; **8**:1683.
20. Nath, R., and Melillo, A. Dosimetric characteristics of a double wall ^{125}I source for interstitial brachytherapy. *Med. Phys.* 1993; **20**(5):1475–1483.
21. Weaver, K. A., Anderson, L. L., and Meli, J. A. Source characteristics. In *Interstitial Brachytherapy: Physical, Biological, and Clinical Considerations*, L. Anderson, R. Nath, K. A. Weaver, Nori, D., Phillips, T. L., Son, Y. H., Chiu-Tsao, S. T., Mciqooni, A. S., Meli, J. A., and Smith, V. (eds.). New York, Raven Press, 1990.
22. Gearheart, D. M., Drogin, A., Sowards, K., Meigooni, A. S., and Ibbott, G. S. Dosimetric characteristics of a new ^{125}I brachytherapy source. *Med. Phys.* 2000; **27**(10):2278–2285.
23. Hedtjarn, H., Carlsson, G. A., and Williamson, J. F. Monte Carlo-aided dosimetry of the Symmetra model 125.S06 ^{125}I, interstitial brachytherapy seed. *Med. Phys.* 2000; **27**:1076–1085.
24. Williamson, J. F. Monte Carlo modeling of the transverse-axis dose distribution of the Model 200 ^{103}Pd interstitial brachytherapy source. *Med. Phys.* 2000; **27**:634–654.
25. Duggan, H. Results using strontium-90 beta-ray applicator on eye lesions. *J. Can. Assoc. Radiol.* 1966; **17**:132.
26. Friedell, H., Thomas, C., and Krohmer, J. Evaluation of clinical use of strontium-90 beta-ray applicator with review of underlying principles. *Am. J. Radiol.* 1954; **71**:25.
27. Deasy, J. O., and Soares, C. G. Extrapolation chamber measurements of ^{90}Sr+ ^{90}Y beta-particle ophthalmic applicator dose rates. *Med. Phys.* 1994; **21**(1):91–99.
28. Hendee, W. R. Measurement and correction of nonuniform surface dose rates for beta eye applicators. *Am. J. Radiol.* 1968; **103**:734.
29. Hendee, W. R. Thermoluminescent dosimetry of the beta depth dose. *Am. J. Radiol.* 1966; **97**:1045.
30. Nag, S., Quivey, J. M., Earle, J. D., Followill, D. S., Fontanesi, J., and Finger, P. The American Brachytherapy Society Recommendations for Brachytherapy of Uveal Melanomas, *Int. J. Radiat. Oncol. Biol. Phys.* 2003; **56**:544–555.
31. Oliver, G., and Wright, C. Dosimetry of an implantable ^{252}Cf source. *Radiology* 1969; **92**:143.
32. Reinig, W. Advantages and applications of ^{252}Cf as a neutron source. *Nucl. Applic.* 1968; **5**:24.
33. Wright, C., et al. Implantable californium-252 neutron sources for radiotherapy, *Radiology* 1967; **89**:337.
34. Hendee, W. R., and Lohlein, S. Handling radium in a hospital. *Radiol. Technol.* 1968; **39**:221.
35. Johns, H., and Cunningham, J. *The Physics of Radiology*, 3rd edition. Springfield, III, Charles C Thomas, 1969.
36. Morgan, J., and Nunnally, J. Report on a radium safe and leak testing system. *Radiology* 1969; **92**:161.
37. National Council on Radiation Protection and Measurements. *Protection against radiation from brachytherapy sources*, Report No. 40. Washington, DC, NCRP Publications, 1972.
38. Webb, H. An improved radium safe. *Br. J. Radiol.* 1960; **33**:654.
39. Pochin, E. E., and Kermode, J. C. Protection problems in radionuclide therapy: The patient as a gamma ray source. *Br. J. Radiol.* 1975; **48**:299.
40. Glasgow, G. P., and Dillman, L. T. Specific γ-ray constant and exposure rte constant of ^{192}Ir. *Med. Phys.* 1979; **6**:49.
41. Glasgow, G. P. The specific γ-ray constant and exposure rate constant of ^{182}Ta. *Med. Phys.* 1982; **9**:250.
42. Anderson, L. L., Kaum, H. M., and Ding, I. Y. Clinical dosimetry with I-125. In *Modern Interstitial and Intracavitary Radiation Cancer Management*, F. W. George (ed.). New York, Masson Publishing, 1981.

13

BRACHYTHERAPY TREATMENT PLANNING

OBJECTIVES   296

RADIATION DOSE FROM BRACHYTHERAPY SOURCES   296

SIEVERT INTEGRAL   297

ISODOSE DISTRIBUTIONS FROM INDIVIDUAL
SEALED SOURCES   300

DESIGN OF IMPLANTS   300

Intracavitary Implant Applicators   300
Interstitial Implant Applicators   301

DISTRIBUTION RULES FOR INTERSTITIAL IMPLANTS   302

The Quimby System   303
The Manchester System   305
The Paris System   311

AIR-KERMA STRENGTH CALCULATION   313

DOSE OVER TREATMENT DURATION   316

PLAQUES   316

REMOTE AFTERLOADING   317

RADIOGRAPHIC LOCALIZATION OF IMPLANTS   318

THREE-DIMENSIONAL IMAGE-BASED IMPLANTS   322

Prostate Seed Implants   322
Prostate HDR   325
LDR Gynecologic Interstitial Implant   327
Breast Brachytherapy   327

THERAPY WITH RADIOPHARMACEUTICALS   327

INTRAVASCULAR BRACHYTHERAPY   328

SUMMARY   329

PROBLEMS   329

REFERENCES   330

Radiation Therapy Physics, Third Edition, by William R. Hendee, Geoffrey S. Ibbott, and Eric G. Hendee
ISBN 0-471-39493-9 Copyright © 2005 John Wiley & Sons, Inc.

■ OBJECTIVES

By studying this chapter, the reader should be able to:

- Compute the dose at a specified distance from a brachytherapy source.
- Describe different interstitial and intracavitary implant systems.
- Calculate the dose delivered for temporary and permanent implants.
- Discuss methods for localizing brachytherapy sources from planar images.
- Give examples of volumetric imaging techniques for high and low dose rate brachytherapy.

■ RADIATION DOSE FROM BRACHYTHERAPY SOURCES

Early prescriptions for brachytherapy treatments were expressed in terms of radiation exposure, and they neglected the effects of photon scatter and attenuation in tissue. For many sources, the contributions of scattered radiation to a point very nearly compensate for the tissue attenuation of radiation reaching the same point. Consequently, calculations that neglect the presence of tissue can be reasonably accurate. The exposure rate (in R/hr) at some distance r (cm) from a "point source" of radioactive material is

$$\dot{X} = \frac{\Gamma_\infty A}{r^2} \tag{13-1}$$

where A is the activity of the source, and Γ_∞ is the exposure rate constant for the nuclide (Table 12-1). For radium filtered by 0.5-mm Pt(Ir) and in equilibrium with its decay products,

$$\Gamma_\infty = \frac{8.25 \text{ R} \cdot \text{cm}^2}{\text{mCi} \cdot \text{hr}}$$

Example 13-1

What is the exposure rate at a distance of 100 cm from a 50-mCi point source of radium filtered by 0.5 mm of Pt(Ir)?

$$\dot{X} = (8.25 \text{ R} \cdot \text{cm}^2/\text{hr} \cdot \text{mCi})\frac{A}{r^2}$$

$$\dot{X} = (8.25 \text{ R} \cdot \text{cm}^2/\text{hr} \cdot \text{mCi})\frac{50 \text{ mCi}}{(100 \text{ cm})^2}$$

$$\dot{X} = 41.2\frac{\text{mR}}{\text{hr}}$$

The exposure rate $\dot{X}$ at a location P at a distance r from a radioactive source of short length L and linear density ρ is described by the equation

$$\dot{X} = \frac{\Gamma_\infty \rho L e^{-\mu t/\cos\theta}}{r^2} \tag{13-2}$$

where μ is the attenuation coefficient of the wall of thickness t for the x and γ rays emitted by the source (Figure 13-1). The absorption of radiation from the source is greatest in directions at small angles with respect to the source axis, and least in directions perpendicular to the source axis. This "self-absorption" of radiation leads to an anisotropic dose distribution around the source. To facilitate "point-source" calculations, small sources are frequently characterized in terms of their "effective activity," which takes into account the anisotropy.

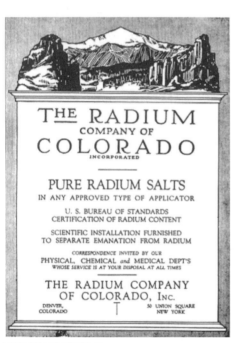

MARGIN FIGURE 13-1
Advertisement for the Radium Company of Colorado.

In the early 1900s, radium was popular as the desired prophylaxis for: gout, rheumatism, enhanced urine secretion, stimulation of digestive tract activity, blood vessel dilation, hypertension, insomnia, increased sexual activity, neuralgia, sciatica, diabetes, and catarrh.

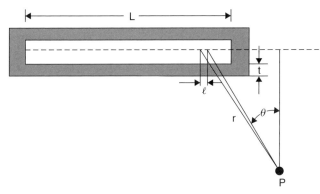

FIGURE 13-1
Geometry for calculating the exposure rate at location P near a radium source of active length L. (From Hendee, W. R. *Medical Radiation Physics,* 1st edition. St. Louis, Mosby–Year Book, 1970.)

SIEVERT INTEGRAL

For a source of greater length L, the exposure rate $\dot{X}$ is computed by integrating Equation (13-2) over the length L. The equation cannot be integrated in closed form, but may be approximated by a technique using the Sievert integral.[1] With this approach, Meredith[2] compiled data for radium sources with different active lengths and wall thicknesses. The data describe the product of the amount of radium in milligrams and the exposure time in hours required for an exposure of 1000 R at locations along a line perpendicular to the center of a radium source. Quimby[3] expanded these data to include locations described as distances "along" (parallel with) the source axis and "away" (perpendicular to) from the source axis. The "along distance" is the distance from the center of a source to the location where a line coincident with the source axis and a line through the location of interest intersect at a right angle. The "away distance" is the distance between this intersection and the location of interest. Greenfield and associates[4] revised Quimby's tables to furnish data that describe the exposure/mg-hr at locations on a 0.5-cm grid surrounding a source of radium.

Sievert's method for calculating the dose at points around a linear source requires that the relationship between the point of interest and the source be expressed in terms of (a) the angle between a perpendicular from the point to the source longitudinal axis and (b) lines to each of the source elements. The resulting Sievert integral is shown as Equation (13-3).

$$\dot{D}(r, \theta) = \frac{\Gamma_\infty A f}{lr} \int_{\theta_1}^{\theta_2} e^{-\mu t / \cos \theta} d\theta \qquad (13\text{-}3)$$

In this equation, $\dot{D}(r, \theta)$ is the dose rate at point $P(x, y)$, Γ_∞ is the exposure rate constant, A is the activity of a source element, f is the f factor (exposure to dose conversion), l is the source element length, r is the distance from the source element to the point $P(x, y)$, μ is the attenuation coefficient of the wall of thickness t, and θ is the angle between r and a perpendicular from $P(x, y)$ to the source axis.

The geometry of this integral is shown in Figure 13-2.[5] Equation (13-3) applies only in zone I, which includes only those points that the radiation can reach without passing through an end of the source. Hence, only perpendicular or oblique transmission of the radiation through the side wall of the source is considered. In zone II, transmission of radiation at an oblique angle through either the side wall or end wall of the source is considered. At points in zone III, only the end wall is considered, while in zone IV all of the radiation is assumed to pass perpendicularly through the end wall. In all zones, an attenuation correction for the source material itself must be considered. Some contemporary calculations consider additional zones through more complex computations.

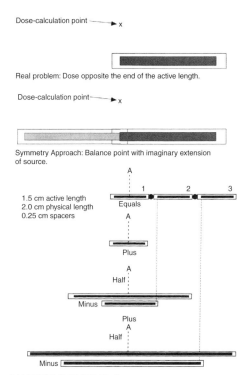

MARGIN FIGURE 13-2
Symmetry in brachytherapy. The dose at a point off the perpendicular bisector can be computed using the principle of symmetry as shown in the diagrams. Illustrations are from Thomadsen, B. R. Brachytherapy radionuclides, dosimetry and dose distributions. In *Biomedical Uses of Radiation,* Part B, W. R. Hendee (ed.). New York, Wiley-VCH, 1999.

The Sievert integral accounts for wall thickness changes as a function of angle for a linear source. The Sievert integral is solved using numerical analytic methods.

$$\int_{\theta_1}^{\theta_2} e^{-\mu t / \cos \theta} d\theta$$

Although no longer in use clinically, radium and its properties have persisted as the foundation for many of the brachytherapy treatments given today with other types of sealed sources. The use of units such as "milligrams radium equivalent," along with conversion of radium dose tables for different radionuclides, was done to ensure consistency of treatment as the replacement sources were implemented clinically.

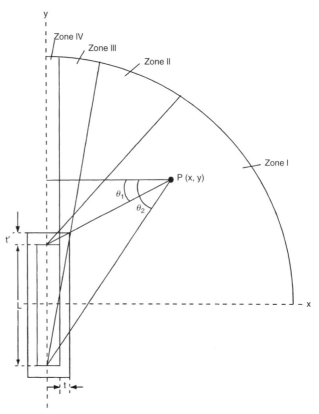

FIGURE 13-2
Geometry used for calculating the dose rate at a point near a line source, according to the Sievert integral.

The Sievert integral, with corrections for attenuation and scatter in soft tissue around the source,[6] has been used by Shalek and Stovall[7] to compute tables of dose rates similar to those prepared by Quimby. An excerpt of these data is shown in Tables 13-1 and 13-2. The data are corrected for oblique filtration of the γ rays in the radium salt and in the walls of the needles. Calculated dose rates around the sources appear in Table 13-3.

TABLE 13-1 Dose (cGy) per mg · hr in Tissue Delivered at Various Distances by Linear Radium Sources[a]

Perpendicular Distance from Source (cm)	Distance Along Source Axis (cm from Center)										
	0.0	0.5	1.0	1.5	2.0	2.5	3.0	3.5	4.0	4.5	5.0
0.25	50.67	43.75	11.94	3.34	1.48	0.81	0.50	—	—	—	—
0.5	20.26	16.95	8.18	3.38	1.70	1.00	0.64	0.44	0.31	0.23	0.18
0.75	10.84	9.29	5.67	2.99	1.67	1.03	0.69	0.48	0.35	0.27	0.21
1.0	6.67	5.89	4.10	2.52	1.55	1.01	0.69	0.50	0.37	0.28	0.22
1.5	3.20	2.96	2.38	1.74	1.24	0.89	0.65	0.48	0.37	0.29	0.23
2.0	1.85	1.76	1.52	1.23	0.96	0.74	0.57	0.45	0.35	0.28	0.23
2.5	1.20	1.15	1.04	0.89	0.74	0.60	0.49	0.40	0.32	0.26	0.22
3.0	0.83	0.81	0.75	0.67	0.58	0.49	0.41	0.34	0.29	0.24	0.21
3.5	0.61	0.60	0.57	0.52	0.46	0.40	0.35	0.30	0.26	0.22	0.19
4.0	0.47	0.46	0.44	0.41	0.37	0.33	0.29	0.26	0.23	0.20	0.17
4.5	0.37	0.36	0.35	0.33	0.30	0.28	0.25	0.22	0.20	0.18	0.16
5.0	0.30	0.29	0.28	0.27	0.25	0.23	0.21	0.19	0.17	0.16	0.14

[a] Filtration = 0.5-mm Pt (lr). Active length = 1.5 cm.

Source: Shalek, R. J., and Stovall, M. Dosimetry in implant therapy. In *Radiation Dosimetry*, F. H. Attix and E. Tochin (eds.). New York, Academic Press, 1969, p. 776. Used with permission.

TABLE 13-2   Dose (cGy) per mg · hr in Tissue Delivered at Various Distances by Linear Radium Sources[a]

Perpendicular Distance from Source (cm)	Distance Along Source Axis (cm from Center)										
	0.0	0.5	1.0	1.5	2.0	2.5	3.0	3.5	4.0	4.5	5.0
0.25	45.87	39.70	10.19	—	—	—	—	—	—	—	—
0.5	18.56	15.51	7.25	2.88	1.39	0.78	0.49	—	—	—	—
0.75	10.01	8.54	5.10	2.60	1.43	0.86	0.56	0.38	0.27	0.20	0.16
1.0	6.20	5.44	3.72	2.23	1.35	0.86	0.58	0.41	0.30	0.22	0.17
1.5	2.99	2.75	2.18	1.57	1.10	0.78	0.56	0.41	0.31	0.24	019
2.0	1.73	1.64	1.40	1.12	0.86	0.65	0.50	0.39	0.30	0.24	0.20
2.5	1.12	1.08	0.97	0.82	0.67	0.54	0.43	0.35	0.28	0.23	0.19
3.0	0.78	0.76	0.70	0.62	0.53	0.44	0.37	0.31	0.26	0.21	0.18
3.5	0.57	0.56	0.53	0.48	0.42	0.37	0.31	0.27	0.23	0.19	0.17
4.0	0.44	0.43	0.41	0.38	0.34	0.31	0.27	0.23	0.20	0.17	0.15
4.5	0.34	0.34	0.33	0.31	0.28	0.26	0.23	0.20	0.18	0.16	0.14
5.0	0.28	0.27	0.26	0.25	0.23	0.22	0.20	0.18	0.16	0.14	0.13

[a] Filtration = 1.0-mm Pt (lr). Active length = 1.5 cm.

Source: Shalek, R. J., and Stovall, M. Dosimetry in implant therapy. In *Radiation Dosimetry*, F. H. Attix and E. Tochin (eds.). New York, Academic Press, 1969, p. 776. Used with permission.

Example 13-2

What is the dose rate at point P in Figure 13-2? The source is a 10-mg radium tube with an active length of 1.5 cm, filtered by 0.5-mm Pt(Ir). Point P is located at $x = 2$ cm, $y = 2$ cm (the midpoint of the source is at the origin).

The "along" and "away" distances are both 2 cm, so from Table 13-1 the dose rate = (0.96 cGy/mg hr)(10 mg) = 9.6 cGy/hr.

What is the dose rate at P if the source is a cesium tube of 10 mg-Ra-eq, with active length = 1.4 cm and filtration = 1-mm stainless steel?

From Table 13-3,

$$\text{Dose rate} = (0.975 \text{ cGy/mg-Ra-eq hr})(10 \text{ mg-Ra-eq}) = 9.75 \text{ cGy/hr}$$

A Monte Carlo analysis of the Sievert integral has been performed for radium sources.[8] The analysis indicates that while the Sievert integral overestimates dose rates in tissue per unit activity, the error is reduced if the source intensity is expressed in units of exposure rate rather than activity.

Rolf Sievert was a prominent Swedish physicist who was very active for many years in the International Commission on Radiological Protection.

TABLE 13-3   Dose (cGy) per mg · hr in Tissue Delivered at Various Distances by Linear [137]Cs Sources[a]

Distance Along Length of Source (cm from Center)	Transverse Distance from Center of Source (cm)									
	0.5	1.0	1.5	2.0	2.5	3.0	3.5	4.0	4.5	5.0
0.0	21.052	6.808	3.241	1.866	1.204	0.837	0.614	0.468	0.368	0.296
0.5	17.445	5.997	2.996	1.773	1.162	0.816	0.602	0.461	0.364	0.293
1.0	8.404	4.177	2.409	1.536	1.051	0.758	0.569	0.441	0.351	0.285
1.5	3.663	2.597	1.777	1.245	0.902	0.676	0.521	0.411	0.331	0.271
2.0	1.943	1.639	1.275	0.975	0.750	0.585	0.464	0.375	0.307	0.255
2.5	1.187	1.093	0.925	0.757	0.613	0.498	0.407	0.336	0.280	0.236
3.0	0.794	0.768	0.686	0.591	0.500	0.420	0.353	0.298	0.253	0.216
3.5	0.566	0.564	0.522	0.466	0.408	0.353	0.304	0.262	0.226	0.196
4.0	0.422	0.429	0.407	0.374	0.336	0.298	0.262	0.230	0.202	0.177
4.5	0.326	0.335	0.325	0.304	0.279	0.252	0.226	0.201	0.179	0.159
5.0	0.258	0.268	0.263	0.250	0.233	0.214	0.195	0.177	0.159	0.143

[a] Filtration = 1.0-mm stainless steel. Active length = 1.4 cm.

Source: Reprinted with permission from Krishnaswamy, V. Dose distributions about ^{137}Cs sources in tissue. *Radiology*, 1972; **105**:181–184.

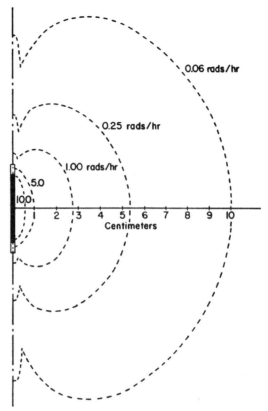

FIGURE 13-3
Isodose distribution for a 1 mg radium needle. (Reprinted with permission from Rose, J., Bloedorn, F., and Robinson, J. A computer dosimetry system for radium implants. *Am. J. Radiol.* 1966; **97**:1032.)

■ ISODOSE DISTRIBUTIONS FROM INDIVIDUAL SEALED SOURCES

Isodose curves for a sealed source may be measured, or may be computed with data such as those in Tables 13-1, 13-2, and 13-3. An isodose distribution computed for a 1-mg radium needle is shown in Figure 13-3. The dose rate is reduced near the ends of the needle because γ rays emitted at a slight angle with respect to the source axis are filtered by a greater thickness of the platinum–iridium wall. Measurement of isodose distributions has been accomplished using ionization chambers,[9,10] diodes,[11] thermoluminescent dosimeters,[12,13] and film dosimetry.[14] Because many brachytherapy sources emit a spectrum of x and γ rays, attention must be paid to the response of the detector to different photon energies.

■ DESIGN OF IMPLANTS

Intracavitary Implant Applicators

Cancer of the uterus and cervix often is treated with an applicator designed to hold sealed radioactive sources in a fixed position against the cervix and in the uterine canal. One to four sealed sources are contained within a central tube ("tandem"), which is inserted into the uterine canal. Additional sources are placed in capsules or "ovoids" positioned against the cervix. The ovoids may be separated from each other by rubber or plastic spacers. One of the first applicators designed for treatment of the cervix is shown in Figure 13-4.[15] Several modern intracavitary applicators are shown in Figure 13-5.

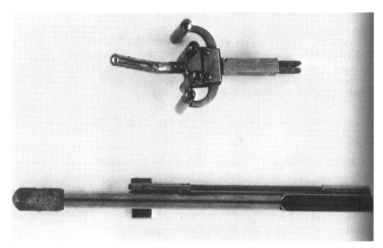

FIGURE 13-4
Expanding Ernst applicator for sealed source therapy of cancer of the cervix and uterus. (Reprinted with permission from Hendee, W. R. *Medical Radiation Physics*, 1st edition. St. Louis, Mosby–Year Book, 1970.)

When cancer of the cervix or uterus is treated with sealed sources, the absorbed dose is generally calculated at points identified as A and B. Point A is located 2 cm laterally from the uterine canal and 2 cm above the lateral fornix. Point B is located on the pelvic wall 3 cm lateral to point A (MF 13-3). The absorbed dose to these points from each source in the applicator may be computed with data such as those in Tables 13-1, 13-2, and 13-3. The total dose to points A and B is the sum of the contributions from each source. The total dose also should be computed for the anterior wall of the rectum and the posterior wall of the bladder. If the computed doses are excessive, gauze inserted between the applicator and the rectum or bladder may be repacked to provide greater separation. Dose rates along the anterior wall of the rectum and in the bladder may be measured with lithium fluoride or with a dosimeter such as a cadmium sulfide probe. Modern brachytherapy applicators incorporate lead or tungsten shielding to provide additional protection to the rectum and bladder. The influence of the shielding material on the dose distribution has been measured (Figure 13-6), but corrections are rarely applied in clinical practice.[16,17] Clinical techniques for low-dose-rate brachytherapy in the treatment of cervical cancer have been summarized by the American Brachytherapy Society.[18]

Personnel involved in brachytherapy implants are potentially subject to high radiation exposures. "Afterloading" techniques have been developed to reduce these exposures.[19–21] Some afterloading applicators are shown in Figure 13-5. Sources are not introduced into the applicator until the applicator itself has been positioned inside the patient and packed into position. The sources are then installed quickly and in a manner that minimizes the radiation exposure to personnel.

Interstitial Implant Applicators

Early interstitial applications were administered by inserting radium needles directly into tissue. Today, interstitial implants may be temporary (the sources are removed after a few hours or days of treatment) or permanent (the sources remain in the patient permanently). Permanent implants are practical only when sources with a short half-life are used. The sources are inserted directly into the tissue being treated, and they generally are positioned with an applicator such as that shown in Figure 13-7. When a temporary interstitial implant is used, catheters may be introduced into the tissue, and radioactive sources encased in nylon ribbons are passed through the catheters and fixed into place for the duration of treatment. For both permanent and temporary implants, rules are available for positioning the sources to achieve a desired dose distribution.

Institutions frequently differ in their designations of points A and B. The Gynecologic Oncology Group has recommended a method to identify these points. An alternate recommendation for identifying reproducible calculation points is described in ICRU Report No. 39.[24] With the increased use of CT and MRI in treatment planning for brachytherapy, these definitions may eventually be replaced by patient-specific treatment volumes much like three-dimensional conformal treatment planning for external beam radiotherapy.

Note that there are two points A and two points B, with one A and one B on each side of the uterus.

One of the most durable contributions of the Manchester system is the definition of points A and B. Point A simultaneously represents two treatment-limiting conditions: (1) the lateral aspect of the target organ (the cervix) that must receive at least the minimum target dose and (2) the location of dose-sensitive normal structures, the ureter and the uterine artery, that limit the maximum dose tolerated.

The procedure for identifying points A and B changed in 1953. On x-ray images, the ovoids often cast very little shadow, making the baseline difficult to establish. Instead of a line connecting the tops of the sources to the ovoids, the new origin became the bottom of the most inferior tandem source. Due to the construction of the spacer that separates the ovoids and holds the tandem in place, this origin usually falls near the original baseline. When afterloading tandems became prevalent, the origin frequently was defined by the position of the flange abutting the external cervical os to prevent the tandem from perforating the top of the uterus.

While each of the definitions of points A and B (and others that have appeared in the literature from time to time) yields points A that fall close together, they are not exactly aligned. The general location of point A lies near a steep gradient in dose rate. Hence, small changes in the definition of point A can produce large variations in the delivered dose.

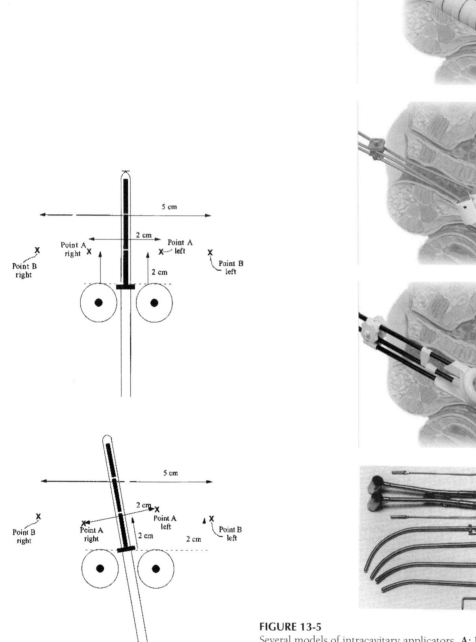

MARGIN FIGURE 13-3
Point A is 2 cm lateral from the uterine canal and 2 cm above the lateral fornix. Point B is on the pelvic wall 3 cm lateral to Point A.

FIGURE 13-5
Several models of intracavitary applicators. **A:** HDR segmented cylinders. **B:** HDR Fletcher/Williamson tandem and ovoids. **C:** HDR CT/MR compatible tandem and ring. **D:** LDR Fletcher–Suit–Delclos tandem and ovoids. (Parts A–C courtesy of Nucletron Corporation; Part D courtesy of Mick Radio-Nuclear Instruments, Inc.)

■ DISTRIBUTION RULES FOR INTERSTITIAL IMPLANTS

Three approaches have been widely used for determining the amount and distribution of activity required for a surface mold or interstitial implant. These approaches were developed with radium sources but are widely used for radium substitutes such as cesium and iridium. To some extent, the rules can be used without modification so long as the source activities are expressed in mg-Ra-eq.

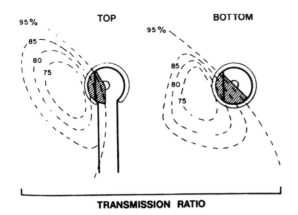

FIGURE 13-6
Effect of bladder and rectal shields in the coronal plane above and below a Fletcher–Suit colpostat. The dashed curves indicate the transmission of the tungsten shielding. (Reprinted with permission from Haas, J. S., Dean, R. D., and Mansfield, C. M. Fletcher–Suit–Delclos gynecologic applicator: Evaluation of a new instrument. *Int. J. Rad. Oncol. Biol. Phys.* 1983; **9**:763–768.)

The Quimby System

With the approach described as the Quimby system, the implant is composed of one or more planes containing a uniform distribution of sealed sources. The radiation dose to tissue near the center of the plane is much greater than that delivered to tissue near the edges. With the Quimby system, a uniform distribution of sealed sources is used to produce a nonuniform distribution of radiation dose to the treated region. Listed in Table 13-4 are the number of milligram-hours of radium required to deliver an absorbed dose of 1000 cGy to locations along a line drawn perpendicular to the center of the implant plane. At any distance from the implant plane, the dose decreases with lateral displacement from this perpendicular line. Data in Table 13-4 may be used for surface molds and for one- and two-plane interstitial implants, provided that sealed sources are distributed uniformly over the implant plane(s).

Example 13-3

Using the Quimby approach, determine the amount and distribution of radium (0.5-mm Pt(Ir)) required for a treatment mold 2 cm above a 4 × 6 area. A dose

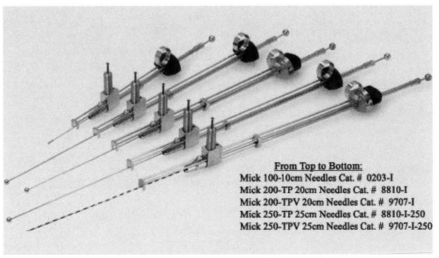

From Top to Bottom:
Mick 100-10cm Needles Cat. # 0203-I
Mick 200-TP 20cm Needles Cat. # 8810-I
Mick 200-TPV 20cm Needles Cat. # 9707-I
Mick 250-TP 25cm Needles Cat. # 8810-I-250
Mick 250-TPV 25cm Needles Cat. # 9707-I-250

FIGURE 13-7
Instrument for interstitial implants. (Courtesy of Mick Radio-Nuclear Instruments, Inc.)

TABLE 13-4   Milligram-Hours Required for Absorbed Dose of 1000 cGy at Locations Along a Line Perpendicular to Center of Applicator or Implant Plane[a,b]

| Distance (cm) | Circular Applicators (Diameter in cm) | | | | | |
	1	2	3	4	5	6
0.5	47	80	110	181	234	319
1.0	145	187	234	319	394	482
1.5	301	345	426	506	598	725
2.0	528	577	646	745	846	977
2.5	782	846	920	1016	1229	1346
3.0	1160	1224	1298	1404	1522	1665

| Distance (cm) | Square Applicators (Length of side in cm) | | | | | |
	1	2	3	4	5	6
0.5	49	85	122	210	266	372
1.0	150	200	253	348	431	544
1.5	314	367	442	544	638	782
2.0	532	606	686	795	910	1064
2.5	777	846	952	1075	1213	1458
3.0	1160	1224	1351	1479	1617	1777

| Distance (cm) | Rectangular Applicators (Dimensions in cm) | | | | | |
	1 × 1.5	2 × 3	3 × 4	4 × 6	6 × 9	8 × 12
0.5	54	110	152	305	606	1016
1.0	157	228	291	453	772	1181
1.5	317	394	496	664	1005	1442
2.0	538	628	761	930	1319	1777
2.5	767	894	1053	1213	1617	2128
3.0	1181	1266	1420	1617	2054	2660

[a] Modified from data of Quimby, E. In *Physical Foundations of Radiology*, 4th edition. P. Goodwin, E. Quimby, and R. Morgan, New York, 1970. Harper & Row.

[b] The radium sources are distributed uniformly across the plane and filtered by 0.5-mm Pt(lr).

of 6000 cGy in 72 hr is desired at the center of the area. What is the dose 1 cm below the skin?

From Table 13-4, 930 mg-hr is required for 1000 cGy. The number of milligram hours required for 6000 cGy is

$$\text{mg} \cdot \text{hr} = \frac{930 \text{ mg} \cdot \text{hr}}{1000 \text{ cGy}} \cdot 6000 \text{ cGy}$$

$$= 5580 \text{ mg} \cdot \text{hr}$$

The number of milligrams of radium required is

$$\text{mg} = \frac{5580 \text{ mg} \cdot \text{hr}}{72 \text{ hr}}$$

$$= 77 \text{ mg}$$

The radium is distributed uniformly over the mold.

From Table 13-4, the fractional depth dose FDD 1 cm below the surface is the ratio of mg· hr at 2 cm and 3 cm.

$$\text{FDD} = \frac{930 \text{ mg} \cdot \text{hr}}{1617 \text{ mg} \cdot \text{hr}}$$

Fractional depth dose = 0.57

Edith Quimby was a prominent medical physicist who worked in radiation oncology for many years at Columbia University.

TABLE 13-5   Milligram-Hours Required for Absorbed Dose of 1000 cGy at Locations Along Line Perpendicular to Center of Applicator or Implant Plane[a,b]

Area (sq. cm)	Treatment Distance (cm)									
	0.5	1.0	1.5	2.0	2.5	3.0	3.5	4.0	4.5	5.0
0	32	127	285	506	792	1139	1551	2026	2566	3166
1	72	182	343	571	856	1204	1625	2100	2636	3295
2	103	227	399	632	920	1274	1697	2172	2708	3349
3	128	263	448	689	978	1331	1760	2241	2772	3383
4	150	296	492	743	1032	1388	1823	2307	2835	3450
5	170	326	531	787	1083	1436	1881	2369	2896	3513
6	188	354	570	832	1134	1495	1938	2432	2956	3575
7	204	382	603	870	1182	1547	1993	2490	3011	3634
8	219	409	637	910	1229	1596	2047	2548	3067	3694
9	235	434	667	946	1272	1645	2099	2605	3123	3752
10	250	461	697	982	1314	1692	2149	2660	3178	3809
12	278	511	755	1053	1396	1780	2247	2769	3284	3917
14	306	557	813	1120	1475	1865	2341	2870	3389	4027
16	335	602	866	1184	1553	1947	2429	2968	3490	4131
18	364	644	918	1245	1622	2027	2514	3063	3585	4240
20	392	682	968	1303	1690	2106	2601	3155	3682	4341
22	418	717	1021	1362	1755	2180	2683	3242	3777	4441
24	444	752	1072	1420	1821	2252	2764	3326	3872	4540
26	470	784	1122	1477	1881	2328	2841	3405	3962	4634
28	496	816	1170	1530	1943	2398	2917	3484	4047	4730
30	521	846	1215	1582	2000	2468	2997	3562	4131	4824
32	546	876	1261	1635	2060	2532	3073	3639	4220	4915
34	571	909	1305	1688	2119	2598	3145	3713	4306	5000
36	594	935	1349	1743	2179	2662	3215	3787	4389	5089
38	618	967	1392	1793	2234	2726	3285	3859	4466	5174
40	642	994	1432	1843	2290	2787	3351	3931	4546	5258
42	664	1024	1472	1894	2344	2848	3421	4003	4626	5341
44	685	1053	1511	1942	2399	2908	3484	4071	4706	5422
46	708	1080	1550	1990	2452	2966	3548	4139	4781	5505
48	729	1110	1585	2037	2504	3025	3612	4207	4857	5586
50	750	1141	1619	2083	2556	3082	3676	4275	4929	5668
60	851	1283	1790	2319	2815	3362	3974	4605	5288	6054
70	947	1426	1944	2532	3059	3628	4257	4913	5632	6419
80	1044	1567	2092	2726	3301	3891	4532	5213	5958	6756

[a] Modified from data of Meredith, W. (ed.). *Radium Dosage: The Manchester System*, 2nd edition. Baltimore, Williams & Wilkins, 1967.

[b] Radium sources are distributed in a nonuniform manner across the plane to provide a dose rate which varies by less than ±10% across the plane. The sources are filtered by 0.5-mm Pt(lr).

Consequently, the absorbed dose 1 cm below the surface is

$$(6000 \text{ cGy})(0.57) = 3420 \text{ cGy}$$

The Manchester System

With the Manchester system for the construction of surface molds and interstitial implants, the sealed sources are arranged in a nonuniform manner to furnish a distribution of radiation dose that varies by less than ± 10% across the implant plane(s). Shown in Table 13-5 is the number of milligram-hours of radium required to deliver an absorbed dose of 1000 cGy to locations along a line perpendicular to the center of the implant plane. Rules for distributing the activity across the implant are described in Table 13-6.

Manchester interstitial implant rules—Planar Implants

Area (cm²)	On Periphery	Over the Interior
<25	2/3	1/3
25–100	1/2	1/2
>100	1/3	2/3

The Manchester system (Manchester, England) is also known as the "Paterson–Parker" system after its developers R. Paterson and H. Parker.

TABLE 13-6   Systems for Interstitial Brachytherapy

	Paterson and Parker IManchester)	Quimby	Paris
Representative dose and dose rate	6000–8000 R in 6–8 days 1060 R/day or 40 R/hr)	5000–6000 R in 3–4 days (60 R/hr to 70 R/hr is expected to be biologically equivalent to Manchester system)	6000–7000 cGy in 3–11 days (25–90 cGy/hr); usually in 3–6 days
Dose prescription point(s)	Effective minimum dose is 10% above the absolute minimum dose in a plane or volume	Planar implants: on the perpendicular bisector to the plane. Volume implants: to the periphery point receiving a minimum dose, the minimum in the actual implanted region	Basal dose is the average of the minimum doses in the central plane in the region defined by the source; reference dose is 85% of the basal dose and encompasses the target plane, or volume
Dose gradient	Does not vary by more than 10%, except in localized hot spots around the source	No stated goal; the intent was to determine the increased dose gradients resulting from using sources all with the same linear activity; gradient frequently approaches 100% with twice the dose in the center as at the edge of the region	15% between reference dose and basal dose (average minimum) by definition
Linear activity	Variable (0.66 mg Ra/cm, 0.50 mg Ra/ cm, 0.33 mg Ra/cm)	Constant (1.0 mg Ra/cm used historically; 0.20–0.70 mg Ra eq/cm commonly used)	Constant 0.8 to 0.6 mg Ra eq/cm commonly used
Activity distribution: single plane	Areas smaller than 25 cm^2; 2/3 activity on periphery, 1/3 activity in center Areas 25–100 cm^2; 1/2 activity on periphery, 1/2 activity in center Areas >100 cm^2; 1/3 activity on periphery, 2/3 activity in center	Uniform distribution over implant plane	Uniform distribution over implant plane
Activity distribution: volume	Cylinder: 4/8 of the activity in the belt; 2/8 of the activity in the core 1/8 of the activity on each end. Sphere: 6/8 of the activity in the rind 2/8 of the activity in the core. Cube: 1/8 of the activity in each face 2/8 of the activity in the core	Uniform distribution of activity throughout the volume	For volume, the sources are arranged in planes such that the sources in adjacent planes form either equilateral triangles or squares. Spacing between planes is about 0.87 times the spacing between sources for equivalent triangles.
Source implant pattern and spacing between sources as a function of implant volume	Constant uniform spacing; 1-cm separation between sources recommended	Variable but uniform spacing with up to 2-cm separation allowed between sources; spacing between sources determined by implant target dimensions	Variable but uniform spacing. Spacing determined by implant target dimensions; larger source separation in larger volumes; 5-mm minimum to 20-mm maximum separation
Crossing needles	Perpendicular to and at the active ends of the plane of sources; if placed beyond the active ends of the needles, should be double strength. Crossing needles required; if one end uncrossed, then area of implant for calculation is decreased by 10%. Twenty percent area reduction. Correction (10% each end) for both ends uncrossed	Same as Paterson and Parker	Not used; active sources are 20% to 30% longer than the target volume at *both* ends to compensate for uncrossed ends
Elongation factors	Area: long side/short side ratio and % correction: 2/1 (+ 5%); 3/1 (+ 9%); 4/1 (+ 12%) Volume: length/diameter ratio and % correction: 1.5/1 (+ 3%); 2/1 (+ 6%); 2.5/ 1 (+ 10%); 3/1 (+ 15%)	Same as Paterson and Parker	Not used
Relation of source length to target (volume) length	Active length determines target length (or vice versa); inner needles (not periphery) determine target width	Same as Paterson and Parker	Active source lengths 20% to 30% longer than the target dimensions at both ends to compensate for uncrossed ends

Example 13-4

Repeat Example 13-3 using the Manchester system. The area of the implant is 4×6 cm $= 24$ cm^2.

From Table 13-5, 1420 mg · hr is required for a uniform ($\pm 10\%$) dose of 1000 cGy over the entire treated area. The number of milligram hours required for 6000 cGy is

$$\text{mg} \cdot \text{hr} = \frac{1420 \text{ mg} \cdot \text{hr}}{1000 \text{ cGy}}(6000 \text{ cGy})(1.025)$$

$$= 8750 \text{ mg} \cdot \text{hr}$$

where 1.025 is an elongation correction obtained from Table 13-5. The number of milligrams of radium is

$$\text{mg} = \frac{8750 \text{ mg} \cdot \text{hr}}{72 \text{ hr}}$$

$$= 121 \text{ mg}$$

The radium is evenly distributed entirely on the periphery of the implant plane, because the short side of the rectangular implant is not greater than twice the treatment distance (Table 13-6). The linear density of the radium around the 20-cm periphery of the implant plane is

$$\frac{121 \text{ mg}}{20 \text{ cm}} \approx 6 \text{ mg/cm}$$

Therefore, 36 mg of radium should be distributed along each 6-cm side and 24-mg along each of the shorter sides. This distribution is achieved approximately by placing four 10-mg sources along each 6-cm side and two 10-mg sources along each 4-cm side.

From Table 13-5, the fractional depth dose 1 cm below the skin is the ratio of the mg · hr at 2 cm and 3 cm.

$$\text{FDD} = \frac{1420 \text{ mg} \cdot \text{hr}}{2252 \text{ mg} \cdot \text{hr}}$$

Fractional depth dose $= 0.63$

Consequently, the absorbed dose 1 cm below the surface is

$$(6000 \text{ cGy})(0.63) = 3780 \text{ cGy}$$

By comparing Examples 13-3 and 13-4, it is apparent that more activity is required for an implant designed according to the Manchester system than for one designed by the Quimby system, provided that the doses are equal at the center of the treated area. However, the radiation dose is more uniform with the Manchester System.

Data in Tables 13-4, 13-5, and 13-6 may be used to compute the number of milligram-hours of radium or radium substitute required for one- and two-plane interstitial implants. A single-plane implant is adequate if the thickness of the region to be treated does not exceed 1 cm. For this type of implant, the sources are inserted in the center of the treated region and a treatment distance of 0.5 cm is used for computation (Example 13-5). If the thickness of the treated region is greater than 1 cm but less than 2.5 cm, a two-plane implant may be used (Example 13-6). Volume implants are necessary for regions more than 2.5 cm thick (Example 13-7).

British standard radium needles, those associated with the Manchester system, came in two linear radium densities: "full strength" of 0.66 mg/cm, and "half strength" of 0.33 mg/cm.

For a planar implant, the Manchester system always specifies the dose in a plane 0.5 cm from the plane containing the needles.

Example 13-5

Using the Manchester system, determine the amount and distribution of radium required to treat a 3×6 cm region 1 cm thick with a single plane implant with one uncrossed end. The absorbed dose should be 5000 cGy in approximately 120 hr.

With correction for the uncrossed end (Table 13-6), the area of the implant plane is

$$(3 \text{ cm})(6 \text{ cm})(1.10) = 20 \text{ cm}^2$$

From Table 13-5, the number of milligram-hours required for an actual treated area of 18 cm², increased by an elongation factor of 1.05, is

$$\text{mg} \cdot \text{hr} = (364 \text{ mg} \cdot \text{hr}/1000 \text{ cGy})(5000 \text{ cGy})(1.05)$$
$$= 1920 \text{ mg} \cdot \text{hr}$$
$$\text{mg} = 1920 \text{ mg} \cdot \text{hr}/120 \text{ hr}$$
$$= 16.0 \text{ mg}$$

The short side (3 cm) of the implant is greater than twice the treatment distance of 0.5 cm. Hence, two extra lines of radium spaced 1 cm apart should be added parallel to the long side of the implant (Table 13-6). The linear density desired for these lines is $2\rho/3$, where ρ is the linear density of the outside lines. To calculate ρ, use the equation

$$6.6\rho + 6.6\rho + \left(\frac{2}{3}\rho\right)6.6 + \left(\frac{2}{3}\rho\right)6.6 + 3.0\rho = 16.0 \text{ mg}$$
$$25\rho = 16.0 \text{ mg}$$
$$\rho = 0.64 \text{ mg/cm}$$

The implant could be made according to the diagram below.

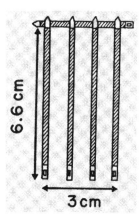

The needles on the periphery of this implant have a linear density of 0.66 mg/cm, and the needles along the inner lines have a linear density of 0.5 mg/cm. The total activity of the implant is 18.3 mg. The treatment time is

$$\text{Treatment time} = (120 \text{ hr})\frac{16.0 \text{ mg}}{18.3 \text{ mg}} = 104.9 \text{ hr}$$

Example 13-6

A two-plane implant designed according to the Manchester system is used to treat a volume of tissue 2.5 cm thick and 5 × 5 cm². One end of the implant is uncrossed. The minimum absorbed dose is 5000 cGy to the treated tissue. The treatment time is roughly 120 hr. What are the amount and distribution of radium on each plane?

The treated region is diagrammed below.

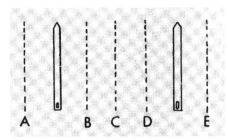

If the implant planes are placed 0.25 cm from the margins of the tissue volume to be treated, then the minimum dose occurs along plane C, 1 cm from each implant plane. The area of the implant plane, corrected for the uncrossed end, is

$$\text{Area} = (5 \text{ cm})(5 \text{ cm})(1.10) = 27.5 \text{ cm}^2$$

From Table 13-5, the number of milligram hours required for an area of 25 cm^2 and an absorbed dose of 5000 cGy to locations in plane C is

$$\text{mg} \cdot \text{hr} = (770 \text{ mg} \cdot \text{hr}/1000 \text{ cGy})(5000 \text{ cGy}) = 3850 \text{ mg} \cdot \text{hr}$$

For a treatment time of 120 hr, the number of milligrams of radium is

$$\text{mg radium} = 3850 \text{ mg} \cdot \text{hr}/120 \text{ hr} = 32.0 \text{ mg}$$

Half of the radium (16 mg) is distributed across each of the two planes. To satisfy the rules in Table 13-6, the following distribution might be used for each plane.

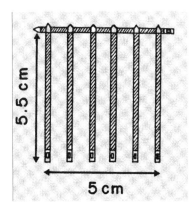

To calculate the linear density ρ, use the equation

$$2(5.5 \text{ cm})\rho + 4(5.5 \text{ cm})\left(\frac{2}{3}\rho\right) + (5 \text{ cm})\rho = 16 \text{ mg}$$

$$30.7\rho = 16 \text{ mg}$$

$$\rho \approx 0.5 \text{ mg/cm}$$

The needles along the periphery should possess a linear density of 0.5 mg/cm, and the needles along the internal lines should possess a linear density of 0.33 mg/cm. The total activity in each plane of the implant is 15.3 mg. The treatment time should be increased slightly.

$$\text{Treatment time} = (120 \text{ hr})\frac{16 \text{ mg}}{15.3 \text{ mg}} = 125 \text{ hr}$$

The dose to locations on planes B and D is

$$\left(\frac{5000 \text{ cGy}}{2}\right)\left(\frac{770 \text{ mg} \cdot \text{hr}}{458 \text{ mg} \cdot \text{hr}}\right) + \left(\frac{5000 \text{ cGy}}{2}\right)\left(\frac{770 \text{ mg} \cdot \text{hr}}{1100 \text{ mg} \cdot \text{hr}}\right)$$

$$= 4190 \text{ cGy} + 1750 \text{ cGy}$$

$$= 5940 \text{ cGy}$$

The dose to locations on planes A and E is

$$\left(\frac{5000 \text{ cGy}}{2}\right)\left(\frac{770 \text{ mg} \cdot \text{hr}}{458 \text{ mg} \cdot \text{hr}}\right) + \left(\frac{5000 \text{ cGy}}{2}\right)\left(\frac{770 \text{ mg} \cdot \text{hr}}{1850 \text{ mg} \cdot \text{hr}}\right)$$

$$= 4190 \text{ cGy} + 1040 \text{ cGy}$$

$$= 5230 \text{ cGy}$$

An improved implant might be achieved by separating the implant planes by 1.5 cm rather than by 2.0 cm.

Rules for interstitial implants must be modified if one or both ends of the implant are not crossed with additional sources. If one end of an implant is uncrossed, then the area of the implant plane over which radium is distributed should be increased by 10%, with the increased area located at the uncrossed end. The implant area is increased by 20% if both ends are uncrossed. The original area is used to determine the amount of radium required for the implant.

In the situation where an implant has been performed and the dose is to be determined retrospectively, the rules for uncrossed ends are modified. Rather than using the actual area of the implant when referring to the tables, the area is reduced by 10% if one end is uncrossed and by 20% if both ends are uncrossed.

If the thickness of tissue to be treated exceeds 2.5 cm, a volume implant should be used. Volume implants usually are made in the shape of a sphere, cylinder, or cube and may be considered as a "rind" (surface) with an inner "core." With the Manchester system, the sealed sources are arranged by rules to furnish a relatively uniform absorbed dose throughout the treated region. With the Quimby approach, the sources are distributed uniformly and the absorbed dose at the center of the treated region is about twice that at the edges.

In Table 13-7, the milligram-hours required to deliver a uniform absorbed dose of 1000 cGy are tabulated as a function of the volume of the treated region. Included in Table 13-7 are elongation factors, to be applied if the treated volume is not symmetric. According to the Manchester system, distribution rules for a volume implant are:

Sphere: Rind, 6 parts; core, 2 parts.
Cylinder: Belt, 4 parts; ends, 1 part each; core, 2 parts.
Cube: Each side 1 part; ends, 1 part each; core, 2 parts.

Most volume implants with sealed sources are cylindrical. If one end of a cylindrical implant is not crossed, the volume of tissue over which the sources are distributed should be increased by 7.5%, with the extra volume added to the uncrossed end. If both ends of the implant are uncrossed, the implant volume should be increased by 15%. The original volume is used to determine the activity required for the implant. The sealed sources on each surface of the implant are spaced evenly, with at least seven or eight needles on the belt of a cylinder.

Data in Table 13-8 furnish the milligram-hours required for a volume implant designed by the Quimby method. The minimum absorbed dose to the treated region is 1000 cGy, and the dose at the center is much greater than 1000 cGy. Elongation factors should be employed if the treated volume is not symmetric. The number of milligram-hours required for an absorbed dose of 1000 cGy is higher with the Quimby approach to volume implants, because with this approach the minimum

---

"Effective area"—the area used to look up R_A values for an implant, when one or both of the ends is uncrossed.

$A_{\text{eff}} = (0.9) \times (\text{width}) \times (\text{length})$ for one end uncrossed

$A_{\text{eff}} = (0.8) \times (\text{width}) \times (\text{length})$ for both ends uncrossed

Manchester system volume implants

$R_V = 3.78 \cdot V^{2/3} e^{0.07(E-1)}$ in mg Ra eq $\cdot$ h/Gy

$R_V = 27.3 \cdot V^{2/3} e^{0.07(E-1)}$ in mCi $\cdot$ h/Gy (^{137}Cs)

where V is the volume of the implant and E is the longest principal axis/shortest principal axis.

TABLE 13-7   Milligram-Hours Required for a Uniform Absorbed Dose of 1000 cGy Throughout a Volume Implant[a,b]

Volume (cc)	mg-hr/1000 cGy (0.5-mm Pt(Ir))	Length/Diameter	Elongation Correction
1	36.3	1.5	+3%
3	75.4	2.0	+6%
5	106	2.5	+10%
10	168	3.0	+15%
15	220		
20	267		
30	350		
40	425		
50	493		
60	556		
80	673		
100	782		
140	979		
180	1156		
220	1322		
260	1479		
300	1672		

[a] Modified from data of Meredith, W. (ed.). *Radium Dosage: The Manchester System*, 2nd edition. Baltimore, Williams & Wilkins, 1967.

[b] For asymmetric volumes, the number of milligram-hours should be increased by an elongation correction.

dose is 1000 rad. With the Manchester system, the absorbed dose is approximately 1000 cGy throughout the treated region.

The Paris System

In the early 1970s, the availability of radioactive iridium wire led to the development of the *Paris system* for interstitial implant calculations. The system was designed

TABLE 13-8   Milligram-Hours Required for Minimum Absorbed Dose of 1000 rad in Volume Implant[a,b]

Volume (cc)	mg-hr for 1000 cGy	Diameter of Sphere (cm)	mg-hr for 1000 cGy
5	213	1.0	43
10	340	1.5	106
15	415	2.0	192
20	468	2.5	298
30	575	3.0	415
40	660	3.5	505
60	798	4.0	612
80	926	4.5	718
100	1064	5.0	841
125	1192	6.0	1138
150	1330	7.0	1490
175	1479		
200	1596		
250	1788		
300	1915		

[a] Modified from data of Quimby, E. In P. Goodwin, E. Quimby, and R. Morgan (eds.). *Physical foundations of radiology*, 4th edition. New York, Harper & Row, 1970.

[b] The radium sources are distributed uniformly and filtered by 0.5-mm Pt(Ir).

originally for use with continuous wires of iridium, but was later adapted for implants constructed with iridium seeds in nylon ribbons, with the assumption that the linear activity (mCi/cm) is constant. The Paris method does not permit use of crossing sources; instead, the length of the sources is chosen to extend beyond the target volume at both ends of the implant (Table 13-6). The spacing between sources, which may vary from 5 mm to 20 mm, is kept uniform for a given implant. For volume implants, the sources are arranged in parallel planes, with the spacing between planes equal to 0.87 times the spacing between sources in a plane. The planes may be arranged so that the sources form a rectilinear pattern, or the sources in alternate planes may be offset by half the distance between sources.

Several parameters must be quantified when the Paris system is used (Figure 13-8). The *basal dose rate* is the average of the dose rates at points intermediate between the sources, in a central plane perpendicular to the sources. From this value, a *reference dose rate* is computed as 85% of the basal dose rate. If the implant is designed according to the rules of the Paris method, the reference dose rate corresponds to an isodose curve that encompasses the target volume. The length of the volume encompassed by the reference dose rate isodose line is shorter than the length of the sources, which should be chosen to exceed the dimensions of the target volume

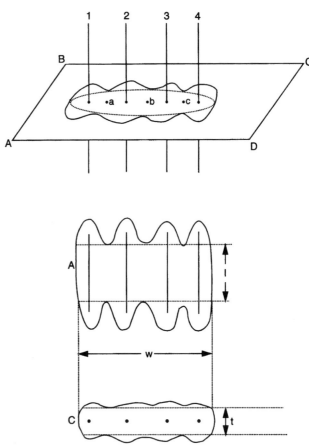

FIGURE 13-8

Some definitions used in the Paris system of interstitial implants. Four ribbon or wire sources (1, 2, 3, 4) transect the central plane (A, B, C, D) on which the dose calculation is carried out. The basal dose rate (BD) is the mean of the dose rates a, b, and c midway between the sources. The reference dose rate (0.85 BD) has an irregular contour (wavy line) and totally encloses the target volume. The length (l) of the treatment volume is the separation between the minimum indentations in the reference isodose curves; the width (w) is determined by the maximum extent of the reference dose rate curve. The reference dose rate and length and width are specified in the plane containing the sources. (Redrawn with permission from Pierquin, B., Dutreix, A., Paine, C. H., Chassagne, D., Marinello, G., and Ash, D. The Paris system in interstitial radiation therapy. *Acta Radiol. Oncol.* 1978; **17**:33.)

by 20% to 30%. The width and thickness of the volume encompassed by the reference dose rate isodose line are determined by the number of sources and the number of planes, respectively.[22] The Paris system has been compared with the Manchester system and offers several advantages.[23]

AIR-KERMA STRENGTH CALCULATION

Brachytherapy sources sometimes are specified in terms of their *air-kerma strength* (S_k), expressed in units of μGy-m^2/hr or cGy-cm^2/hr. When these units are used, the dose rate $\dot{D}(r, \theta)$ in the vicinity of the source is expressed as[24]

$$\dot{D}(r, \theta) = S_k \cdot \Lambda \cdot \frac{G(r, \theta)}{G(r = 1 \text{ cm}, \theta = \pi/2)} \cdot g(r) \cdot F(r, \theta) \qquad (13\text{-}4)$$

where Λ is the dose-rate constant for the source and surrounding medium defined at 1 cm away from the source on its perpendicular bisector.[25] The dose-rate constant is expressed in units of cGy/hr per unit air-kerma strength. In other words,

$$\Lambda = \frac{\dot{D}(1, \pi/2)}{S_k}$$

The value of the dose-rate constant Λ depends on the medium surrounding the source, because it indicates the rate at which energy is absorbed by the medium. It also depends on the design and construction of the source, because these factors influence the scattering of photons in the medium. Values of the dose-rate constant are available from the literature, source manufacturers, and calibration laboratories. Source strength conversion factors for several sources are given in Table 13-9.

$G(r, \theta)$, the *geometry function* with units of cm^{-2}, describes the decrease in dose as a function of distance from the source. For a point source, $G(r, \theta) = r^{-2}$. For a line source of significant length and uniform distribution of activity, $G(r, \theta) = (\theta_2 - \theta_1)/Ly$ (see Figure 13-2). By dividing by the value of G at 1 cm and 90°, the units cancel. Representative values of $G(r, \theta)$ are shown in Table 13-10.

Paris system "basal dose"—A local minimum in the dose distribution, identified as the point midway between the needles in the implant. Averaging of all basal doses within an implant gives the overall basal dose, or BD.

Paris system "reference dose"—The prescription is to the reference dose, which is 85% of the basal dose.

RD = 0.85 BD

The earliest use of implants by Regaud in Paris was widely referred to in the past as the "Paris" system. This system was supplanted by the Manchester system. This earlier terminology should not be confused with the "Paris" system discussed in this chapter.

Batho and Young developed a single table for use with all sources of a given filtration based on "relative coordinates." The relative coordinate $J = z/L$, where L is the active length of the source.

TABLE 13-9 Source Strength Conversion Factors for Interstitial Brachytherapy Source[a]

Sources	Source Strength Quantity	Units	Exposure Rate Constant $(\Gamma\delta)_x$ or Exposure Rate Constant for Filtration $(\Gamma\delta)_{x,t}$ R cm$^2 \cdot$ m Ci$^{-1} \cdot$ hr^{-1}	Air-kerma Strength Conversion Factor (S/Quantity)[c]
All	Equivalent mass of Radium	mg $\cdot$ Ra $\cdot$ eq	8.25	7.227 U mg-Ra-eq^{-1}
All	Reference exposure rate	mR $\cdot$ m$^2 \cdot$ hr^{-1}	—	8.760 U/mR m$^2 \cdot$ hr^{-1}
		nR $\cdot$ m$^2 \cdot$ sec^{-1}	—	3.154×10^{-2} U/nR m^2 sec^{-1}
		C $\cdot$ kg^{-1} m$^2 \cdot$ sec^{-1}	—	1.222×10^{11} U/C kg$^{-1} \cdot$ m$^2 \cdot$ sec^{-1}
^{192}Ir seed $t = 0.2$-mm Fe	Apparent activity	mCi	4.60	4.030 U mCi^{-1}
^{192}Ir seed $t = 0.05$-mm Pt-Ir	Apparent activity	mCi	4.80[b]	4.205 U mCi^{-1}
^{125}I seeds	Apparent activity	mCi	1.45	1.270 U mCi^{-1}
^{103}Pd seeds	Apparent activity	mCi	1.48	1.293 U mCi^{-1}

[a] Data from Williamson and Nath (reference 69)

[b] See the explanation for using 4.80 versus 4.60 in reference 69. Briefly the manufacturer uses 4.80 in calibrating the sources; therefore the user must also use the same number.

[c] 1u = 1 unit of Air Kerma Strength = 1uGy $\cdot$ m^2, h^{-1} = 1cGy $\cdot$ cm$^2 \cdot$ h^{-1}

TABLE 13-10   The Geometry Factor, $G(r, \theta)$, for a 3.0-mm Line Source (^{125}I, model 6711)

$\theta(degrees)$	$r = 0.5\ cm$	$r = 1.0\ cm$
0	4.396	1.023
10	4.377	1.022
20	4.23	1.019
30	4.246	1.015
90	3.885	0.993

Source: Reproduced with permission from Meli, J. A., Anderson, L. L., and Weaver, K. A. Dose distribution. In: *Interstitial Brachytherapy.* Interstitial Collaborative Working Group, New York, Raven Press, 1990.

The *radial dose function* $g(r)$, accounts for absorption and scatter along the transverse axis of the source, normalized to the value at 1 cm from the source. $g(r)$ is determined from depth dose measurements along the transverse axis of the source. Representative measurements are shown in Figure 13-9 for a model 6711 ^{125}I seed.

$F(r, \theta)$ is an *anisotropy factor* that accounts for absorption and scatter in the medium and in the source encapsulation. This function is obtained from relative dose measurements, and it is normalized to the measurement at $\theta = 90°$ for each value of r. Representative values of $F(r, \theta)$ are given in Table 13-11 for a model 6711 ^{125}I seed.

Example 13-7

What is the dose rate at a point near a model 6711 ^{125}I seed, if the point is located as shown in the diagram below:

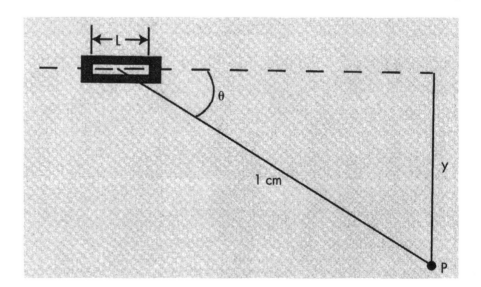

$$L = 0.3\,\text{cm}, \theta = 30°, y = 0.5\,\text{cm}, r = 1.0\,\text{cm}$$

The air-kerma strength S_k of the source is 1.0 cGy·cm^2/hr.
From Equation (13-4) we obtain

$$\dot{D}(r, \theta) = S_k \cdot \Lambda \cdot \frac{G(r, \theta)}{G(1, \pi/2)} \cdot F(r, \theta) \cdot g(r)$$

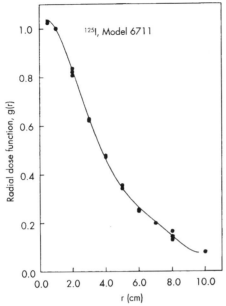

FIGURE 13-9
The radial dose function, $g(r)$, for model 6711 ^{125}I seed. The solid curve is the polynomial fit to the data. (Reprinted with permission from Meli, J. A., Anderson, L. L., and Weaver, K. A. Dose distribution. In *Interstitital Brachytherapy*, Interstital Collaborative Working Group, New York, Raven Press, 1990.)

where

$$S_k = 1.0 \text{ cGy cm}^2/\text{hr}$$

$$\Lambda = 0.847 \text{ cGy/hr per unit air-kerma strength}$$

$$G(1 \text{ cm}, 30°) = 1.015$$

$$G(1 \text{ cm}, \pi/2) = 0.993$$

$$F(1 \text{ cm}, 30°) = 0.799$$

$$g(1 \text{ cm}) = 1.0$$

Therefore,

$$\dot{D}(1 \text{ cm}, 30°) = 0.69 \text{ cGy/hr}$$

TABLE 13-11 The Anisotropy Factor, $F(r, \theta)$, for ^{125}I Model 6711 Calculated from Equation 3 Using Ling's Matrix Fit Dose Anisotropy Polynomial Up to a Distance of 5 cm from the Source.

r(cm)	0°	10°	20°	30°	90°
0.5	0.376	0.448	0.627	0.783	1.00
1.0	0.369	0.464	0.658	0.799	1.00
2.0	0.419	0.503	0.683	0.791	1.00
3.0	0.474	0.551	0.715	0.800	1.00
4.0	0.493	0.579	0.736	0.813	1.00
5.0	0.478	0.583	0.743	0.823	1.00

Source: Ling, C. C., Yorke, E. D., Spiro I. J., Kubiatowicz, D., S Bennett D. Physical dosimetry of ^{125}I seeds of a new design for interstitial implant. *Int. J. Radiat. Oncol. Biol. Phys.* 1983; **9**:1747–1752.

■ DOSE OVER TREATMENT DURATION

The total dose delivered over a treatment time t is determined by integrating the instantaneous dose rates over the treatment time, where the dose rate at a given time is simply the initial dose rate corrected for radioactive decay.

$$D = \int_0^t \dot{D}(t)\, dt = \int_0^t \left(\dot{D}_0 \cdot e^{-\lambda t} \right) dt$$

Since the decay constant is equal to $0.693/T_{1/2}$, solving the integral gives

$$D = 1.44 \cdot T_{1/2} \cdot \dot{D}_0 \left(1 - e^{-0.693 t / T_{1/2}} \right)$$

In clinical practice for temporary treatments, one is often interested in finding the treatment duration. Solving for t gives

$$t = -1.44 \cdot T_{1/2} \cdot \ln \left(1 - \frac{D}{1.44 \cdot T_{1/2} \cdot \dot{D}_o} \right) \tag{13-5}$$

For permanent implants, the duration continues through total decay of the implanted radioactive material. Thus, $t \gg T_{1/2}$ and the equation for total dose reduces to

$$D = 1.44 \cdot T_{1/2} \cdot \dot{D}_0$$

This equation can be solved for the initial dose rate to determine the required activity of the seeds.

Also, for temporary applications where $t \ll T_{1/2}$, such as applications with cesium or iridium, the dose equation reduces to

$$D = \dot{D}_o \cdot t$$

In general practice, if the treatment duration is less than about 8% of the half-life (e.g., 5 days for ^{192}Ir), the change in dose rate due to decay is ignored, and this simpler equation is used.

■ PLAQUES

Tumors of the eye are notoriously difficult to treat effectively without injuring normal structures such as the lens, macula, and optic nerve. One approach for treating ocular tumors is use of an ophthalmic irradiator as discussed in Chapter 12. Ophthalmologic conditions such as pterygium and vascularization or ulceration of the cornea may be treated effectively with a small radioactive applicator positioned on or near the cornea for a short period of time.[26,27] Although early applicators used sources of radium or ^{210}Pb–^{210}Bi, most applicators now contain ^{90}Y ($T_{1/2} = 64$ hr) in secular equilibrium with its parent ^{90}Sr ($T_{1/2} = 28$ yr). The front surface of the applicator absorbs most of the low-energy beta particles from ^{90}Sr (0.54-MeV E_{max}), but permits the high-energy beta particles from ^{90}Y (2.27-MeV E_{max}) to enter the eye. The dose rate at the center of the applicator surface may be as high as 100 cGy/s, and it may vary greatly across the surface of the applicator. The dose rate may be made more uniform by constructing a compensating filter designed to fit over the end of the applicator.[28] The dose rate from a beta applicator decreases to about 5% of the surface dose rate at a depth of 4 mm, the depth of the lens below the cornea.[29,30]

Radioactive sources contained in plaques have been used for many decades to treat superficial disease. Since the 1940s, ophthalmic plaques have been used as an attractive alternative to implantation of radioactive sources directly into the eye,[31] as well as for external beam therapy with heavy charged particles.[32] A study of the effectiveness of plaque therapy compared with enucleation is presently being conducted by the Collaborative Ocular Melanoma Study.[33] The plaque consists of a bowl-shaped outer shell made of an attenuating material such as a gold alloy, along with a means for attaching radioactive seeds (typically ^{125}I) inside the plaque. The gold shell is

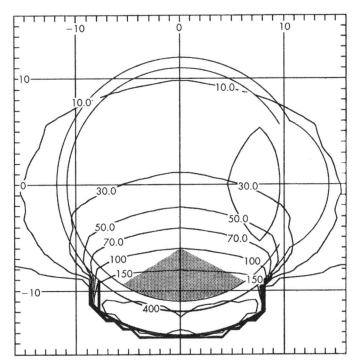

FIGURE 13-10
Treatment of an eye lesion about 5.5 mm thick with an eye plaque. (Diagram produced using BEBIG plaque simulators V2.15, distributed by BEBIG Trade GmbH.)

constructed to match the curvature of the orbit, and it includes eyelets to permit the plaque to be sutured to the orbit. By providing some limited collimation (Figure 13-10), the gold shell limits the dose to uninvolved structures of the eye. The plaque also protects other organs, as well as persons in the vicinity of the patient. The plaque is usually left in place for up to a week while the treatment is delivered. Often the treatment is planned with software developed for ophthalmic plaque radiotherapy.[34]

REMOTE AFTERLOADING

The benefits of brachytherapy *afterloading* have been discussed earlier in this chapter. These benefits are exploited further through the use of *remote afterloading*. Remote afterloading devices consist of a mobile shielded safe that can be connected by a tube to an implant applicator previously placed in the patient (Figure 13-11). One or more radioactive sources can be moved by remote control from the shielded safe, through the tube, and into the implanted applicator. A programmable timer in the console of the unit causes the sources to be retracted when treatment is complete.

Remote afterloading systems may use low-activity sources that provide dose rates in the range of 0.4 to 2 Gy/hr. This approach is called low-dose-rate (LDR) brachytherapy. Low-dose-rate systems are intended to replace conventional implants, with the added benefit that the sources can be retracted into the safe at the touch of a button, thereby permitting medical personnel to attend to the patient without risk of exposure.

Higher-activity sources are used in medium-dose-rate (MDR) units for dose rates of 2 to 12 Gy/hr, and in high-dose-rate (HDR) units that provide dose rates greater than 12 Gy/hr, typically in the range of 150 Gy/hr. High-dose-rate units permit the delivery of brachytherapy treatments on an outpatient basis. That is, the patient is fitted with an interstitial or intracavitary applicator, and a treatment lasting only a few seconds or minutes is delivered. The treatment is repeated on several occasions, perhaps 1 or 2 weeks apart. The biological equivalence of HDR and LDR treatments is being evaluated.[35,36]

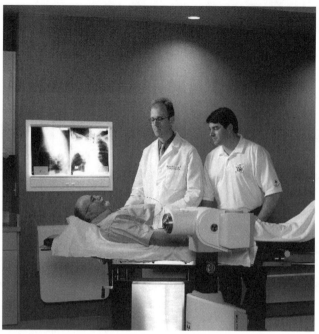

FIGURE 13-11
A high-dose-rate remote afterloader depicting a patient setup for endobronchial treatment. (Courtesy of Rapid City Regional Hospital.)

Recently, the use of pulsed brachytherapy (PDR) has been introduced.[37] It offers the benefits of LDR brachytherapy combined with the radiation safety advantages of a remote afterloader. Moderately high activity sources are used (typically 1 Ci of ^{192}Ir), and the dose is protracted over several days by delivering the treatment in small fractions at hourly intervals. By delivering the dose over several days, a radiobiological response similar to LDR brachytherapy is achieved, while providing almost unlimited access to the patient by healthcare staff. Monitoring of a PDR system requires the continuous availability of a knowledgeable operator to ensure safe treatment.

A remote afterloading unit offers the advantage of great flexibility in the design of the dose distribution. The unit can be programmed to position the source at a large number of locations and to pause at each location for a pre-selected time ("dwell" time). Careful selection of dwell times permits duplication of implants designed according to the Quimby system, the Manchester system, or the Paris system. Software has recently become available for optimization of implants using remote afterloading systems.[38]

■ RADIOGRAPHIC LOCALIZATION OF IMPLANTS

In the planning of interstitial and intracavitary implants, rules and conventions are followed for placing the sources in the tissue to be treated. When the sources are inserted into tissue, however, their placement often is different from that planned. Hence, the area or volume of the actual implant may be significantly more or less than that used to compute the activity and treatment time required for the implant. After the sources have been inserted, the treatment time should be altered to correct for this difference in area or volume. Several methods have been devised for determining the actual area or volume of an implant.[39–49] One common approach to this problem is described here.

The actual area or volume of an implant may be determined from radiographs exposed at right angles to each other ("orthogonal films"). Usually, anteroposterior (AP) and lateral radiographs are used. The lengths of the borders of the implant are

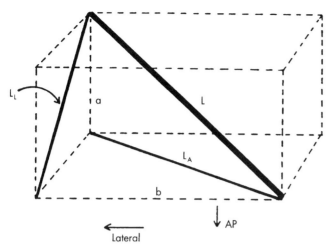

FIGURE 13-12
Geometry for calculating the actual borders of an interstitial implant. (Reprinted with permission from Hendee, W. R. *Medical Radiation Physics*, 1st edition. St. Louis, Mosby–Year Book, 1970.)

found by the Pythagorean theorem. Consider a line of length L and its projections L_A and L_L, on AP and lateral radiographs, respectively (Figure 13-12). The length L is

$$L = \sqrt{L_A^2 + a^2}$$

or

$$L = \sqrt{L_L^2 + b^2}$$

where a and b equal the sides of a right triangle with L_L as the hypotenuse. In Figure 13-12, a is parallel to the AP direction in the lateral radiograph, and b is parallel to the lateral direction in the AP radiograph.

Projections L_A and L_L for each border of the implant are determined with the AP and lateral radiographs. The true length of each border is found by one of the expressions above. The projections of the borders must be corrected for magnification of the radiographic image. The magnification correction may be determined by placing a metal ring at the same level as the implant before each radiograph is exposed. The ratio of the largest diameter of the ring image to the actual diameter of the ring furnishes a magnification correction by which each projection of an implant border is divided before the actual border of the implant is computed.

Example 13-8

A single-plane implant in the base of the tongue appears as shown in Figure 13-13 in AP and lateral radiographs. The magnification corrections M_A and M_L for the AP and lateral radiographs are determined by measuring the diameter of the ring image in the radiographs. The diameter of the ring is 4.0 cm. What activity and treatment time are required to deliver a dose of 4000 cGy at 0.5 cm from the implant plane?

$$M_A = \frac{4.5 \text{ cm}}{4.0 \text{ cm}}$$
$$= 1.13$$
$$M_L = \frac{5.0 \text{ cm}}{4.0 \text{ cm}}$$
$$= 1.25$$

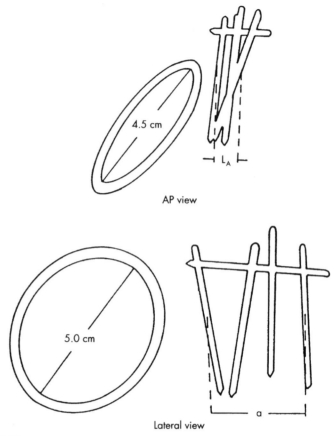

FIGURE 13-13
AP and lateral views of a single-plane radium implant in the base of the tongue. (Reprinted with permission from Hendee, W. R. *Medical Radiation Physics*, 1st edition. St. Louis, Mosby–Year Book, 1970.)

The width a of the implant on the lateral radiograph is 3.7 cm, and the projection L_A on the AP radiograph is 1.1 cm. The needles have an active length of 3 cm. The actual length of the implant is

$$\text{Length} = \sqrt{\left(\frac{3.7 \text{ cm}}{1.25}\right)^2 + \left(\frac{1.1 \text{ cm}}{1.13}\right)^2}$$

$$= 3.12 \text{ cm}$$

The area of the single-plane implant is

$$\text{Area} = (\text{Length})(\text{Height})$$
$$\text{Area} = (3.12 \text{ cm})(3 \text{ cm})$$
$$= 9.36 \text{ cm}^2$$

The area, corrected for one uncrossed end, is

$$\text{Area} = (9.36 \text{ cm}^2)/(1.10)$$
$$= 8.50 \text{ cm}^2$$

From Table 13-5, the number of milligram-hours per 1000 cGy is 228 for an area of 8.5 cm². Three of the needles in the implant possess an activity of 2 mg, and two have 1 mg of radium. All needles are shielded by 0.5-mm Pt(Ir). The number of

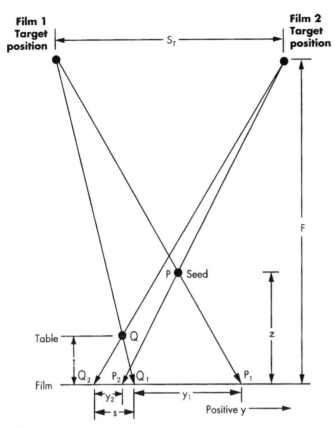

FIGURE 13-14
The geometry of stereoshift radiographs. The coordinates of radioactive seeds (labeled P and Q) may be determined from the position of their shadows (P_1, P_2, Q_1, Q_2) on films exposed with a tube shift S_T between exposures. (Redrawn with permission from Feldman A: Brachytherapy implant coordinates from stereoradiographs: a modified technique giving high accuracy, *Int. J. Radiat. Oncol. Biol. Phys.* 1979; **5**(Suppl. 2):2.)

hours required to deliver 4000 cGy is

$$\text{Number of hours for treatment} = (4000 \text{ cGy}) \left(228\frac{\text{mg} \cdot \text{hr}}{1000 \text{ cGy}}\right) \Big/ 8 \text{ mg} = 114 \text{ hr}$$

In some situations, radioactive sources are difficult to identify on lateral radiographs. This is particularly true for seed implants of the prostate. Under these circumstances, the stereo-shift method may be used. The geometry of stereo-shift radiographs is shown in Figure 13-14.[44,45] The tube shift S_T required for accurate localization of the radioactive sources should be at least 20 cm, when a source-to-film distance of 100 cm is used. A radiation therapy simulator may be used to obtain stereo-shift films. The technique is known as the "variable angle" method, because the films are obtained at different angles of the simulator gantry.[50] In addition, the use of computed tomographic images to determine the locations of brachytherapy sources has been introduced, as discussed in the next section.[51]

Example 13-9

A simplified conventional Fletcher–Suit implant of the cervix is shown in Figure 13-15. The diagram indicates source locations as they appear on AP and lateral radiographs superiorly and 2 cm laterally from the cervical os, as identified by a flange on the cervical tandem. Determine the dose rate at Point A. The source activities are shown in the diagram, and all sources are radium, 1.5-cm active length, 0.5-mm Pt(Ir) filtration (refer to Table 13-1).

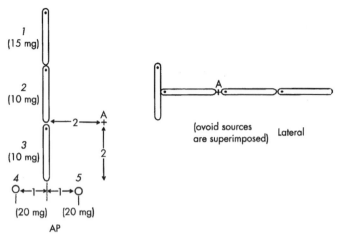

FIGURE 13-15
A simplified conventional Fletcher-Suit implant of the cervix as seen on AP and lateral radiographs.

From source 1: "along" distance = 3 cm, "away" distance = 2 cm

Dose rate = (0.57 cGy/mg · hr)(15 mg) = 8.6 cGy/hr

From source 2: "along" distance = 1 cm, "away" distance = 2 cm

Dose rate = (1.52 cGy/mg · hr)(10 mg) = 15.2 cGy/hr

From source 3 (same geometry as source 2):

Dose rate = 15.2 cGy/hr

From source 5: "along" distance = 0 cm, "away" distance = $\sqrt{2^2 + 1^2}$ = 2.2 cm

Dose rate = (1.59 cGy/mg · hr)(20 mg) = 31.8 cGy/hr

From source 4: "along" distance = 0 cm, "away" distance = $\sqrt{2^2 + 3^2}$ = 3.6 cm

Dose rate = (0.58 cGy/mg · hr)(20 mg) = 11.6 cGy/hr

Total dose rate = 8.6 + 15.2 + 15.2 + 31.8 + 11.6 = 82.4 cGy/hr

■ THREE-DIMENSIONAL IMAGE-BASED IMPLANTS

Prostate Seed Implants

Imaging methods used in external-beam treatment planning are employed in brachytherapy to aid in structure definition and catheter/source reconstruction.[52–55] One of the more common methods is use of axial ultrasound images in the planning of permanent prostate seed implants. The patient is positioned in the lithotomy position, and a rectal ultrasound probe is used to visualize the prostate. Axial images are obtained at fixed increments (e.g., 0.5 cm) by use of an indexed positioning system called a "stepper." With these images, a three-dimensional (3-D) volume of the prostate is reconstructed for treatment planning. A template is used to identify needle locations in a grid pattern. The template is superimposed on the ultrasound images, and the displayed positions should match the positions of the physical template used for the actual implant. The planning system uses the template to define allowable needle locations.

Most dedicated prostate seed programs have commercially available sources characterized in terms of physical properties such as source strength, geometry, and

Memorial system prostate implant source strength specification for ^{125}I for an absorbed dose of 139 Gy, where the average diameter d_a of the target is greater than 3 cm:

Activity = $1.33 d_a^{2.2}$ (mCi)

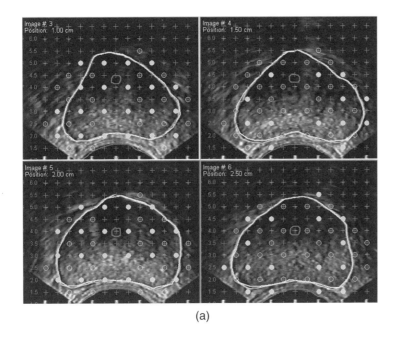

(a)

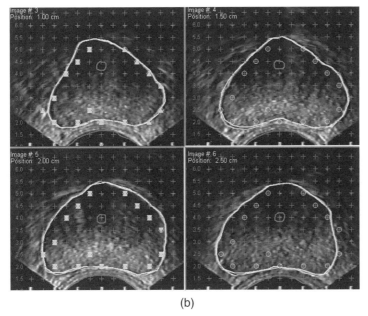

(b)

FIGURE 13-16

A: Modified peripheral loading example. Planes are 5 mm apart and sources are 1 cm apart on a given plane, with an alternating pattern of needles used between planes. Loading is interior on one plane, peripheral on the next, and so on. **B:** Peripheral loading example. Seeds are loaded only on the periphery of alternating planes.

attenuation properties. Often, they allow seeds to be automatically placed in prostate locations according to certain "rules." Two common rules are "peripheral loading" and "modified peripheral loading" (Figure 13-16).[56] Clinicians can adopt either of these techniques for their patients, and they may include their own source-loading rules such as excluding sources within 1 cm of the urethra.

At the time of implant, the physician must position the patient to match the images obtained during the volume study and also must accurately identify the base of the prostate. Then special needles are inserted to anchor the prostate. To deposit the sources, the ultrasound is positioned at a *retraction plane* that corresponds to the plane of the first seed in the needle. The needle is inserted until it appears on the ultrasound

Peripheral loading—Seeds placed only on the periphery of the prostate, needles 1 cm apart.

Modified peripheral loading—Seeds alternately placed on the periphery and interior of the prostate. Needles often shifted by 0.5 cm in alternate slices. Compared with the peripheral loading technique, more needles are used for a modified peripheral loading implant.

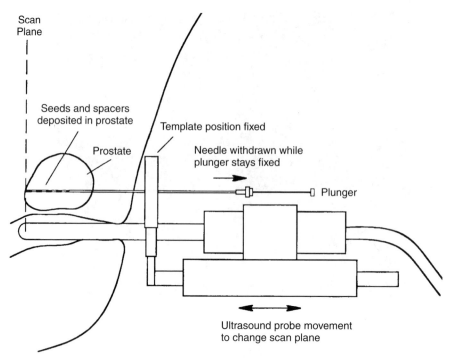

Scan
Plane

Seeds and spacers
deposited in prostate

Template position fixed

Prostate

Needle withdrawn while
plunger stays fixed

Plunger

Ultrasound probe movement
to change scan plane

FIGURE 13-17

Prostate seed implant. The needle is advanced to the plane of the ultrasound image as
determined from the treatment plan. The needle is retracted while the plunger stays fixed,
depositing seeds and spacers in the prostate gland.

image, and it may be further advanced slightly to account for material in the end of
the needle holding the source in place. The needle is then retracted while holding the
stylette (or plunger) in place to deposit the seeds (Figure 13-17 and Table 13-12).

Example 13-10

A prostate implant patient has a transureteral resection of the prostate (TURP) procedure 6 months after a prostate seed implant. If the specimen contains 10 seeds that
had an activity of 0.3 mCi each at the time of implant, what is the exposure rate to
the pathologist at a distance of 50 cm from the specimen?

The specimen is taken approximately 3 half-lives after the implant, so the activity
in the specimen is

$$\text{Activity} = (10 \text{ seeds}) \times (0.3 \text{ mCi})/2^3 = 0.375 \text{ mCi}$$

**TABLE 13-12   Memorial System Source Strength Recommendations for a Prostate
Seed Implant**

Radionuclide	Dose (TG43) [Gy]	Range of d_a [cm]	Strength [mCi$_{apparent}$]	[U]
^{125}I	139	≤3 cm	$5d_a$	$6.35(d_a)$
		>3 cm	$1.33(d_a)^{2.2}$	$1.69(d_a)^{2.2}$
^{103}Pd	120	≤3 cm	$17.78(d_a)$	$23(d_a)$
		>3 cm	$3.2(d_a)^{2.56}$	$4.14(d_a)^{2.56}$
^{198}Au	$D = \dfrac{1.344}{\sqrt{V}}$	All	$50.4(d_a)$	$1.344(d_a)$

Source: Hendee, W. R. (Ed.). *Biomedical Uses of Radiation*, Vol. 1 and 2. New York: VCH Publishers, 1999.
The recommended activity is based on the average prostate gland diameter obtained from the volume
study.

For ^{125}I seeds, the exposure rate constant is $1.45\ \mathrm{R\cdot cm^2/(mCi\cdot hr)}$. The exposure rate is then

$$\dot{X} = (0.375\ \mathrm{mCi})\left(1.45\frac{\mathrm{R\cdot cm^2}}{\mathrm{mCi\cdot hr}}\right)\left(\frac{1}{50\ \mathrm{cm}}\right)^2 = 2.18\times10^{-4}\ \mathrm{R/hr} = 0.2\ \mathrm{mR/hr}$$

Post-implant brachytherapy dosimetry often uses CT images to identify the location of the sources.[57] The sources can be clearly seen in the axial images, although there may be some uncertainty about exact location and orientation because of the finite thickness of the CT slice. Using a table increment that approximates the seed length limits duplication of sources, but gives poor resolution in the axial direction. Comparison of planar film images with 3-D source positions reconstructed from CT images can be helpful in evaluating the accuracy of seed location. If the structures of interest are outlined in the CT images (prostate, bladder, and rectum), then post-implant dosimetry values can be computed to evaluate the effectiveness of the implant. For example, V200 is the volume of the prostate receiving at least 200% of the prescription dose, and D90 is the dose that covers at least 90% of the prostate volume.

Example 13-11

A prostate gland measures 5 cm superior to inferior, 4.5 cm left to right, and 3.5 cm anterior to posterior. The treatment plan calls for 92 ^{125}I seeds, with an activity of 0.35 mCi/seed, to deliver 139 Gy (TG43) to the target. How does this plan compare with the Memorial system source strength recommendations for volume implants described in Table 13-12?

The average diameter for this implant is $(5 + 4.5 + 3.5)/3 = 4.3$ cm. The total activity used is

$$(92\ \mathrm{seeds})\times(0.35\ \mathrm{mCi/seed}) = 32.2\ \mathrm{mCi}$$

From Table 13-12, the recommended strength is

$$A_{\mathrm{app}} = 1.33d_a^{2.2} = 1.33(4.3)^{2.2} = 33.5\ \mathrm{mCi}$$

Thus, the treatment plan calls for about 4% less activity.

Prostate HDR

Treatment of prostate cancer with high-dose-rate (HDR) remote afterloading techniques has increased dramatically, in part because of the supposition that the alpha–beta ratio is lower than previously thought, particularly for high-grade tumors. This finding means that patients with high-grade disease could potentially benefit from shorter overall treatment times. Also, use of HDR to boost the prostate dose can shorten the overall course of treatment by a few weeks. Prostate HDR involves placement of several plastic catheters in the prostate gland under ultrasound guidance, much like a permanent seed implant.[58] The catheters are initially placed halfway into the gland, then advanced using a flexible cystoscope that is retroflexed back to look at the wall of the bladder (Figure 13-18). When the catheters "tent" the bladder wall, the physician stops the advancement. Care has to be taken for posterior catheters, because they can end up posterior to the bladder and tenting will not occur.

After tenting, the patient is imaged with a CT scanner, first using scout films with steel stylets in place and contrast in the bladder to evaluate catheter positions. A few axial cuts may help determine if further advancement of any of the catheters is desired. A complete series of axial images is then obtained, and the images are transferred to the HDR treatment planning system. The plastic catheters appear as dark holes in the prostate and are easily identified. CT slices close to the template provide information to track the catheters into the patient for proper numbering when connected to the afterloader. With the CT images, a treatment plan is generated to produce dwell times

Alpha–beta ratio. In the linear quadratic model of cellular response to radiation, "alpha" (α) is the coefficient for the linear portion of the response, and "beta" (β) is the quadratic coefficient. The alpha–beta ratio, (α/β), can be used to predict how cells may respond to radiation. In general, normal tissues have a higher ratio and benefit from dose fractionation. A tumor with a high ratio would be better treated by prolonged irradiation, as in permanent seed implants for prostate cancer. If the ratio is low, however, then the tumor would be expected to respond favorably to a shorter treatment duration as in high-dose-rate brachytherapy.

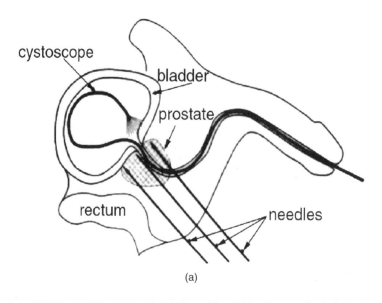

(a)

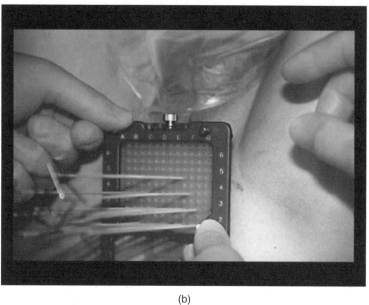

(b)

FIGURE 13-18
High-dose-rate (HDR) prostate implant. The flexible cystoscope is inserted through the urethra and into the bladder. It is then retroflexed to observe the bladder wall as the needles are advanced to avoid puncturing the bladder.

for active dwell positions of the sources. Several methods, including inverse planning techniques based on dose objectives, are available to identify ideal dwell positions (e.g., activate all dwells within the target, but stay at least 1 cm from the urethra) and to optimize dwell times. A common treatment prescription is 3 or 4 fractions of 400–600 cGy, each over a 24- to 30-hr period. A Radiation Therapy Oncology Group (RTOG) multi-institutional study is underway to develop a protocol for treatment of prostate cancer with HDR alone ("HDR prostate monotherapy").

Example 13-12

A treatment plan using ^{192}Ir produces an isodose surface that adequately covers a target volume with 0.55 Gy/hr. Calculate the duration to deliver a 25-Gy dose.

From Equation (13-5), the time to deliver the treatment is

$$t = -1.44 \cdot 73.8 \text{ day} \cdot 24 \text{ hr/day} \cdot \ln \left(1 - \frac{25 \text{ Gy}}{1.44 \cdot 73.8 \text{ day} \cdot 24 \text{ hr/day} \cdot 0.55 \text{ Gy/hr}} \right)$$

$$= 45.9 \text{ hr} = 1 \text{ day } 21 \text{ hr } 54 \text{ min}$$

Using the simpler equation, we obtain

$$t = \frac{D}{\dot{D}_0} = \frac{25 \text{ Gy}}{0.55 \text{ Gy/hr}} = 45.45 \text{ hr} = 1 \text{ day } 21 \text{ hr } 27 \text{ min}$$

Note that because of the short implant duration compared with the half-life of ^{192}Ir, there is only a 1% difference between these two methods.

LDR Gynecologic Interstitial Implant

Template-based interstitial implants for gynecologic tumors may be used when intracavitary techniques are unable to treat the full extent of the disease.[59] Image-based virtual simulation is a useful aid in determining the number, source strength, and position of needles to implant within a template. For a gynecologic implant (e.g., a Syed implant based on a particular concentric needle geometry named for Dr. Nisar Syed), the patient is simulated with the template in position and with the vaginal obturator used to provide a reproducible position. The physician contours the tumor and other structures of interest, possibly with the aid of MRI image-fusion techniques. The dosimetrist or physicist then places "virtual needles" to determine the best locations on the template to implant. Various source loadings can be tried, with the resulting dose distribution presented to the physician for approval. Sources are then ordered for the surgical implant. With the treatment plan as a guide, including how far to insert the needles, the physician is able to perform the implant. The patient can be imaged after surgery to verify needle placement. The planning system may allow these images to be fused into the original planning CT image for comparison. After making necessary adjustments, the clinical team can load the sources into the needles for treatment.

Breast Brachytherapy

Templates may also be used for interstitial volume implants of the breast. The treatment may be either low dose rate or high dose rate.[60-63] In some cases, a multi-plane implant is used with an applicator as shown in Figure 13-19. Cosmesis is an important consideration for these patients, and dose homogeneity is a treatment planning objective. In other cases where a tumor is well-localized and the margins are negative, a small balloon may be inserted into the tumor site for treatment with a single high-dose-rate dwell position. A device that can be used in these cases is shown in Figure 13-20. Note that there must be adequate distance between the skin surface and balloon to reduce the chance of an undesirable skin reaction.

◼ THERAPY WITH RADIOPHARMACEUTICALS

Unsealed radioactive materials have been used in radiation therapy for many decades. Iodine-131 has long been used to treat diseases of the thyroid (hyperthyroidism and thyroid carcinoma), and ^{32}P has been used for treatment of hematologic malignancies (polycythemia vera and leukemia) as well as malignant bone lesions. Radioactive phosphorus-32 in colloidal form has been used to treat malignancies in serosal cavities (particularly ovarian carcinoma).[64] Very little has been published regarding the dosimetry of ^{32}P used for intraperitoneal radiotherapy. Prescriptions are generally based on historical evidence showing, for example, that an activity of 15 mCi of ^{32}P sulfur colloid injected into the peritoneal cavity is effective and causes minimal complications.

Several organizations exist to support and promote multi institutional research efforts. Among them are the Radiation Therapy Oncology Group (RTOG), Eastern Cooperative Oncology Group (ECOG), Gynecological Oncology Group (GOG), and North Central Cancer Treatment Group (NCCTG).

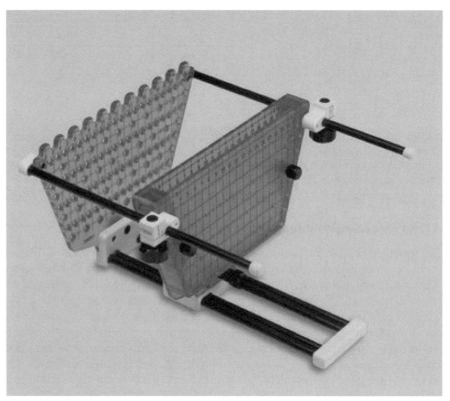

FIGURE 13-19
Application for a multiplane interstitial implant for breast cancer.

■ INTRAVASCULAR BRACHYTHERAPY

Coronary artery disease is the leading cause of death in the United States, and it is responsible for nearly 1 million interventional procedures each year. These procedures include bypass surgery and percutaneous transluminal coronary angioplasty (PTCA). Angioplasty may include deployment of a mesh wire stent to aid in keeping the vessel open. Nearly half of the patients who receive PTCA will return within 6 months with a re-narrowing of the vessel. This re-narrowing is known as restenosis, and it is caused by the body's response to the strain done to the vessel during angioplasty.

During angioplasty, balloon inflation can cause cracks in the atherosclerotic plaque that extend into the vessel, thus damaging the vessel wall. The body's natural response is to promote smooth muscle cell growth to repair the damage. However, the new growth (neointimal hyperplasia) can eventually result in vessel obstruction or "restenosis."

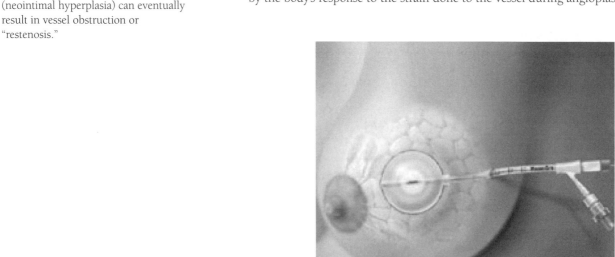

FIGURE 13-20
Single-dwell treatment of a localized breast tumor using a balloon and source applicator.

Ionizing radiation delivered at the time of angioplasty is effective in preventing restenosis.[65-67] Dose levels on the order of 12–20 Gy to the vessel wall appear to be effective. Several devices have been used to deliver the radiation, including hand-held and remote afterloaders. Radioisotopes include both gamma and beta emitters. The sources must be small enough to fit into the narrow coronary arteries (3 to 4-mm diameter), be able to navigate tortuous vessels, and have a high specific activity to keep treatment times short. Gamma emitters have the advantage of better penetration of the target, but require more stringent radiation safety precautions for the staff and yield higher doses to the patient's normal tissues. Beta emitters have a rapid falloff and present a reduced radiation hazard, but are more sensitive to nonuniformity in treatment geometry (such as dense plaque material and noncentered delivery). Clinical trials for commercial devices using beta sources have demonstrated considerable success. Many other methods to combat the restenosis problem are under investigation, including drug-coated stents and ultrasonic treatments. As these are developed, clinicians will have several options to choose among in aiding their patients.

■ SUMMARY

- Early dose calculations for brachytherapy sources were based on the exposure rate at a distance from the source.
- The Sievert integral predicts the exposure at a point from a source based on source geometry, particularly oblique filtration through the jacket or wall material.
- To facilitate treatment planning, away/along tables provide normalized dose values.
- Intestitial implants use needles for source placement, while intracavitary implants utilize applicators within an existing body cavity or opening.
- Implant rules or "systems" were developed by several institutions to aid in needle/applicator placement, source loading, and dose prescription.
- The dose for temporary implants must account for the duration of the implant and possibly source decay (unless the half-life is long compared to the implant duration).
- The dose from permanent implants is determined from the initial dose rate and the half-life of the isotope.
- Remote afterloading brachytherapy reduces the radiation exposure to staff.
- The availability of three-dimensional image-based treatment planning allows customized implants and dose distributions.
- Low-dose-rate brachytherapy is characterized by dose rates on the order of Gy/hr, whereas high-dose-rate brachytherapy dose rates are expressed in units of Gy/min.
- Intravascular brachytherapy is used to reduce the chance of restenosis by lowering the proliferation rate of vascular endothelial cells in response to damage during angioplasty.

PROBLEMS

13-1. What is the exposure rate 20 cm from a 10-mg point source of radium filtered by 1.0-mm Pt(Ir)?

13-2. For a 1-mg Ra-eq cesium source with an active length of 1.4 cm and filtered by 1-mm stainless steel, compare the dose rates at locations 2 cm and 5 cm from the source along a line perpendicular to the center of the source. Compute the dose rates:
   a. Using the inverse square expression and an f-factor of 0.96
   b. Using data in Table 13-3

Explain why the dose rates computed by the two methods do not agree. Would the agreement be improved if the active length of the needle were 0.5 cm?

13-3. Two 2-mg radium needles [0.5-mm Pt(Ir)] with active lengths of 1.5 cm are positioned in line with each other. The centers of the needles are 5 cm apart. A third needle is placed between the two needles. This needle also has an active length of 1.5 cm and is filtered by 0.5-mm Pt(Ir). What activity should the third needle possess to provide equal dose rates at locations 2 cm from the center of each source? What treatment time is necessary for an absorbed dose of 5000 cGy at each location?

13-4. The projection of a radium needle is 2.2 cm in an AP radiograph. In a lateral radiograph, the projection of the needle is 0.8 cm in the AP direction. Magnifications are 1.1 in the AP direction and 1.2 in the lateral direction. What is the true length of the needle?

13-5. What are the amount and distribution of radium in a surface applicator designed to treat:
   a. A circular area 4 cm in diameter at a treatment distance of 1.5 cm, if an absorbed dose of 6000 cGy is desired in 5 days?
   b. A rectangular area 12 cm × 4 cm at a treatment distance of 2 cm, if an absorbed dose of 5000 cGy is desired in 72 hr?

13-6. Design an interstitial iridium wire implant to treat a 6-cm × 6-cm volume of tissue 0.8 cm thick. Both ends of the implant may be crossed, and a dose of 4500 cGy is desired.

13-7. Design an interstitial radium implant to deliver 5000 cGy to a 5-cm × 5-cm volume of tissue 2 cm thick. Only one end of the implant may be crossed. What is the dose rate at the center of the treated volume?

13-8. Design a cylindrical volume radium implant for a region 4 cm in diameter and 6 cm long. One end of the implant cannot be crossed. An absorbed dose of 6000 cGy is desired in about 72 hr.

13-9. Repeat problem 13-8, using ^{192}Ir seeds instead of radium.

13-10. Iodine-125 seeds with an activity of 0.5 mg-Ra-eq are used for a two plane permanent implant for a region of tissue 4 cm × 6 cm × 2.5 cm thick. A uniform absorbed dose of 5000 cGy is desired for the treated volume. Design the implant.

13-11. Repeat problem 13-10, substituting 1 mCi ^{103}Pd for the ^{125}I sources.

13-12. A lesion is treated with fifteen 1-mCi ^{125}I seeds distributed uniformly over the surface of a sphere 2 cm in diameter. What is the absorbed dose at the center of the sphere during complete decay of the sources?

13-13. What is the treatment time necessary for the loaded Fletcher–Suit applicator diagrammed in Figure 13-14 to deliver 2000 cGy to point A? What is the dose at point B, 3 cm lateral to point A? All sources are cesium and are 1.4 cm in active length filtered by 0.5-mm stainless steel.

Source	Activity
1	20 mg-Ra-eq
2	15 mg-Ra-eq
3	10 mg-Ra-eq
4	15 mg-Ra-eq
5	15 mg-Ra-eq

13-14. A prostate ^{125}I implant patient has 90 seeds at 0.35 mCi/seed. Assuming that the patient's body effectively acts like two half-value layers of attenuator, determine the expected exposure rate at 1 m?

13-15. A prostate boost implant using ^{125}I is to deliver a total dose of 108 Gy. What is the initial dose rate in cGy/hr? How long does it take to deliver 90% of the dose?

REFERENCES

1. Sievert, R. Die Gamma-strahlungsintensitat an der ober Fläche and in der nächsten Umgebang von Radium-Nadeln. *Acta Radiol.* 1930; **11**:249.
2. Meredith, W. (ed.). *Radium Dosage: The Manchester System*, 2nd edition. Baltimore, Williams & Wilkins, 1967.
3. Quimby, E. Dosage table for linear radium sources. *Radiology* 1944; **43**:572.
4. Greenfield, M., Fichman, M., and Norman, A. Dosage tables for linear radium sources filtered by 0.5 and 1.0 mm of platinum. *Radiology* 1959; **73**:418.
5. Rose, J., Bloedorn, F., and Robinson, J. A computer dosimetry system for radium implants. *Am. J. Radiol.* 1966; **97**:1032.
6. Meisberger, L. L., Keller, R. J., and Shalek, R. J. The effective attenuation in water of the gamma rays of gold-198, iridium-192, cesium-137, radium-226, and cobalt-60. *Radiology* 1968; **90**:953.
7. Shalek, R. J., and Stovall, M. Dosimetry in implant therapy. In *Radiation Dosimetry*, F. H. Attix and E. Tochlin (eds.). New York, Academic Press, 1969.
8. Williamson, J. F., Morin, R. L., and Khan, F. M. Monte Carlo evaluation of the Sievert integral for brachytherapy dosimetry. *Phys. Med. Biol.* 1983; **28**:1021–1032.
9. Baltas, D., Kramer, R., and Loffler, E. Measurements of the anisotropy of the new iridium-192 source for the microSelectron-HDR. Special Report No. 3. In *Activity selectron*, R. F. Mould (ed.). Veenendaal, Nucletron International BV, 1993.
10. Walstam, R. The dosage distribution in the pelvis in radium treatment of carcinoma of the cervix. *Acta Radiol.* 1954; **42**:237.
11. Ling, C. C., Yorke, E. D., Spiro, I. J., Kubiatowicz, D., and Bennett, D. Physical dosimetry of ^{125}I seeds of a new design for interstitial implant. *Int. J. Radiat. Oncol. Biol. Phys.* 1983; **9**:1747–1752.
12. Muller-Runkel, R., and Cho, S. H. Anisotropy measurements of a high dose rate Ir-192 source in air and in polystyrene. *Med. Phys.* 1994; **21**:7:1131–1134.
13. Nath, R., Meigooni, A. S., Muench, P., and Melillo, A. Anisotropy function for ^{103}Pd, ^{125}I, and ^{192}Ir interstitial brachytherapy sources. *Med. Phys.* 1993; **20**(5):1465–1473.
14. Chiu-Tsao, S., et al. High-sensitivity GafChromic film dosimetry for ^{125}I seeds. *Med. Phys.* 1994; **21**:651–657.
15. Ernst, E. Probable trends in irradiation of carcinoma of cervix uteri with improved expanding type of radium applicator. *Radiology* 1949; **52**:46.
16. Haas, J. S., Dean, R. D., and Mansfield, C. M. Fletcher–Suit–Delclos gynecologic applicator: Evaluation of a new instrument. *Int. J. Radiat. Oncol. Biol. Phys.* 1983; **9**:763–768.
17. Ling, C. C., Spiro, I. J., Kubiatowicz, D. O., Gergen, J., Peksens, R. K., Bennet, J. D., and Gagnon, W. F. Measurement of dose distribution around Fletcher–Suit–Delclos colpostats using a Therados radiation field analyzer (RFA-3). *Med. Phys.* 1984; **11**(3):326–330.
18. Nag, S., Chao, C., Erickson, B., Fowler, J., Gupta, N., Martinez, A., and Thomadsen, B. The American Brachytherapy Society recommendations for low-dose-rate brachytherapy for carcinoma of the cervix. *Int. J. Radiat. Oncol. Biol. Phys.* 2002; **52**(1):33–48.
19. Fishman, R., and Citrin, L. New radium implant technique to reduce operating room exposure and increase accuracy of placement. *Am. J. Radiol.* 1956; **75**:495.
20. Henschke, U., Hilaris, B., and Mahan, G. Afterloading in interstitial and intracavitary radiation therapy. *Am. J. Radiol.* 1963; **90**:386.
21. Simon, N. (ed.). Afterloading in radiotherapy. Proceedings of a conference held in New York City, May 6–8, 1971. Department of HEW Publication No. (FDA)72-8024 (BRH/DMRE 72-4).
22. Pierquin, B., Dutreix, A., Paine, C. H., et al. The Paris system in interstitial radiation therapy. *Acta Radiol. Oncol.* 1978; **17**:33.

23. Gillin, M. T., Kline, R. W., Wilson, J. F., and Cox, J. D. Single and double plane implants: A comparison of the Manchester system with the Paris system. *Int. J. Radiat. Oncol. Biol. Phys.* 1984; **10**:921.

24. Meli, J. A., Anderson, L. L., and Weaver, K. A. Dose distribution. In *Interstitial Brachytherapy*, Interstitial Collaborative Working Group (eds.). New York, Raven Press, 1990.

25. Nath, R., Anderson, L. L., Luxton, G., Weaver, K. A., Williamson, J. F., and Meigooni, A. S. Dosimetry of interstitial brachytherapy sources: Recommendations of the AAPM Radiation Therapy Committee Task Group No. 43. American Association of Physicists in Medicine. *Med. Phys.* 1995; **22**(2):209–234.

26. Duggan, H. Results using strontium-90 beta-ray applicator on eye lesions. *J. Can. Assoc. Radiol.* 1966; **17**:132.

27. Friedell, H., Thomas, C., and Krohmer, J. Evaluation of clinical use of strontium-90 beta-ray applicator with review of underlying principles. *Am. J. Radiol.* 1954; **71**:25.

28. Hendee, W. R. Measurement and correction of nonuniform surface dose rates for beta eye applicators. *Am. J. Radiol.* 1968; **103**:734.

29. Coffey, C., Sayeg, J., Beach, J. L., Song, S., Landis, C., and Connor, A. Calibration of surface dose rate for a Sr-90 beta applicator: Comparison of experimental, theoretical, and biological methods. *Med. Phys.* 1981; **8**:558.

30. Hendee, W. R. Thermoluminescent dosimetry of beta depth dose. *Am. J. Radiol.* 1966; **97**:1045.

31. Stallard, H. B. Malignant melanoma of the coroid treated with radioactive applicators. *Ann. R. Coll. Surg. Engl.* 1961; **29**:170.

32. Gragoudas, E. S., Goitein M., Verhey, L., Munzenreider, J., Urie, M., Suit, H., and Koehler, A. Proton beam irradiation of uveal melanomas: Results of a 5 1/2 year study. *Arch. Ophthalmol.* 1982; **100**:928–934.

33. Collaborative Ocular Melanoma Study, COMS Coordinating Center, The Wilmer Ophthalmological Institute, The Johns Hopkins School of Medicine, Baltimore, MD, 1989.

34. Astrahan, M. A., Luxton, G., Jozsef, G., Kampp, T. D., Liggett, P. E., Sapozink, M. D., and Petrovich, Z. An interactive treatment planning system for ophthalmic plaque radiotherapy. *Int. J. Radiat. Oncol. Biol. Phys.* 1990; **18**:679–687.

35. Brenner, D. J., and Hall, E. J. Fractionated high dose rate versus low dose rate regimes for intracavitary brachytherapy of the cervix. 1. General considerations based on radiobiology. *Br. J. Radiol.* 1991; **64**:133–144.

36. Orton, C. G., Seyedsadr, M., and Somnay, A. Comparison of high and low dose rate remote afterloading for cervix cancer and the importance of fractionation. *Int. J. Radiat. Oncol. Biol. Phys.* 1991; **21**:1425–1434.

37. Fowler, J. F., and Mount, M. Pulsed brachytherapy: The conditions for no significant loss of therapeutic ratio compared with traditional low dose rate brachytherapy. *Int. J. Radiat. Oncol. Biol. Phys.* 1992; **23**:661–669.

38. Edmundson, G. K. Volume optimization: An American viewpoint. In *Brachytherapy from Radium to Optimization*, R. F. Mould et al. (eds.). Veenendaal, Nucletron International BV, 1994.

39. Egan, R., and Johnson, G. Multisection transverse tomography in radium implant calculations. *Radiology* 1956; **74**:402.

40. Hidalgo, J. U., Spear, V. D., Garcia, M., Maduell, C. R., and Burke, R. The precision reconstruction of radium implants. *Am. J. Radiol.* 1967; **100**:852.

41. Holt, J. A nomographic wheel for three dimensional localization of radium sources and calculation of dose rate. *Am. J. Radiol.* 1956; **75**:476.

42. Johns, H., and Cunningham, J. *The Physics of Radiology*, 3rd edition. Springfield, IL, Charles C Thomas, 1969.

43. Kligerman, M., Vreeland, H., and Havinga, J. A graphical method for the localization of radium sources for dosage calculation. *Am. J. Radiol.* 1956; **75**:484.

44. Mussel, L. E. The rapid reconstruction of radium implants: A new technique. *Br. J. Radiol.* 1956; **29**:402.

45. Nuttal, J. R., and Spiers, F. W. Dosage control in interstitial radium therapy. *Br. J. Radiol.* 1946; **19**:133.

46. Shalek, R. J., and Stovall, M. Dosimetry in implant therapy. In *Radiation Dosimetry*, Vol. III (31), F. H. Attix and W. C. Roesch (eds.). New York, Academic Press, 1969.

47. Smith, M. A graphic method of reconstructing radium needle implants for calculation purposes. *Am. J. Radiol.* 1958; **79**:42.

48. Terta, E. Methods of dosage calculation for linear radium sources. *Radiology* 1957; **69**:558.

49. Vaeth, J., and Meurk, J. Use of Rotterdam radium reconstruction device. *Am. J. Radiol.* 1963; **89**:87.

50. Feldman, A. Brachytherapy implant coordinates from stereoradiographs: A modified technique giving high accuracy. *Int. J. Radiat. Oncol. Biol. Phys.* 1979; **5**(Suppl 12):80.

51. Schoeppel, S. L., LaVigne, M. L., Martel, M. K., McShan, D. L., Fraass, B. A., and Roberts, J. A. Three-dimensional treatment planning of intracavitary gynecologic implants: Analysis of ten cases and implications for dose specification. *Int. J. Radiat. Oncol. Biol. Phys.* 1991; **28**:277–283.

52. Nag, S., Beyer, D., Friedland, J., Grimm, P., and Nath, R. American Brachytherapy Society (ABS) recommendations for transperineal permanent brachytherapy of prostate cancer. *Int. J. Radiat. Oncol. Biol. Phys.* 1999; **44**(4):789–799.

53. Yu, Y., Anderson, L. L., Li, Z., Mellenberg, D. E., Nath, R., Schell, M. C., Waterman, F. M., Wu, A., and Blasko, J. C. Permanent prostate seed implant brachytherapy: Report of the American Association of Physicists in Medicine Task Group No. 64. *Med. Phys.* 1999; **26**(10):2054–2076.

54. Nag, S. Brachytherapy for prostate cancer: Summary of American Brachytherapy Society recommendations. *Semin. Urol. Oncol.* 2000; **18**(2):133–136.

55. Blasko, J. C., Mate, T., Sylvester, J. E., Grimm, P. D., and Cavanagh, W. Brachytherapy for carcinoma of the prostate: Techniques, patient selection, and clinical outcomes. *Semin. Radiat. Oncol.* 2002; **12**(1):81–94.

56. Butler, W. M., Merrick, G. S., Lief, J. H., and Dorsey, A. T. Comparison of seed loading approaches in prostate brachytherapy. *Med. Phys.* 2000; **27**(2):381–392.

57. Nag, S., Bice, W., DeWyngaert, K., Prestidge, B., Stock, R., and Yu, Y. The American Brachytherapy Society recommendations for permanent prostate brachytherapy postimplant dosimetric analysis. *Int. J. Radiat. Oncol. Biol. Phys.* 2000; **46**(1):221–230.

58. Demanes, D. J., Rodriguez, R. R., and Altieri, G. A. High dose rate prostate brachytherapy: The California Endocurietherapy (CET) method. *Radiother. Oncol.* 2000; **57**(3):289–296.

59. Tewari, K. S., Cappuccini, F., Puthawala, A. A., Kuo, J. V., Burger, R. A., Monk, B. J., Manetta, A., Berman, M. L., Disaia, P. J., and Nisar, A. M. Primary invasive carcinoma of the vagina: Treatment with interstitial brachytherapy. *Cancer* 2001; **91**(4):758–770.

60. Edmundson, G. K., Weed, D., Vicini, F., Chen, P., and Martinez, A. Accelerated treatment of breast cancer: Dosimetric comparisons between interstitial HDR brachytherapy, mammosite balloon brachytherapy, and external beam quadrant radiation. *Int. J. Radiat. Oncol. Biol. Phys.* 2003; **57**:S307–308.

61. Vicini, F., Baglan, K., Kestin, L., Chen, P., Edmundson, G., and Martinez, A. The emerging role of brachytherapy in the management of patients with breast cancer. *Semin. Radiat. Oncol.* 2002; **12**(1):31–39.

62. Keisch, M., Vicini, F., Kuske, R., Hebert, M., White, J., Quiet, C., Arthur, D., Scroggins, T., and Streeter, O. Two-year outcome with the mammosite breast brachytherapy applicator: Factors associated with optimal cosmetic results when performing partial breast irradiation. *Int. J. Radiat. Oncol. Biol. Phys.* 2003; **57**:S315.

63. Keisch, M., Vicini, F., Kuske, R. R., Hebert, M., White, J., Quiet, C., Arthur, D., Scroggins, T., and Streeter, O. Initial clinical experience with the MammoSite breast brachytherapy applicator in women with early-stage breast cancer treated with breast-conserving therapy. *Int. J. Radiat. Oncol. Biol. Phys.* 2003; **55**:289–293.

64. Spencer, R. P. (ed.). *Therapy in Nuclear Medicine*, New York, Grune & Stratton, 1978.

65. Apisarnthanarax, S., and Chougule, P. Intravascular brachytherapy: A review of the current vascular biology. *Am. J. Clin. Oncol.* 2003; **26**:E13–E21.

66. Nath, R., Amols, H., Coffey, C., Duggan, D., Jani, S., Li, Z., Schell, M., Soares, C., Whiting, J., Cole, P. E., Crocker, I., and Schwartz, R. Intravascular brachytherapy physics: Report of the AAPM Radiation Therapy Committee Task Group No. 60. American Association of Physicists in Medicine, *Med. Phys.* 1999; **26**(2):119–152.

67. Nguyen-Ho, P., Kaluza, G. L., Zymek, P. T., and Raizner, A. E. Intracoronary brachytherapy. *Catheter Cardiovasc. Interv.* 2002; **56**:281–288.

68. International Commission on Radiation Units and Measurements, Report No. 39: *Determination of Dose Equivalents Resulting from External Radiation Sources.* Bethesda, MD, ICRU Publications, 1985.

69. Williamson, J. F., and Nath, R. Clinical implementation of AAPM Task Group 32 recommendations on brachytherapy source strength specification. *Med. Phys.* 1991; **18**:439–448.

CHAPTER

14

RADIATION PROTECTION

OBJECTIVES   334

INTRODUCTION   334

EFFECTS OF RADIATION EXPOSURE   336

Stochastic Radiation Effects   336
Nonstochastic Effects   336

HISTORY OF RADIATION PROTECTION STANDARDS   337

CURRENT LIMITS ON RADIATION EXPOSURE   338

PROTECTIVE BARRIERS FOR RADIATION SOURCES   341

Protection from Small Sealed Gamma-Ray Sources   341
Design of Structural Shielding   343
Primary Radiation Barriers   343
Secondary Barriers for Scattered Radiation   346

Secondary Barriers for Leakage Radiation   347
Door Shielding   349
Neutron Shielding   351

PROTECTION FOR SEALED RADIOACTIVE SOURCES   352

RADIATION SURVEYS   352

Ionization Chambers   353
G–M Counters   353
Neutron Detectors   353

PERSONNEL MONITORING   353

SUMMARY   354

PROBLEMS   354

REFERENCES   355

Radiation Therapy Physics, Third Edition, by William R. Hendee, Geoffrey S. Ibbott, and Eric G. Hendee
ISBN 0-471-39493-9 Copyright © 2005 John Wiley & Sons, Inc.

■ OBJECTIVES

By studying this chapter, the reader should be able to:

- Explain the philosophy of risk underlying radiation protection, including the linear, non-threshold model of radiation injury.
- Describe the stochastic and nonstochastic effects of radiation exposure.
- Depict the history of radiation protection, including the evolution and definition of radiation units.
- Define the current recommended limits for radiation exposure.
- Demonstrate a conceptual understanding of computations of shielding requirements for primary, secondary, and neutron radiation, including variables that influence the computations.
- Employ the radiation protection principles important to the safe use of sealed brachytherapy sources.
- Delineate the uses and limitations of various devices for radiation surveys and personnel monitoring.

■ INTRODUCTION

For a few years after their discovery, x rays and radioactive materials were used with little knowledge of their biologic effects. Soon, however, the consequences of excessive exposure to radiation became apparent, including skin burns (erythema), hair loss (epilation), and, later, skin cancer (squamous and basal cell carcinoma). Persons affected included several physicians, physicists, and technicians who pioneered the early applications of ionizing radiation in medicine.[1]

By this time, ionizing radiation was proving to be helpful in medical diagnosis and therapy. The issue facing radiation experts was whether radiation could be used to benefit patients and society without exposing radiation users to unacceptable hazards. This issue is phrased today as a question of risk versus benefit. To reduce the risk, advisory groups were formed to establish upper limits for the exposure of radiation users, with the recognition that the risk to individual patients must always be balanced against medical benefits. Advisory groups have reduced the upper limits many times since the first limits were promulgated, as discussed later in this chapter. These reductions reflect the use of radiation by greater numbers of persons, the implications of new data concerning the sensitivity of biologic organisms to radiation, and improvements in the design of radiation devices and the architecture of facilities where radiation sources are used.

The philosophy underlying the control of radiation hazards is described as a *philosophy of risk*. In this approach, advisory groups attempt to establish standards for radiation protection that maintain radiation risks at an acceptable level to individuals and society without unnecessarily impeding the useful applications of radiation.[2] The philosophy of risk is portrayed in Figure 14-1. The total biological damage (the *radiation detriment*) to a population is the sum of various effects, such as mortality, morbidity, genetic damage, shortened life span, and reduced vitality, that may result from receipt of a particular dose rate of radiation averaged over the lifetime of individuals in the population. The total damage is assumed to increase gradually as the average dose rate increases to a value of perhaps 0.01 Sv per week. Above this dose rate, the biologic damage is assumed to increase more rapidly. The *area of uncertainty* shown in Figure 14-1 is the region of greatest concern in radiation protection because it encompasses the dose rates typically encountered by radiation users. It is also the region where data are most limited. As indicated by curve *c*, the damage may remain at zero for dose rates below some threshold level, suggesting that biologic repair of radiation injury may occur, provided that the damage does not take place so rapidly that repair mechanisms are overwhelmed. Considerable evidence supports this *threshold model of radiation injury* for certain types of exposures, including the induction of

Cable news releases announced Röntgen's 1895 discovery to several developed countries. Within a few months, x rays were being used in hospitals and physicians' offices in these countries. Several cases of radiation-induced dermatitis soon followed.

The first fatality caused by radiation exposure was Clarence Dally, an assistant to Thomas Edison. After several surgeries, including amputation of his arm, Dally died in 1904 from x-ray induced cancer.

Initial concern about radiation exposure focused more on the operator than on the patient because (1) patient exposures are intermittent while operators are exposed continuously and (2) the patient benefits directly from the exposure.

William Collins, a Boston dentist, was a major early influence on radiation protection practices. He was the first to propose a "tolerance dose" limit for occupational radiation exposure.

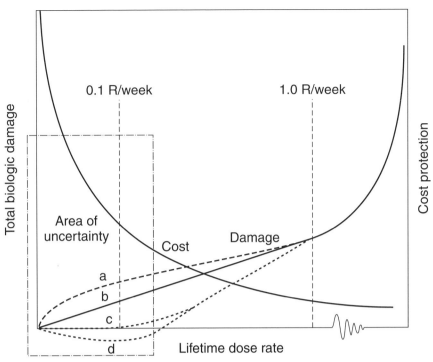

FIGURE 14-1

Total biological damage to a population expressed as a function of the average dose rate to individuals in the population. The cost of protection is reduced as greater biological damage is tolerated. (From W. Claus.[3])

osteogenic carcinoma in individuals with significant bone concentrations of radium.[4] Conceivably the curve for biologic effects might follow path *d*, suggesting that low dose rates are beneficial, a hypothesis known as *radiation hormesis*. Although considerable experimental evidence supports this hypothesis,[5] it continues to generate considerable controversy among radiation experts. Some persons suggest that the curve for total biologic damage follows curve *a*[6], but this *superlinearity theory of radiation damage* is not strongly supported by experimental data. Curve *b* suggests that the total biologic damage to a population is linearly proportional to the average dose rate to individuals in the population down to a dose rate approaching zero. This model, known as *the linear hypothesis of radiation injury*, is the model usually employed to estimate radiation risks and establish standards for radiation protection.[7]

Data are inadequate to identify which of the models for predicting biologic damage is most appropriate within the area of uncertainty depicted in Figure 14-1. Consequently the cost of radiation protection (e.g., for shielding, remote control techniques, monitoring procedures, and personnel restriction) must be balanced against uncertain biologic effects that may result at any given level of protection. The cost increases from almost zero for no restrictions on radiation exposure to a high cost if attempts are made to reduce exposures to a level approaching zero. Somewhere within the area of uncertainty, an upper limit must be established for permissible radiation exposures. This limit should reflect a risk that is acceptable to the exposed individuals and to society in general, without depriving society of the benefits derived from judicious use of ionizing radiation. In addition, it should be recognized that exposures should always be kept *as low as reasonably achievable (ALARA)* consistent with reasonable costs and convenience and without compromising the benefits of radiation to society.

The estimation of radiation risk at low exposures is controversial. Use of curve *b* (the linear, non-threshold model of radiation injury) yields risk estimates at low exposures (e.g., 5 cases of cancer over a lifetime in 10,000 persons exposed whole-body to 1 rem (0.01 Sv). Such risk estimates lead to substantial numbers of calculated cancers for circumstances such as medical procedures where many people are exposed.

ALARA was preceded by the protection philosophy of "As Low as Possible (ALAP)." It was soon recognized, however, that exposures can always be reduced further if enough resources are dedicated to the task. The substitution of "Reasonably Achievable" for "Possible" was intended to reflect the need for common sense in resource allocation to radiation protection.

Example 14-1

The lifetime risk of adverse biologic effects from radiation exposure is approximately 5×10^{-2} Sv^{-1} for radiation workers. Using the linear hypothesis, estimate the lifetime risk for a whole-body x-ray dose equivalent of 0.01 Sv (1 rem):

$$\text{Lifetime risk} = (\text{Risk/Sv})[\text{Dose equivalent (Sv)}]$$
$$= (5 \times 10^{-2}\,\text{Sv}^{-1})(0.01\,\text{Sv})$$
$$= 5 \times 10^{-4}$$

That is, there is a risk of 5 chances in 10,000 that the radiation dose will cause an adverse biological effect over the lifetime of the exposed individual.

■ EFFECTS OF RADIATION EXPOSURE

Exposure to ionizing radiation can produce several effects in an individual, depending on (1) the type and amount of radiation producing the exposure, (2) the fraction of the body that is exposed, (3) the general health of the exposed individual, and (4) the quality of medical care available in the event of a relatively high exposure. If the exposure is relatively high, adverse effects may occur almost immediately or within several days or weeks. These effects are referred to as *immediate effects* of radiation exposure. At lower exposures, the effects, termed *delayed effects* of radiation exposure, may not appear for several years.

Stochastic Radiation Effects

It is well understood today that the incidence of leukemia and several forms of solid cancers began to increase in the atomic bomb survivors in Hiroshima and Nagasaki several years after the explosions occurred. This increase has been associated with exposure of the survivors to ionizing radiation released during the explosions. Increased likelihood of cancer *carcinogenesis* is the principal delayed (long-term) effect of exposure to radiation. Other delayed effects include *teratogenesis* (the induction of birth defects by irradiation of the fetus) and *mutagenesis* (the induction of genetic disorders in future generations by irradiation of germ cells).

Biological effects that appear several months or years after exposure to radiation have several characteristics in common: (1) The probability of occurrence of the effect (i.e., the number of persons in an exposed population who exhibit the effect) increases with dose; (2) the severity of the effect in a single individual is unrelated to the magnitude of the dose (i.e., the effect is an "all or none" response); and (3) no definitive threshold exists below which it can be said with certainty that the effect will not occur. These effects are probabilistic in nature and probably reflect the action of radiation to trigger mechanisms in the body that may lead ultimately to the appearance of an effect. Whether an effect actually does appear may depend on the presence of other "promoting" factors in the body. Such effects are known as *probabilistic or stochastic effects*, in which the probability of occurrence but not the severity of the disorder is related to the dose of radiation received.

Precise estimates of the role of an initiating agent such as radiation in producing stochastic effects are difficult to obtain because the effects also occur in the absence of radiation. That is, there is a *natural incidence* of the effects related to causes other than radiation exposure. Cancer, birth defects, and genetic mutations all occur naturally at relatively high rates in human populations, and identifying an increase in these rates caused by exposure to small amounts of ionizing radiation is subject to considerable uncertainty.

Nonstochastic Effects

The short-term (acute) effects of radiation are associated with levels of radiation far above those received by persons working in a modern radiation facility. These acute effects, known as *acute radiation syndromes*, are divided into three categories that differ in the relative radiation sensitivities of the involved organ systems and in the time

---

Immediate effects of radiation exposure are also referred to as *early effects*; Delayed effects are frequently termed *late effects* of radiation exposure.

Stochastic radiation effects are those effects for which there is no threshold dose. Stochastic effects are sometimes called *probabilistic effects*.

Of the three stochastic effects, available data suggest that carcinogenesis presents the greatest risk to a population. These data include studies of cell cultures, experimental animals, and human populations exposed to medical procedures, fallout from nuclear test explosions, and survivors of Hiroshima and Nagasaki.

The impact of stochastic radiation effects in a population depends on the dose and the number of persons exposed. These factors are combined in the concept of *collective dose*, sometimes called *population dose*, expressed in units of person-sieverts.

Exposure of a population to a dose-equivalent of 1 rem (0.01 Sv) would increase the incidence of cancer by about 0.1% over the lifetime of the exposed individuals.

Nonstochastic radiation effects are those effects that exhibit a dose threshold. Nonstochastic effects are sometimes called *deterministic effects*.

required for the effects to occur. The three categories are the *hematopoietic syndrome*, *gastrointestinal syndrome*, and *cerebrovascular syndrome*.

The stem cells of the hematopoietic system, residing primarily in the bone marrow as precursors of mature blood cells, can be inactivated in significant numbers at a dose level of a few gray. Loss of stem cells may not become apparent until the time arrives for the precursor cells to reach maturity, when the body may lose its ability to combat infection. This latency period of a few weeks provides an opportunity to reestablish the stem cell population by a bone marrow transplant.

Cells in the gastrointestinal tract, particularly epithelial cells that line the intestinal surface, are highly vulnerable to radiation injury. Following an absorbed dose of several gray, diarrhea, hemorrhage, electrolyte imbalance, dehydration, and other gastrointestinal effects may appear within a few days as a consequence of cell damage.

At doses above about 50 Gy, cellular injury may be severe in the relatively radiation-insensitive neurologic and cardiovascular compartments of the body. This effect may produce life-threatening changes almost immediately after exposure. Death in a few hours or days usually is caused by destruction of blood vessels in the brain, fluid accumulation, and neuronal damage.

Fertility can also be impaired at relatively high doses of ionizing radiation. Temporary sterility occurs in the male at single doses above about 0.15 Gy to the testes, and permanent sterility may occur at doses above about 3.5 Gy.[8] Single ovarian doses above about 0.65 Gy may cause temporary sterility in the female, and permanent sterility has been observed at doses above 2.5 Gy.[9] Doses required to produce temporary or permanent sterility are increased by orders of magnitude if delivered in fractions or continuously at low dose rates.[2]

HISTORY OF RADIATION PROTECTION STANDARDS

As appreciation of the adverse effects of radiation exposure grew in the early years of the century, advisory groups of radiation experts were established to develop upper limits of exposure for radiation users (referred to as radiation workers or occupationally exposed individuals). In 1921, the British X-Ray and Radium Protection Committee developed the recommendations delineated in the margin for physicians and other radiation workers.[10] Numerical limits for radiation exposure required a quantitative measure of radiation, however, and were not proposed until the roentgen was defined in 1931. In 1934, the International Committee on X-Ray and Radium Protection, later renamed the International Commission on Radiological Protection (ICRP), established a limit of 0.2 R/day for exposure of persons using radiation sources.[11] Two years later, the U.S. Advisory Committee for X-Ray and Radium Protection (now the National Council on Radiation Protection and Measurements [NCRP]) recommended a tolerance dose of 0.1 R/day. Both groups believed that the recommended limits were well below exposure levels at which immediate (deterministic) effects might occur. Initially the standards were intended only for x-ray exposure. However, the NCRP standard was later applied to gamma rays from radium and served as a protection standard for workers on the atomic bomb (Manhattan) project during World War II.[12]

In 1949, the NCRP substituted the concept of *maximum permissible dose (MPD)* for tolerance dose in response to the growing recognition of the leukogenic and mutagenic effects of ionizing radiation and the possibility that these effects might not exhibit a dose threshold. An MPD of 0.3 R/week (15 R/year) was established for radiation workers, principally in response to concerns about the genetic effects of radiation, the dependence of the extent of occurrence of these effects on the number of individuals exposed, and the growing number of persons employed in the postwar nuclear industry.[13]

In 1956, the first of several reports on radiation effects was released by the Committee on the Biological Effects of Atomic Radiation (BEAR) of the U.S. National Academy of Sciences' National Research Council.[14] This report suggested that the total

The cerebrovascular syndrome is sometimes referred to as the central nervous system (CNS) syndrome, because the effects are experienced in the CNS.

Radiation-induced changes in the vascular endothelium are thought to be the underlying cause of most nonstochastic radiation effects.

Radiation-induced edema in the brain may be caused by a breakdown in the blood–brain barrier. This effect is reversible over a few days if the dose is not too high.

Recommendations for Protection Against Radiation Hazards Developed in 1921 by the British X-Ray and Radiation Protection Committee

> No more than 7 working hours/day Sundays and two half-days off per week
>
> As much leisure time as possible spent outdoors
>
> Annual holiday of 1 month or two 2-week holidays annually.
>
> Personnel working full-time in x-ray and radium departments should not be expected to perform other hospital services

(Adapted from British X-Ray and Radium Protection Committee. X-ray and radium protection, *J. Roentgen Soc.*[10] Used by permission)

Both the ICRP and NCRP are voluntary efforts, and their recommendations are purely advisory. In the United States, NCRP recommendations are frequently codified into radiation regulations by federal and state agencies, including the Nuclear Regulatory Commission and the Environmental Protection Agency.

The possibility of a dose threshold for radiation-induced cancer is an ongoing controversy which is ultimately impossible to resolve.

The assumption underlying the importance of cumulative dose is that at least some radiation-induced bioeffects are irreversible.

Several later committees of the National Academy of Sciences have guided the estimation of radiation risk over the years. These committees are referred to as BEIR committees (BEIR—Biological Effects of Ionizing Radiation.)

The use of Hiroshima–Nagasaki data for generalization of radiation-induced cancer risks has been criticized because

- Cancer incidence varies with population groups, and Japanese data may not describe other groups.
- Exposures at Hiroshima and Nagasaki were acute, not chronic, exposures.
- Social support and medical care were severely compromised in Hiroshima and Nagasaki, and they may have affected cancer incidence and mortality.

The publication of Silent Spring by Rachel Carson in 1962 reinforced the public's awareness about the potential health consequences of environmental agents such as fallout and pesticides.

Responses to concerns over radioactive fallout in the 1950s and early 1960s led to an effort to reduce the much greater exposures for medical radiation. One consequence of this effort was passage of the Radiation Control for Health and Safety Act of 1968. This act established manufacturing performance standards for radiation-emitting devices.

The effective quality factor $\overline{Q_r}$ is usually referred to as the *radiation weighting factor* w_r.

dose accumulated by an individual is more important than the dose received over any limited period in terms of effects on the health of the individual or the individual's progeny. A year later, the NCRP established a limit of $5(N - 18)$ rad ($0.05[N - 18]$ Gy) as the *maximum cumulative dose* for a radiation worker, with N = age in years.[15] This limit implies that a person less than 18 years of age could not be considered a radiation worker. A person was permitted to receive up to 12 rad/year, provided that the cumulative dose limit of $5(N - 18)$ was not exceeded. In 1959, the ICRP adopted the same limit,[16] and this protection standard remained in place for the next 18 years.

In 1977, the ICRP introduced a conceptual change in protection standards by restating radiation limits in terms of the *effective dose equivalent* (H_e) expressed in units of rem, now redefined in units of sievert.[17] The (H_e) was intended to permit summation of external and internal exposures in evaluating the overall risk to an exposed individual, and the unit rem (now sievert) was used to express differences in the capacity of various types of radiation to affect the overall well-being of exposed individuals. A numerical limit of 5 rem/year (0.05 Sv/year) was recommended consistent with the cumulative dose limit of $5(N - 18)$, and radiation-induced cancer (carcinogenesis) replaced genetic effects (mutagenesis) as the principal health concern. This shift in concern reflected data from studies of the survivors of the atomic explosions at Hiroshima and Nagasaki revealing that the cancer risk of radiation exposure significantly exceeds the genetic risk. The ICRP also recommended that radiation protection standards should be based on acceptable health risks rather than on arbitrary dose limits, and that these risks should be determined by comparison with the health risks of individuals working in "safe" industries that do not employ radiation. The 1977 recommendations of the ICRP established a risk-oriented philosophy of radiation protection standards that continues to guide the work of both the ICRP and the NCRP.[18] In 1987, the NCRP recommended discontinuance of the $5(N - 18)$ cumulative dose limit, and its replacement by a cumulative limit of $N/100$ sievert, where N is the age of the exposed individual in years.[19]

In the early years of radiation protection, exposure standards were developed principally for the protection of radiation workers. With expansion of the nuclear weapons industry in the early 1950s and because of growing concern about exposure to fallout from atmospheric weapons tests, advisory groups began to consider *protection standards for the general public*. In 1955, the ICRP suggested that no member of the public (i.e., anyone other than a radiation worker) should be exposed to more than 1/10 of the MPD for an occupationally exposed person.[20] A lower limit was justified for members of the public because these individuals receive no direct benefits from radiation exposure (i.e., their jobs do not require radiation exposure), and they constitute a much greater population group compared with radiation workers. In 1957, the NCRP restated the ICRP recommendation as a dose limit of 0.5 rem/year (5 mSv/year) for individual members of the public, consistent with its standard of 5 rem/year for radiation workers.[15] The ICRP later added a population dose limit of 5 rem over 30 years averaged over the entire population, principally in response to concern about the possible genetic consequences of radiation exposure of large populations.[16] In 1977, the ICRP reinforced the 0.5-rem/year (5-mSv/year) limit for members of the public but added that the cumulative dose to these individuals should not exceed 0.1 rem/year (1 mSv/year) averaged over a lifetime.[17] The NCRP officially adopted the ICRP recommendation in 1987.[19]

■ CURRENT LIMITS ON RADIATION EXPOSURE

In Chapter 5, the *mean dose equivalent* $\overline{H}$ (sometimes termed the *equivalent dose*) was defined as the average absorbed dose to a region of tissue multiplied by an effective quality factor $\overline{Q}$ that depends on the linear energy transfer (LET) of the radiation averaged over the region of exposed tissue. When the radiation dose is delivered by more than one type of radiation, the total $\overline{H}$ is the sum of the average absorbed dose

TABLE 14-1   Weighting Factors w_t for Different Tissues

0.01	0.05	0.12	0.20
Bone surface	Bladder	Bone marrow	Gonads
Skin	Breast	Colon	
	Liver	Lung	
	Esophagus	Stomach	
	Thyroid		
	Remainder[a,b]		

[a] The remainder includes the following additional tissues and organs: adrenals, brain, small intestine, large intestine, kidney, muscle, pancreas, spleen, thymus, and uterus.

[b] In exceptional cases in which one of the remainder tissues or organs receives an equivalent dose in excess of the highest dose in any of the 12 organs for which a weighting factor is specified, a weighting factor of 0.025 should be applied to that tissue or organ and a weighting factor of 0.025 should be applied to the average dose in the other remainder tissues or organs.

Source: National Council on Radiation Protection and Measurements: *Limitation of Exposure to Ionizing Radiation*, NCRP Report no. 116. Bethesda, MD, NCRP, 1993.

$\overline{D}_r$ times the effective quality factor $\overline{Q}_r$ for each type of radiation ($\overline{H} = \sum \overline{D}_r \cdot \overline{Q}_r$), where $\overline{Q}_r$ is a function of the LET of the radiation. The mean dose equivalent is a measure of the biologically effective radiation dose averaged over a tissue region of interest. However, it does not address the need for a dose unit that considers the different sensitivities of specific tissues for the expression of radiation-induced biologic effects. Hence, a unit is needed that accounts for nonuniform exposures of tissues and their significance in terms of the overall biologic effect on the exposed organism. The effective dose equivalent has been created to address this need.

The *effective dose equivalent* H_e (sometimes referred to as the *effective dose*, although the two quantities are not numerically identical) to an irradiated organism (i.e., an exposed person) is the sum over all exposed tissues of the mean dose equivalent $\overline{H}$ to each region multiplied by a *weighting factor* w_t (see margin), for the tissue in the region. The effective dose equivalent is $H_e = \sum \overline{H} \cdot w_t$, where the weighting factor w_t accounts for influences such as the probability of cancer morality and morbidity linked to irradiation of a specific tissue, the risk of hereditary effects related to irradiation of the tissue, and the relative length of life lost per unit dose caused by exposure of the specific tissue. The H_e is the sum of the absorbed doses to various regions multiplied by the weighting factors Q_r and w_t appropriate for each region:

$$H_e = \sum w_t \cdot \sum Q_r \cdot D_{t,r} = \sum Q_r \cdot \sum w_t \cdot D_{t,r}$$

As implied in this equation, the effective quality factor Q_r is independent of the tissue or organ, and the tissue weighting factor w_t is independent of the radiation type or energy. Weighting factors w_t for different tissues and organs are shown in Table 14-1.

The establishment of *an effective dose equivalent limit* on radiation exposures to workers and the general public is based on several assumptions. First, no exposure is justified unless there is a commensurate benefit to the exposed person, other individuals, or society at large. The benefit must always outweigh the risk, no matter how small the risk may be. Second, radiation exposures must be kept ALARA, consistent with sound economic and administrative practice. Third, no specific individual or group should be subjected to a risk greater than that judged acceptable. Fourth, a lower limit of radiation exposure also exists for individuals, below which the risk is negligible and does not warrant extensive administrative control. Although most radiation advisory groups subscribe philosophically to this last assumption, referred to as a *negligible individual dose* (NID), or *negligible individual level* (NIL), identification of a specific value for the lower level has not been possible to date. Efforts to establish a NIL of 0.01 mSv/year have been unsuccessful.[19]

Finally, upper limits of radiation exposure should be established to restrict the maximum risk to individuals in terms of both immediate and long-term effects of

Radiation Weighting Factor W_r

Type and Energy	W_r
X and gamma rays, electrons,[a] positrons, muons	1
Neutrons, energy	
<10 keV	5
>10–100 keV	10
>100 keV–2 MeV	20
>2–20 MeV	10
>20 MeV	5
Protons other than recoil protons, energy >2 MeV	2[b]
Alpha particles, fission fragments, nonrelativistic heavy nuclei	20

Note: All values apply to radiation incident on the body or, if internal sources, emitted from the source.

[a] Excluding Auger electrons emitted from nuclei bound to DNA.

[b] For body irradiated by protons of >100-MeV energy, W_r of unity applies.

Source: Adapted from NCRP Report 116, 1993.[21]

ALARA, an acronym for As Low As Reasonably Achievable, is a philosophy that espouses exposures as low as reasonably achievable consistent with practical and economic considerations.

Although virtually everyone agrees that the benefit of radiation exposure must outweigh the risk, considerable disagreement exists concerning the magnitude of benefit and risk. Furthermore, benefit and risk should be expressed in identical terms (e.g., the numbers of lives saved and lost per unit exposure) if a comparison of benefit and risk is to be meaningful.

In the United States, recent attempts to establish a NIL have been stymied by Congress.

radiation exposure. An upper limit of radiation exposure should ensure that risks to which radiation workers are exposed are no greater than those encountered by workers in other "safe" industries. Radiation risks should be based on the *total biological detriment* resulting from radiation exposure, including the risk of fatal cancer, hereditary defects caused by genetic mutations, relative length of life lost, and the contribution of nonfatal cancer to compromised quality of life.

The current guidance of the NCRP concerning radiation limits for occupationally exposed persons can be summarized as[19,21]:

- The lifetime total effective dose equivalent in mSv should not exceed 10 times the individual's age in years.
- Occupational exposure to radiation should not be permitted for persons below age 18.
- The annual total effective dose equivalent should be limited to 50 mSv, provided that the limit on lifetime total effective dose equivalent is not exceeded.
- Exposures should always be maintained at levels ALARA.

Expression of radiation protection standards in terms of effective dose equivalent reduces the need to identify dose limits for specific regions of the body. Use of such standards, however, could conceivably permit doses of several Sv/year to certain body regions that have relatively small values of w_t. To prevent excessive doses to these regions, additional dose limits have been established:

- 150 mSv to the crystalline lens of the eye.
- 500 mSv to all other tissues and organs, including the red bone marrow, breast, lung, gonads, extremities, and localized areas of the skin. These limits on total effective dose equivalent are generally consistent with recommendations of the ICRP.[17,20,22]

Reports suggest that mental retardation may be the greatest risk of radiation exposure of the human fetus, especially if exposures are received 8–15 weeks following conception. The risk of radiation-induced mental retardation during this period is estimated as 0.4/Sv, which has also been expressed as a reduction in IQ of about 30%/Sv.[23] Some investigators have suggested that mental retardation may not occur for doses below about 0.4 Sv, although a mechanism has not been delineated to explain a dose threshold for this effect. Some evidence also exists that the risk of adult cancer may be significantly greater in persons exposed to radiation in utero compared with unexposed individuals.[24] The NCRP recommends that exposures to the embryo–fetus be limited to no more than 0.5 mSv/month once pregnancy is known.[19] Both the NCRP and the ICRP suggest that restrictions beyond those appropriate for radiation workers in general should not be applied to workers who are fertile women but are not known to be pregnant.

Circumstances such as planned special exposures and emergency situations may arise occasionally during the course of a radiation worker's career. Specific guidelines for control of radiation exposures during these circumstances have been developed by the NCRP.[19] For planned special exposures, a few workers may be allowed to exceed 50 mSv for essential tasks planned well in advance. In emergency situations, no guidelines are intended to inhibit actions necessary to save lives in the event of a catastrophe. Exposures greater than 100 mSv, however, must be justified in any postcatastrophe review of actions of individuals confronted with a life-saving situation.

Radiation limits for members of the public are proposed as a maximum H_e of 5 mSv/year and an H_e of 1 mSv/year averaged over a lifetime. This average H_e is comparable to the average exposure to natural background radiation excluding exposure to radon. In 1992, the U.S. Nuclear Regulatory Commission adopted a revision of the Code of Federal Regulations (10CFR20) in which public exposure to reactor-produced radioactive sources is limited to 1 mSv/year (0.02 mSv/week). In

One drawback to the comparison of radiation workers to those in other "safe" industries is the difficulty of comparing the somewhat hypothetical risks of radiation exposure to the documented hazards of accidents.

Recommendations of the ICRP are slightly different. Rather than 10 mSv × (age in years), the ICRP recommends a limit of 100 mSv over 5 years cumulative.

The ICRP recommends a limit of 2 mSv to the woman's abdomen over the course of pregnancy once pregnancy is known.

1994, the Conference of Radiation Control Program Directors recommended in its Suggested State Regulations for Control of Radiation that the same limit should be applied for exposure of the public to all sources of radiation.

If an exposure exceeds the limit for an individual by a small amount, the expectation of harm to the individual is small. Nevertheless, this occurrence should be investigated to identify the reason for the excessive exposure. Questions such as whether there was a lapse in institutional safety procedures and what will be done to prevent a reoccurrence of the exposure should be answered. To permit identification of problems before a significant exposure occurs, institutions should set action levels based on review of personnel exposure records. These action levels are below effective dose equivalent limits but above exposures thought to be necessary to perform typical tasks requiring radiation exposure.[25] Many institutions set action levels at 1/10 of the limits on effective dose equivalent. If an individual's exposure falls between the action level and the effective dose equivalent limit, an investigation is conducted to determine the cause while the individual continues to function as a radiation worker.

The NCRP has stated that a higher limit of 5 mSv/year is permissible for a small group within the general public, provided that it is not repeated in subsequent years for the same group.

For the general public, the NCRP recommends an annual limit of 50 mSv to the lens of the eye, skin, and extremities.

PROTECTIVE BARRIERS FOR RADIATION SOURCES

The walls, ceiling, and floor of a room containing an x-ray or radioactive source may be constructed to permit use of adjacent rooms when the x-ray source is energized or the radioactive source is exposed. With an effective dose equivalent limit of 50 mSv/year for occupational exposure, the maximum permissible average dose equivalent equals 1 mSv/week. This dose rate is used in computations of the thickness of radiation barriers required for controlled areas. For uncontrolled areas (i.e., areas outside of direct supervision) a value of 0.1 mSv/week is usually used. Because $Q_r = 1$ for x rays and gamma rays and because radiation around shielded facilities usually is assumed to produce whole-body exposures ($w_t = 1$), exposure limits for shielding purposes can be expressed as 1 mGy/week (0.1 rad/week) in controlled areas and 0.1 mGy/week (0.01 rad/week) in uncontrolled areas. Finally, the conversion from roentgens to rads is nearly unity for x rays and gamma rays. Hence, the exposure limits sometimes are still expressed as 0.1 R/week in controlled areas and 0.01 R/week in uncontrolled areas around rooms containing an x-ray or gamma-ray source. In a shielded room, *primary barriers* are designed to attenuate the primary (useful) beam from a radiation source, and *secondary barriers* are constructed to reduce scattered and leakage radiation from the source.

Controlled areas are areas under the direct supervision of a radiation safety officer [RSO], sometimes called a radiation protection officer [RPO].

NCRP Report no. 116[21] recommends that a limit of 50 mSv/year [1 mSv/week] for controlled areas "... should be utilized only to provide flexibility required for existing facilities and practices. The NCRP recommends that all new facilities and the introduction of all new practices should be designed to limit annual exposures to individuals to a fraction of the 10 mSv per year limit implied by the cumulative dose limit by occupation."

Protection from Small Sealed Gamma-Ray Sources

The dose in Gy to an individual in the vicinity of a point source of radioactivity is

$$D = \Gamma_\infty AtB/d^2$$

where Γ_∞ is the dose rate constant in units of (Gy-m²/hr-MBq) at 1 m, A is the activity of the source in Mbq, t is the time in hours spent in the vicinity of the source, d is the distance from the source in meters, and B is the fraction of radiation transmitted by a protective barrier between the source and the individual. Dose rate constants for several gamma-emitting sources are given in Table 14-2. The dose may be reduced by (1) decreasing the time t spent in the vicinity of the source, (2) increasing the distance d between the source and the individual, and (3) increasing the attenuation (reducing the transmission B) of the protective barrier. The thickness of lead required to provide a given transmission factor B can be determined from Figure 14-2 for three radionuclide sources (^{182}Ta, ^{60}Co, and radium).

The three factors (*time, distance, and shielding*) are often referred to as the *three options for radiation protection*. The exposure to an individual varies directly with the activity of the source and the time spent in its vicinity, and inversely with the square of the distance between the source and the individual.

Example 14-2

What is the dose rate at a distance of 1 m from a 50-mCi (1.85 × 10⁵ MBq) point source of radium filtered by 0.5-mm Pt(lr) with a dose rate constant of 2.15 ×

TABLE 14-2 Dose Rate Constants Γ_∞ for Selected Radionuclides

Radionuclide	Exposure Rate Constant (R-m²/hr Ci)	Dose Rate Constant ($\times 10^7$) [Gy-m²/hr-MBq]
^{60}Co	1.31[a]	3.41
^{125}I	0.1.45[a]	0.378
^{137}Cs	0.328[a]	0.856
^{192}Ir	0.462[a]	1.21
^{198}Au	0.238[a]	0.619
^{222}Rn	1.02[a,b]	2.65
^{225}Ra	0.825[b,c]	2.15

[a] Unfiltered.

[b] In equilibrium with progeny.

[c] Filtered by 0.5-mm Pt.

10^{-7}-Gy-m²/hr-MBq? What thickness of lead is required to reduce the dose rate to less than 1 mGy/hour if the HVL is 8-mm lead for radium?

$$D = \Gamma_\infty AtB/d^2$$

$$= (2.15 \times 10^{-7}\text{ Gy-m}^2/\text{hr-MBq})(1.85 \times 10^5\text{ MBq})(1\text{m})^2$$

$$= 39.8\text{ mGy/hr}$$

Six half-value layers (6×8 mm $= 4.8$ cm) of lead are required to reduce the dose rate to less than 1 mGy/hr.

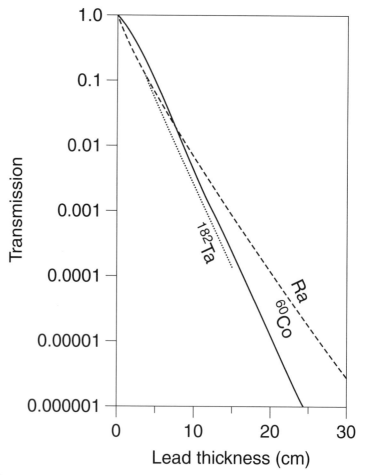

FIGURE 14-2

Transmission of gamma radiation through lead for three radionuclides (^{182}Ta, ^{60}Co, ^{226}Ra).[26]

TABLE 14-3 Typical Use Factors for a Radiation Therapy Installation

Full use ($U = 1$)	Floors of radiation rooms except dental installations, doors, walls, and ceilings of radiation rooms exposed routinely to the primary beam.
Partial use ($U = 1/4$)	Doors and walls of radiation rooms not exposed routinely to the primary beam; also, floors of dental installations.
Occasional use ($U = 1/16$)	Ceilings of radiation rooms not exposed routinely to the primary beam. Because of the low use factor, shielding requirements for a ceiling are usually determined by secondary rather than primary beam considerations.

Source: International Commission on Radiological Protection.[26]

Design of Structural Shielding

The design of shielding for radiation sources is discussed extensively in several reports of the NCRP.[21,27–29] The fundamental considerations of shielding design are presented in this section; published reports should be consulted for technical details important to the design of specific shielding configurations.

Several factors are important to the design of shielded facilities for x-ray sources used in radiation therapy. Among the factors to be considered are the following:

- The *workload W* describes the "output" of the x-ray unit. For units operating below 500 kVp, the workload is usually expressed as milliampere-minutes per week (0.01 mA-min/week), computed as 1/100 times the average mA per treatment multiplied by the approximate minutes/week of beam "on time." The factor of 1/100 reflects the observation that the dose rate is approximately 0.01 Gy/min (1 R/min) at a distance of 1 m from an x-ray tube. For units above 500 kVp, the workload is described as a weekly dose (Gy/week) delivered at 1 m from the source, estimated as the number of patient treatments per week multiplied by the dose in Gy delivered per treatment at 1 m.
- The *use factor U* is the fraction of the operating time during which the primary radiation beam is directed toward a particular protective barrier. Typical values of U are given in Table 14-3. The use factor is always unity for scattered and leakage radiation because these radiations impinge on the barrier for all orientations of the primary beam.
- The *occupancy factor T* is the fraction of the operating time of the x-ray unit that a particular area to be shielded is occupied. Representative values of T are given in Table 14-4. The occupancy factor is always unity for a controlled area.
- The distance *d* is the separation in meters between a source of radiation and a protective barrier. In calculating shielding requirements, the factor d asserts that the radiation intensity decreases as the square of the distance from a radiation source (inverse square fall-off of intensity with distance).

The room surfaces (e.g., walls, floor, and ceiling) that are exposed to the primary beam are known as *primary barriers*. Other surfaces are termed *secondary barriers* because they are exposed only to secondary (scatter and leakage) radiation.

Values of T in Table 14-4 are suggested values in areas where occupancy factors specific for the facility are not known.

The rule that radiation intensity decreases with $(1/\text{distance})^2$ applies exactly for only a point radiation source under conditions of good (narrow beam) geometry.

In barrier calculations for radiation sources in medicine, Q_r (w_r) and w_t are all assumed to equal unity. Hence, dose limits can be expressed as mGy/week because such limits are numerically equal to effective dose equivalent limits in mSv/week.

Primary Radiation Barriers

For a maximum permissible dose *P* in a protected area (1 mGy/week [0.001 Gy/week] in a controlled area, 0.1 mGy/week [0.0001 Gy/week] in an uncontrolled area), the required transmission *B* of a primary barrier is

$$P = (WUTB)/d^2$$

$$B = Pd^2/(WUT)$$

By consulting broad-beam attenuation curves for the radiation energy of the primary beam, the required barrier thickness can be determined (Example 14-3). Typical broad-beam attenuation curves are shown in Figures 14-3 and 14-4. A full range of attenuation curves is available in the literature.[27,28]

TABLE 14-4 Typical Occupancy Factors for a Radiation Therapy Installation

Full occupancy ($T = 1$)	Control spaces, offices, corridors, and waiting spaces large enough to hold desks, darkrooms, workrooms and shops, nurse stations, rest and lounge rooms used routinely by occupationally exposed personnel, living quarters, children's play areas, and occupied space in adjoining buildings
Partial occupancy ($T = 1/4$)	Corridors too narrow for desks, utility rooms, rest and lounge rooms not used routinely by occupationally exposed personnel, wards and patients' rooms, elevators with operators, and unattended parking lots
Occasional occupancy ($T = 1/16$)	Closets too small for future occupancy, toilets not used routinely by occupationally exposed personnel, stairways, automatic elevators, pavements, and streets

Source: International Commission on Radiological Protection.[26]

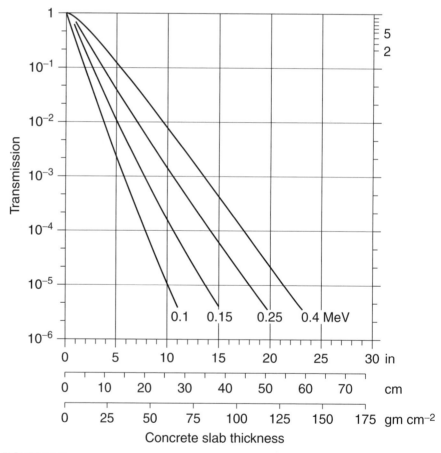

FIGURE 14-3
Broad-beam transmission through concrete (density 2.35 g/cm³) of x rays produced by 0.1- to 0.4-MeV electrons.[28]

Example 14-3

A 6-MV linear accelerator delivers up to 300 treatments per week, with each treatment averaging 2 Gy tumor dose at a distance of 1 m from the target. The unit is pointed no more than $1/4$ of the time toward a particular wall 4 m from the target. The laboratory on the other side of the wall is a controlled area. What thickness of concrete is required for the wall?

With an estimated average tissue–air ratio of 0.7, the workload W of the therapy unit is

$$(2 \text{ Gy/treatment})(300 \text{ treatments/week})/0.7 = 860 \text{ Gy/week at } 1 \text{ m}$$

For a controlled area, $P = 0.001$ Gy/week and $T = 1$. The distance $d = 4$ m and $U = 1/4$:

$$B = Pd^2/WUT$$
$$= [0.001][4^2]/[860][1/4][1]$$
$$= 7.4 \times 10^{-5}$$

From Figure 14-4, the required thickness is 140-cm concrete.

In Example 14-3 and in following examples, shielding computations are designed to limit occupational exposures to 50 mSv/year (1mSv/week). To shield to lower limits, the value of P should be reduced (e.g., from 0.001 Gy/week to 0.0002 Gy/week to achieve a lower limit of 10 mSr/year).

Some isocentric therapy machines are equipped with a counterweight that intercepts the primary beam after it exits the patient. This counterweight, usually referred to as a "beam stopper," greatly reduces the primary beam intensity (often by a factor of 0.001). When a beam stopper is present, its attenuation factor F_{BS} would appear in the primary beam equations as

$$P = (WUTBF_{BS})/d^2$$
$$B = Pd^2/(WUTF_{BS})$$

In shielding computations, attenuation of the beam by the patient is neglected.

The TVL is the thickness of a material required to reduce the beam intensity to 1/10. TVL = 3.32 HVL. The number N of TVLs required to achieve a barrier transmission B is $N = \log(1/B)$.

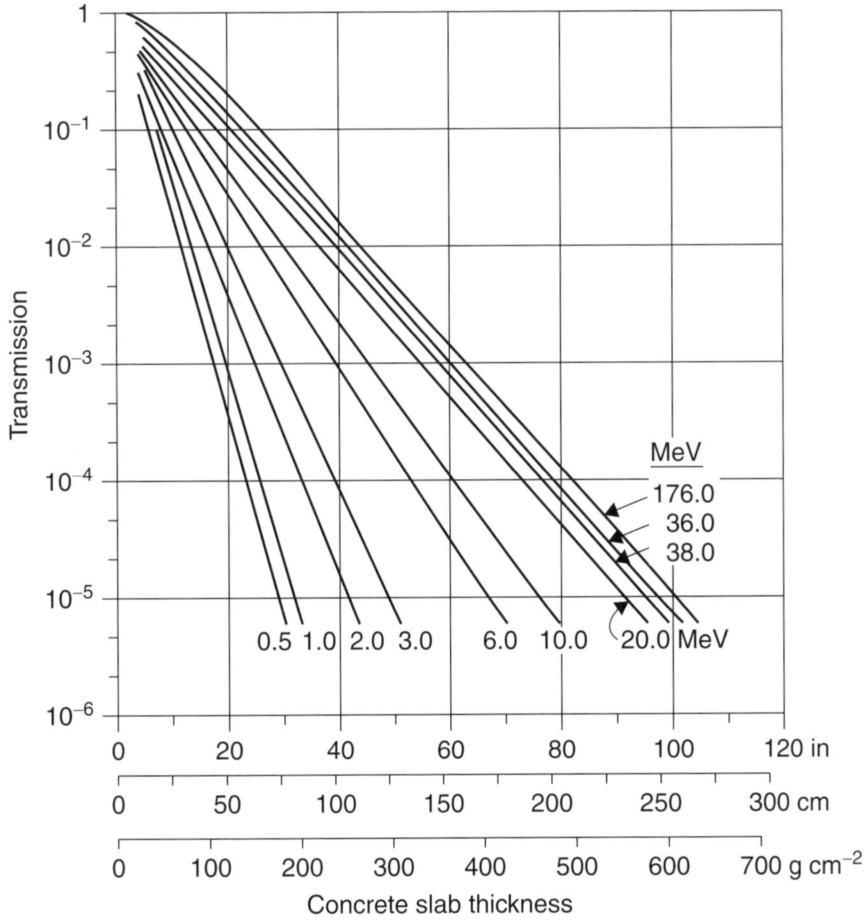

FIGURE 14-4
Broad-beam transmission of x rays through concrete, density 2.35 g/cm^3. Energy designations refer to monoenergetic electrons incident on a thick x-ray target.[28]

TABLE 14-5 Physical Densities and Tenth-Value Layers (TVLs) for Various Materials and Beam Energies

Peak Voltage (kV)	Lead (mm) $\rho = 11.36$ g/cm^3		Concrete (cm) $\rho = 2.35$ g/cm^3		Iron (cm) $\rho = 7.8$ g/cm^3	
	HVL	TVL	HVL	TVL	HVL	TVL
50	0.06	0.17	0.43	1.5		
70	0.17	0.52	0.84	2.8		
100	0.27	0.88	1.6	5.3		
125	0.28	0.93	2.0	6.6		
150	0.30	0.99	2.24	7.4		
200	0.52	1.7	2.5	8.4		
250	0.88	2.9	2.24	7.4		
300	1.47	4.8	3.1	10.4		
400	2.5	8.3	3.3	10.9		
500	3.6	11.9	3.6	11.7		
1000	7.9	26	4.4	14.7		
2000	12.5	42	7.4	24.5		
3000	14.5	48.5	7.4	24.5		
4000	16	53	8.8	29.2	2.7	9.1
6000	16.9	56	10.4	34.5	3.0	9.9
8000	16.9	56	11.4	37.8	3.1	10.3
10,000	16.6	55	11.9	39.6	3.2	10.5
Cesium-137	6.5	21.6	4.8	15.7	1.6	5.3
Cobalt-60	12	40	6.2	20.6	2.1	6.9
Gold-198	3.3	11.0	4.1	13.5		
Iridium-192	6.0	20	4.2	14.7	1.3	4.3
Radium	16.6	55	6.9	23.4	2.2	7.4

The type of barrier material to be employed (e.g., concrete, lead, or steel) depends on several factors, including structural, space, and cost considerations and the efficiency with which different materials attenuate radiation of a particular energy. For radiation therapy units, concrete is usually employed except in cases in which space is at a premium, in which case steel or lead may be preferred. For megavoltage x rays, the equivalent thickness of various materials can be estimated by comparing tenth value layers (TVL). A coarse approximation can be obtained by comparing physical densities. Densities and TVLs for various materials and beam energies are given in Table 14-5.

Secondary Barriers for Scattered Radiation

In radiation therapy, the patient is the principal source of scattered radiation. The amount of scattered radiation varies with the dose rate, beam energy, beam area incident on the patient, and the angle of scatter. The ratio of radiation scattered at various angles at 1 m from the patient to the amount of radiation incident on the patient is denoted as α. Values of α for different scattering angles and beam energies are given in Table 14-6 for an incident beam area of 400 cm^2. For megavoltage x-ray beams, α is usually taken as 0.1% for 90° scatter from a 400-cm^2 beam. The value of α increases with decreasing scattering angle. Values of α for incident beam areas other than 400 cm^2 can be estimated by multiplying α by area/400.

Scattered radiation is usually lower in energy than the primary beam. At relatively low energies (<500 kVp), however, the difference is not great, and the scattered energy is usually assumed to be equal to the energy of the primary beam. For higher-energy x-ray beams (>500 kVp), the energy of the x rays scattered at 90° cannot exceed 511 keV (Example 3-8), and the required barrier thickness can be determined with the transmission curve for 500-kVp x rays. The energy of scattered radiation increases as the scattering angle decreases.

TABLE 14-6 Ratio α of Scattered to Incident Radiation, with the Scattered Radiation Measured 1 m from a Phantom with a Field Area of 400 cm^2, and the Incident Radiation Measured at the Center of the Field 1 m from the Source in the Absence of the Phantom

	Scattering Angle (from Central Ray)					
Source	30	45	60	90	120	135
X rays						
50 kV[a]	0.0005	0.0002	0.00025	0.00035	0.0008	0.0010
70 kV[a]	0.00065	0.00035	0.00035	0.0005	0.0010	0.0013
100 kV[a]	0.0015	0.0012	0.0012	0.0013	0.0020	0.0022
125 kV[a]	0.0018	0.0015	0.0015	0.0015	0.0023	0.0025
150 kV[a]	0.0020	0.0016	0.0016	0.0016	0.0024	0.0026
200 kV[a]	0.0024	0.0020	0.0019	0.0019	0.0027	0.0028
250 kV[a]	0.0025	0.0021	0.0019	0.0019	0.0027	0.0028
300 kV[a]	0.0026	0.0022	0.0020	0.0019	0.0026	0.0028
4 MV[b]	—	0.0027	—	—	—	—
6 MV[c]	0.007	0.0018	0.0011	0.0006	—	0.0004
Gamma rays						
^{137}Cs[d]	0.0065	0.0050	0.0041	0.0028	—	0.0019
^{60}Co[e]	0.0060	0.0036	0.0023	0.0009	—	0.0006

Source: National Council on Radiation Protection and Measurements.[27]

[a] Average scatter for beam centered and beam at edge of typical patient cross-section phantom. Peak pulsating x-ray tube potential. (From Trout and Kelley. *Radiology* 1972; **104**:161.)

[b] Cylindrical phantom. (From Greene and Massey. *Br. J. Radiol.* 1961; **34**:389.)

[c] Cylindrical phantom. (From Karzmark and Capone. *Br. J. Radiol.* 1968; **41**:222.)

[d] These data were obtained from a slab placed obliquely to the central ray. A cylindrical phantom should give smaller values. (Interpolated from Frantz and Wyckoff. *Radiology* 1959; **73**:263.)

[e] Modified for $f = 400$ cm^2. (From Mooney and Braestrup. Atomic Energy Commission Report NYO 2165, 1967.)

For a maximum permissible dose rate P in Gy/week from radiation scattered from a patient, the required transmission B of a secondary barrier can be estimated as

$$P = [(\alpha \cdot W \cdot U \cdot T)/d^2(d')^2] \cdot [F/400] \cdot B$$
$$B = [P/(\alpha \cdot U \cdot W \cdot T)] \cdot [400/F] \cdot d^2 \cdot (d')^2$$

where α is the fractional scatter at 1 m for a beam area of 400 cm^2, F is the actual beam area in cm^2, d is the source–patient distance in meters, and d' is the distance in meters from the patient to the barrier. For radiation scattered at 90°, U is usually assumed to be unity. The barrier thickness that provides the required transmission is determined from the appropriate attenuation curve in Figures 14-3 and 14-4 (primary energy curve for beams <500 kVp and the 500-kVp curve for beams >500 kVp for scatter at 90 degrees; curves such as those in Figure 14-5 are used for radiation scattered at angles other than 90°).

Secondary Barriers for Leakage Radiation

For therapy x-ray units operating below 500 kVp, the maximum leakage of radiation from the tube housing is 1 rad/hour (0.01 Gy/hour) at a distance of 1 m. For therapy units above 500 kVp (i.e., ^{60}Co gamma-ray and megavoltage x-ray units), the maximum leakage radiation at 1 m in any direction from the source is confined by regulatory statute to 0.1% of the dose rate from the useful beam at 1 m from the source. The required secondary barrier B for leakage radiation to yield a permissible dose rate P (Gy/week) at 1 m from the source is determined as follows:

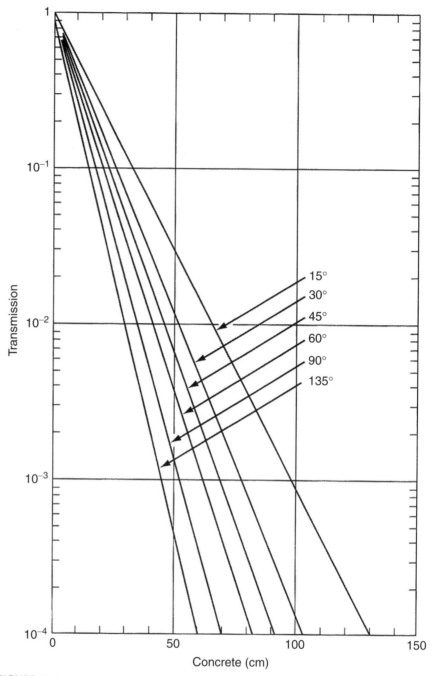

FIGURE 14-5
Broad-beam transmission of 6-MV x rays scattered at various angles.

For therapy units <500 kVp, we obtain

$$P = WTB/(d^2 \cdot 60I)$$

$$B = Pd^2 \cdot 60I/WT$$

where I is the maximum tube current for continuous operation of the x-ray source, W is the workload expressed as 0.01 mA-min/week, the number *60* converts minutes to hours, and d is the distance from the source to the barrier.

For therapy units > 500 kVp, we obtain

$$P = 0.001WTB/d^2$$

$$B = Pd^2/(0.001WT)$$

where 0.001 is the 0.1% leakage through the source housing measured at 1 m.

The energy of leakage radiation is approximately the same as the energy of the primary beam, and the transmission curve for primary radiation should be used to determine the barrier thickness for leakage radiation.

For therapy x-ray beams, a barrier thickness for primary radiation greatly exceeds that for secondary radiation. Hence, secondary radiation can be ignored when barrier thicknesses are determined for primary radiation because a primary barrier also reduces secondary radiation to a negligible level. For megavoltage x-ray beams, shielding requirements for leakage radiation usually significantly exceed those for scattered radiation because the leakage radiation is more energetic. Hence, requirements for secondary barriers are usually dominated by leakage radiation except in situations in which small scattering angles must be considered. For lower-energy beams, differences may be small between the requirements for scattered and leakage radiation. Shielding requirements for secondary barriers are computed separately for scattered and leakage radiation. If the difference in shielding requirements exceeds 3 HVLs (or 1 TVL) for the primary beam, the greater of the two thicknesses provides adequate shielding for both. If the difference is less than 3 HVLs, one HVL of shielding thickness should be added to the larger thickness to provide adequate shielding against both scattered and leakage radiation.

Door Shielding

Unless the entrance to a room housing a radiation therapy unit is constructed as a maze, the room door must provide radiation shielding equivalent to the contiguous wall. For higher-energy therapy beams, the door contains massive quantities of lead or steel and requires a motor drive for opening and closing. A manual means of moving the door must be available in the event that electrical power fails. In most cases, a maze entranceway is preferable to a motorized door because it greatly reduces the shielding requirements for the door. The maze is designed so that radiation must be scattered at least once, and usually multiple times, before it reaches the door (Figure 14-6). With each scattering, the intensity and energy of the radiation is decreased, and the required door shielding is reduced. The shielding requirements of the door can be determined by using the equation given earlier for the intensity of scattered radiation for each scattering angle in the pathway from the radiation source to the door. In most cases, the use of an entrance maze can reduce the required door shielding to a few millimeters of lead.

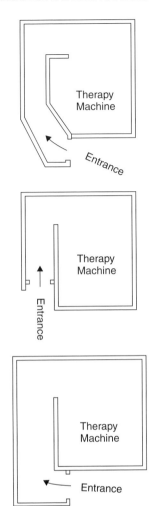

MARGIN FIGURE 14-1
Typical designs for maze entrances to radiation therapy rooms. (From Jayaraman and Lanzl, with permission.[30])

Example 14-4

The 6-MV linear accelerator described in Example 14-3 is equipped with a primary beam stopper that transmits less than 0.1% of the primary beam. Radiation scattered by the patient through angles up to 30° is also intercepted by the beam stopper. Under these conditions and for use and occupancy factors of unity, what thickness of concrete is required for the wall described in Example 14-3?

From Table 14-6, the fraction of the incident radiation scattered at 1 m through a scattering angle of 30° is 0.007 for a 400-cm^2 field. With the patient 1 m from the target, the distance d' from the patient to the wall is

Leakage radiation is isotropic (equal intensity in all directions), so $U = 1$ in barrier computations for leakage radiation.

$$d' = (3\,\text{m})/(\cos 30°) = (3\,\text{m})/(0.866)$$

$$= 3.46\,\text{m}$$

If the average field size for patient treatment is 400 cm^2, the required attenuation factor B is

$$B = [P/(\alpha W U T)][400/F]d^2/d'^2)^2$$

$$= [0.001/(0.007)(860)(1)(1)][400/400][(1)^2/(3.46)^2]$$

$$= 2.0 \times 10^{-3}$$

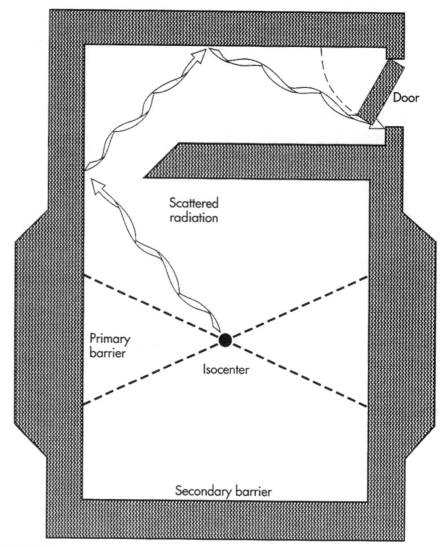

FIGURE 14-6
Entrance maze for a high-energy accelerator used in radiation therapy. The maze is designed so that only multiply-scattered radiation can reach the door.

From Figure 14-5, 70 cm of concrete is required to provide an attenuation factor of 2.0×10^{-3} for 6-MV x rays scattered through 30°. This thickness provides more than adequate protection against scattered radiation because scattered radiation skims past the beam stopper and strikes the wall only when the therapy unit is oriented toward the wall (i.e., $U = \frac{1}{4}$ could have been used in this computation). The remainder of the time the unit is oriented in a different direction in which the scattering angle is greater, and both α and the average energy of scattered photons are reduced.

Example 14-5

For the 6-MV accelerator described in Example 14-3, a wall perpendicular to the axis of rotation of the unit is never exposed to the primary beam. The wall is 4 m from the patient, and the average field size at the patient is 20 × 20 cm. What thickness of concrete is required to shield nonoccupationally exposed individuals ($P = 0.0001$ Gy/week) in the adjoining room from scattered radiation, if the occupancy factor for the room is $1/4$?

$$B = [P/(\alpha W 400/F)]d^2/d')^2$$
$$= \frac{(0.0001)(400/400)(1)^2/(4)^2}{(0.0006)(860)(1/4)}$$
$$= 1.2 \times 10^{-2}$$

From the 500-kVp curve in Figure 14-4, 33 cm of concrete is required to reduce scattered radiation to an acceptable level.

Example 14-6

For the wall described in Example 14-5, determine the thickness of concrete required to protect the nonoccupationally exposed individuals from leakage radiation:

$$B = \frac{P d^2}{0.001 W T}$$
$$= \frac{(0.0001)(4)^2}{(0.001)(860)(1/4)}$$
$$= 7.4 \times 10^{-3}$$

Leakage radiation has essentially the same energy as primary radiation, so attenuation curves for the primary beam are consulted when leakage is considered. The required thickness of concrete is 70 cm.

Example 14-7

For the wall described in Examples 14-5 and 14-6, 33 cm of concrete is required to shield against scattered radiation, and 70 cm is needed to shield for leakage radiation. The difference of 37 cm in these thicknesses slightly exceeds the 35 cm of concrete described as 1 TVL—hence, the required barrier thickness is 70 cm of concrete. If the difference had been less than 35 cm, 1 HVL (11 cm of concrete) would have to be added to the 70-cm thickness of concrete.

Neutron Shielding

Neutrons are released when electrons and x rays produced in a high-energy accelerator interact with the target, flattening filter, collimator, patient, and materials in the accelerator room. Hence, the x-ray beam from a high-energy (>10 MV) accelerator is contaminated with neutrons. The electron beam from a high-energy accelerator is contaminated with neutrons to a much smaller degree than the x-ray beam because electrons produce neutrons with a much lower efficiency compared with x rays. The neutron contamination increases rapidly with increasing x-ray energy from 10 to 20 MV and remains relatively constant above 20 MV.[31] For x rays between about 15 and 25 MV, the neutron dose equivalent rate along the central axis of the beam is about 0.5% of the x-ray dose-equivalent rate and falls to about 0.1% outside the primary beam.[32] The energy of the neutrons extends over a wide range with a maximum of about 1 MeV. The neutron energy is rapidly degraded by multiple scattering. Neutrons are attenuated efficiently in concrete, and concrete barriers for x-ray shielding almost always provide adequate shielding against neutrons.

The door to a treatment room for a high-energy accelerator often presents a special challenge with regard to neutron shielding.[33] A maze entranceway can be designed to reduce greatly the quantity and energy of neutrons reaching the door. In most cases, a few inches of a hydrogenous material such as polyethylene in the door are sufficient to reduce the neutron dose equivalent to an acceptable level outside the treatment room. However, as the neutrons are absorbed by (n, γ) reactions in the

The degradation ("moderation") of neutron energy occurs most efficiently by elastic scattering with hydrogen nuclei (protons) and other light nuclei. Heavy nuclei such as lead are poor moderators because they deflect neutrons with little energy loss.

Boron is a strong absorber (i.e., it has a high cross section) for low-energy neutrons. Hence, polyethylene impregnated with boron is often used to shield the treatment-room door.[34]

NCRP Report no. 79 provides the following expressions for computation of TVLs for reduction of absorbed dose for neutrons of average energy $\bar{E}$ in MeV:

Concrete: TVL (cm) $= 15.5 + 5.6\bar{E}$
Polyethylene:
TVL (cm) $= 6.2 + 3.4\bar{E}$

An accurate inventory of long-lived brachytherapy sources must be maintained. An inventory is especially challenging when radioactive wires (e.g., ^{192}Ir, ^{182}Ta, or ^{198}Au) are present that can be cut into segments of variable length.

Beta-emitting sources such as ^{90}Sr–^{90}Y ophthalmic applicators should be manipulated behind a low-Z shield such as acrylic. High-Z shielding materials such as lead are undesirable for β sources because they generate more bremsstrahlung during absorption of β particles.

Brachytherapy sources should be sterilized only by chemical treatment. They should never be subjected to heat or steam sterilization methods.

Radium sources are particularly hazardous and subject to radon leakage. Although these sources are no longer recommended for brachytherapy, they are still occasionally found in storage receptacles in medical facilities.

door, gamma rays (called neutron-capture gamma rays) are released with energies in the range of a few MeV. These gamma rays must be attenuated by lead in the door so that dose rates outside the room do not exceed acceptable levels.

The determination of shielding barriers for high-energy accelerators required to reduce x rays, neutron-capture rays, and neutrons to acceptable levels outside a treatment room is a complex process. Several references are available to aid these computations.[28–34] However, the computations should be performed by persons who are expert in shielding design for high-energy accelerators.

■ PROTECTION FOR SEALED RADIOACTIVE SOURCES

The safe handling, transport, and storage of sealed radioactive sources used for brachytherapy (*brachy*, Greek for "short distance") require supervision by an individual with extensive knowledge of radiation protocols and safety. A few principles are discussed in this section, but detailed safety procedures are required for the safe use of high-activity sealed sources of radioactivity in radiation therapy.[35–37]

Long-lived brachytherapy sources are stored in a lead-lined "safe" with lead-filled drawers designed to hold sources in the shape of needles, capsules, and other configurations. The safe should be designed to facilitate rapid removal and return of sources. A shielded area, often equipped with an *L-block* of lead with a lead-glass window, should always be used when sealed sources are handled. The shielded area may be equipped with mirrors to permit handling of the sources under conditions in which direct viewing of the sources is undesirable.

Sealed sources should always be handled with forceps and never with the hands. A sink trap should always be present in the sink used to clean brachytherapy applicators to prevent loss of a sealed source that has been left accidentally in the applicator. Afterloading procedures should be used whenever possible to reduce the exposure to personnel engaged in brachytherapy. The three principles of radiation protection (time, distance, and shielding) are particularly applicable in the handling and transport of sealed radioactive sources.

Brachytherapy sources should always be transported in a lead-shielded container, often a cart that can be rolled to the application site. The cart should be well balanced so that it cannot tip over and spill its contents. The container should display a radiation warning sign and should never be left unattended while radioactive sources are inside. The container should be used only to transport brachytherapy sources and should not be used for permanent storage of sources.

Sealed radioactive sources must be *leak tested* at periodic intervals, not to exceed 6 months by regulation. Most sealed sources are tested by wiping the surface with a moistened cloth or cotton swab and determining if any radioactivity has been transferred to the wiping material. A source is considered "leaky" if 0.005 μCi (185 Bq) or more activity is present on the material. A leaking source should be sealed in a container and returned to the supplier.

■ RADIATION SURVEYS

After installation or modification of radiation equipment, a radiation survey must be performed to verify that exposure levels in all occupied areas are within acceptable limits and that the integrity of the shielding material has not been compromised. The survey also should ensure that the equipment is functioning properly and that safety interlocks and emergency procedures are appropriate, functional, and well understood by all employees. Three instruments commonly employed in radiation protection surveys are the portable ionization survey meter, G–M counter, and neutron detector.

Ionization Chambers

Exposure rates in the range of a few mR/hour can be measured with a portable survey meter such as that depicted in Margin Figure 14-2. This instrument contains an ionization chamber as the radiation-sensitive component and is often referred to as a *cutie pie*. Air inside the large (~600 cm^3) ionization chamber is ionized during exposure to radiation, and an electrical current is measured as this ionization is collected. The measured current is displayed directly on a meter scale denoting radiation units such as mR/hour. The response of the chamber must be calibrated periodically against a standard source, such as ^{137}Co and an energy-dependence correction applied if the measured photons differ significantly in energy from those used for instrument calibration. A correction may also be required if the instrument varies in sensitivity with the direction of impinging radiation. Most ionization-chamber survey instruments are unsealed, and corrections may be necessary for the ambient temperature and pressure if the chamber is calibrated under conditions greatly different from those encountered during routine use.

G–M Counters

The *Geiger–Mueller (G–M) counter* uses a sealed cylindrical detector filled with an inert gas containing small amounts of impurities (Margin Figure 14-3). When radiation interacts with the gas, an avalanche of ionization is created as a result of the relatively high voltage (~ 1000 V) applied across the chamber. As this ionization is collected, a voltage pulse is produced across the detector electrodes that indicates that an ionization event has occurred inside the detector. This indication is displayed by a meter with units of counts/min. The G–M counter records individual interactions and is not useful for measurement of actual exposure or dose rates around a radiation unit. It is much more sensitive than a cutie pie, however, and is helpful in identifying the presence of small amounts of radioactivity or small voids in radiation shields.

Neutron Detectors

Various types of instruments are available to detect and measure the presence of neutrons in occupied areas outside the treatment room. A common instrument is an ionization chamber or proportional counter filled with BF$_3$ gas or composed of walls coated with lithium, boron, or a hydrogenous material. A BF$_3$ proportional counter is shown in Margin Figure 14-4 in which the detector is surrounded by a 9-inch cadmium-loaded polyethylene sphere to slow (moderate) the neutrons so that they interact efficiently with the detector. Measurements with the chamber are recorded in units of mrem/hour or mSv/hour.

■ PERSONNEL MONITORING

Radiation exposures must be monitored for persons working with or near sources of ionizing radiation. Individuals who have a potential of receiving doses of one-tenth or more of the permissible limit must wear one or more radiation monitors that can be read out periodically (e.g., biweekly or monthly) to determine their actual exposure to radiation. Over the years, the monitor used most often has been the film badge containing two or more dental-size x-ray films in a sealed packet. The films differ in sensitivity to permit measurement over a wide range of exposures. A film badge is worn on the collar or trunk of the body, or sometimes in both locations during each workday. Periodically the films are replaced, and the optical densities of the exposed films are measured as an index of the exposure received by the person wearing the badge. Radiations detectable with the film badge include x rays, gamma rays, high-energy electrons, and neutrons. In many "film badges" in use

The name cutie pie, originated as a code name assigned during the Manhattan Project, refers to three of the variables (charge [Q], time [t], and volume [π]) that affect the instrument's sensitivity.

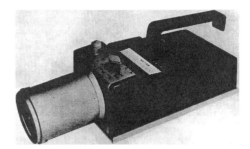

MARGIN FIGURE 14-2
Cutie-pie ionization-chamber survey meter. (Courtesy of Nuclear Associates Inc.)

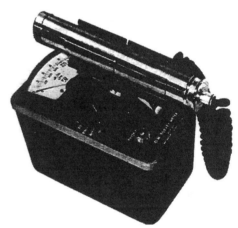

MARGIN FIGURE 14-3
Geiger–Mueller survey meter. (Courtesy of Nuclear Associates Inc.)

G–M counters have a relatively long resolving time (50–300 μsec). Hence, high activities can paralyze a G–M counter, resulting in suppression of the count rate.

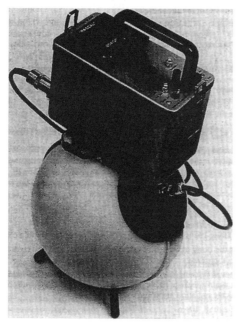

MARGIN FIGURE 14-4
BF$_3$ proportional counter used for surveys of neutron levels. (Courtesy of Eberline, Santa Fe, New Mexico.)

Modifications of the TLD whole-body monitor have yielded wrist and finger dosimeters to monitor the radiation exposure to the extremities. These monitors are especially useful in angiography and nuclear medicine.

today, thermoluminescent dosimeters (TLDs) have replaced x-ray film as the sensitive element in the monitor.

Small ionization chambers about the size of a fountain pen can be worn in the pocket while an individual is engaged in a procedure involving exposure to ionizing radiation. Many of these pocket chambers can be read at any time by the individual and permit periodic assessment of exposure as the procedure progresses. Pocket chambers are sometimes used by persons engaged in brachytherapy procedures.

■ SUMMARY

- Standards for radiation are based on estimates of risk derived from the linear non-threshold model of radiation injury.
- Stochastic effects of radiation exposure include carcinogenesis, teratogenesis, and mutagenesis.
- Nonstochastic effects of radiation exposure include the hematopoietic syndrome, gastrointestinal syndrome, and cerebrovascular syndrome.
- Organizations important to the evolution of radiation protection standards include the International Commission on Radiological Protection and the U.S. National Council on Radiation Protection and Measurements.
- Radiation limits expressed as effective dose equivalents are influenced by the average absorbed dose to tissue and weighted by factors that account for the LET of the radiation and for mortality and morbidity linked to irradiation of specific tissues.
- Shielding barriers for x rays include (a) primary barriers to protect against the primary beam and (b) secondary barriers to protect against secondary radiation (scatter and leakage).
- Factors that influence the thickness of primary and secondary barriers include the workload W, use factor U, occupancy factor T, and distance from the radiation source to the barrier.
- Shielding against neutrons may be required for high-energy accelerators (>10 MV). Instruments used for radiation surveys include cutie pies, G–M counters and, for high-energy accelerators, a neutron survey instrument.

PROBLEMS

14-1. The lifetime risk of a particular form of radiation-induced cancer is estimated as 10^{-3} Sv^{-1}. What is the lifetime risk for a whole-body dose equivalent of 0.05 Sv? Does your estimate assume that the dose response follows a linear, non-threshold model?

14-2. For a 45-year-old radiation worker, what is the maximum cumulative dose limit recommended by the NCRP? If the worker's cumulative dose were below this limit, what would be the dose limit for the next year? What would be the maximum cumulative dose limit if the individual were a member of the general public?

14-3. What is the dose rate at a distance of 2 m from a 200-mCi (7.4×10^3 MBq) point source of ^{137}Cs ($\Gamma_\infty = 8.5 \times 10^{-8} \frac{Gy-m^2}{hr-MBq}$). What thickness of lead (HVL 7 mm) is required to reduce the dose rate to less than 0.02 mGy/hr (2 mR/hr)? What additional thickness of lead would keep the dose rate at the same level if the source activity were increased to 800 mCi (29.6×10^4 MBq)?

14-4. A therapy facility is designed to treat as many as 60 patients per week with a 6-MV linear accelerator. Treatments will deliver a tumor dose of 2 Gy on the average with a tissue air ratio of approximately 0.7. For an uncontrolled adjacent room at a distance of 6 meters and full occupancy, what is the required thickness of concrete wall for a use factor of ¼? If 4 inches of lead (attenuation factor 10^{-2}) are placed along the wall, how much additional concrete would be needed?

14-5. Repeat the computation in Problem 14-4 for a wall 6 m away that never receives the primary beam ($P = 10^{-4}$ Gy/wk, $T = 1$).

14-6. For the wall described in Problem 14-3, what thickness of concrete is required to protect against leakage radiation? Is additional shielding required when scattered and leakage radiation are considered together?

REFERENCES

1. Stannard, J. N. *Radioactivity and Health: A History.* Springfield, VA, Department of Energy, National Science and Technology Information Service, (DOE/RL101830-759), 1988.

2. Moeller, D. History and perspective on the development of radiation protection standards. In *Radiation Protection Today: The NCRP at 60 Years,* W. K. Sinclair (ed.). Proceedings of the 25th Annual Meeting. Bethesda, MD, National Council on Radiation Protection and Measurements, 1990.

3. Claus, W. The concept and philosophy of permissible dose to radiation. In *Radiation Biology and Medicine,* W. Claus (ed.). Reading, MA, Addison-Wesley, 1958.

4. Stebbings, J. H., Lucas, H. F., and Stehney A. F. Mortality from cancers of major sites in female radium dial workers. *Am. J. Ind. Med.* 1984; **5**:435–459.

5. Luckey, T. D. *Hormesis with Ionizing Radiation.* Boca Raton, FL, CRC Press, 1980.

6. Gofman, J. W. *Radiation and Human Health.* San Francisco, Sierra Club, 1981.

7. Edwards, F. M. Development of radiation protection standards. *Radiographics* 1991; **11**:699-712.

8. International Commission on Radiological Protection. *Nonstochastic Effects of Ionizing Radiation,* ICRP Publication No. 41. Oxford, Pergamon Press, 1984.

9. United Nations Scientific Committee on the Effects of Atomic Radiation. (UNSCEAR). *Ionizing Radiation: Sources and Biological Effects Report E.82.1X.8.* New York, United Nations, 1982.

10. British X-Ray and Radium Protection Committee. X-ray and radium protection. *J Roentgen Soc.* 1921; **17**:100.

11. International Commission on Radiological Protection (ICRP). International recommendations for x-ray and radium protection. *Radiology* 1934; **23**:682 and *Br. J. Radiol.* 1934; **7**:695.

12. Taylor, L. S. The development of radiation protection standards (1925–40). *Health Phys.* 1981; **41**:227–232.

13. Taylor L. S. Organization of radiation protection. *The Operations of the ICRP and NCRP—1928–1974,* DOE/TIC-10124. Washington, DC, U.S. Department of Energy, Office of Technical Information, 1979.

14. National Academy of Sciences, National Research Council. *The Biological Effects of Atomic Radiation—Summary Report.* Washington, DC, National Academy of Sciences Press, 1956.

15. National Council on Radiation Protection and Measurements (NCRP). Maximum permissible radiation exposure to man: A preliminary statement of the National Committee on Radiation Protection and Measurements. *Am. J. Roentgenol.* 1957; **68**:260–267.

16. International Commission on Radiological Protection. *Recommendations of the ICRP,* ICRP Publication No. 1. London, Pergamon Press, 1957.

17. International Commission on Radiological Protection: *Recommendations of the ICRP,* ICRP Publication No. 26. London, Pergamon Press, 1977.

18. Kocher, DC. Perspective on the historical development of radiation protection standards. *Health Phys.* 1991; **61**:519–527.

19. National Council on Radiation Protection and Measurements. *Recommendations on Limits for Exposure to Ionizing Radiation.* NCRP Report No. 91. Bethesda, MD, NCRP, 1987.

20. International Commission on Radiological Protection. *Statement and Recommendations of the 1980 Brighton Meeting of the ICRP,* ICRP Publication No. 30. Elmsford, NY, Pergamon Press, 1980.

21. National Council on Radiation Protection and Measurements: *Limitations of Exposure to Ionizing Radiation,* NCRP Report No. 116. Bethesda, MD, NCRP, 1993.

22. International Commission on Radiological Protection. *Nonstochastic Effects of Ionizing Radiation.* ICRP Publication No. 41. Elmsford, NY, Pergamon Press, 1984.

23. Meinhold C. Past-President, National Council on Radiation Protection and Measurements: Personal communication, 1992.

24. United Nations Scientific Committee on the Effects of Atomic Radiation. *Genetic and Somatic Effects of Ionizing Radiation: UNSCEAR Report to the General Assembly with Annexes.* New York, United Nations, 1981.

25. National Council on Radiation Protection and Measurements. *Implementation of the Principle of as Low as Reasonably Achievable (ALARA) for Medical and Dental Personnel.* NCRP Report No. 107. Bethesda, MD, NCRP, 1990.

26. International Commission on Radiological Protection. *Report of Committee III on Protection Against X Rays Up to Energies of 3 MeV and Beta and Gamma Rays from Sealed Sources,* ICRP Publication No. 3. New York, Pergamon Press, 1960.

27. National Council on Radiation Protection and Measurements. *Structural Shielding Design and Evaluation for Medical Use of X Ray and Gamma Rays of Energies Up to 10 MeV,* NCRP Report No. 49. Bethesda, MD, NCRP, 1976.

28. National Council on Radiation Protection and Measurements. *Radiation Protection Design Guidelines for 0.1–100 MeV Particle Accelerator Facilities,* NCRP Report No. 51. Bethesda, MD, NCRP, 1977.

29. National Council on Radiation Protection and Measurements. *Medical X-ray, Electron Beam and Gamma-Ray Protection for Energies Up to 50 MeV (Equipment Design, Performance and Use),* NCRP Report No. 102, NCRP, Bethesda, MD, 1989.

30. Jayaraman, S. and Lanzl, L. (eds.). *Clinical Radiotherapy Physics,* Vol II. Bethesda, MD, CRC Press, 1996, p. 171.

31. Sohrabi, M., and Morgan, K. Z. Neutron dosimetry in high-energy x-ray beams of medical accelerators. *Phys. Med. Biol.* 1979; **24**:756–766.

32. Axton, E., and Bardell, A. Neutron production from electron accelerators used for medical purposes. *Phys. Med. Biol.* 1972; **17**:293–298.

33. Kersey, R. Estimation of neutron and gamma radiation doses in the entrance mazes of SL 75-20 linear accelerator treatment rooms. *Medicamundi* 1979; **24**:151.

34. National Council on Radiation Protection and Measurements: *Neutron Contamination for Medical Linear Accelerators,* NCRP Report No. 79. Bethesda, MD, NCRP, 1984.

35. National Council on Radiation Protection and Measurements. *Protection Against Radiation from Brachytherapy Sources,* NCRP Report No. 40. Bethesda, MD, NCRP, 1972.

36. American Association of Physicists in Medicine. *Remote Afterloading Technology,* AAPM Report No. 41. New York, American Institute of Physics, 1993.

37. International Electrotechnical Commission. *Particular Requirements for the Safety of Remote Controlled Automatically Driven Gamma-Ray Afterloading Equipment,* International Standard IEC 601, Medical Electrical Equipment, Part 2. Geneva, Bureau de la Commission Electrotechnique Internationale, 1989.

CHAPTER

15

QUALITY ASSURANCE

OBJECTIVES 358

INTRODUCTION 358

COMPONENTS OF A QUALITY ASSURANCE PROGRAM 359

PERSONNEL 360

RECOMMENDED QUALITY ASSURANCE PROCEDURES 360

PHYSICS INSTRUMENTATION 361

Ionization Chambers and Electrometers 361
Beam Scanning Systems 363
Ancillary Equipment 363
Relative Dose Measuring Equipment 363
Survey Meters 363

MEGAVOLTAGE TREATMENT EQUIPMENT 364

Safety Procedures 365
Mechanical Alignment 367
Beam Alignment Tests 370
Multi-Leaf Collimator Quality Assurance 372
Calibration 375
Photon Beam Characterization 377
Electron Beam Characterization 379

QUALITY ASSURANCE PROCEDURES FOR RADIATION THERAPY SIMULATORS 380

Mechanical Alignment Tests 380
Safety Procedures 380
Beam Alignment Tests 382

Focal Spot Size 382
X-Ray Beam Performance 383

CT SIMULATOR QUALITY ASSURANCE 385

Lasers 385
Couch 386
Image Orientation 386
Image Quality 386
CT to Density Table 387

IMAGE QUALITY ASSURANCE 387

Film Processor 387
Portal Imaging and Computed Radiography 388

TREATMENT PLANNING COMPUTER 389

QUALITY ASSURANCE FOR INTENSITY-MODULATED RADIATION THERAPY (IMRT) 394

Radiation Safety 394
Treatment Planning 395
Machine Characteristics 395
Patient-Specific Dose Verification 396

STEREOTACTIC RADIOSURGERY AND RADIOTHERAPY 397

BRACHYTHERAPY QUALITY ASSURANCE PROCEDURES 399

SUMMARY 409

PROBLEMS 409

REFERENCES 410

Radiation Therapy Physics, Third Edition, by William R. Hendee, Geoffrey S. Ibbott, and Eric G. Hendee
ISBN 0-471-39493-9 Copyright © 2005 John Wiley & Sons, Inc.

■ OBJECTIVES

By studying this chapter, the reader should be able to:

- Describe the importance of an effective quality assurance program in radiation therapy.
- Identify standard equipment for performing quality assurance measurements.
- List resources for recommended testing procedures and tolerances for relevant equipment.
- Differentiate between commissioning tests and patient-specific tests for intensity modulated radiation therapy.
- Describe the components of a quality assurance program for high-dose-rate brachytherapy.

■ INTRODUCTION

"Technology confers wonderful benefits on society, but it also makes society dependent on the continuing performance and good behavior of technological goods and services. This is 'life behind the quality dikes'—a form of securing benefits but living dangerously. Like the Dutch who have reclaimed much land from the sea, we secure benefits from technology but we need good dikes—good quality—to protect us against the numerous service interruptions and occasional disasters."
Dr. Joseph M. Juran

A carefully developed and maintained program of quality assurance is an essential component of any radiation oncology department. The Joint Commission on Accreditation of Healthcare Organizations (JCAHO) has used the term quality assurance to describe those processes that are related to the correct treatment of a patient. Others have used the term to refer specifically to physician peer review. Although peer review is an important component of a quality assurance program, this text will deal primarily with the technical factors of importance in radiation therapy. The recommendations presented here are limited to the equipment and procedures commonly found in contemporary radiation oncology departments. They may be used as a guide for developing a quality assurance program, in conjunction with institution specific procedures.

The emphasis on quality assurance programs in radiation therapy that has evolved over the past several decades has spawned a vocabulary peculiar to this field. The developers of methods of assessing the quality of healthcare delivery frequently consider the framework of health care to be divisible into three broad areas.[1,2] *Structure* encompasses the adequacy of facilities, the credentials of staff, and the administrative organization. *Process* entails the appropriateness of care, including issues such as the thoroughness of physical exams and diagnostic tests, the technical competence with which procedures are performed, and the medical justification for tests and therapies administered. Finally, *Outcome* describes the quality of the care provided; it is gauged in terms of recovery, restoration of function, and survival.

Quality assurance (QA) generally refers to deliberate actions necessary to provide confidence that a service or product will satisfy established requirements for quality. This term is closely related to Quality control (QC), which generally refers specifically to measurement aspects of a quality assurance program. It is now generally accepted that a comprehensive QA program must include mechanisms for analyzing the results of quality measurements, utilizing these results to improve the quality of the product or service, and monitoring the effects of the program (i.e., outcomes) on a continuing basis. These efforts collectively can be characterized as accountability in healthcare delivery.

Quality control generally refers to systems of checks in a process to prevent errors from passing beyond a certain point (i.e., "controlling" the quality of the product or service). Quality assurance generally refers to identifying the source of error and preventing its occurrence (i.e., "assuring" that the product or service is of high quality).

The goal of radiation therapy is to achieve the greatest possible local and regional tumor control, with the fewest complications. The response of most tissues to radiation is characterized by a sigmoid curve as shown in Figure 15-1. Relatively little response is seen until the dose reaches some threshold value, after which the response is quite rapid.[3,4] In the latter region, relatively small variations in dose can yield significant differences in the response of both tumors and normal tissue.[5] To minimize the variability of tissue response, the ICRU has recommended that the uncertainty in dose delivery be maintained below approximately 5%.[6,7] Delivering a dose to a patient within a tolerance of 5% is no simple task.[8] It has been estimated that the equipment used by most medical physicists to calibrate therapeutic radiation

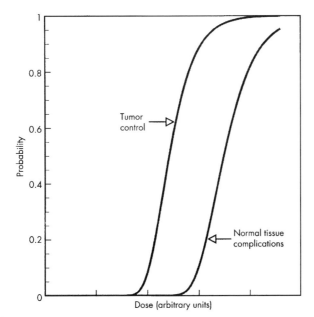

FIGURE 15-1
The response of most tissues to ionizing radiation is thought to be characterized by a sigmoid curve.

beams is accurate to an overall uncertainty (expressed at the 95% confidence level) of approximately 1.5%.[9]

Uncertainties associated with the characterization of radiation beams, patient anatomy and location of the target volume, and reproducibility of the treatment from day to day must also be considered.[10,11] A comprehensive quality assurance program should address all sources of variability in the treatment of patients, in an effort to minimize the overall uncertainty of treatment.

While this text and others make recommendations for quality assurance procedures and tolerance levels, a good quality assurance program should be designed specifically for each facility. Differences in equipment design and reliability, staffing levels, patient mix, and other variables may justify a tightening or possibly a relaxation of the recommendations presented here. The development of a good QA program is an evolutionary process. As experience is gained with particular items of equipment and staffing circumstances, measurement frequencies and tolerances may need to be adjusted to balance assurance of quality against effective use of resources.

COMPONENTS OF A QUALITY ASSURANCE PROGRAM

To be effective, a quality assurance program must address all aspects of a department's operation. Advice and recommendations concerning clinical issues may be found in a number of publications.[12–17] These would normally include items such as physician peer review, chart review conferences, and an analysis of indicators related to treatment outcome.

Technical aspects of quality assurance address a wide array of issues, including performance of simulation and treatment, treatment planning equipment, stability of measurement and test equipment, accuracy and appropriateness of treatment planning calculations, and accuracy and completeness of documentation. Recommendations are available that offer advice on the design of the radiation therapy treatment chart.[18–20] The patient's treatment chart is a legal document and must meet several requirements for clarity, unambiguity, and accuracy. A QA program should consider how well the chart meets these requirements, and it should address any

RMS error—The root mean square error is determined by considering all sources of error. Suppose when calibrating a source, the error in chamber calibration is 2%, the error in electrometer calibration is 3%, the error in temperature reading is 0.5%, and the error in pressure reading is 1%. Since the measurements are independent variables, the final error is determined as the RMS error. For this example, it is

$$RMS\ error = \sqrt{(2^2 + 3^2 + 0.5^2 + 1^2)} = 3.8\%$$

When adding or subtracting values with associated error, the error values are determined as the square root of the sum of the squares of the errors. For example,

$$(4 \pm 1) + (7 \pm 3) = (4 + 7) \pm \sqrt{(1)^2 + (3)^2}$$
$$= 11 \pm \sqrt{10} = 11 \pm 3.16$$

and

$$(4 \pm 1) - (7 \pm 3) = (4 - 7) \pm \sqrt{(1)^2 + (3)^2}$$
$$= -3 \pm \sqrt{10} = -3 \pm 3.16$$

The endpoint of radiation therapy is successful patient treatment. Quality assurance programs must be balanced against the needs of the institution to provide quality care. With rapidly advancing technologies, systems in place must be adaptable to new techniques and must permit obsolete processes to be abandoned. For example, one of the recent technology pushes is intensity modulated radiation therapy. Without an efficient and adaptable framework for quality assurance, implementation of this technology can be overburdensome, reducing its potential benefits to patients.

Quality assurance should be reflected in the patient's chart through continuity of process. When auditing a chart, the person performing the audit should be able to trace the treatment delivered through all aspects of the QA program. For example, there should be continuity among the monitor units delivered, the dose determined from the treatment plan, quality assurance of the planning system, and quality assurance of the treatment machine.

As a department wide commitment, the personnel requirements for a successful quality assurance program must be understood and supported by administration. With rapidly changing technologies, the time required for maintaining existing programs and adopting new programs can be overwhelming to staff. In cases where resources in the department are lacking, outsourcing is a viable option to help alleviate the problem.

The first person to notice an equipment problem is usually the person who uses it the most. For linear accelerators and simulators, this is commonly the radiation therapist. For treatment planning, the dosimetrist is on the front line to notice problems with the planning system. A nurse may take note of patient responses and make suggestions for quality improvements in patient care. The physician closely monitors the treatment and its effects on the patient. The administrator is in touch with program development and competitive services. The physicist oversees technical aspects of the quality assurance program. The front desk is the front line for a significant portion of the patient's impression of the department and the treatment. That is, all members of the radiation therapy staff are highly involved in providing quality patient care and contributing to quality improvement initiatives. Treating quality assurance and process improvement as a department-wide initiative helps ensure a successful program.

The timing and frequency of quality assurance tests should be designed to reduce the risk of errors going undetected.

deficiencies. The quality assurance of some technical aspects of treatment delivery, such as patient positioning and immobilization, are not described here but may be found elsewhere.[21–24]

■ PERSONNEL

A critical part of a quality assurance program is the dedication of involved personnel and their commitment to excellence. To help foster such an attitude, a quality assurance program must be maintained as a department-wide effort, to which all staff members contribute.

It is customary for the medical director of a radiation oncology department to assume overall responsibility for the quality assurance program. A quality assurance committee should be established to develop procedures and policies, review program effectiveness, and develop appropriate responses upon receipt of results. All other department personnel should be encouraged to contribute to the quality assurance program. Radiation therapists (previously known as radiation therapy technologists) often are most familiar with the operation and idiosyncrasies of treatment equipment, and they may be the first to recognize unusual behavior. A comprehensive QA program should not only take advantage of the therapists' intimate knowledge of the equipment, but also ensure that the therapists are integral members of the quality assurance team.

■ RECOMMENDED QUALITY ASSURANCE PROCEDURES

The recommendations summarized in Tables 15-1 through 15-5 have evolved over a number of years as a product of the authors' experience in several institutions, combined with publications of several organizations.[12,14,15,21,25–31] Recommended frequencies agree with those in contemporary publications. However, the frequency of QA procedures should be determined individually by each institution for each piece of equipment. Equipment that demonstrates instability, or that has not yet demonstrated a record of stability, should be tested frequently. Once a piece of equipment has demonstrated stability, or aspects of its performance have been shown to be stable, consideration might be given to reducing the frequency of certain testing procedures. Any proposed reduction in test frequency must always be balanced against the risk of failure to detect poor performance. For example, the output of many linear accelerators has been shown to be very stable. However, the failure to detect an unexpected change in output could be catastrophic. Therefore, daily measurements of output constancy are recommended.

Quality assurance procedures are most conveniently performed at regular intervals. Recommendations are made here for tests to be conducted biennially, annually, semiannually, quarterly, monthly, and daily. To reduce the time required to perform annual tests, some procedures may be distributed among the monthly or quarterly checks. If this approach is taken, the procedures should be designed carefully to ensure that none of the measurements are overlooked. Daily QA procedures should always be performed at the beginning of the day, before patient treatments are delivered. This is because malfunctions sometimes occur as equipment is being turned off at the end of the day, or at the beginning of the day, possibly due to a change in power status or to the time interval since last usage. In this manner, malfunctions can be detected before any patients are treated. Performing QA tests during the day or at the end of the treatment day not only carries an increased risk that patients might be treated with malfunctioning equipment, but also yields the additional risk that procedures will have to be interrupted or postponed at times when the workload is heavy, or when a patient arrives unexpectedly for treatment.

Continuous quality improvement (CQI) requires careful documentation of the results of a quality assurance program, as well as action whenever the results are outside the stated tolerance. Determining the action to be taken requires experience and reasoned judgment.

Clearly, when a measured parameter falls outside the tolerance limits, action should be taken that is commensurate with the deviation from the stated tolerance and with the impact that the corrective action might have. For example, a recommendation is made later in this chapter that measurements of photon beam symmetry should be made on a regular basis. Daily constancy measurements should indicate that beam symmetry is constant to within 3%. If beam symmetry on a particular day disagrees with previous measurements by, say, 15%, patient treatments should be interrupted until asymmetry is corrected. On the other hand, if the measured value disagrees with previous values by 4% (only 1% outside tolerance), one could argue that patient treatments should not be suspended immediately, and that service work could be postponed until the end of the treatment day. Naturally, more careful, comprehensive measurements should be obtained before taking action on the basis of measurements made with a simple daily QA test.

PHYSICS INSTRUMENTATION

Instruments used to perform quality assurance procedures should be incorporated into a comprehensive QA program. Clearly, the reliability of major pieces of radiation therapy equipment cannot be demonstrated satisfactorily with instruments of questionable reliability. Quality assurance procedures should address not only ionization chambers used for calibrations, but also the instruments used for determining other beam characteristics, such as water phantom scanning systems, film scanners, diodes, and thermoluminescent dosimetry systems (TLDs). Ancillary devices such as thermometers and barometers should also be incorporated into the QA program. This section offers advice on procedures and frequencies for the quality assurance of these devices. The recommendations are summarized in Table 15-1.

Ionization Chambers and Electrometers

Under normal conditions, the instruments used for calibration of therapy equipment are very stable.[32] Unless careful QA procedures are followed, a change in response might not be detected. The Nuclear Regulatory Commission (NRC) and several states require that instruments used to calibrate treatment units must themselves be calibrated at intervals of no more than 2 years by a dosimetry laboratory that has been accredited by the American Association of Physicists in Medicine (AAPM). These accredited dosimetry calibration laboratories (ADCLs) have been established to transfer calibration factors from instruments calibrated by the National Institute for Standards and Technology (NIST) to a customer's instrument. The ADCLs are supervised by the AAPM, to which they provide frequent reports of their workload and experiences, and by which they are inspected on a regular basis.[33,34] Through the use of carefully designed equipment and well-defined procedures, the ADCLs are able to assign a calibration factor to a customer's instrument with only a slight increase in the uncertainty associated with national standards maintained at NIST.[9]

It is recommended that an institution submit an ionization chamber and electrometer system to an ADCL for calibration at intervals of no more than 2 years. However, biennial calibrations should not be substituted for regular QA procedures. The instrument submitted for calibration, hereafter referred to as the *local standard*, cannot be assumed to maintain its calibration factor throughout the 2-year interval. Instead, twice-yearly intercomparisons with another instrument or an isotope source are recommended. Intercomparisons also should be performed before and after an instrument is sent to an ADCL, to reveal damage sustained during shipping. An ideal redundant system can be assembled from two ionization chamber/electrometer systems and an isotope source.[34] An institution should make available a second ionization chamber and electrometer, as well as some type of isotope source (either a

Some confusion exists in many fields over the difference between "quality assurance" and "quality control." The term "assurance" relates to confidence and certainty, whereas "control" relates to evaluation and corrective measures. Thus, when combined with the word quality, "quality assurance" refers to the systems and processes in place to provide confidence or certainty in the product or service, and "quality control" refers to the techniques used to measure the level of quality and take necessary corrective actions. Both expressions are in use in radiation therapy, and an institution should use both techniques in providing quality healthcare to its patients.

Quality assurance tests must allow for reasonable judgment. There can be adverse effects when strict quality assurance guidelines interrupt patient treatment. The program must be able to adapt to normal fluctuations in measured values to detect problematic errors, but not to shut down treatment due to a statistical fluctuation that may simply require monitoring.

The characteristics of all equipment used to directly or indirectly measure properties of the radiation delivery must be understood and documented. The use of independent, external services to help with this task, such as an Accredited Dosimetry Calibration Laboratory (ADCL), provides a link to national standards and reduces the chance that internal measurement systems may propagate error. For constancy checks of system performance, internal checks may be used.

The Accredited Dosimetry Calibration Laboratories participate in a "Round Robin" where a device such as an ion chamber or radioactive source is sent to each center to calibrate without knowing the actual calibration value. The results are compared to make sure there is consistency among the ADCLs, and that they agree with the National Standard calibration for the device.

TABLE 15-1 QA Procedures for Physics Instrumentation

Measurement Equipment	Procedure	Frequency	Comments
Calibration Equipment			
Ionization chamber and electrometer (local standard)	ADCL calibration	Biennially	Should include a measurement of linearity (within 0.5%) and venting
All ionization chambers and electrometers used clinically	Intercomparison	Semiannually	With a radioactive source or another instrument
Scanning Equipment			
Detectors	Linearity	Annually	Document and apply correction
	Stem effect	Annually	Document and apply correction
	Leakage current	Initial use	Document and apply correction
	Short term stability	Initial use	Document and apply correction
	Energy dependence	Initial use	For diode detectors only, document and apply correction within 1 mm
Positioner	Accuracy and reproducibility	At each use	
Dosimetry Accessories			
Solid phantom materials	Inspect for damage	At each use	Pay particular attention to development of voids or cracks, or damage to recess for detector.
Thermometer (mercury in glass)	Intercomparison with calibrated standard	Initial use	Less than 0.1°C error
Thermometer (electronic)	Intercomparison with calibrated standard	Monthly	Less than 0.5°C error
Barometer (aneroid or electronic)	Intercomparison with calibrated standard	Monthly	Less than 2 mmHg error
Linear rule	Intercomparison with calibrated standard	Initial use	0.3%
Miscellaneous Dosimetry Devices			
TLD system	Calibration	At each use	Document and apply correction
	Linearity	Initial use	Document and apply correction
Film	Dose response	Initial use	Test each batch of box of film, for each modality and energy. Test includes the response of the densitometer and processor

The calibration factor for an ionization chamber is determined by its geometry, collecting volume, and composition. Since these factors should remain constant over time, the calibration factor should not change significantly. Any change in the calibrated value by more than 1–2% should be investigated to determine the reason. Having a chamber calibrated by more than one calibration laboratory, or performing an internal comparison of the relative response of two calibrated chambers, may provide added assurance of the value used. For the same measurement conditions, for example, the signal detected in two similar chambers (i.e., same model number) should be equal to the ratio of their calibration values.

^{60}CO treatment unit or a so-called "chamber checker" containing a ^{90}Sr source) to establish this redundant system. An ongoing record should be kept of intercomparisons of the components of this redundant system, so that the behavior of each component can be monitored over time.

Several other performance indicators for ionization chambers and electrometer systems should be evaluated. Before the initial use of each piece of equipment, the *stem effect* should be determined. The stem effect is a measurement of extracameral signal resulting from ionization events occurring in the chamber stem and cable.[35,36] Each ionization chamber should also be tested for losses due to ionic recombination (see Chapter 5). This measurement should be made for each beam modality and energy for which the ionization chamber is used.

Each time an ionization chamber and electrometer system is used, a simple capacitance test should be performed as a quick check of the constancy of response of the system.

The capacitance check is made by measuring the charge integrated by the electrometer as the chamber bias is applied or removed. The quotient of measured charge over applied collecting potential indicates the capacitance of the chamber/electrometer system. This value should remain constant from one use to the next. At the same time, the applied collecting potential should be noted. With many electrometer systems, this potential is provided by a battery that can slowly discharge. The presence of adequate collecting potential should be confirmed before measurements are made.

Beam Scanning Systems

Instruments used to characterize radiation beams are not generally used to calibrate these beams. Instead, they are used to make measurements of relative dose or ionization distributions, and the resulting data are used for treatment planning calculations. The detectors associated with these systems need not be calibrated, but tests should be performed to evaluate their reliability and constancy of response over the time interval required to make a full set of measurements. Upon receipt, the detectors should be investigated to verify that, over the course of a day, their response is constant, they remain waterproof, and the leakage current does not change significantly or exceed acceptable values. Their linearity and stem effect should be tested yearly. These tests should be documented and corrections applied to the chamber readings when appropriate. The mechanical integrity of the detectors should be tested at each use. Scanning mechanisms should be tested to ensure that they move smoothly and reliably and that the detector can be positioned reproducibly. The linearity of positioning and of readout devices should be ensured. Similar procedures should be applied to scanning film densitometers.

Ancillary Equipment

Accurate calibration of a treatment unit depends as much on careful placement of the detector and accurate measurements of environmental conditions as it does on the calibration of the ionization chamber. Devices used to position the calibration instrument in a phantom should be inspected for wear and damage on a regular basis. These devices include rulers, chamber positioning devices, and solid phantom materials.

Devices for determining environmental conditions should be tested regularly. Thermometers, particularly electronic devices, should be compared with a reference instrument on a regular basis. The frequency of comparison depends on the type of instrument. Electronic devices should be intercompared frequently; weekly or monthly intervals are recommended. Mercury-in-glass thermometers should be intercompared with a similar instrument before their initial use. Barometers should be intercompared regularly; again, the frequency of comparison depends on the type of instrument. Aneroid and electronic devices should be intercompared at weekly or monthly intervals. Mercury barometers should be compared with a similar device before first use. A suitable instrument for comparison may be located at a nearby weather station.

Positioning and scanning equipment should be reproducible to within 1 mm and should report the detector position to within 1-mm accuracy.

Relative Dose Measuring Equipment

Dosimeters used for measurement of relative dose (e.g., diodes and TLDs) or dose distributions (e.g., film) do not require calibration. However, their performance should be monitored as part of the ongoing quality assurance program. The response of devices such as TLDs and radiographic film should be measured frequently, even at each use, and appropriate corrections applied. Similarly, behavior that can affect the response of these devices, such as the linearity of response, should be evaluated before their initial use, and corrections (if necessary) should be applied when measurements are taken.

Survey Meters

Devices used to measure dose levels around patients, such as Geiger counters and survey meters, should be calibrated yearly. This is often a state or NRC requirement, and it is likely that the calibration status of these instruments will be verified during an inspection. If they are battery operated, the batteries must be operational and tested prior to use. A check source is a reliable method for verifying operation of these devices.

Beam scanning systems can directly affect dose calculations. Therefore, correct operation is critical. These systems are expected to provide accurate distance measurements, and to respond appropriately in regions of high dose rate, low dose rate, and high dose gradients. To remove the effects of linac dose-rate variations, a reference chamber is often used. For the same linear accelerator, the dose profiles and depth dose curves should be the same when measured with two systems. It may be wise to spot check measured profiles for accuracy using a system other than the primary system employed for collecting data (e.g., film, diode array, another scanner, or point measurements with ion chamber). For systems that allow disabling of the reference chamber, a sample profile without the reference chamber may be noisy, but it will indicate if the ratio is correctly accounted for, particularly in low dose regions outside of the field. This will help detect any systematic errors in the data.

"It is not enough to do your best; you must know what to do, and THEN do your best." W. Edwards Deming, Quality pioneer.

■ MEGAVOLTAGE TREATMENT EQUIPMENT

Quality assurance procedures are described here for megavoltage treatment units. As most treatment units in service today are linear accelerators, at least in the United States, no specific mention will be made of ^{60}Co units. However, most of the procedures described here apply equally to ^{60}Co units, as do recommended frequencies. Likewise, procedures specific to superficial and orthovoltage x-ray units are not presented, but the recommendations here should be followed where applicable. Modern treatment units are considerably more complex than earlier devices, and they rely increasingly on computer technology. The application of advanced technology may eliminate some sources of error but may introduce other sources, and the risk of injury to the patient must be guarded against.[37] A comprehensive QA program can help to reduce these risks. Recommended procedures and measurement frequencies are summarized in Tables 15-2 and 15-3.

TABLE 15-2 Frequency of Quality Assurance Procedures and Recommended Tolerances for Megavoltage Treatment Units

Procedure	Annually	Monthly	Daily
Safety Procedures			
Protection survey	Limited survey	—	Watch for signs of deterioration. Be aware of changes in design/use of adjacent space.
Test of interlocks	Test safety interlocks.	Test safety interlocks.	Test door interlocks.
Patient monitoring device operation	—		Check for proper operation.
Mechanical Alignment			
Collimator isocenter	1-mm radius circle (test with mechanical pointer)	1-mm radius circle (test with light field)	—
Jaws parallel and orthogonal, and symmetrical about collimator axis	Parallel 0.5°, orthogonal 0.5°, symmetrical about collimator axis ±2 mm	—	—
Light field versus indicators	±2 mm each jaw, 2 mm overall for field sizes 5 × 5 to 20 × 20, 1% overall for fields > 20 × 20	Meet specifications of annual test at selected field sizes.	±2 mm overall in a single field size. Central axis indicator ±2 mm from center of light field at one field size.
Collimator angle indicator	±1° mechanical, ±0.5 digital over full range of motion	±1° mechanical, ±0.5° digital at selected angles	—
Gantry isocenter	1-mm radius sphere	—	—
Gantry angle indicator	1° mechanical, ±0.5° digital over full range of motion	±1° mechanical, ±0.5° digital at selected angles	—
Couch isocenter	1-mm radius circle	—	—
Couch angle	±1° mechanical, ±0.5° digital over full range of motion	±1° mechanical, ±0.5° digital at selected angles	—
Couch position indicators	2 mm	±2 mm	Couch height 2 mm
Couch top sag	2 mm	—	—
Range light	±1 mm at isocenter, ±5 mm elsewhere	±1 mm at isocenter, ±5 mm elsewhere	±2 mm at isocenter
Localizing laser	±1 mm	±1 mm	±2 mm
Beam Alignment Tests			
Light versus radiation field congruence	±2 mm each jaw, ±2 mm overall for field sizes 5 × 5 to 20 × 20, ±1% overall for fields > 20 × 20	Meet specifications of annual test at selected field sizes	—
Collimator rotation	1-mm radius circle	—	—
Gantry rotation	1-mm radius circle	—	—
Couch rotation	1-mm radius circle	—	—

(Continued)

TABLE 15-2 (*Continued*)

Procedure	Annually	Monthly	Daily
Calibration			
Output calibration	±2% (dose to water)	±2% (constancy check)	±3% (constancy check)
Monitor chamber linearity	≤1%	—	—
Output variation with gantry angle	≤1% at selected angles	—	—
Photon Beam Characterization			
Field size dependence of output	±2% constancy over full range of field sizes	±2% constancy at selected field	—
Percent depth dose (or TPR)	±2% constancy over full range of depths and field sizes	±2% constancy at selected depths and field sizes	—
Beam flatness	±3% over central 80% of fields up to 30 × 30 cm at 10-cm depth, for selected gantry angles	±2% constancy in selected field sizes	—
Beam symmetry	≤2% difference between points equidistant from the beam axis for selected gantry angles	±2% constancy in selected field sizes	±3% constancy in a single field size
Transmission factor of wedge filters and treatment accessories	2% constancy over applicable range of field sizes	2% constancy at a single field size, or check of alignment	—
Electron Beam Characterization			
Dependence of output on applicator size	±2% constancy over full range of applicator sizes	—	—
Percent depth dose	±2% constancy over full range of depths and applicator sizes (2 mm in region of steep dose gradient)	±2-mm constancy with selected applicator size in region of steep dose gradient	—
Beam flatness	±3% over central 80% of fields up to 30 × 30 cm at 10-cm depth, for selected gantry angles	±2% constancy in selected field sizes	—
Beam symmetry	±2% difference between points equidistant from the beam axis	±2% constancy in selected field sizes	±3% constancy in a single field size

Safety Procedures

1. Radiation Protection Survey. At the time of installation of new megavoltage equipment, a complete radiation protection survey should be performed.[38] It is not necessary to repeat the survey unless changes in the equipment, treatment facility, workload, or use of the space surrounding the facility are made. On an annual basis, it is advisable to review the conditions under which the original protection survey was performed and to determine whether or not the conditions are still applicable. For example, it is not unusual for the workload of a megavoltage treatment unit to increase with time. If the present workload exceeds that anticipated at the time of installation, the original protection survey and associated calculations may no longer be valid. At the same time, the use of space around the treatment facility should be reviewed and compared with the conditions at the time of installation. One should be alert not only for changes in construction but also for changes in the use and duration of occupancy of the space. Finally, the review should include an inspection of the physical condition of the facility. Any indication of deterioration in the construction warrants a repeat protection survey. The physical condition of the treatment unit itself should not be overlooked, although a thorough inspection can rarely be accomplished without removing the covers of the equipment. In a few reported instances, sections of shielding in the treatment head of a megavoltage treatment unit that were inadvertently removed during service procedures were not replaced. Should one suspect an event of this type, a leakage survey of the accelerator head should be performed.[38,39] Regions exhibiting high radiation leakage can be identified by covering the head of

TABLE 15-3   Sample Monthly QA Mechanical Checks Based on AAPM Task Group 40 Recommendations

MECHANICAL (per AAPM TG 40, Table II)	
Safety Interlocks	Tolerance
Emergency off switches	Functional
Wedge interlocks	Functional
Electron cone interlocks	Functional
Door interlock	Functional
Mechanical Checks	
Gantry	
Digital: 180°	±1 degree
Digital: 90°	±1 degree
Digital: 0°	±1 degree
Digital: 270°	±1 degree
Collimator	
Digital: 0°	±1 degree
Digital: 270°	±1 degree
Digital: 90°	±1 degree
Optical Distance Indicator	
SSD: 90 cm	±2 mm
SSD: 100 cm	±2 mm
SSD: 110 cm	±2 mm
Couch Extents	Nominal values ±1 cm
Lateral	±2 mm
Vertical	±2 mm
In/out	±2 mm
Couch Rotation	
Digital: 0°	±1 degree
Digital: 270°	±1 degree
Digital: 90°	±1 degree
Couch Position @ isocenter	
Isocenter at "O" in NO step @ 100-cm table height:	±2 mm
Light/Radiation Field	2 mm or 1%
Wedge Position	2 mm or 2% change in wedge factor
Tray Position	±2 mm
Applicator Position	±2 mm
Field Size Indicators	±2 mm
Crosshair Centering	2-mm diameter
Wedges/Blocks Latches	Functional
Jaw symmetry	±2 mm
Field Light Intensity	Functional
LASERS	
Sagittal	±2 mm
Ceiling	±2 mm
Backpointer	±2 mm
Wall laser (XI)	±2 mm
Wall laser (X2)	±2 mm

the accelerator with film enclosed in paper "ready-pack" envelopes. For this procedure the collimator should be closed, and any residual aperture should be blocked. A long exposure should be made; and after processing, the films should be replaced on the accelerator to indicate areas of leakage. Measurements of leakage from these areas may be made with a large-volume ionization chamber instrument placed 1 m from the path of the electron beam.

2. Interlocks. Modern computerized linear accelerators are equipped with software to test many of the interlocks. Some, such as the treatment room door interlock,

are not easily tested automatically. They are of such great importance to safe operation that they should be tested manually on a regular basis. Interlocks that directly affect the safety of the patient or staff, as well as those that indicate the dose and uniformity of the beam, should be tested at least annually. The door interlock should be tested daily. The daily test should not be conducted with the beam on, because such a test creates a slight risk of exposure to personnel. Instead, most linear accelerators indicate the state of the door interlock switch at the console, when the accelerator is in the "ready" mode (that is, in a state in which irradiation can be initiated following a single action, such as pressing a button). The operation of the indicator can be monitored while the door is opened. A radiation-on test of the interlock can be conducted on a monthly or less frequent basis.

3. Patient Monitoring Equipment. Megavoltage treatment rooms are required by the NRC and by state regulations to be equipped with closed circuit television and audio monitoring systems. These devices should be checked every day for proper operation.

Mechanical Alignment

1. Collimator Rotation Stability. At the time of acceptance testing, sophisticated mechanical tests are conducted to ensure that the collimator axis of rotation is stable and deviates from intersection with the gantry axis of rotation by no more than a specified small amount. On an annual basis, the deviation of the collimator axis of rotation should be tested, again with a mechanical device. This is most conveniently done with the mechanical front pointer provided with most linear accelerators (Figure 15-2). It should be possible to adjust (shim) the mechanical pointer so that its tip moves in a circle of radius less than 1 mm during rotation of the collimator over its full range of motion. (When performing annual QA procedures, it is most convenient to proceed immediately to the test of gantry isocenter, once the mechanical pointer has been correctly shimmed.)

On a monthly basis, this test may be conducted using the crosshairs projected within the light field. Again, the center of the crosshairs should not wander outside a circle of 1-mm radius during rotation of the collimator.

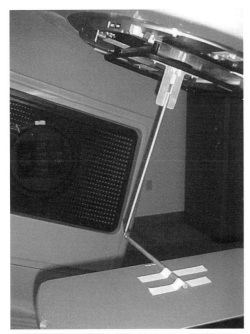

FIGURE 15-2
The use of mechanical pointers to measure the stability of rotation of the collimator, the gantry, and the patient treatment couch.

Misalignment of the radiation/light fields can be due to:

- Misalignment of the transmission mirror
- Misalignment of the light source or fiber optics
- Movement of the film over the period between marking the light field and exposing the radiation field

2. Collimator Jaws. Collimator jaws should be parallel, orthogonal, and symmetrical about the collimator axis. Collimator jaw orientation should be tested annually using the light field. Opposing jaws should be parallel to within 0.5 degrees, and adjacent jaws should be orthogonal to within 0.5 degrees. The jaw positions (when operated in the symmetrical field mode) should be symmetrical about the collimator axis of rotation to within 2 mm.

3. Light Field Indicators. With most megavoltage therapy units, the dimensions of the radiation field are indicated by a light field projected through the collimator by a light source mounted inside the collimator. The shape and dimensions of the treatment field are frequently determined during simulation or treatment planning, and these dimensions are reproduced at the time of treatment. Therefore it is essential that the displays that indicate the dimensions of the light field agree precisely with the light field. The indicated position of each edge of the light field should agree with the actual position of the edge to within 2 mm. This is particularly important for treatment units with collimator jaws that move independently of each other. In addition, the overall dimensions of the light field must be indicated correctly. At field sizes less than 20 × 20 cm, the indicated dimension should agree with the measured dimension to within 2 mm. At field sizes greater than 20 × 20 cm, the indicated dimension should agree with the measured dimension to within 1% of the field size.

In some previously published recommendations, specifications on collimator indicator accuracy below a certain field size, such as 5 × 5 cm, are relaxed or removed.[15] In recent years, however, interest in delivering treatments with smaller field sizes has increased. Therefore, relaxing the alignment specifications at small field sizes is not recommended.

Tests should be conducted annually to ensure that collimator indicator accuracy is maintained over the full range of available field sizes. At monthly intervals, the test may be performed at a few selected field sizes. Because of the importance of the accuracy of collimator indicators, a daily test should be performed at a single representative field size, say 10 × 10 cm.

4. Collimator Angle Indicator. There has been a recent increase in sophisticated field-matching techniques, particularly for tumors of the head and neck. These techniques often take advantage of the availability of independent collimator jaw motions on some linear accelerators, to provide nondiverging beam edges at field junctions. When such techniques are used, the angle of collimator rotation must be known precisely. Digital displays of collimator angle should agree with the actual angle to within 0.5 degrees. Where only mechanical scales are available, they should be accurate to within 1 degree. The accuracy of the angle indicator can easily be assessed by (a) rotating the gantry of the accelerator to the horizontal position and (b) positioning a digital level against either the collimator jaw or a machined surface that is parallel to one of the jaws. Once each year, the accuracy of the angle indicator should be tested over the full range of collimator rotational motion. Monthly tests of accuracy should be made at a few selected angles.

5. Gantry Isocenter. The increasing use of dynamic therapy, intensity modulation, and treatment with multiple small fields places stringent demands on the stability of the treatment unit isocenter. Beams directed toward the tumor from multiple angles must coincide to within a small tolerance. This is ensured in part by measuring the gantry isocenter variation using mechanical methods. The mechanical pointer adjusted under Step 1 (above) can be used to demonstrate the isocenter variation. For reference, a metal pointer such as a small-diameter drill bit should be taped to the treatment couch and raised to the approximate location of the isocenter. The collimator pointer should be extended until it almost touches the couch pointer. The gantry should be rotated throughout its entire range of motion while observing the variation in position of the tip of the collimator pointer (Figure 15-2). If necessary, the length of the collimator pointer should be adjusted to reduce the motion of the tip to a minimum. Variations both within and perpendicular to the gantry plane of rotation should be observed. The motion of the tip of the pointer should be confined within a sphere of 1-mm radius. The center of this sphere is the isocenter. A

more demanding tolerance, perhaps 0.5 mm, might be appropriate for an accelerator used for delivering radiosurgery treatments. This test should be repeated annually. With the collimator and couch pointers still in place, it is convenient to proceed directly to Step 7 to test the couch isocenter position.

6. Gantry Angle Indicator. For the same reasons that field size and collimator angle indicators must be accurate, the gantry angle indicator also must be accurate. Because most linear accelerators offer sharply collimated beams, field edges are often placed close to normal tissue structures. A small error in gantry angle can result in unplanned irradiation of a normal structure or exclusion of a portion of the tumor from the irradiated volume. Digital angle indicators should be accurate to within 0.5 degrees, while mechanical scales should be accurate to within one degree. The accuracy should be tested annually over the full range of motion, and monthly at selected angles.

7. Couch Isocenter. The stability of the couch axis of rotation is most conveniently tested with the pointers previously positioned for the gantry and collimator isocenter tests. The collimator pointer should be adjusted so that it indicates the center of the sphere containing the gantry isocenter. The couch should be rotated through its complete range of motion while observing the movement of the pointer attached to the couch top (Figure 15-2). The tip of the couch pointer should describe a circle of radius no more than 1 mm. This test should be performed annually.

8. Couch Angle. Until recently, it was unusual for treatments to be delivered with the treatment couch angled away from the central position. However, with the increasing use of noncoplanar fields, and the frequent need to carefully match the borders of adjacent fields, couch rotation has become more common. In these situations, an error in couch position can have consequences as serious as those caused by an error in gantry or collimator angle. Therefore, the tolerances on couch angle must be just as stringent. Digital scales should be accurate to within 0.5 degrees, and mechanical scales should be accurate to within 1 degree. The couch angle indicators should be tested over their full range once each year, and at selected angles every month.

9. Couch Top Sag. Almost all treatment couches are of a cantilevered design. Consequently, the extension of the couch top combined with the patient's weight causes the table top to sag slightly. A measurement of the couch top sag should be made by extending the couch fully toward the gantry and by raising the couch top to the level of the isocenter. A small amount of weight such as 10 kg (22 lb) should be placed at the gantry end of the couch top. The position of the couch top relative to a point of reference should be noted. The alignment lasers or the collimator front pointer can be used for this purpose. Additional weight should then be added to the couch top to simulate the distributed weight of a 75-kg (170-lb) patient. It is acceptable to add 25 kg (55 lb) to the gantry end of the couch for this purpose. The displacement of the couch top relative to the reference point should be noted. The displacement should not exceed 2 mm. This test should be performed once each year.

10. Couch Position Indicators. The use of couch position indicators can greatly speed and enhance patient positioning.[11,40,41] In some circumstances, positioning is facilitated by first placing the patient so that external anatomic landmarks align with the localizing laser lights. For treatment, the couch and patient are moved a prescribed distance in each of three orthogonal directions. In other cases, the patient position may be reproduced through use of a mold or mask at a position keyed to a particular location on the couch top. This ensures that reproducing the couch position reproduces the patient position for treatment each day. Even when the techniques just mentioned are not used, the use of the couch height indicator is a valuable aid in confirming patient position in the vertical direction. When available, couch position indicators should be accurate to within 2 mm. The accuracy of the indicators should be tested over their full range each year and at selected positions every month. A test of couch height indicator accuracy should be performed on a daily basis at one location, perhaps as part of another test.

There are many ways of testing mechanical positioning and rotation. By using a combination of techniques, the consistency between systems can be checked. For example, if the field light crosshairs are set accurately to indicate the isocenter, then they can project onto the floor to identify a point for testing couch rotation. Care must be taken that the gantry is level and pointing straight down when performing this test. The couch angle indicator on the floor can then be used as a scale to check collimator rotation accuracy.

Radiation therapists often set patients up using the "table top," where the distance from the surface of the table to the laser line is measured using a ruler. If the table is not level, the table-top values will be different from one side to the other.

The ODI should be most accurate over the range of common use. For most clinical situations with 100-cm SAD linacs, this range is 80–100 cm.

The use of lasers in patient alignment is commonplace. When performing quality assurance tests, one must be aware of how the lasers are used in daily patient alignments so that they can be accurate under those conditions. For example, it may be intuitive to check the lasers at the isocenter. With the patient on the table, however, the radiation therapists most often perform alignment up to 30 cm or more from the isocenter. Thus, the accuracy of alignment lasers over the range of use must be verified.

Projection of the light field is sensitive to the position of the transmission mirror within some linacs. If the mirror is replaced or if it is moved while repairs take place, it is important to verify the light/radiation field alignment immediately.

When physicians evaluate port films, shifts are often made based on the position of the graticule markers, which are assumed to correctly identify the central axis. If the graticule markers are off, then the field may be set up correctly, but the patient may be shifted based on the positions of the markers, resulting in incorrect patient treatment. Accessories (such as the graticule) that are used for patient alignment should be included in quality assurance checks. Radiation therapists and/or physicists can easily check the graticule by verifying that the bb's line up with the crosshairs.

11. Optical Distance Indicator. The optical distance indicator (or "range light") is one of several valuable aids for ensuring correct patient positioning. Its accuracy should be determined by comparison with a mechanical front pointer, or by measurements made from a reference point on the collimator. The design of most optical indicators permits the greatest accuracy at the position of the isocenter; at this location the optical distance indicator should be accurate to within 1 mm. At other distances, an error of ±5 mm is acceptable. Optical indicators may lose accuracy with time and should be tested over their full range on an annual as well as monthly basis. A daily test of accuracy at the level of the isocenter should be performed.

12. Localizing Laser Alignment. In most radiation oncology departments, the reproducibility of daily patient positioning depends greatly on the accuracy of alignment of the localizing laser lights. The accuracy of these devices is crucial. With the collimator front pointer still in place from previous tests, the alignment of the localizing lasers with the isocenter can easily be verified and adjusted. The position of the laser should be within 1 mm of the isocenter, and a test of the position should be performed monthly. On a daily basis, a simpler test can be performed to confirm that the laser alignment is within 2 mm of the isocenter.[42] It should be noted that the lasers should be mounted on a solid structure such as the concrete wall of the treatment room, in a location that avoids having the lasers bumped by personnel, patients, or moveable items such as stretchers. In many treatment rooms, the localizing lasers are recessed into the wall.

Beam Alignment Tests

1. Light Versus Radiation Field Congruence. On most megavoltage therapy units, the dimensions of the radiation field are indicated by a light field projected through the collimator by a light source mounted inside the collimator. The light source may be positioned at the location of the x-ray target by a rotating carousel or a sliding drawer assembly, or it may be positioned to one side of the collimator axis of rotation, with the light reflected from a mirror. In either case, the location of the light source must agree with the actual or virtual location of the radiation source. The agreement of the light field with the radiation field can most easily be verified through the use of film in a paper ("ready pack") envelope. The film should be taped to the treatment tabletop, which has been positioned at the level of the isocenter. The field should be set to a convenient size such as 10 × 10 cm, and the location of the edges of the light field should be marked on the paper film packet either through use of high-density markers, by pricking the paper packet with a pin, or by making an impression with a ballpoint pen. The film should then be irradiated sufficiently to enable comparison between the irradiated field and the marks indicating the light field. Bolus material may be placed over the film before irradiation to increase the dose to the film, but this is not essential. The agreement between the light and radiation fields can be evaluated at several field sizes on the same piece of film. The light field should agree with the radiation field to within 2 mm along each edge. In addition, the overall dimensions of the light field should agree with the dimensions of the radiation field to within 2 mm for field sizes up to 20 × 20 cm, and to within 1% of the field dimension for fields larger than 20 × 20 cm.

At the same time, the agreement between the radiation field and the collimator size indicators should be checked. The specifications indicated above should apply to the agreement between the field size indicators and the radiation field size. Otherwise, errors between the field size indicators, the light field size, and the radiation field size could accumulate to unacceptable levels.[43]

The test of light field and radiation field congruence should be performed annually over the full range of field sizes, and monthly at selected field sizes.

2. Collimator Rotation Stability. The mechanical test described earlier ensures that the collimator axis of rotation is stable. However, it does not ensure that the radiation beam also rotates about the same axis. Failure of the radiation beam and mechanical axes of rotation to coincide may indicate that the radiation source is not

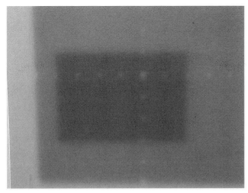

FIGURE 15-3
Sample monthly symmetric and asymmetric field size test. Graticle bb markers show up as small light circles and identify the central axis of the beam.

positioned properly on the collimator axis of rotation. A test of collimator rotation stability is easily performed by positioning the treatment couch top at isocenter and taping a film in a light-tight envelope to the couch top. One pair of collimator jaws should be opened to a moderate size (say, 15 cm) while the other pair should be closed to the minimum achievable symmetrical position. Several exposures should then be made on a single film, with the collimator rotated between exposures. The collimator angle should be chosen so that exposures do not overlap one another. Exposures should be made throughout the entire range of collimator motion; making five or six exposures usually yields an adequate test.

After processing, the film should exhibit a pattern reminiscent of the spokes of a wheel (Figure 15-4). If the spokes are more than 1–2 mm wide, a pencil line should be drawn carefully down the center of each spoke. Ideally, the spokes should all intersect at a single point. In most circumstances, the spokes will pass within a short distance of a point representing the collimator axis of rotation. The spokes should all fall within 1 mm of the collimator axis of rotation, indicating a circle of radius no more than 1 mm. The test should then be repeated with the jaw positions reversed. This test should be repeated annually.

3. Couch Rotation Stability. As in the previous test, a "spoke image" is generated. This time, however, the collimator position is fixed, and the couch is rotated between exposures. Variation in the position of the spokes on the developed film indicates the variation in rotation of the couch axis. This test should be repeated annually.

4. Gantry Rotation Stability. A spoke image of gantry rotation can be generated by positioning a film upright on the table top so that it is perpendicular to the gantry axis of rotation. The collimator jaws whose edges are parallel to the gantry axis of rotation are closed to their minimum symmetrical setting, while the opposite jaws

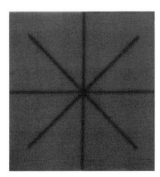
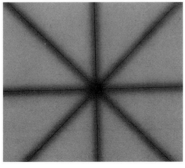

FIGURE 15-4
A "spoke film" indicating good stability of collimator ratation. (Courtesy of Rich Goodman, Waukesha Memorial Hospital.)

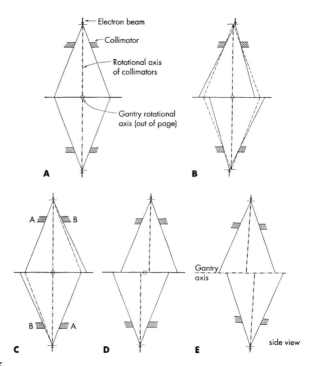

FIGURE 15-5
Correct (**A**) and incorrect (**B–E**) treatment beam alignment as shown by two opposing fields. A lateral shift between the fields can be caused by a lateral focal spot displacement (**B**), asymmetric collimators (**C**), or nonintersecting collimator and gantry rotational axes (**D**). A longitudinal shift between the field can be due to a flexing head support (**E**). (From Lutz, W. R., Larsen, R. D., and Bjarngard, B. E. Beam alignment tests for therapy accelerators, *Int. J. Radiat. Oncol. Biol. Phys.* 1981; **7**:1727–1731.

are opened to an intermediate size. Exposures are made with the gantry at several different angles, with care taken to avoid overlapping exposures. For this test, it is important that the film be located exactly in the plane described by the beam central axis as the gantry is rotated. In addition, it is important that the collimator be rotated so that the edges of the jaws closed to minimum setting be exactly parallel to the gantry axis of rotation. The film is evaluated as before. The spokes should all pass within 1 mm of the gantry axis of rotation. This test should be repeated annually.

An alternative test using equipment found in most therapy departments is called the "split-field" test.[42] This test evaluates misalignment of the x-ray target with the collimator axis of rotation, collimator asymmetry, and movement of either the collimator rotation axis or the gantry rotation axis. Figure 15-5 displays these sources of misalignment. Irradiating a single film from opposite directions can assist in identifying such misalignment.

Multi-Leaf Collimator Quality Assurance

Most modern linear accelerators incorporate tertiary field-shaping in the form of multi-leaf collimators in their design. In many treatment applications, multi-leaf collimators eliminate the need for cerrobend blocking and are able to conform to relatively complex shapes. Several configurations are available, depending on the manufacturer, as either intrinsic to the treatment device or as an add-on accessory. A sample configuration is shown in Figure 15-6 to illustrate a possible mechanical arrangement. As mechanical devices, the radiation properties of multi-leaf collimators in treatment delivery are largely dependent on their physical design.

The original intent of the multi-leaf collimator was to provide an outer field boundary to eliminate the hazards and tedious work of creating custom cerrobend blocks. With the delivery of intensity modulated radiation therapy using multi-leaf

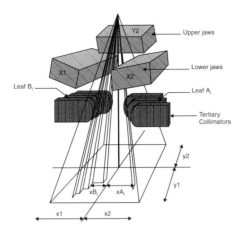

FIGURE 15-6
Generic configuration for multi-leaf tertiary collimators. This figure shows double-focused leaves in addition to primary collimation jaws X and Y (note jaw Y2 not shown for clarity). (From AAPM Report No. 72, Basic Application of Multileaf Collimators, Report of Task Group No. 50, July 2001.)

collimators, their physical characteristics are now integral to therapeutic dose delivery. Now a more thorough understanding of the design of multi-leaf collimators is required for treatment planning and quality assurance. For example, whether the path of the radiation follows beam divergence or is linear creates differing penumbra effects (Figure 15-7).

Some basic properties of multi-leaf collimators are presented in this text. For more information, one may refer to the manufacturer's documentation. Developing a quality assurance program for multi-leaf collimators should be consistent with the institution's program for treatment delivery.[44] Initial tests should characterize the mechanical and radiation properties, whereas components for daily, monthly, and annual tests generally involve ensuring proper operation and monitoring for any changes.

While it is true that custom cerrobend blocking was traditionally not subject to stringent quality control testing, the nature of computer-controlled multi-leaf collimators, along with the highly technical aspects of their use, suggests that multi-leaf collimators should be included in the quality assurance program. Some of the important

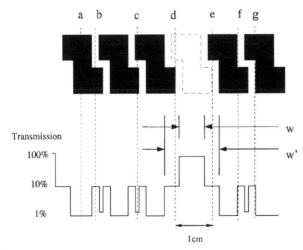

FIGURE 15-7
MLC QA. Effects of interleaf transmission and the effect of leaf geometry on penumbra. (From AAPM Report No. 72, Basic Applications of Multileaf Collimators, Report of Task Group No. 50, July 2001.)

tests and characteristics of MLCs include leaf calibration, leaf transmission, light field versus radiation field congruence, the tongue and groove effect, and stability with gantry and collimator rotation.

1. MLC Leaf Calibration. MLC leaf positions are computer controlled by optical encoders and/or stepping motors, for example. The accuracy of leaf positioning over the range of motion should be tested by comparing the set leaf position to the observed position. By placing a piece of graph paper on the treatment couch at the nominal SSD, the shadow of leaf positions can be marked on the paper. Individual leaves should not vary by more than 2 mm from the programmed position. Exposing a piece of film to leaf calibration fields provides an accurate record of leaf positions.

2. Leaf Transmission. MLCs incorporate a tongue and groove design to reduce inter-leaf leakage. A profile of leaf transmission perpendicular to the direction of leaf motion indicates variable leaf transmission due to the different thicknesses of attenuator encountered. Any significant change in this profile over time can indicate a developing problem with leaf motion, or possible interlocking of the leaves, either of which requires investigation.

3. Light Field Versus Radiation field. The standard definition for the radiation field is the full-width, half-maximum distance (FWHM). For divergent jaws or blocks, this value is very close or equal to the radiation light field. For double-focused MLCs, where the ends are rounded to correct for the lack of divergence in their linear travel direction (Figure 15-8), the radiation field width is larger than the light field width. Combined with any physical gap to prevent the leaves from colliding when fully closed, there exists an offset between the radiation field width and light field width on the order of a millimeter or two. Since the FWHM is dependent on the radiation transmission through the rounded leaf ends, the offset is also a function of beam energy. For an outer field boundary, this error may be insignificant. For IMRT, however, where there may be many junctions within the treatment field, the error can affect the observed fluence map for a particular field. The result is regions of higher dose perpendicular to the direction of leaf travel.

4. Tongue and Groove Effect. Consider the case of two adjacent leaves that are either fully open or fully closed. As shown in Figure 15-9, when leaf A is closed and leaf B is open, the central portion is partially blocked by the tongue of leaf A. Then, when leaf A is open and leaf B is closed, the center is still partially blocked by the groove of leaf B. Therefore, the center is always blocked, resulting in a region of lower dose in the direction of leaf travel. This particular effect is of concern for IMRT treatment, and many MLC conversion algorithms attempt to minimize it.

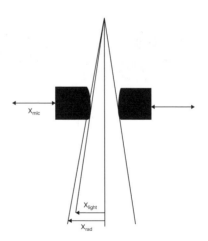

FIGURE 15-8
MLC light-field versus radiation-field edge for rounded end leaves. (From Graves, M. N., Calibration and quality assurance for rounded leaf-end MLC systems. *Med. Phys.* 2001; **28**(11):2227–2233.)

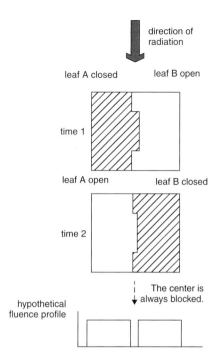

direction of
radiation

leaf A closed   leaf B open

time 1

leaf A open   leaf B closed

time 2

The center is
always blocked.

hypothetical
fluence profile

FIGURE 15-9

Tongue and Groove effect. In either case adjacent leaves are open/closed, the center is always blocked, resulting in lower dose. (From Balog, J. P., Mackie, T. R., Wenman, D. L., Glass, M., Fang, G. and Pearson, D. Multileaf collimator interleaf transmission. *Med. Phys.* 1999; **26**(2): 176–186.)

5. MLC Stability with Gantry and Collimator Rotation. The effects of gravity on leaf operation should be investigated by testing patterns over a variety of gantry and collimator angles. For example, attaching a sheet of film to the head of the treatment unit and exposing a uniformly moving pattern (such as a slit) should yield a predictable and uniform pattern on the film. Any deviations are likely to be due to gravity effects on the MLC.

In addition to initial tests, MLCs are subject to periodic testing. A summary of recommended tests and frequency from the American Association of Physicists in Medicine is shown in Table 15-4. Patient-specific tests include verifying the blocking against the simulation field, as one would do with cerrobend blocks, but also double-checking the blocking before every fraction. This is because the computer controlling the MLC could produce a change in the MLC pattern. Quarterly tests include checking the leaf position (light versus radiation field), communications, and interlocks. For institutions with IMRT programs in place, it may be wise to check MLC calibration more frequently as part of the monthly machine QA. Annual QA should include leaf position checks for a variety of gantry and collimator angles, leakage and transmission tests, and profile analysis (e.g., water scans or film profiles).

Calibration

1. Output Calibration. The procedures described in Chapter 6 of this text should be followed to verify accurate calibration of the output monitoring system. The AAPM has recommended that the monitor chamber indicate dose to water at the depth of maximum dose in a 10×10 field, with the phantom surface positioned at the normal treatment distance (usually 100 cm).[45] Once each year, the accuracy of the output monitoring system should be determined from fundamental measurements. Accuracy to within 2% is required. On a monthly basis, a constancy check of output should be performed. This check may be performed using a solid phantom material, to help

TABLE 15-4 Multi-leaf Collimator Quality Assurance

Frequency	Test	Tolerance
Patient specific	Check of MLC-generated field versus simulator film (or DRR) before each field is treated	2 mm
	Double check of MLC field by therapists for each fraction	Expected field
	On-line imaging verification for patient on each fraction	Physician discretion
	Port film approval before second fraction	Physician discretion
Quarterly	Setting versus light field versus radiation field for two designated patterns	1 mm
	Testing of network system	Expected fields over network
	Check of interlocks	All must be operational
Annually	Setting versus light versus radiation field for patterns over range of gantry and collimator angles	1 mm
	Water scan of set patterns	50% radiation edge within 1 mm
	Film scans to evaluate interleaf leakage and abutted leaf transmission	Interleaf leakage <3%, abutted leakage <25%
	Review of procedures and in-service with therapists	All operators must fully understand operation and procedures

Source: AAPM Report No. 72, Basic applications of Multileaf Collimators, Report of Task Group No. 50, July 2001; and Klein, E. E., Low D. A., and Purdy, J. A. A quality assurance program for ancillary high-technology devices on a dual-energy accelerator. *Radiother. Oncol.* 1996; **38**:51–60.

ensure reproducible geometry. A high-quality ionization chamber should be used to perform this test. The measurement should be constant to within 2% from one month to the next. Because the accuracy of the radiation output of a treatment machine is of consummate importance, a daily measurement of output constancy should be made. Numerous commercial devices are available for such tests (Figure 15-10); these are

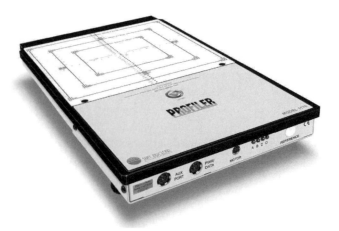

FIGURE 15-10
Daily QA measurement device.

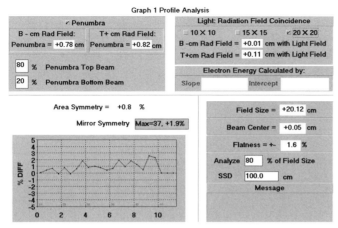

FIGURE 15-11
Measurements obtained with daily QA measurements device shown in Figure 15-10.

designed to facilitate the measurement, as well as to perform several other routine QA measurements, as shown in Figure 15-11.[46,47] The daily constancy check should be reproducible to within 3%.

2. Monitor Chamber Linearity. Monitor output calibration is generally performed at a single representative monitor unit setting such as 100 MU. Because patient treatments may involve the delivery of monitor unit settings over a wide range, the linearity of the monitor system must be verified. Readings with an ionization chamber may be made at a number of different monitor unit settings, and the output is graphed as a function of monitor unit setting. A straight line fit to the data should fall within 1% of all the data points and pass within 1% of the origin.

As an alternative, the *monitor end effect* can be determined through the use of a single–multiple exposure technique.[48] The ionization chamber reading for a single exposure of, say, 200 MU should be determined. Next, the exposure should be integrated as four identical exposures of 50 monitor units each. The end effect is determined as.

$$\text{End effect} = \frac{MU_1 (R_2 - R_1)}{n R_1 - R_2}$$

where MU_1 is the meter setting for the long exposure (200 MU in the example above); R_1 is the ionization reading measured for a meter setting of MU_1; R_2 is the *integrated* reading for n exposures of MU_2 each; MU_2 is the shorter meter setting (50 MU in the example above); and n is the number of times the shorter exposure is repeated ($n = 4$ in the example above). Note that $nMU_2 = MU_1$. When measured this way, the end effect should be less than 1 monitor unit. This test should be performed annually.

3. Output Variation with Gantry Angle. Output calibration measurements are most often made with the beam oriented in the vertical-downward position. Many treatments, however, are delivered with the gantry at other angles, and it is essential that the output not vary significantly as the gantry is rotated. The output calibration test is not easily performed with a water phantom at other gantry angles, but a solid phantom or even a suitable buildup cap may be used to measure the radiation output for other gantry angles. It is important only to ensure that the ionization chamber is located at the same distance from the source for each measurement. The variation with gantry angle should not exceed 1%. The variation should be measured once each year.

Photon Beam Characterization

1. Output Dependence on Field Size. The dose rate (measured in terms of cGy/MU) from a linear accelerator beam generally varies with field size, as was described in

Chapter 7. It is customary to characterize this variation at the time a linear accelerator is commissioned. At regular intervals following commissioning, the variation of output with field size should be reevaluated. Measurements at representative field sizes should be made annually to confirm that output dependence has not changed by more than 2% from original measurements. Changes of more than 2% indicate that data used for treatment planning calculations may require revision.

2. Percent Depth Dose. Complete measurements of percent depth dose or tissue phantom ratio (TPR) are ordinarily made at the time of equipment commissioning, or following repair. Periodically, the constancy of the beam energy should be checked, to ensure both consistent operation of the treatment unit and that the data in use for treatment planning calculations remain valid. Modern electrical treatment machines can vary in rather subtle ways, so that a change in the beam energy might not easily be detected. Percent depth dose should be checked annually at a large number of depths and field sizes to verify that the data remain within 2% of the original measurements. Once a month, a limited set of such measurements should be made.

3. Beam Flatness. To ensure that the target volume identified by the radiation oncologist receives a uniform dose, the treatment beam must itself be uniform. At the time of acceptance testing, measurements are ordinarily made of beam flatness to ensure proper design of the flattening filter and proper operation of the accelerator.[29,30] These measurements should be repeated annually, again not only to ensure proper operation of the treatment unit, but also to verify that the data in use for treatment planning remain valid. Beam flatness is specified at 10-cm depth in water or water equivalent material, at field sizes up to 30 × 30 cm. Over the central 80% of the field width along the major axis of the field, the maximum and minimum dose values should be determined. The difference between these values divided by their sum should be less than 0.03. Expressed differently, the variation should not be more than ± 3% of the mean. At monthly intervals, measurements should be made to ensure constancy of beam flatness. These measurements may be made in one or a few field sizes and should demonstrate that the flatness remains constant to within 2%.

4. Beam Symmetry. Acceptance testing procedures generally include measurements of beam symmetry, as well as adjustment of the devices that monitor and display beam symmetry. Continued proper operation of the symmetry monitoring device should be verified annually. Several different methods for measuring and describing beam symmetry have been recommended.[29,31,49] An accepted procedure consists of (a) measuring the beam profile at the depth of maximum dose and (b) examining the dose at points equidistant from the central axis. Corresponding points on each side of the central axis should not vary by more than 2% of the central axis value. Measurements should be made in large, medium, and small field sizes, as well as at representative gantry angles.

Beam symmetry can be altered by a change in the position of the flattening filter, as well as by electrical changes in the operation of the treatment unit. Such asymmetries can introduce distortions into the dose distribution throughout a patient's target volume, particularly when multiple field treatments are delivered.

Monthly spot checks of beam symmetry constancy should be made to verify continued agreement with initial commissioning measurements. Daily or weekly measurements of beam symmetry should also be made. Several commercially available devices that permit making such measurements with minimal effort are available (Figure 15-10). Measurements made on a daily basis should indicate constancy of the beam symmetry to within 3%.

5. Transmission Factor of Treatment Accessories. Treatment accessories such as blocking trays and wedge filters are unlikely to change in ways that would affect the transmission of radiation through them. However, periodic measurements of the transmission factors of these devices are important because they can expose two important sources of error. First, devices such as blocking trays are subject to wear and breakage, and they must periodically be replaced. Blocking trays have on occasion unintentionally been replaced with trays having a different thickness or made from

Beam flatness is largely a physical parameter determined by the flattening filter used and not readily adjustable. Symmetry, on the other hand, can be controlled by beam steering and needs to be watched to make sure the beam has not drifted off target.

different material, so that the transmission factor in use is no longer applicable. Second, removable "hard" wedge filters are mounted on trays that can occasionally become damaged; this necessitates their replacement, possibly with a tray having different transmission characteristics. In addition, damage to the wedge tray can result in a misalignment of the wedge. A measurement of the wedge transmission factor is often the most straightforward way to uncover such misalignment. Annually, measurements should be made of wedge and tray transmission factors in selected field sizes covering the applicable range. Constancy to within 2% of measurements made at the time of commissioning should be demonstrated. Wedges and other devices should be inspected monthly to ensure their proper alignment. As indicated previously, a transmission measurement indicating constancy within 2% may be the best way to demonstrate continued alignment.

Electron Beam Characterization

1. Output Dependence on Applicator Size. As is the case with photon beams, electron beams should be thoroughly characterized at the time of treatment unit commissioning. Electron beam output varies with field size; depending on the design of the collimation system; however, the variation may not be straightforward. Linear accelerators that employ electron applicators or "cones" frequently adjust the setting of the collimator jaws for different applicators. Small variations in the setting of the collimator jaws, or minor damage to the electron applicators, might result in a change in the electron beam output. It is recommended that periodic measurements be made of electron beam output as a function of applicator size. The agreement between annual measurements and the original commissioning data should be within 2%.

2. Percent Depth Dose. Percent depth dose (or relative ionization) is generally the means by which electron beam energy is characterized. Radiation oncologists frequently select an electron beam energy by matching the depth of the 80% or 90% depth dose with the deepest extent of the target volume. This choice is sometimes made through the use of a "rule of thumb," or by familiarity with data obtained at the time of accelerator commissioning. Consequently, it is important that the electron beam characteristics not vary from the data used for treatment planning by more than a small amount. Measurements should be made annually of percent depth dose or percent ionization at a wide variety of depths and field sizes. Agreement with original measurements should be (a) within 2% in regions of low-dose gradient and (b) within 2 mm in regions of high-dose gradient. Monthly relative ionization measurements should be acquired at a point corresponding to the depth of maximum dose, as well as at a second point located in the region of steep dose gradient. The relative reading at the deeper point should be compared with the original depth-ionization data to ensure that the curve has not shifted by more than 2 mm. This test is easily conducted by use of a parallel plate ionization chamber in a solid phantom, but other techniques are acceptable.[50] The test should be combined with the monthly check of output calibration.

3. Beam flatness. Electron beam flatness should meet the same specification as does photon beam flatness, with the exception that measurements are made at the depth of maximum dose. Annual measurements should be made to ensure that the beam flatness continues to meet the original specifications, in a range of field sizes and throughout the range of gantry angles. Monthly, the constancy of beam flatness should be tested in selected field sizes. This measurement might easily be made by exposing a film at the depth of maximum dose in a solid phantom, or by moving an ionization chamber off the central axis of the beam to representative locations. Commercially available devices discussed earlier may also be used. Constancy within 2% of the original measurements should be demonstrated.

4. Beam Symmetry. As with photon beams, several procedures for determining electron beam symmetry have been recommended, including the procedure described

For physical wedges, the transmission factor can vary as much as 1–2% per mm in the wedge direction. This is apparent in the cross-beam profiles for the wedge. Therefore, small shifts of the wedge (or of the patient) can affect the delivered dose significantly. For example, suppose that in a breast treatment using a physical wedge the physician decides that not enough margin is included medially. The physician can either (a) open the field or (b) shift the patient. Shifting the patient effectively puts the breast under a thicker part of the wedge, whereas opening the field does not.

above for photon beams. The ionization at representative points equidistant from the beam central axis should be measured; the difference in readings at these points should be less than 2% of the average reading. Complete measurements of beam symmetry for a variety of field sizes and gantry angles should be made annually. The constancy of beam symmetry should be checked monthly, to ensure less than 2% variation from measurements obtained at the time of commissioning. This test can easily be combined with the previous measurement of beam flatness. A verification of the constancy of beam symmetry should also be made on a daily or weekly basis, with an instrument sufficiently reliable to indicate constancy within 3% of the original commissioning measurements. These tests should be designed to ensure that the measurements are made at or near the depth of maximum dose.

■ QUALITY ASSURANCE PROCEDURES FOR RADIATION THERAPY SIMULATORS

Radiation therapy simulators are intended to reproduce the geometry and motions of treatment units. Their mechanical specifications are similar, if not identical, to those of megavoltage units. Consequently, they are subject to comparable quality assurance procedures. Advice regarding simulator QA procedures is available from several sources.[15,49,51,52]

Mechanical Alignment Tests

As indicated in Table 15-5, QA procedures for the mechanical alignment of radiation therapy simulators should be conducted with the same techniques and at the same frequencies recommended for megavoltage treatment units. Two additional tests of mechanical alignment are recommended for radiation therapy simulators:

   1. Target to Axis Distance. Most simulators are equipped with a variable target (or focus) to axis distance (TAD). The TAD indicator should be accurate to within 2 mm. Most simulator manufacturers provide a permanent reference mark to indicate the standard target-to-axis distance, generally 100 cm. Measurements can be made from this reference mark to facilitate positioning of the gantry at other target-to-axis distances. A test of the indicator accuracy should be made annually, at distances covering the full range of motion. Once each month the accuracy of the TAD indicator should be tested at selected distances; the consistency between the TAD indicator and the optical distance indicator should be verified daily.
   2. Image Intensifier Radial Position (Target to Film Distance). The distance from the x-ray target of a simulator to the image intensifier determines the magnification of images produced by the simulator. The magnification of fluoroscopic images is not of great concern during simulation, but the magnification of radiographic images often has a bearing on both treatment planning procedures and the design of treatment aids. Many simulators provide an indication not only of the intensifier radial distance, usually measured from isocenter, but also the target to film distance (TFD). The TFD indicator should be tested for accuracy over its full range once each year. It should be accurate to within 2 mm. Once each month, the accuracy should be tested at one or more representative locations.

Safety Procedures

1. Protection Survey. The x-ray tube of a radiation therapy simulator is regarded as a diagnostic x-ray device; therefore it must meet the same standards as conventional diagnostic x-ray equipment. A measurement of tube leakage radiation should be made annually to ensure that the ICRP recommendation of 0.1 R/hr at 1 m is not exceeded. The measurement is to be made at the highest-rated kVp setting for the

TABLE 15-5 Frequency of Quality Assurance Procedures and Recommended Tolerances for Radiation Therapy Simulators

Procedures	Annually	Monthly	Daily
Safety Procedures			
Protection survey	Limited survey	Watch for signs of deterioration. Be aware of changes in design/use of adjacent space	—
Test of interlocks	Test safety interlocks	Test safety interlocks	Test door interlock
Patient monitoring device operation	—	—	Check for proper operation
Mechanical Alignment			
Collimator isocenter	1-mm radius circle. Test with mechanical pointer	1-mm radius circle. Test with light field	±2 mm from center of light field at one field size
Delineators and blades parallel and orthogonal, and symmetrical about collimator axis	Parallel ±0.5°, orthogonal ±0.5°, symmetrical about collimator axis ±2 mm	—	—
Light field versus indicators	±2 mm each delineator and each blade, ±2 mm overall for field sizes 5 × 5 to 20 × 20, ±1% for fields > 20 × 20.	Meet specifications of annual test at selected field sizes	±2 mm overall in a single field size
Collimator angle indicator	±1° mechanical, ±0.5° digital over full range of motion	±1° mechanical, ±0.5° digital at selected angles	—
Gantry isocenter	1-mm radius sphere	—	—
Gantry angle indicator	±1° mechanical, ±0.5° digital over full range of motion	±1° mechanical, ±0.5° digital at selected angles	—
Target-to-axis indicator	±2 mm over full range	±2 mm at selected distances	Test agreement with range light at one distance
Couch isocenter	1-mm radius circle	—	—
Couch angle	±1° mechanical, ±0.5° digital over full range of motion	±1° mechanical, ±0.5° digital at selected angles	—
Couch position indicators	±2 mm	±2 mm	Couch height ±2 mm
Couch top sag	2 mm	—	—
Image intensifier radial position indicator (TFD indicator if available)	±2 mm over full range	±2 mm at selected location	—
Range light	±1 mm at isocenter, ±5 mm elsewhere	±1 mm at isocenter, ±5 mm elsewhere	±2 mm at isocenter
Localizing laser	±1 mm	±1 mm	±2 mm

x-ray tube, as well as with the largest mA permitted for continuous operation. It is advisable to verify that scattered or primary radiation reaching the position of the operator at the control console does not exceed acceptable limits. As is the case with treatment units, it is advisable to inspect the equipment itself as well as the facility construction for evidence of deterioration, building modifications, or changes in use of the surrounding occupiable space.

2. Safety Interlocks. Interlocks affecting the safe operation of the simulator should be tested on an annual basis. This includes the door interlock as well as the interlocks that limit mechanical motions of the simulator in order to avoid damage to the equipment. In addition, the interlocks that prevent damage to the x-ray system, such as the tube overload indicator, should be tested. The equipment limit switches and the door interlocks should be tested monthly, and a test of the door interlock should be performed each day as part of the warm-up procedure. Interlocks intended to prevent collisions between parts of the equipment should be tested annually, as should software that prohibits machine configurations that could lead to a collision.

3. Patient Monitoring device operation. The devices used to monitor the patient during simulation procedures should be checked every day for proper operation. This includes a closed-circuit TV system and an intercom.

4. Emergency Off Buttons. As is true of a treatment unit, a simulator must be equipped with emergency off buttons with which the operator can immediately remove all power from the equipment. The operation of all emergency off buttons should be tested annually.

Beam Alignment Tests

The beam alignment tests described previously for linear accelerators should be performed also for radiation therapy simulators. In the case of simulators equipped with dual focus x-ray tubes, the tests should be repeated for each focal spot. If the simulator is equipped with fluoroscopy, several of the tests may conveniently be performed using the fluoroscopy system rather than film. For example, the test of gantry isocenter stability can be performed by mounting a metallic pointer, visible under fluoroscopy, to the table top and observing its position on the fluoro monitor relative to the x-ray beam crosshair as the collimator is rotated. Once the stability of collimator rotation has been demonstrated, as well as the stability of the x-ray crosshairs, a similar procedure may be used to test the gantry-isocenter stability and the couch rotation stability.

Focal Spot Size

The focal spot size is most conveniently determined through the use of a "star pattern."[53] Before performing this test, it is advisable to remove all easily removable graticules and alignment devices from the collimator. The star pattern is positioned at an intermediate location between the x-ray tube and a film placed on the table top. It is important to use film in a ready pack envelope rather than a cassette for this test. A radiographic exposure is made to produce an image similar to the image shown on the right in Figure 15-12. In each quadrant of the image, the largest diameter at which the image is blurred is noted. The diameter of the blur pattern is recorded, and the effective focal spot size may be computed. The focal spot dimensions calculated

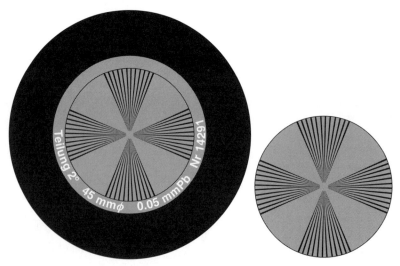

FIGURE 15-12
Contact radiograph (**left**) and x-ray image (**right**) of a star test pattern. The effective size of the focal spot may be computed from the diameter of the blur zone in the x-ray image. (From Hendee, W., Chaney, E., and Rossi, R. *Radiologic Physics, Equipment and Quality Control.* St. Louis, Mosby–Year Book, 1977.)

in this fashion should agree with the manufacturer's specification of focal spot size. This test should be performed annually.

X-Ray Beam Performance

Essentially a diagnostic x-ray unit, the simulator should be subjected to the same quality assurance tests that would be performed on any other piece of diagnostic x-ray equipment. Specific recommendations for diagnostic x-ray QA procedures can be found in a number of publications.[54–56] Measurements should be made of several parameters that indicate x-ray beam performance: Equipment is now available that permits measurement of a number of parameters and the opportunity to determine considerably more information about the x-ray beam and the operation of the generator. These measurements, which can be made in a noninvasive fashion, can make the performance of routine quality assurance procedures considerably more efficient.

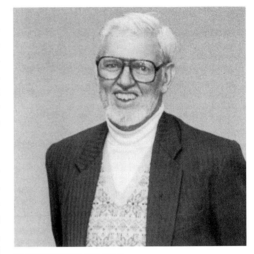

MARGIN FIGURE 15-1
John R. Cameron is one of the early pioneers of quality assurance in radiology and radiation oncology. In 1974, he and his wife Von founded Radiation Measurements Incorporated (RMI), a nonprofit company to manufacture and sell specially designed quality assurance tools. Many of the employees were medical physics graduate students who also performed research on these devices.

    1. X-Ray Beam Half-Value Layer. Half-value layer measurements should be performed at least annually. The measurement of half-value layer is straightforward; it can be made with the equipment frequently found in a radiation oncology department. An ionization chamber with a flat energy response in the diagnostic range should be used. Exposure measurements should be made under easily reproduced conditions, with all removable graticules and trays removed from the beam. Aluminum filters are added until the exposure is reduced to half the original value. From a graph on semilogarithmic paper, the beam half-value layer can be determined. Reproducible measurements of half-value layer ensure that both the x-ray beam and the x-ray generator are stable.

    2. kVp Accuracy. A noninvasive test device such as the instrument shown in Figure 15-13 can be used to determine the effective kVp of the x-ray beam. This value should be compared with the kVp selected at the operator's control panel. The measured kVp should not disagree with the selected kVp by more than 5 kVp.

    3. mA linearity. As the x-ray tube current (measured in mA) increases, the exposure rate should increase proportionally. Measurements should be made periodically of the exposure for several different mA settings. During these measurements, the kVp and timer settings should be kept constant. When plotted on graph paper, the radiation exposure as a function of mA setting should fall on a straight line that passes through the origin.

    4. Timer Accuracy and Linearity. Noninvasive QA instruments can be used to measure the duration of x-ray exposures. The measured duration should agree with the timer setting to within 5%. At the same time, radiation exposure can be measured. The radiation exposure should vary linearly with the timer setting, and a

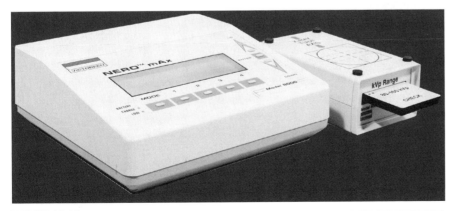

FIGURE 15-13
A representative instrument for noninvasive measurements of x-ray beam performance. (Courtesy of Victoreen, Inc.)

graph of exposure as a function of timer setting should yield a straight line passing through the origin.

5. mAs Linearity. Because radiation exposure depends both on the tube current and the timer setting, exposure should vary linearly with the product of tube current and timer setting (mAs). Measurements of radiation exposure should be made as the mAs is changed, for constant settings of kVp. For convenience and future use, these measurements should be made at the location of the x-ray film cassette, under easily reproduced geometry.

6. Automatic Exposure Control. Most modern simulators are equipped with a *phototimer* that can switch off the x-ray beam when a predetermined radiation exposure has been reached at the film cassette. The proper operation of an automatic exposure control (AEC) system should be verified on a regular basis. The evaluation is performed by making a series of x-ray exposures on radiographic film. Lucite phantoms of several different thicknesses should be used, with a different-size phantom for each exposure. Exposures should be made at kVp settings that span the range commonly used in clinical practice. After processing, the films should all indicate approximately the same optical density. Significant variations among the films indicate that the phototimer is not properly terminating the beam.

7. Fluoroscopic System Quality Assurance. The quality of the fluoroscopic image is frequently an important factor in a radiation oncology department. Simulations often are performed by staff members who have little or no training in diagnostic radiology. Poor image quality, or even the absence of an image, may be blamed on malfunctioning equipment, when in fact the poor results are caused by operator error or misunderstanding. The following short checklist should be followed whenever the performance of a fluoroscopic system is questioned.

- Is the video monitor properly adjusted? Many video monitors have controls for brightness and contrast on the front panel. It is tempting to adjust these controls in an effort to improve image quality, but sometimes the opposite effect occurs.
- Is a grid being used? An x-ray grid can improve image quality, but only if it is the proper grid for the simulator geometry. The target-to-film distance (TFD) of a simulator is frequently much longer than that of a conventional diagnostic x-ray unit. Grids "borrowed" from the diagnostic radiology department may be intended for shorter TFDs and demonstrate *grid cutoff* at the longer TFD of the simulator. Grid cutoff occurs when the angle of the lead strips in the grid is not matched to the divergent x rays from the x-ray target. If a grid is to be used, it should be a general-purpose grid, with a grid ratio of no more than 6.
- Are the collimator blades open? As the dimensions of a radiation field are increased, the amount of scatter generated within the patient increases rapidly. The scatter reaches the image intensifier and degrades the image. In addition, the portions of the beam that do not intercept the image intensifier are "wasted"; the patient receives additional exposure, but no useful image information is produced. The dimensions of the collimator blades should be close to those of the image intensifier. Many radiation therapy simulators provide an automatic tracking feature that adjusts the collimator blades during fluoroscopy.
- Does the simulator have automatic brightness control? An automatic brightness stabilization (ABS) system can adjust kVp and/or mA to achieve the optimal image. The ABS system often performs this function more rapidly and more effectively than do manual adjustments of the controls. When available, this system should be used.

To help ensure proper operation of a fluoroscoic system, two straightforward tests should be performed on a regular basis. The *spatial resolution* can be evaluated with a line pair test tool. Several types of test tools are available; any tool that provides a high-contrast pattern with variable spacing can be used. A measurement of *contrast resolution* also is a useful indicator of fluoroscopic system performance. Test tools are available that provide objects of various sizes and amounts of contrast. The reproducible performance of the fluoroscopic system should be determined with these devices.

■ CT SIMULATOR QUALITY ASSURANCE

Simulation of patients using computed tomography is now commonplace in many centers. Features of these systems, such as moving lasers (either wall-mounted or internal CT lasers), must be evaluated with a quality control program to ensure accuracy in patient alignment. In addition, differences in geometry between the CT scanner and the treatment unit must be correctly accounted for. For example, in cases where the patient is scanned feet first but treated head first, the transformation of patient data in treatment planning is critical. For centers that have a dedicated CT simulator in radiation oncology, routine image quality evaluation will likely be the responsibility of the radiation oncology physicist. Changes in Hounsfield units (CT numbers) may affect image quality slightly, but could affect dose calculation significantly. Radiation therapists performing simulation are often required to adapt quickly to an entirely new piece of equipment. With relatively few simulations compared to CT procedures in radiology for a typical scanner, it may take some time for the therapists to become proficient. Finally, with replacement of high-quality x-ray simulation films by digitally reconstructed radiographs (DRR), therapists and dosimetrists must also learn how to generate clinically acceptable DRR images.

Lasers

With a conventional simulator, marking a reference point on the patient can be accomplished with fluoroscopy and fixed wall-mounted lasers, after which the patient is sent for a CT scan (usually in radiology). To identify the reference point on the CT images, small fiducials (bb's) are often used. This approach eliminates reliance on the laser localizing lights of the CT scanner, other than perhaps to level the patient. In the absence of a conventional simulator, or when pure CT simulation is performed, an accurate laser marking system is required. One complicating factor is any physical shift between the wall laser isocenter and the isocenter of the CT gantry. In addition, the CT scanner internal laser localizers need to be accurate if used, and the wall lasers may in fact be "movable" to assist in marking the patient. Obviously, laser quality assurance for CT simulators is more involved than for conventional simulators. To verify that the laser isocenter matches the CT isocenter, a phantom is used that is first aligned to the lasers using crosshairs with corresponding fiducials, then the phantom is shifted to the gantry isocenter using the couch and a known shift increment (see Figure 15-14). A single scan at this point should have the fiducial markers intersecting the gantry isocenter. For movable lasers, positioning should be accurate to within ± 2 mm. This can be verified using a ruler or graph paper positioned on the treatment couch.

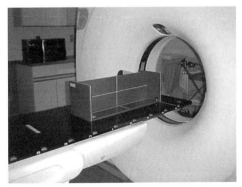

FIGURE 15-14
Phantom for quality assurance of a CT simulator.

Couch

Key parameters in CT imaging studies include slice thickness and table increment. For diagnostic studies, slight inaccuracies in table increment may not affect diagnosis. For radiation therapy, however, an inaccurate table increment will produce a false data set, notably in the superior/inferior direction. The result is incorrect tumor volumes, beam blocking, jaw positions, and DRRs. Patient anatomy on portal films will not match, even though the isocenter may be exact. Accurate couch positioning and calibration is important and must be verified for axial and helical modes. Since the flat couch top is often removable to allow conventional CT scanning using a rounded table top, a check is required to ensure that the flat couch top is level when reinstalled. Finally, couch sag should be evaluated, particularly when the couch is extended far into the gantry (e.g., scanning a prostate patient head first). Progressive couch sag on the images will appear as a slight table angle when viewed in a sagittal plane.

Image Orientation

The correct translation of imaging coordinates to treatment coordinates is critical. Since axial images are often symmetric, an incorrect transformation of coordinates may not be apparent. One simple solution to this problem is to create a known asymmetric geometry by placing a wire on one side of the treatment couch. This marker should always be on the same side of the image set, regardless of patient position. To evaluate correct tranformation of patient position, a cube with imagable markers (A, anterior; P, posterior; L, left; R, right; S, superior; I, inferior) can be scanned in various treatment positions (Figure 15-15).

Image Quality

While not specifically used for diagnostic radiology, a CT simulator in radiation therapy is still obliged to produce high-quality images. The physician defines target volumes and critical structures using these images, and any deterioration in the images

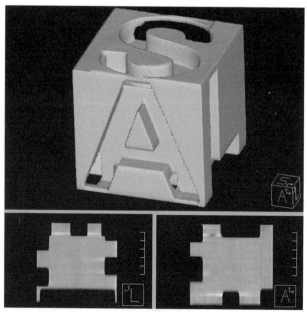

FIGURE 15-15
Reconstruction of an orientation phantom to verify proper patient position in the treatment planning system.

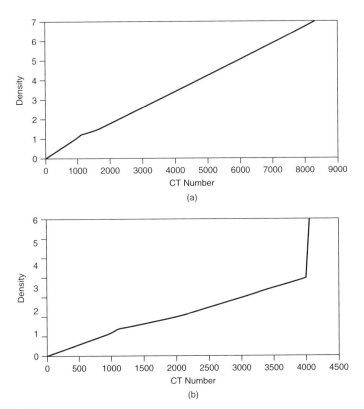

FIGURE 15-16
A, B: Measured CT to density graphs for a treatment planning system. For this system, the pixel values became saturated at a value of 4096 and data were extrapolated to a density of 7. In Part B, it is assumed that any pixel values that are saturated most likely reflect the presence of a metal prosthesis, and a density of 6 is used as an estimation of the object's density.

will adversely affect the ability to delineate the structures. Use of a standard CT phantom to test variables such as spatial resolution, low contrast resolution, slice positioning, and spatial accuracy can accomplish this task.

CT to Density Table

Correct mapping of Hounsfield numbers to physical densities contributes to accurate treatment planning calculations. By scanning a phantom of known densities, a table or graph can be generated for the treatment planning computer (Figure 15-16). Care must be taken to scan objects that adequately represent the range of densities encountered within the body, including high-density objects such as dense bone or a hip prosthesis. One should avoid objects that have an unnaturally high atomic number since the photoelectric effect in these objects will inflate the observed CT number.

▦ IMAGE QUALITY ASSURANCE

Film Processor

Regardless of how well an x-ray system performs and how appropriate the x-ray technique is, the final radiographic image may not be acceptable unless the film processor is functioning properly. In radiation oncology, there is a tendency to dismiss the importance of image quality as being a requirement only in diagnostic radiology. Although it is true that simulator films are rarely used for diagnosis, the correct placement of radiation fields often depends on the ability of the radiation oncologist to visualize the patient's anatomy without difficulty. Under some circumstances, the

Phantoms for IMRT. Since quality assurance in IMRT often requires transfer of the treatment plan to a phantom, the phantom must be scanned so the dose can be calculated. This is a new application of phantom materials in radiation oncology, namely that phantoms intended for megavoltage dose measurement are imaged on a CT scanner. One must be careful that the phantom properties are correctly accounted for in treatment planning. For example, the physical density and chemical makeup of some phantoms are designed so they are water equivalent at megavoltage energies. Photoelectric and density effects may yield higher or lower CT numbers for these phantoms, and the planning system may interpret these numbers as representing materials different from water for the purpose of dose calculation. One simple solution is to use only phantoms that are truly water equivalent at megavoltage energies.

TABLE 15-6 CT Simulator Daily, Monthly and Annual QA Tests

	Item Tested	Description
Daily	Lasers	Verify isocenter location on wall lasers and correct transformation to CT coordinates.
	Tube warm-up	CT simulator in radiation oncology often not used continually as in radiology. May require warmup prior to patient scanning.
	Water phantom	Verify CT number of water.
	Interlocks	Test scanner interrupt button.
	Patient viewing and intercom	Test functionality.
Weekly	Detector calibration	Run calibration routine for CT detector ring.
	Isocenter shift	For movable lasers, correct translation to new isocenter coordinates.
	Couch	Accuracy of travel.
Monthly	Lasers	Verify isocenter and transformation of coordinates from CT simulation software.
	Density check	Verify density of water, low density object, and high density object.
	Interlocks	Test safety interlocks and interrupt.
	Slice thickness	Verify slice thickness using phantom.
	Table increment	Verify table increment by scanning object of known length.
Annual	Resolution	Check high and low contrast resolution. Check spatial resolution.
	Tube parameters	Measure kVp and mAs.
	CT density table	Verify CT to density table or graph over full range of densities encountered.
	Exposure rate	Check exposure rates for commonly used scanning configurations.

quality of the image determines whether an important structure is visible. Measurements of the processor chemistry, the developer temperature, and the reproducibility of the film characteristic curve should be made on a regular basis. Measurements should be made weekly and whenever there is a question about the performance of the processor. Specific recommendations for performing processor QA procedures may be found in several publications.[54–57]

Portal Imaging and Computed Radiography

Digital "filmless" techniques such as computed radiography and portal imaging are finding a place in radiation therapy. For these systems, performance characteristics should be compared against product specifications as part of acceptance testing. For computed radiography systems, tests may include dark noise, uniformity, exposure response, laser beam function, spatial resolution, low-contrast resolution, spatial accuracy, erasure thoroughness, and throughput.[58] In addition, tests related to sensitivity, modulation transfer function (MTF), noise power spectra (NPS), and detective quantum efficiency (DQE) have been performed, as shown in Figure 15-17.[59] With the adoption of new digital imaging techniques, concepts familiar to diagnostic radiological physicists become integral to quality assurance in radiation therapy. The tests should ensure that the equipment performs its intended function, i.e. the equipment produces comparable or better portal images. Comparing the image obtained on a phantom using film vs portal imaging or CR will provide the information needed to make an overall assessment of image quality.

Modulation transfer function: A measure of how well information presented to the imaging system in the form of a sine wave is represented in the image. As the frequency of the sine wave increases, the ability of the system to represent the information in the image decreases.

Detective quantum efficiency: A measure of the detection efficiency that includes the effects of noise. It may be defined as the ratio of the signal-to-noise at the output of the system to the signal-to-noise at the input of the system.

$$DQE = \frac{SNR_{OUT}}{SNR_{IN}}$$

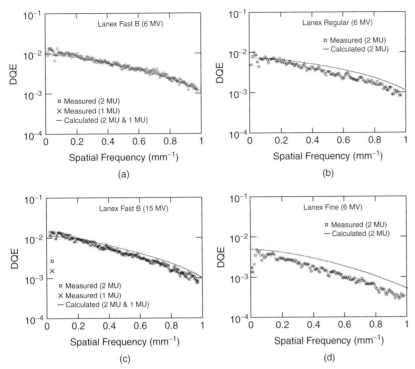

FIGURE 15-17
Megavoltage MTF and DQE data at megavoltage energies for an active matrix, flat panel imager. (From EL-Mohri, Y., Jee, K. W., Antonuk, L. E., Maolinbay, M., and Zhao, Q. Determination of the detective quantum efficiency of a prototype, megavoltage indirect detection, active matrix flat-panel imager. *Med. Phys.* 2001; **28**(12): 2538–2550, with permission.)

■ TREATMENT PLANNING COMPUTER

Treatment planning computers are widely used in radiation therapy departments. Most departments are equipped with a computer capable of generating isodose distributions for multiple rectangular beams. Treatment planning systems are also available that can determine the dose at selected points in irregular fields, and that can calculate complete isodose distributions throughout such irregular fields. Other programs are available to calculate the dose throughout a complete three-dimensional volume, making corrections for the patient contour as well as for the presence of inhomogeneities. Fully three-dimensional treatment planning programs consider the effects of tissue densities throughout the irradiated volume and thus permit the entry of beams whose central axes do not lie in the same plane (*noncoplanar* beams). Some of these treatment planning computers are equipped with programs that calculate the monitor unit setting (or treatment time) required to deliver the prescribed dose according to the treatment plan.

Treatment planning computer programs are quite complex, and the user is likely to have neither access to, nor a complete understanding of, the computational methods involved. Because of the complexity of the software, it is virtually impossible to test every conceivable computational situation. Therefore, a QA program for treatment planning computers can only address a finite range of treatment situations, computational requirements, and specific calculations (see Tables 15-7 to 15-9). It is possible, however, to design a QA program that gives the user confidence that the treatment planning system provides acceptable accuracy over a clinically useful range of situations.[15,60–62]

As described in Chapter 11, most treatment planning computer systems require the entry of measured beam data. These measured data may be so detailed that the

TABLE 15-7 QA for Treatment Planning Systems and Monitor Unit Calculations

Frequency	Test	Tolerance[a]
Commissioning and following software update	Understand algorithm	Functional
	Single field or source isodose distribution	2%[a] or 2 mm[b]
	MU calculations	2%
	Test cases	2% or 2 mm
	I/Q system	1 mm
Daily	I/O devices	1 mm
Monthly	Checksum	No change
	Subset of referece QA test set (when checksums not available)	2% or 2 mm[c]
	I/Q	1 mm
Annual	MU calculations	2%
	Reference QA test set	2% or 2 mm[d]
	I/O sytem	1 mm

[a] Percent difference between claculation of the computer treatment planning system and measurement (or independent calculation).

[b] In the region of high dose gradients the distance between idodose lines is more appropriate than percent difference. In addition, less accuracy may be obtained near the end of single sources.

[c] These limits refer to the comparison of dose calculations at commissioning to the same calculations subsequently.

[d] These limits refer to comparison of calculations with measurement in a water tank.

Source: Comprehensive QA for radiation oncology: Report of AAPM Radiation Therapy Committee Task Group 40. Med. Phy. 1994; **21**(4):581–618.

computer needs only to perform minor computations in order to display dose distributions for many clinical situations. Often, interpolation between closely spaced field sizes is all that is required. Other treatment planning systems require only a small amount of data to be entered; from these data, the computer calculates dose distributions for a wide variety of treatment conditions. In this case, it is up to the user to confirm that the measured data entered into the computer represent the range of clinical conditions likely to be encountered, and that the computer is able to successfully mimic these situations from the small amount of data provided. The commissioning of a treatment planning system therefore requires the following steps:

1. Understanding, in a broad sense, the treatment planning software algorithms and their dependence on measured data.
2. Collection of appropriate data required by the treatment planning system, and entry of these data.
3. Collection of additional data (a) fully characterizing the beams for which treatment planning will be done and (b) representing a range of clinical situations.
4. Calculation of dose distributions, point doses, and monitor unit or treatment time settings, along with comparison of these calculations with the measured data.

The steps described above are complex and may be quite time-consuming. The collection and analysis of large amounts of data cannot be avoided if a treatment planning system is to be thoroughly evaluated. Even if a treatment planning system operates on a limited set of measured data, the user must still make extensive measurements to fully evaluate the system. A complete set of measured data and test cases has been prepared to assist in the commissioning of treatment planning systems.[63]

Once the initial commissioning and evaluation of a treatment-planning system has been completed, an ongoing program of quality assurance is required to ensure the

TABLE 15-8 Periodic Treatment Planning Process QA Checks

Recommended Frequency	Item	Comments/Details
Daily	Error log	Review report log listing system failures, error messages, hardware malfunctions, and other problems. Triage list and remedy any serious problems that occur during the day.
	Change log	Keep log of hardware/software changes.
Weekly	Digitizer	Review digitizer accuracy.
	Hard-copy output	Review all hard-copy output, including scaling for plotter and other graphics-type output.
	Computer files	Verify integrity of all RTP system data files and executables using checksums or other simple software checks. Checking software should be provided by the vendor.
	Review clinical planning	Review clinical treatment planning activity. Discuss errors, problems, complications, difficulties. Resolve problems.
Monthly	CT data input into RTP system	Review the CT data within the planning system for geometrical accuracy, CT number consistency (also dependent on the QA and use of the scanner), and derived electron density.
	Problem review	Review all RTP problems (both for RTP system and clinical treatment planning) and prioritize problems to be resolved.
	Review of RTP system	Review current configuration and status of all RTP system software, hardware, and data files.
Annual	Dose calculations	Annual checks. Review acceptability of agreement between measured and calculated doses for each beam/source.
	Data and I/O devices	Review functioning and accuracy of digitizer tablet, video/laser digitizer, CT input, MR input, printers, plotters, and other imaging output devices.
	Critical software tools	Review BEV/DRR generation and plot accuracy, CT geometry, density conversions, DVH calculations, other critical tools, machine-specific conversions, data files, and other critical data.
Variable	Beam parameterization	Checks and/or recommissioning may be required due to machine changes or problems.
	Software changes, including operating system	Checks and/or recommissioning may be required due to changes in the RTP software, any support/additional software such as image transfer software, or the operating system.

Source: American Association of Physicists in Medicine Radiation Therapy Committee Task Group 53: Quality assurance for clinical radiotheraphy treatment planning. *Med. Phys.* 1998; **25**(10): 1773–1829.

continued reliable operation of the system. Computer systems have been characterized as being both unlikely to fail at all, and unlikely to fail in any but obvious and catastrophic ways. This statement is probably true for most computer hardware such as the central processing unit (CPU), memory, and disk-storage devices. Failures are rare, and when they do occur, they are generally obvious. This rule does not always hold, however. A highly publicized failure of the Intel Pentium processor chip resulted in frequent incorrect calculations.[64–67] The magnitude of the error was so small as to be negligible except when iterative calculations were performed.

Other computer components may be subject to failure in a more insidious and less easily detectable fashion. Graphics tablets, for example, have failed in ways that yield results that are in error by only a small amount. Under such conditions, a patient contour can be digitized that is incorrect enough to cause significant errors in the final calculations, even though the contour error may not be obvious to the user.

Output devices may also fail in ways that are not immediately obvious to the user. For example, a printer connected to a treatment planning computer was observed to fail so that the letter W was printed when the printer was instructed to print the letter R. Although this particular failure provided an endless source of amusement for the staff and did not present much risk of erroneous calculations, one must consider the impact of a similar error in which the number 2 is printed instead of the number 5.

A QA program for treatment planning computer systems must address several major sources of uncertainty[68] (the operator as a source of inaccuracy is not considered

TABLE 15-9 Criteria of Acceptability for Photon and Electron Beam Dose Calculations

Descriptor	Criterion
I. Photon beams	
A. Homogeneous calculation (no shields)	
1. Central ray data (except in buildup region)	2%
2. High dose region-low dose gradient	3%
3. Large dose gradients (>30%/cm)	4 mm
4. Small dose gradients in low dose region (ie., <7% of normalization dose)	3%
B. Inhomogeneity corrections	
1. Central ray (slab geometry, in regions of electron equilibrium)	3%
C. Composite uncertainty, anthropomorphic phantom	
Off axis	
Contour corrections	
Inhomogeneities	
Shields	
Irregular feilds	
In regions of electronic equilibrium	
Attenuators	
1. High dose region–low dose gradient	40%
2. Large dose gradient (>30%/cm)	4 mm
3. Small dose gradients in low dose region (i.e., <7% of normalization dose)	3%
II. Electron beams	
A. Homogeneous calculation (no shields)	
1. Central ray data (except in buildup region)	2%
2. High dose region-low dose gradient	4%
3. Large dose gradients (>30%/cm)	4 mm
4. Small dose gradients in low dose region i.e., <7% of normalization dose	4%
B. Inhomogeneity corrections	
1. Central ray (slab geometry, in regions of electron equilibrium)	5%
C. Composite uncertainty, anthropomorphic phantom	
Contour correction	
Inhomogeneities	
Shields	
Irregular fields	
Off axis	
1. High dose region-low dose gradient	7%
2. Large does gradient (>30%/cm)	5 mm
3. Small dose gradients in low dose region (i.e., <7% of central ray dose)	5%

Note: Percentages are quoted as a percent of the central ray normalization dose.

Source: Van Dyk, J. Commissioning and Quality Assurance of Treatment Planning Computers, *Int. J. Radiat. Oncol. Biol. Phys.* 1993; **26**(2):261–273.

here): some specific recommendations for test frequencies and tolerances are shown in Table 15-7.

1. Inaccuracies in Measured Data. Measured data fall into two categories: (a) measurements of beam data and (b) measurements of patient specific data. Inaccuracies in measured beam data may be caused by incorrect or inappropriate measurements, or by changes in the treatment beam or beam parameters that have occurred

since the original measurements were made. Uncertainties in patient-specific data may include erroneous caliper measurements, as well as the incorrect interpretation of imaging data such as that obtained from CT scans. This last category would include an incorrect relationship between CT information and electron densities.

Under certain conditions, measured data stored in a computer can be changed unintentionally by the user. Some computer systems use computational techniques called *checksums* to detect changes in stored values, but many systems do not have such safeguards. Other treatment planning systems fail to clearly indicate stored data that are used in calculations, and this may alter the result. As an example, a recent version of a particular treatment planning system permitted the user to store the wedge transmission factor with the measured data characterizing the wedged beam profile. The wedge transmission factors were used in the calculation of monitor unit settings, but this fact was not clearly indicated on the printout. Consequently, it was possible for the user to correct a second time for the presence of a wedge, without recognizing that the transmission correction had already been applied.

To guard against the risk of undetected changes in stored data, careful records should be kept of data entry sessions and software upgrades. In addition, calculations should be repeated on a regular basis to test the veracity of stored data. A subset of the dose calculations performed during commissioning of the planning system would ensure consistency and accuracy.

2. Inaccuracies of Data Entry. Many beam scanning systems provide software for direct electronic transfer of data from the scanning system to the treatment planning computer. Such systems are generally reliable. Without such software, it is necessary to plot the data obtained by the scanning system and then digitize it manually into the treatment planning system. Opportunities for error exist in the digitizing and storing of these data.[69] In addition, patient-specific data, such as contours or data taken from CT hard copies, must generally be digitized by hand with the use of a graphics tablet. Again, opportunities for error exist.

The accuracy of a graphics digitizer tablet can be evaluated by entering a standard patient contour (even a rectangular shape), printing the output, and comparing the printed output with the original contour. This procedure is a test of both the graphics input device and the output device, but it cannot distinguish a source of errors if it exists. All data entry devices should be tested in this fashion, including data input electronically from CT scanners and other imaging devices. All output devices should be tested simultaneously. Such tests are generally simple to perform, yet they assess important functions of the treatment planning system. The tests should be performed weekly, and the output should agree with the input data to within 2 mm.

3. Inaccuracies of Data Output. The output of a treatment planning system may be in the form of graphic isodose plots or numerical printouts. Either type of output may be produced on a video monitor or on a hard-copy device such as a printer or plotter. Graphic output data must be accurate, regardless of its means of production, because they are used frequently to position the patient relative to the treatment beam. Alphanumeric data must likewise be accurate because this information is often used to program the treatment unit. Tests for evaluating the accuracy of data output devices may be conducted simultaneously with the tests of input devices, as described in item 2 above. In addition, it is advisable to retain a standard test case on the computer's hard disk; this case should be printed on occasion to test the output device independently of the source of input data.

4. Algorithm Inaccuracy. Inaccuracies in the computational algorithm are not easily detected or controlled by the operator of the system. Radiation therapy treatment planning presents complicated situations that can only be approximated by computational techniques. Although these techniques may prove sufficiently accurate over a range of frequently encountered treatment techniques, they may not always perform satisfactorily as the limits to these approximations are approached. Evaluation of the software should therefore cover the full range of complexity encountered in the clinic. Inaccuracies may also result from decisions made in implementing the

software. For example, selection of a large grid spacing for the computational algorithm may yield increased computational speed, but also isodose lines that show a scalloped appearance, and rounding or truncation errors when multiple beams are used.

Two types of computational accuracy tests should be performed. A test of reproducibility involves repeating a standard treatment plan on a regular basis. All input information should be identical, so that the output is expected to be identical from one test to the next. Several simple tests should be devised to test calculations using single beams, multiple fields, wedges, and the presence of inhomogeneities. Comparable tests should be devised for verifying the repeatability of calculations using implanted sources, both singly and in arrays.

The second type of test should evaluate the accuracy of calculations. For such a test, it is preferable that the input data not be identical from one test to the next, so that the ability of the system to perform well under different circumstances can be tested. Such a test is not easily devised, and it may be cumbersome and time-consuming to perform. One suitable test consists of comparing calculations with measured data. Field sizes or measurement points should be used that were not included in the measured data originally stored in the computer. This forces the computer to calculate the dose expressly for the test, rather than to simply retrieve stored data. To provide a valid test, the data used for comparison should have been measured at the same time as the data used in the computations. Similar tests can be conducted to compare measured data with calculated doses at points irradiated by two or more fields. Note that if isodose curves are generated, it may be adequate to determine the dose at only a small number of points and then to examine the calculated isodose curves for consistency with these few values. Tests of computational reproducibility should be performed frequently, and monthly intervals are suggested. Tests of computational accuracy need be performed less frequently, but should be performed at no less than yearly intervals, or whenever changes are made to the stored data or software. The ICRU recommends that calculated data agree with measured values to within 2%, or to within 2 mm in regions of high dose gradient.[7]

■ QUALITY ASSURANCE FOR INTENSITY-MODULATED RADIATION THERAPY (IMRT)

As with other specialty procedures, IMRT has its own specific quality assurance procedures. The procedures encompass radiation safety, treatment planning calculations, machine characteristics, and patient-specific dosimetric verification. The primary goals of IMRT QA are to identify safe parameters for treatment and to verify that the dose intended is the dose delivered.

Radiation Safety

Generally speaking, a given treatment field using IMRT will have more monitor units than a comparable conformally shaped field. Depending on the amount of modulation (roughly corresponding to the complexity of the fluence map or the number of segments), it is common to use three to four times the number of monitor units to deliver an IMRT field. Since there are often more beam directions with IMRT, the effect on primary barriers is not a major concern. However, the ability of secondary barriers to handle leakage radiation becomes an issue, particularly if higher energies are used.[70] The calculations used in evaluating secondary barriers for the original vault design should be re-visited using the increased workload for an IMRT patient volume. Also, increased neutron dose to the patient should be considered when x rays above 10 MeV are used.

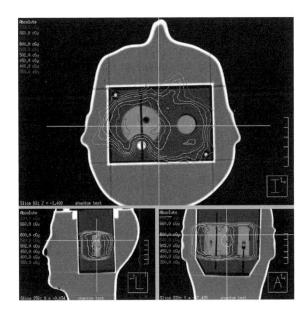

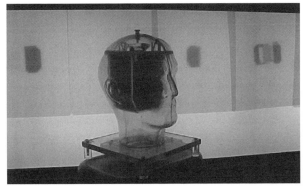

FIGURE 15-18
IMRT head and neck phantom from the Radiological Physics Center at MD Anderson. This phantom is designed to independently test the ability of the institution to deliver IMRT treatments for participation in the RTOG IMRT head and neck protocol. The top figure shows the planned dose distribution, and the bottom figure shows the phantom and delivered fluence maps.

Treatment Planning

The planning system should be commissioned for IMRT by verifying that the dose predicted by the planning system is accurate to within acceptable limits. Since actual patient plans are quite complex, it may be best to start with geometric test patterns with a predictable or known dose. For example, computing the expected dose on a segment as shown in Figure 15-18, and then measuring the delivered dose in a phantom, will illustrate the ability of the planning system to predict dose in a simple geometry. Then, by combining several segments, one can determine if the cumulative dose for multiple segments is correctly computed, accounting for such parameters as MLC transmission within the field. Finally, a complex dose distribution using multiple segments from several beam directions can simulate an actual patient treatment.

Machine Characteristics

There are two general classifications of machine characteristics to investigate: (a) multi-leaf collimators (MLC) and (b) dose delivery. Parameters to be tested for MLC characteristics are detailed earlier in this chapter in the section for MLC quality assurance; they refer to the mechanical properties of MLC leaf design, and monitoring them for any abberant behavior. With heavily blocked segments where the jaws remain fixed for each segment, the jaws move with each segment, or the MLCs replace one set of jaws, leaf and jaw transmission contribute to the therapeutic dose delivery. This must be correctly calculated in the planning system. With the potential for segments with small numbers of monitor units, the ability of the treatment unit to deliver the correct dose must be investigated.

Patient-Specific Dose Verification

The ASTRO/ACR guidelines for IMRT treatment delivery specify "the dose delivery must be documented for each course of treatment by irradiating a phantom that contains either calibrated film to sample the dose distribution, or an equivalent measurement system to verify that the dose delivered is the dose planned." This guideline implies that each and every IMRT plan must be verified by measuring the dose delivered. There are several techniques available to accomplish this task, including point dose or planar dose measurements for individual fields and for all fields.[71,72]

1. Point Dose Measurements for a Single Field. Can be measured using film, ion chamber, or diodes. Film measurements may involve sampling locations specified on the planar dose map. Ion chamber measurements in a phantom are generally acquired at a single specified point such as the isocenter. Diode measurements can be done directly on the patient, as is common in external beam treatment. One must be careful when measuring the dose for a single field since high dose gradients may exist.
2. Point Dose Measurements for All Fields. A composite film can be used to sample the dose at a specified point (or points), or an ion chamber may be used.
3. Planar Dose Measurements for a Single Field. Dose is computed at a specified depth in the phantom, perpendicular to the central axis of the beam. It may be

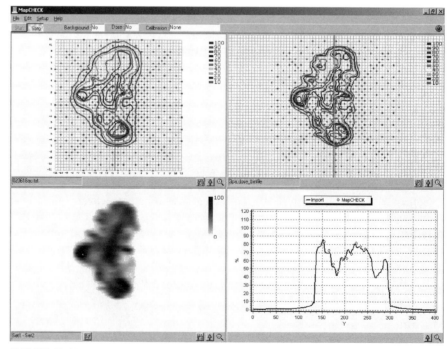

FIGURE 15-19
Quality assurance tool consisting of 400 diodes to generate a two-dimensional map of delivered dose. This tool allows instantaneous evaluation of IMRT fields without processing film. (Courtesy of Sun Nuclear.)

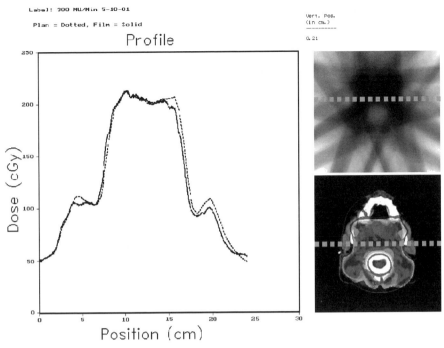

FIGURE 15-20
Composite dose verification for multiple fields. Profiles through the target volume and parotids are compared. (Courtesy of Chester Ramsey, Ph.D.)

measured using film or an array of diodes (e.g., MapCheck from Sun Nuclear Corporation; see Figure 15-19). Dose profiles or isodose lines may be compared quantitatively using specialized software to scan and analyze the film (e.g., RIT, Radiological Imaging Technologies, Inc.; see Figure 15-20).

4. Planar Dose Measurements for Multiple Fields. These are typically measured using film. Dose profiles or isodose lines may be compared to the treatment plan.

The approach implemented in a clinic is largely a matter of personal preference, and it may change over time as a comfort level with IMRT treatment is established. When setting acceptable tolerances for dosimetric measurements, limits should be set for individual fields as well as for overall delivery. These limits may be expressed in terms of absolute error or percentage error. For example, individual field tolerances could be set at 5% or 3 cGy, whichever is less, and the tolerance for overall dose delivery could be set at 3%. There are also several commercially available software systems that can perform an independent monitor unit check for IMRT fields, as well as predicted fluence maps (Figure 15-21). These systems can supplement, or possibly replace, phantom measurements.

Tools available for IMRT analysis are also quite useful for quality assurance of other delivery techniques, such as stereotactic radiosurgery and dynamic wedges. They may also be used to compare a typical 3-D treatment with an IMRT treatment to evaluate the differences between these two techniques. For example, by evaluating a composite dose distribution in phantom for a 3-D CRT prostate patient compared with an IMRT plan for the same patient, the clinician can see the difference between the delivered doses. If there are nonuniformities in the target volume due to segmented delivery of the IMRT plan, these will be readily apparent when compared with uniform delivery of 3-D CRT techniques.

■ STEREOTACTIC RADIOSURGERY AND RADIOTHERAPY

Stereotactic radiosurgery was described in 1951 by Lars Leksell for treatment of brain tumors.[73] This procedure is often utilized for small lesions requiring precision localization and highly conformal dose distributions. It has been used most often for treatment of brain tumors because the patient can be easily immobilized. Advances in internal localization techniques, however, have prompted use of the procedure for other cancers, such as prostate. With stiff requirements for precise localization and accurate dosimetry, quality assurance for stereotactic treatment is quite involved.[74]

The first aspect of quality assurance is immobilization of the target during treatment. In the case of stereotactic radiosurgery of brain tumors, immobilization is often

Stereotactic radiosurgery—Accomplished with a single fraction of radiation. *Stereotactic radiotherapy*—Accomplished with multiple fractions of radiation.

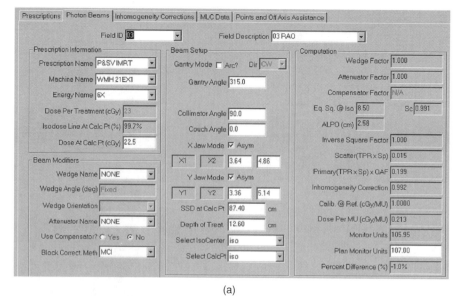

(a)

(b)

FIGURE 15-21

A: Calculation-based evaluation of IMRT fields based on concentric ring evaluation of delivered segments. **B:** This system also provides an independent depiction of the expected fluence map for comparison against a film. (Courtesy of RadCalc, Lifeline Software Inc.)

External Coordinate System: A method of localizing a target based on a coordinate system relative to the immobilization device. For stereotactic radiosurgery, the immobilization device may be a rigid frame mounted to the patient's skull, and the coordinates may be determined by imaged localization rods.

Fiducial Localization: A fixed number of points used to position that target. The points may be seen by a camera system, or may be imaged on portal images of the patient. Localization is done directly on the relative position of the fiducials and target without an intermediate coordinate system.

accomplished by a rigid frame attached to the skull. For stereotactic radiotherapy, where the patient will return for several fractions, a relocatable frame or mask approach may be used. Care must be taken to ensure that the immobilization system is repeatable for fractionated treatments.

The second aspect of quality assurance is localization, accomplished using either an external coordinate system referenced to the immobilization device (e.g., BRW coordinates), or fiducials. In both cases, the location of the target relative to the localization system is known, and it must be accurately positioned on the treatment unit.

The three most common stereotactic treatment units are a linear accelerator, Elekta's Gamma Knife, and Accuray's Cyberknife. Linear accelerators fitted with a stereotactic radiosurgery package and external coordinate system require alignment of the isocenter with the stereotactic treatment fields (cone or multileaf collimator) prior to treatment. Alignment is generally accomplished by setting the treatment coordinates and verifying the treatment field with film in several planes. For fiducial localization, the target is aligned while the patient is on the table, because the fiducials are effectively part of the patient (either implanted or mounted to the patient). For linac-based treatments, one must be careful to monitor any shifts due to couch rotation, because the couch rotational axis may not coincide with the linac's isocenter. If the error is deemed significant, the offsets can be corrected for each couch angle by dialing in a lateral and longitudinal shift. The Gamma Knife is a dedicated mechanical system with precision machining to ensure proper localization. The patient docks into position during treatment with treatment coordinates dialed in. For the Cyberknife, a pair of fluoroscopic images constantly monitor patient position during treatment. The system is completely non-isocentric, so there is no alignment of the isocenter prior to treatment.

■ BRACHYTHERAPY QUALITY ASSURANCE PROCEDURES

As is true of all radiation oncology equipment, brachytherapy equipment and sources should be subjected to routine QA procedures to ensure the safety of patients and staff, as well as to improve the quality of patient treatments.[75,76] In addition, the NRC and many states require that certain QA procedures be performed routinely. Failure to adhere to certain standards can subject an institution to a notice of violation and monetary fine.

Applicators

Applicators for brachytherapy procedures should be inspected and radiographed before their initial use. Frequently these devices are made from several pieces of metal that have been welded together, and there is a risk that flaws can develop and pieces of the applicator can separate. In the case of remote afterloading systems, using radio-opaque dummy markers in conjunction with an autoradiograph of the source in corresponding dwell positions will verify the positional accuracy of the applicator as well as an understanding of the geometry of the applicator for treatment planning purposes. Documentation of this initial inspection and storage of the original films may be valuable for later comparison. After each use, the applicator should be cleaned and then carefully examined for flaws. This inspection can take place before the equipment is sterilized for the next use.

Radioactive Sources

The sources used for radioactive implants should be inspected periodically. Inspection is done most conveniently at the time an inventory is conducted. In most localities, an inventory of radioactive sources is required annually. A systematic program of record-keeping is an essential part of a brachytherapy program.[77] It is also convenient to perform a brief inspection of sources at the time of each use. ^{137}Cs tube sources should be inspected for curvature, because these sources can become caught between the drawers of a safe and bent to the point at which they either begin to leak radioactive material or become difficult to remove from an implant applicator. Leak testing of radioactive sources is required before their initial use and on a regular basis thereafter. Generally, leak testing is required semiannually, but some cesium sources are certified for leak testing only every 3 years.

Remote Afterloading Equipment

As is the case with treatments using any radioactive material, treatments with remote afterloading devices require safety procedures to avoid unintended exposure of the patient or personnel, or the loss of radioactive material. The high activity of sources provided with high-dose rate (HDR) remote afterloading equipment demands that close attention be paid to the whereabouts of the source at all times. Quality assurance procedures must be designed to ensure that the equipment functions as intended. Safety procedures must also be designed and attending personnel must be trained in these procedures, to ensure that the treatments are delivered safely and that employees respond appropriately in emergencies.

The NRC has recently published regulations requiring that a physician and a physicist be nearby whenever HDR treatments are performed. Radiation monitors must be available in the room; they must also be available to personnel entering the room. Following treatment, a survey of the patient is required to ensure that the source has been removed properly from the patient.

Careful documentation of the treatment is required. If multiple applicators are used and are left in place, they must be clearly identified to facilitate connecting the device for subsequent treatment. Finally, all personnel must be adequately trained in emergency procedures. Only properly trained individuals should be permitted to respond in the case of emergencies, and departmental operating procedures should ensure that those trained individuals are available at the time of treatment.

Pulsed-dose-rate (PDR) brachytherapy is an alternative to low-dose-rate (LDR) remote afterloading brachytherapy. As is the case with LDR treatments, the patient must be essentially immobilized for the entire course of treatment. PDR brachytherapy is attractive for a number of logistical and technological reasons. Regardless of the patient's ambulatory status, opportunities increase for medical attention because the radioactive source is extended into the patient for only brief periods each hour. In addition, a source storage facility is necessary, as is frequent source handling and transportation.

Safety Procedures

Whenever brachytherapy is performed, attention must be paid to the use of occupiable space surrounding the treatment room. High-dose-rate brachytherapy generally is performed in a dedicated room, and shielding is designed and installed at the time of equipment installation. However, LDR and PDR brachytherapy treatments are typically given in hospital patient rooms, and it is not always possible or practical to provide radiation shielding. The rooms in which remote afterloading devices are installed must be equipped with a door interlock, to ensure that the source is retracted when the door is opened. The room must be equipped with a functioning radiation area monitor. Staff must be trained in appropriate emergency procedures and must practice these procedures on a regular basis. Recommendations for emergency procedures have been published.[78,79]

The following quality assurance procedures apply equally well to HDR and PDR units. A complete quality assurance program should address not only the treatment unit, but also the treatment planning system and treatment procedures. A QA program for a remote afterloading system can be divided into three phases: (1) procedures associated with a source change, (2) procedures to be performed on a daily basis prior to patient treatments, and (3) procedures to be performed monthly.[78] A summary of the procedures appears in Table 15-10.

Source-Change Quality Assurance

1. Radiation Safety Surveys. A radiation safety survey should be conducted to ensure adequate shielding of the radioactive source when it is housed in the head of the treatment unit. Areas adjacent to the treatment room should be surveyed with the source exposed. In areas where a reading above background is detected, the area should be surveyed with the source retracted as well.
2. Source Calibration. A measurement of the source activity must be made before the source is used for patient treatment. Although no national calibration standard for ^{192}Ir exists, a technique that can be followed by hospital physicists has been developed by the AAPM Accredited Dosimetry Calibration

TABLE 15-10 Brachytherapy QA Procedures and Frequencies

Procedure	At Source Change	Monthly	Daily
Safety Procedures			
Protection survey	Limited survey	—	Watch for signs of deterioration. Be aware of changes in design/use of adjacent space.
Test of interlocks.	Test safety interlocks.	Test safety interlocks.	Test safety interlock.
Applicator integrity	—	Inspect for damage or deterioration.	—
Patient monitoring device operation	—	—	Check for proper operation.
Dose Delivery			
Source activity	Measure source activity.	Perform check of activity and verify agreement with calculated value	—
Stored and computed value	Enter measured source activity.	Check calculated activity for agreement with measured activity.	Verify displays of time, date, and current source activity.
Dwell time accuracy	Performed as part of source calibration.	Performed as part of activity check.	Verify with QA device.
Mechanical Alignment			
Programmed dwell position alignment	Verify with radiograph.	Verify with radiograph.	Verify with QA device.

Laboratories (ADCLs). In addition, the ADCLs calibrate well-type reentrant chambers designed specifically for use with high-activity iridium sources (Figure 15-22).[80,81]

Daily Quality Assurance

Daily quality assurance procedures (Table 15-11) are to be performed every day of patient treatment, and they should be performed prior to initiating a patient treatment

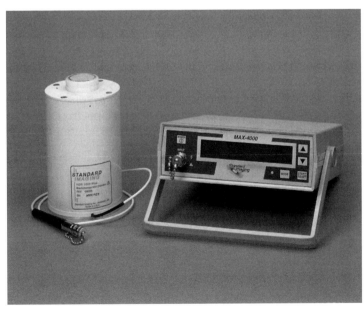

FIGURE 15-22

Well chamber and electrometer for measuring brachytherapy source strength. (Courtesy of Standard Imaging, Middleton Wisconsin.)

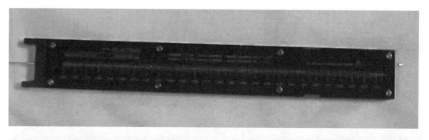

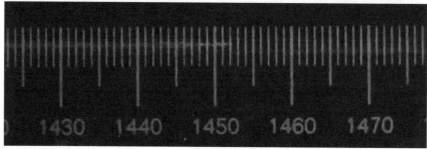

FIGURE 15-23
Source position check ruler. The source is programmed to a given position (1450 mm in this case) and the center of the source as remotely observed should be within 1 mm of the programmed position. (Courtesy of Richard Goodman, Waukesha Memorial Hospital, Wisconsin.)

(for the same reason that daily QA for external beam treatment is done prior to the first patient, as mentioned earlier in this chapter).

1. All monitors and interlocks should be checked, including the door interlocks, emergency off buttons, treatment interrupt buttons, audiovisual monitors, and room radiation monitors. The interlocks that detect missing or misconnected applicators or transfer tubes should be tested.
2. The treatment unit displays of time, date, and current source strength should be verified for accuracy.
3. A test of source-position accuracy, dwell-time accuracy, and normal termination of treatment should be performed. Most HDR and PDR manufacturers provide a test jig to assist in performing this procedure (Figure 15-23).

TABLE 15-11 Sample Daily HDR and PDR Tests

DAILY QA TESTS
Permanent radiation monitor checked for
   proper operation
Viewing and intercom systems verified
Treatment control unit (console) function tests
Printer test
Source status indicators
Treatment room entrance interlocks
Mechanical integrity of applicator(s), source
   guide tubes, and connectors
Source position check
Emergency off
Interrupt
Timer ends treatment
Source activity

TABLE 15-12   Sample Monthly QA Form

Date	
Time	
Operator	
Accuracy of source positioning to within ±1 mm of the programmed position Programmed position Actual position If > ±1 mm, notify authorized physicist and the authorized users	_____ _____
Timer linearity 1. T1 sec reading (nC) 2. Calculated current reading (nA) 3. T2 sec reading (nC) 4. Calculated current reading (nA) 5. Current reading (nA) Ratio 2:4 Ratio average (2,4):5	
Timer accuracy (set 10 sec)	
Measurement of the source guide tubes and connectors (±1 mm)	Pass/Fail
Backup battery test to verify emergency source retraction upon power failure	Pass/Fail

Source Strength Verification
  Manufacturer
  Treatment unit model number and serial number
  Radioactive source serial number
  Well Chamber
    Manufacturer
    Model
    serial number
  Measured source strength	

Source homogeneity (autoradiograph, at source change only)	Pass/Fail
Comments	

Note: T1 and T2 readings have the charge collected during source transit subtracted. The transit charge is determined using a dwell position of zero seconds.

4. The mechanical integrity of applicator connections to the treatment unit should be verified. The availability and integrity of emergency response equipment should be verified daily.

Monthly Quality Assurance Procedures

The following monthly quality assurance procedures (Table 15-12) should be performed at the time of source exchange, and at monthly intervals between source changes.

1. Source positioning accuracy should be checked. This can be done by verifying the alignment of radiographic markers with the programmed source position. This may be accomplished by attaching treatment catheters to ready-pack film or a film cassette, inserting radiographic markers into each catheter, and making an exposure with an x-ray unit. The radiographic markers are

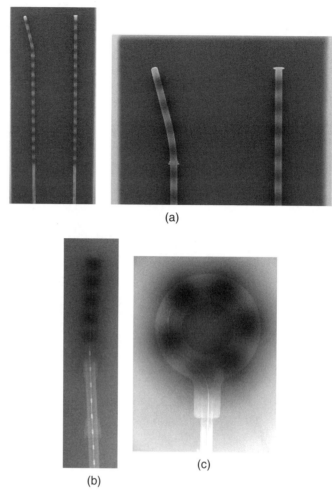

FIGURE 15-24

The positioning of an HDR source can be checked using an autoradiograph of source positions. **A**: Dwell positions relative to the applicator are shown to aid in treatment planning. **B, C**: dummy markers are also visible indicating correlation between expected (light-colored dummy markers) and actual (darkened areas) dwell positions. Note that in C, a slight discrepancy is observed due to the difference in the path of travel between the dummy markers and source cable for a circular path (the dummy markers are 20 and 15 mm apart starting at the tip, while the dwell positions are every 10 mm).

TANDEM AND OVOIDS

FOR POSITION 5:

$$\frac{\text{(Dwell Time For Position 5)} \times \text{(Source Activity)}}{\text{Dose To Point M}}$$

Accepted Range: **34 to 44**

FOR TOTAL TREATMENT:

$$\frac{\text{(Total Dwell Time)} \times \text{(Source Activity)}}{\text{(Dose To Point M)} \times \text{(Number of Dwell Positions)}}$$

Accepted Range: **24 to 30 (2.0 cm ovoids, 31 to 36 corpus)**
28 to 36 (2.5 cm ovoids)

FIGURE 15-25

Sample dosimetry index for tandem and ovoid treatment. Note that Point M in this case is based on the University of Wisconsin system for HDR brachytherapy of the cervix.[82,83] (Courtesy of Bruce Thomadsen, University of Wisconsin.)

TANDEM AND CYLINDERS

FOR POSITION 5:

$$\frac{\text{(Dwell Time For Position 5)} \times \text{(Source Activity)}}{\text{Dose To Point M}}$$

Accepted Range: **34 to 44**

FOR TOTAL TREATMENT:

$$\frac{\text{(Total Dwell Time)} \times \text{(Source Activity)}}{\text{(Dose To Point M)} \times \text{(Number of Dwell Positions)}}$$

Accepted Ranges:
24 to 34 (2.0 cm cylinders)
28 to 36 (2.5 cm cylinders)
27 to 41 (3.0 cm cylinders)
35 to 41 (3.5 cm cylinders)

FIGURE 15-26
Sample dosimetry index for tandem and cylinders. (Courtesy of Bruce Thomadsen, University of Wisconsin.)

OVOIDS

FOR TOTAL TREATMENT:

$$\frac{\text{(Average Dwell Time)} \times \text{(Source Activity)}}{\text{(Dose To Vaginal Surface)}}$$

Accepted Ranges:
21 to 24 (2.0 cm ovoids)
31 to 35 (2.5 cm ovoids)
45 to 48 (3.0 cm ovoids)

FIGURE 15-27
Sample dosimetry index for ovoids. (Courtesy of Bruce Thomadsen, University of Wisconsin.)

SINGLE CATHETER APPLICATION
(e.g. Endobronch)

FOR TOTAL TREATMENT:

$$\frac{\text{(Total Dwell Time)} \times \text{(Source Activity)}}{\text{(Treatment Length)} \times \text{(Dose)}}$$

Accepted Range:
66 to 77 (2 cm radial Tx distance)
for other treatment distances, use the ratio of distances and the
exponent from the graph below

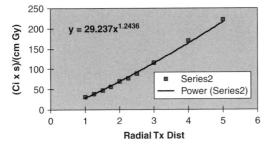

FIGURE 15-28
Sample dosimetry index for single catheter application. The index can apply to endobronchial or cylinder treatments. Either the index or range can be adjusted for other radial treatment distances. (Courtesy of Bruce Thomadsen, University of Wisconsin.)

VOLUME IMPLANTS
(e.g. Prostate)

FOR TOTAL TREATMENT:

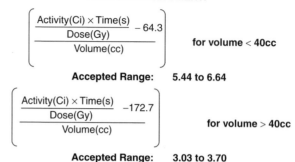

$$\left[\frac{\dfrac{\text{Activity(Ci)} \times \text{Time(s)}}{\text{Dose(Gy)}} - 64.3}{\text{Volume(cc)}}\right] \quad \textbf{for volume} < \textbf{40cc}$$

Accepted Range: **5.44 to 6.64**

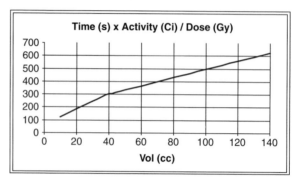

$$\left[\frac{\dfrac{\text{Activity(Ci)} \times \text{Time(s)}}{\text{Dose(Gy)}} - 172.7}{\text{Volume(cc)}}\right] \quad \textbf{for volume} > \textbf{40cc}$$

Accepted Range: **3.03 to 3.70**

Time (s) x Activity (Ci) / Dose (Gy)

FIGURE 15-29
Sample dosimetry index for volume implant. Note that the volume is the volume treated to full dose, obtainable from the dose volume histogram. Adapted from information provided by California Endoenric Institute.

removed and the remote afterloading source is programmed to (a) enter each catheter and (b) stop briefly at each of the positions identified by the radiographic markers. Afterwards, the film is processed to verify that the source positions correspond with the location of the radiographic markers (Figure 15-24). Alternatively, one can check that the programmed position matches the actual dwell position using the room camera or built in treatment unit camera.

2. The source activity should be checked to verify agreement with the calculated activity.

3. The integrity of the applicators used most often should be checked for mechanical damage, ease of coupling, kinks, and mechanical deformation. Transfer tubes should be inspected and measured to verify that they are in proper working condition.

4. The timer should be checked to verify accuracy and linearity.

5. Power failure test. The power to the system should be interrupted to verify that the source retracts.

Brachytherapy Treatment Plan QA
The outline below includes some of the important checks to include in a QA program.

1. Target Coverage. Does the isodose surface selected for the prescription cover the target volume adequately?

SINGLE DWELL POSITION

$$\frac{(\text{Dwell Time}) \times (\text{Source Activity})}{\text{Dose} \times r^2} \times g(r)$$

Note: time in seconds, activity in Ci, distance 'r' in cm, dose in Gy

Accepted Range: 75 to 90 (average anisotropy constant of 0.963)

72 to 87 (anisotropy constant of 1.0, e.g. mammosite)

Radius	g(r)
10	1.000
15	1.003
20	1.007
25	1.008
30	1.008
35	1.007
40	1.004
45	1.000
50	.995
55	.988
60	.981
65	.973
70	.964
75	.953
80	.940
85	.927
90	.913
95	.898
100	.882
105	.864
110	.844
115	.822
120	.799
125	.774
130	.747
135	.716
140	.681

FIGURE 15-30
Sample dosimetry index for single dwell position. For complex geometries that do not fit into any other index, this can be used as a point source approximation so long as the calculation point is relatively distant from the implant. Courtesy of Waukesha Memorial Hospital, Wisconsin.

2. Homogeneity. Does the maximum significant dose remain below the predefined range acceptable at the institution?
3. Dose Prescription. Does the prescribed dose correspond to a protocol for the disease, and does it account for contributions from external beam treatments?
4. Normal Structure Doses. Do the doses to normal structures remain within their tolerances?
5. Consistency. Does the total strength used in the application correspond to that normal for the dose specified to the isodose surface?
6. Duration. Has the total duration of the application been calculated correctly?
7. Independent Dose Check. For a particular type of treatment, it is possible for an institution to develop a set of indices to check that the activity (and time for temporary implants) is appropriate. The units for these tests could be in mCi/Gy for permanent implants, mCi-hr/Gy for LDR temporary implants, or Ci-s/Gy for HDR implants. Sample indices for common treatment sites are included below.

SAMPLE HDR DOSIMETRY CHECK

Date _____ Patient _____ MR# _____ Fraction No. _____

1.   Location and Dose Checks

_____ a. Dose for this fraction on Rx_____ Gy Average dose to Rx points _____ Gy

_____ b Difference between computed and prescribed dose is less than 5%

_____ c Distance of Rx point   Cervical Stopper:_____

Middwell ovoids:_____

        Distance <u>cephalad</u> as defined in Rx _____ mm

        Distance <u>cephalad</u> on films _____ mm

        Distance <u>lateral</u> as defined in Rx _____ mm

        Distance <u>lateral</u> on printout_____ mm

        Distance <u>lateral</u> on coronal plane _____ mm

_____ d Ovoid

        Ovoid Rt   Rt size _____ mm   Rt dist to vaginal dose points _____ mm

        Ovoid Lt   Lt size _____ mm   Lt dist to vaginal dose points _____ mm

_____ e Cylinders

        Cyl 1_____   Cyl 2 _____   Cyl 3 _____   Radius _____ mm

_____ f Dose percentile to surface _____ % of Rx dose = _____ Gy and isodose lines match

_____ g Starting dwell for tandem on plan corresponds to start indicated on film Dwell #:_____

_____ h Bladder _____ Gy (_____%)

        Rectum_____ Gy (_____%)

        _____ Physician alerted if > 70%

2.   Time Checks:

_____ a Time index for dwell 1 cm from first dwell: Range_____ to _____

_____ b Time index for total time: Range _____ to _____

_____ c Total Time Index from previous treatment: Agree within 5% Yes_____ No_____

        Reason for any time variance from previous treatment:

3.   Card/Treatment Unit Check

_____ a Rt. ovoid programmed to channel 1   Length for this channel _____

        Lt. ovoid programmed to channel 2   Length for this channel _____

        Tandem or Cylinders programmed to channel 3   Length for this channel _____

_____ b Step size _____ 2.5 mm   _____ 5.0 mm

_____ c Patient's file has been saved.

4.   Programming of the HDR Unit

_____ Dwell times, positions, and length on print out match that from the computer plan

_____   _____   _____

Physicist   Date   Time

_____   _____   _____

Physician   Date   Time

FIGURE 15-31

Sample treatment plan quality assurance form.

SUMMARY

- The ICRU has recommended that the uncertainty in dose delivery should be no greater than 5%.
- Physics instrumentation includes radiation measuring devices and equipment for evaluating mechanical performance.
- Devices used in the calibration of radiation-producing equipment should be calibrated by a method traceable to national standards.
- The end goal of a quality assurance program in radiation therapy is accurate and safe treatment delivery.
- The quality assurance program should be based on current recommendations such as those provided by Task Group reports from the American Association of Physicists in Medicine.
- Daily checks for linear accelerators emphasize operational safety checks and output constancy. Monthly checks include output and mechanical checks. Yearly checks include output calibration and evaluation of treatment planning parameters.
- Diagnostic x-ray tube performance should be included in the quality assurance tests for simulators (conventional and CT).
- The accuracy of dose calculation in the treatment planning system is evaluated prior to use and anytime there may be a change in software performance, such as during a software version upgrade or change in hardware.
- Provisions should always be in place for quality assurance in intensity-modulated radiation therapy (IMRT) to verify that the dose delivered is the dose intended.
- For precision localization systems, such as external coordinate systems used in stereotactic radiosurgery, stringent quality assurance is required to ensure accurate patient positioning.
- Brachytherapy quality assurance includes source strength verification, treatment plan accuracy, and patient safety. Institutions must abide by state and/or federal regulations for brachytherapy.

PROBLEMS

15-1. Define each of the following terms:
   a. Quality Assurance
   b. Quality Control
   c. Quality Improvement

15-2. The following ionization measurements are made at d_{max} in a 10×10-cm field at 100-cm SSD in a linear accelerator beam:

Monitor Units	Reading
200	196.3
50	49.7
50	49.8
50	49.6
50	49.7

Calculate the end effect. Do these measurements indicate acceptable monitor linearity?

15-3. Calculate the effect of a systematic error in patient source-to-skin distance. Assume that the actual treatment distance is 2 cm greater than the indicated distance and that the patient is being treated with a 6-MV linear accelerator (see data in Tables 7-3 and

7-8). The patient's area of exposure is 20 cm in diameter and is being treated with opposing anterior and posterior 10- × 10-cm fields. Calculate the effect for both (a) 100 cm SSD setup and (b) 100 cm SAD setup.

15-4. It is discovered that a tray factor of 0.95 was not considered in a patient's treatment for the first 15 fractions. If 135 monitor units were given for each of these fractions, and there are 25 fractions remaining, how many monitor units should be used for the remaining fractions?

15-5. The source in an HDR remote afterloader contains 10 Ci of ^{192}Ir. If, during a patient treatment, the source retraction mechanism were to jam, causing the source to remain in the patient for 60 seconds longer than intended, what additional dose would the patient receive at 1 cm from the source? Assume that the exposure to dose conversion factor for iridium is 0.96.

15-6. During the event described in problem 15-5 above, a staff member manually retracts the iridium source from the patient into the remote afterloader. This process takes approximately 15 sec, during which time the staff member is at an average distance of 0.6 m from the source. What is the exposure to the staff member?

15-7. The following measurements are made at 10-cm depth in a water phantom from a 20- × 20-cm field provided by a 6-MV linear accelerator. The maximum reading, found at a point 5 cm to the left of the central axis, is 101.3. The minimum reading, found at a point 8 cm to the right of the central axis, is 94.9. Calculate the beam flatness. Is this flatness acceptable?

15-8. List four parameters of simulator operation that should be checked before a service person is called to address poor fluoroscopic image quality.

15-9. Several afterloading devices are designed as a "closed system." Why is it important to try to maintain a closed system when dealing with an emergency situation?

15-10. What effect results in lines of lower dose parallel to the direction of leaf motion?

15-11. Point dose measurements are performed on an IMRT patient. The calibration field reading of 0.333 nC corresponds to 175.5 cGy. The readings and expected doses for the seven IMRT fields are:

Field 1:	0.040 nC	20.2 cGy
Field 2:	0.031	15.9
Field 3:	0.042	23.4
Field 4:	0.102	53.1
Field 5:	0.044	23.4
Field 6:	0.044	23.5
Field 7:	0.058	31.6

What is the overall error in the delivered dose? Are any fields more than 3 cGy off from their expected value?

REFERENCES

1. Donabedian, A. Evaluating the quality of medical care. *Milbank Memorial Fund Q.*1966; **44**:166–206.
2. O'Leary, M. R. *Lexikon,* Joint Commission on Accreditation of Healthcare Organizations. Oakbrook Terrace, IL, JCAHO, Publishers, 1994.
3. Cunningham, J. R. Development of computer algorithms for radiation treatment planning. *Int. J. Radiat. Oncol. Biol. Phys.*1989; **16**:1367.
4. Fischer, J. J., and Moulder, J. E. The steepness of the dose-response curve in radiation therapy. *Radiology* 1975; **117**:179–184.
5. Hendrickson, F. R. Precision in radiation oncology. *Int. J. Radiat. Oncol. Biol. Phys.* 1981; **8**:311–312.
6. International Commission on Radiation Units and Measurements. *Determination of absorbed dose in a patient irradiated by beams of x or gamma rays in radiotherapy procedures.* ICRU Report No. 24, Washington, DC, 1976.
7. International Commission on Radiation Units and Measurements. *Use of computers in external beam radiotherapy procedure with high energy photons and electrons*, ICRU Report No. 42, Washington, DC, 1988.
8. Leunens, G., et al. Assessment of dose inhomogeneity at target level by in vivo dosimetry: Can the recommended 5% accuracy in the dose delivered to the target volume be fulfilled in daily practice? *Radiother. Oncol.* 1992; **25**:245–250.
9. Ibbott, G. S., et al. Uncertainty of calibrations at the accredited dosimetry calibration laboratories. *Med. Phys.* 1997; **24**(8):1249–1254.
10. Kartha, P. K. I., Chung-Bin, A., and Hendrickson, F. R. Accuracy in clinical dosimetry. *Br. J. Radiol* 1973; **46**:1083–1084.
11. Kartha, P. K. I., Chung-Bin, A., Wachtor, T., and Hendrickson, F. R. Accuracy in patient setup and its consequence in dosimetry. *Med. Phys.* 1975; **2**:331–332.
12. *American College of Radiology: ACR Standard for Radiation Oncology Physics for External Beam Therapy Res.* 15-1994, American College of Radiology Standards, adopted 1995 by the American College of Radiology.
13. *American College of Radiology: ACR Standard for Radiation Oncology Res.* 38-1995, American College of Radiology Standards, adopted 1995 by the American College of Radiology.
14. Joint Commission on Accreditation of Healthcare Organizations. JCAHO *Accreditation Manual for Hospitals, 1995,* Oak Brook Terrace, IL, 1995.
15. Kutcher, G. J., Coia, L., Gillin, M., Hanson, W. F., Leibel, S., Morton, R. J., Palta, J. R., Purdy, J. A., Reinstein, L. E., Svensson, G. K., et al. Comprehensive QA for radiation oncology: Report of AAPM Radiation Therapy Committee Task Group 40. *Med. Phys.* 1994; **21**(4):581–618.
16. Perez, C. A., and Purdy, J. A. Rationale for treatment planning in radiation therapy. In Levitt, and Tapley's *Technological Basis of Radiation Therapy: Practical Clinical Applications,* S. H. Levitt, F. M. Khan, and R. A. Potish (eds.). 2nd edition, Philadelphia: Lea & Febiger, 1992.
17. Perez CA. The critical need for accurate treatment planning and quality control in radiation therapy. *Int. J. Radiat. Oncol. Biol. Phys.* 1977; **2**:815–818.
18. Hanson, W. F., Hahn, P., Shalev, S., Viggars, D., and Therrien, P. Treatment planning for protocol-based radiation therapy. *Int. J. Radiat. Oncol. Biol. Phys.* 1990; **18**:937–939.
19. International Commission on Radiation Units and Measurements: *Prescribing, recording, and reporting photon beam therapy*, ICRU Report No. 50, Washington, DC, 1993.
20. Monti, A. F., Ostinelli, A., Frigerio, M., Cosentino, D., Bossi, A., Cazzaniga, L. F., Scandolaro, L., and Valli, M. C. An ICRU 50 radiotherapy treatment chart, *Radiother. Oncol.* 1995; **35**:145–150.
21. Earp, K. A., and Gates, L. Quality assurance: A model QA program in radiation oncology, *Radiol. Technol.* 1990; **61**(4):297–304.
22. Herring, D. F., and Compton, D. M. J. The degree of precision required in the radiation dose delivered in cancer therapy. In *Computers in Radiotherapy,* Report No. 5, A. S. Glickman, M. Cohen, and J. R. Cunningham (eds.). 1971, p. 51.
23. Heukelom, S., Lanson, J. H., and Mijnheer, B. J. Comparison of entrance and exit dose measurements using ionization chambers and silicon diodes. *Med. Phys. Biol.*1991; **36**(1):47–59.
24. Noel, A., Aletti, P., Bey, P., and Malissard, L. Detection of errors in individual patients in radiotherapy by systematic in vivo dosimetry, *Radiother. Oncol.* 1995; **34**:144–151.
25. Ahuja, S. D. Physical and technological aspects of quality assurance in radiation oncology. *Radiol. Tech.* 1980; **51**(6):759–774.
26. *American College of Radiology: ACR Standards for Brachytherapy Physics: Manually-Loaded Sources Res.* 25-1995, American College of Radiology Standards, adopted 1995 by the American College of Radiology.
27. Annett, C. H. Program for periodic maintenance and calibration of radiation therapy linear accelerators. *Appl. Radiol.*1979; **6**:77–80.
28. Ibbott G. S., Boothe, K. A., Thyfault, P. J., Zunde, A., and Hendee, W. R. Quality assurance workshops for radiation therapy technologists. *Appl. Radiol.* 1977; Issue 2.
29. Bureau Central de la Commission Electrotechnique Internationale. *Medical electrical equipment* International Electrotechnical Commission Report No. 976., Geneva, Switzerland, 1993.
30. Bureau Central de la Commission Electrotechnique Internationale. *Medical electrical equipment: Medical electron accelerators in the range I MeV to 50 MeV. Guidelines for functional performance characteristics,* International Electrotechnical Commission Report No. 977: Geneva, Switzerland, 1993.
31. Nordic Association of Clinical Physics (NACP). Procedures in external radiation therapy dosimetry with electron and photon beams with maximum energies between 1 and 50 MeV. *Acta Radiol* 1980; **19**(1):55–79.
32. Hanson, W. F., Grant, W. 3rd., Kennedy, P., Cundiff, J. H., Gagnon, W. F., Berkley, L. W., and Shalek, R. J. A review of the reliability of chamber factors used clinically in the United States (1968–1976). *Med. Phys.* 1978; **5**:552–554.

33. Lanzl, L. H., Rozenfeld, M., and Wootton, P. The radiation therapy dosimetry network in the United States. *Med. Phys.* 1981; **8**:49–53.

34. Rozenfeld, M., and Jette, D. Quality assurance of radiation dosage: Usefulness of redundancy. *Radiology* 1984; **150**(l):241–244.

35. Campos, L. L., and Caldas, L. V. Induced effects in ionization chamber cables by photon and electron irradiation. *Med. Phys.* 1991; **18**(3):522–526.

36. Ibbott, G. S., et al. Stem corrections for ionization chambers. *Med. Phys.*1975; **2**(6):328–330.

37. Karzmark, C. J. Procedural and operator error aspects of radiation accidents in radiotherapy. *Int. J. Radiat. Oncol. Biol. Phys.* 1987; **13**:1599–1602.

38. National Council on Radiation Protection and Measurements, *Medical x-ray, electron beam and gamma-ray protection for energies up to 50 MeV (Equipment design, performance and use)*, NCRP Report No. 102: Bethesda, MD, 1989.

39. Bureau Central de la Commission Electrotechnique Internationale. *Radiotherapy simulators: Particular requirements for the safety of electron accelerators in the range of I MeV to 50 MeV*, International Electrotechnical Commission Standard No. 601-2-1, Geneva, Switzerland, 1993.

40. Verhey, L. J., et al. Precise positioning of patients for radiation therapy. *Int. J. Radiat. Oncol. Biol. Phys.* 1982; **8**:289.

41. Williamson, T. J. Improving the reproducibility of lateral therapy portal placement. *Int. J. Radiat. Oncol. Biol. Phys.* 1979; **5**:407.

42. Lutz, W. R., Larsen, R. D., and Bjarngard, B. E. Beam alignment tests for therapy accelerators. *Int. J. Radiat. Oncol. Biol. Phys.* 1981; **7**:1727–1731.

43. McCullough EC, McCollough KP. Improving agreement between radiation-delineated field edges on simulation and portal films: The edge tolerance test tool. *Med. Phys.* 1993; **20**(2 Pt 1):375–376.

44. Radiation Therapy Committee, *Basic Applications of Multileaf Collimators*, Report of Task Group No. 50 AAPM Report No. 72, Medical Physics Publishing, 2001.

45. Almond, P. R., Biggs, P. J., Coursey, B. M., Hanson, W. F., Huq, M. S., Nath, R., and Rogers, D. W. AAPM's TG-51 protocol for clinical reference dosimetry of high-energy photon and electron beams. *Med. Phys.* 1999; **26**(9):1847–70.

46. DeWerd, L. A., Price, J., Cameron, J. R., and Goetsch, S. J. Evaluation of a commercial diode monitor for mailed quality control of therapy units. *Int. J. Radiat. Oncol. Biol. Phys.* 1990; **19**:1053–1057.

47. Dixon, R. L., Ekstrand, K. E., Wilenzick R. M., and Williams, K. D. Performance evaluation of a new quality control dose monitor for radiation therapy. *Med. Phys.* 1983; **10**(5):695–697.

48. Orton, C. G., and Siebert, J. B. The measurement of teletherapy unit timer errors. *Phys. Med. Biol.* 1972; **17**(2):198–205.

49. Bureau Central de la Commission Electrotechnique Internationale. *Radiotherapy simulators: Guidelines for functional performance characteristics*, International Electrotechnical Commission Report No. 1170: Geneva, Switzerland, 1993.

50. Rosenow, U. F., Islam, M. K., Gaballa, H., and Rashid, H. Energy constancy checking for electron beams using a wedge-shaped solid phantom combined with a beam profile scanner. *Med. Phys.* 1991; **18**(1):19–25.

51. Bomford, C. K., Dawes, P. J. D. K., Lillicrap, S. C., and Young, J. Treatment simulators. *Br. J. Radiol.* 1989; **23**:1(Suppl 23)1–49.

52. McCullough, E. C., and Earle, J. D. The selection, acceptance testing, and quality control of radiotherapy treatment simulators. *Radiology* 1979; **131**:221–230.

53. Chaney, E., and Hendee, W. Effects of x-ray tube current and voltage on effective focal spot size. *Med. Phys.* 1974; **1**(3):141–147.

54. AAPM Task Force on Quality Assurance Protocol, *Basic Quality Control in Diagnostic Radiology*, AAPM Report No. 4, 1977.

55. AAPM Diagnostic X-Ray Imaging Committee, *Protocols for the Radiation Safety Surveys of Diagnostic Radiological Equipment*, AAPM Report No. 25, TG No. 1, 1988.

56. Bushberg, J. T., Seibert, J. A., Leidholdt, E. M., and Boone, J. M. *The Essential Physics of Medical Imaging*. Baltimore, Williams & Wilkins, 1994.

57. Hendee, W. R., and Ritenour, E. R. *Medical Imaging Physics*, 4th edition. New York, John Wiley & Sons, 2002.

58. Samei, E., et al. Performance evaluation of computed radiography systems. *Med. Phys.* 2001; **28**(3):361–371.

59. El-Mohri, Y., Jee, K. W., Antonuk, L. E., Maolinbay, M., and Zhao, Q. Determination of the detective quantum efficiency of a prototype, megavoltage indirect detection, active matrix flat-panel imager. *Med. Phys.* 2001; **28**(12):2538–2550.

60. Jacky, J., and White, C. P., Testing a 3-D radiation therapy planning program. *Int. J. Radiat. Oncol. Biol. Phys.* 1989; **18**:253–261.

61. Van Dyk, J., Barnett, R. B., Cygler, J. E., and Shragge, P. C. Commissioning and quality assurance of treatment planning computers. *Int. J. Radiat. Oncol. Biol. Phys.* 1993; **26**:261–273.

62. Fraass, B., Doppke, K., Hunt, M., Kutcher, G., Starkschall, G., Stern, R., and Van Dyke, J. American Association of Physicists in Medicine Radiation Therapy Committee Task Group 53: Quality assurance for clinical radiotherapy treatment planning. *Med. Phys.* 1998; **25**(10):1773–1829.

63. American Association of Physicists in Medicine. *Radiation treatment planning dosimetry verification*. AAPM Task Group 23 Test Package, 1987. AAPM Report No. 55, 1995.

64. Cipra, B. How number theory got the best of the Pentium chip. *Science* 1995; **267**:175.

65. Coe, T., Mathisen, T., Moler, C., and Pratt, V. Computational aspects of the Pentium affair. *IEEE Comp. Sci. Eng.* 1995; (Spring):18–30.

66. Edelman, A. The mathematics of the Pentium division bug. *SIAM Review* 1997; **39**:54–67. Available at http://www.siam.org/journals/sirev/39-1/29395.html.

67. Fisher, L. M. Flaw reported in new Intel chip. *New York Times* 1997 (May 5). Available at <http://www.nytimes.com/library/cyber/week/050697intel-chip-flaw.html.

68. McCullough, E. C., and Krueger, A. M. Performance evaluation of computerized treatment planning systems for radiotherapy: External photon beams. *Int. J. Radiat. Oncol. Biol. Phys.* 1980; **6**:1599–1605.

69. Leunens, G., Verstraete, J., Van den Bogaert, W., Van Dam, J., Dutreix, A., and van der Schueren, E. Human errors in data transfer during the preparation and delivery of radiation treatment affecting the final result: "Garbage in, garbage out." *Radiother. Oncol.* 1992; **23**:217–222.

70. Intensity Modulated Radiation Therapy Collaborative Working Group. Intensity-modulated radiotherapy: Current status and issues of interest. *Int. J. Radiat. Oncol. Biol. Phys.*. 2001; **51**(4):880–914.

71. Dong, L., Antolak, J., Salehpour, M., Forster, K., O'Neill, L., Kendall, R., and Rosen, I. Patient-specific point dose measurement for IMRT monitor unit verification. *Int. J. Radiat. Oncol. Biol. Phys.* 2003; **56**(3):867–877.

72. Jursinic, P., and Nelms, B. A 2-D diode array and analysis software for verification of intensity modulated radiation therapy delivery. *Med. Phys.* 2003; **30**(5):870–879.

73. Leksell, L. The stereotaxic method and radiosurgery of the brain. *Acta. Chir. Scand.* 1951; **102**:316–319.

74. Report of Task Group 42. *Stereotactic Radiosurgery*, AAPM Report No. 54, 1995.

75. Nath, R., Anderson, L. L., Meli, J. A., Olch, A. J., Stitt, J. A., and Williamson, J. F. Code of practice for brachytherapy physics: Report of the AAPM Radiation Therapy Committee Task Group No. 56 *Med. Phys.* 1997; **24**(10):1557–1598.

76. Kubo, H. D., Glasgow, G. P., and Pethel, T. D., Thomadsen, B. R., Williamson, J. F. High dose-rate brachytherapy treatment delivery: Report of the AAPM Radiation Therapy Committee Task Group No. 59. *Med. Phys.* 1998; **25**(4):375–403.

77. Slessinger, E., Grigsby, P., and Williams, J. Improvements in brachytherapy quality assurance. *Int. J. Radiat. Oncol. Biol. Phys.* 1988; **16**:497–500.

78. Hicks, J., and Ezzell, G. A. Calibration and quality assurance. In *Activity*, Special Report No. 7. Veenendaal, The Netherlands, Nucletron-Oldelft, 1995.

79. Spicer, B. L., and Hicks, J. A. Safety programs for remote afterloading brachytherapy: High dose rate and pulsed low dose rate. In *Activity*, International Nucletron-Oldelft Radiotherapy Journal, Quality Assurance, Special Report No. 7, Veenendaal, The Netherlands, Nucletron-Oldelft, 1995.

80. Goetsch, S. J., Attix, F. H., DeWerd, L. A., Thomadsen, B. R. A new re-entrant ionisation chamber of the calibration of iridium-192 high dose rate sources. *Int. J. Radiat. Oncol. Biol. Phys.* 1992; **24**:167–170.

81. Goetsch, S. J., et al. Calibration of iridium-192 high dose rate afterloading systems. *Med. Phys.* 1991; **18**:462–467.

82. Stitt, J., et al. High dose rate intracavitary brachytherapy for carcinoma of the cervix: The Madison system: I. Clinical and radiobiological considerations. *Int. J. Radiat. Oncol. Biol. Phys.* 1992; **24**(2):335–348.

83. Thomadsen, B. R., Shahabi, S., Stitt, J. A., Buchler, D. A., Fowler, J. F., Paliwal, B. R., and Kinsella, T. J. High dose rate intracavitary brachytherapy for carcinoma of the cervix: The Madison system: II. Procedural and physical considerations. *Int. J. Radiat. Oncol. Biol. Phys.* 1992; **24**(2):349–357.

C H A P T E R

16

ADVANCES IN RADIATION THERAPY

OBJECTIVES 414

INTRODUCTION 414

HISTORY 414

ALTERED FRACTIONATION 416

BIOLOGICAL MODELING AND PLAN EVALUATION 417

MOLECULAR IMAGING 418

High-Affinity Probes 419
Overcoming Delivery Barriers 419
Amplification Strategies 419
Molecular Imaging Techniques 419

PROTON THERAPY 420

NEUTRON BRACHYTHERAPY 426

NEUTRON CAPTURE THERAPY 427

NEUTRON BEAM THERAPY 428

HEAVY ION AND PION THERAPY 430

CONCLUSIONS 432

REFERENCES 432

Radiation Therapy Physics, Third Edition, by William R. Hendee, Geoffrey S. Ibbott, and Eric G. Hendee
ISBN 0-471-39493-9 Copyright © 2005 John Wiley & Sons, Inc.

■ OBJECTIVES

After reviewing this chapter, the reader should be able to:

- Discuss the evolution of technology employed in radiation therapy.
- Explain the design of treatment delivery schedules to accommodate the biological properties of cancer.
- Identify properties of molecular probes that are important to imaging target molecules.
- Provide an overview of the physics and clinical experience of:
  - Proton therapy
  - Heavy ion and pion therapy
  - Cancer treatment with various neutron sources

■ INTRODUCTION

The objective of curative radiation therapy is delivery of the greatest possible dose of radiation to a tumor while keeping doses to surrounding normal tissues below levels that produce irremediable damage. When this objective is reached, the likelihood of local tumor control is high, the potential for tumor regrowth and metastasis is low, and the probability for normal-tissue complications from the therapy is minimized. How well the objective is attained is described as the therapeutic ratio, expressed as the ratio of cell killing in the tumor divided by the degree of cell killing in normal tissue. An optimum treatment regimen in radiation therapy yields a therapeutic ratio that is as high as possible.

The therapeutic ratio varies with many factors, including the biologic properties of the irradiated tissues (e.g., degree of oxygenation and rate of cell division), the nature of the radiation (e.g., linear energy transfer [LET] and dose rate), the presence of substances (e.g., radiosensitizers and radioprotectors) that modify the response of cells to radiation, the design of the treatment plan, and the precision with which the treatment plan is implemented. The therapeutic ratio also is influenced by chemotherapeutic agents, and their use requires even greater precision in the planning and delivery of radiation treatments.[1] The history of radiation therapy is in part the saga of the search for ways to enhance the therapeutic ratio.

■ HISTORY

For more than 50 years following the discovery of x rays by Röntgen in 1895, external-beam radiation treatments were delivered with x rays generated at a few hundred kVp (orthovoltage x rays) or less. These x-ray beams were not very penetrating, and they delivered a maximum dose to the skin at the location where the x rays entered the body. Often, treatments were limited by skin reactions, referred to as erythemas, that were similar to severe thermal burns. Skin reactions served one useful purpose. They provided a way for the radiation oncologist to monitor the response of patients to radiation treatments.

After World War II, artificially produced radioactive isotopes became available from nuclear reactors built as part of the Project Plowshare effort to identify peaceful applications of nuclear energy. One of these isotopes was ^{60}Co, a nuclide with a half-life of 5.3 years that releases two energetic gamma rays (1.17 and 1.33 MeV) during radioactive decay. This source was promising for external-beam radiation therapy, and the first ^{60}Co teletherapy units were introduced into clinical practice in the 1950s.[2] Over the 1960s and early 1970s, ^{60}Co teletherapy (teletherapy means "therapy at a long distance") units were the mainstay of external-beam radiation therapy. In addition to providing more penetrating photons, the units had another distinct advantage over orthovoltage x rays. They provided a dose buildup region which displaced the maximum dose from the skin surface to a depth of a few millimeters below the surface. This feature greatly alleviated the limitations in dose that could be administered because of skin reactions in external-beam radiation therapy. However, it also eliminated skin reactions as a visible sign of how well the patient was tolerating radiation treatment.

In the absence of skin reactions, the radiation oncologist was forced to rely on indirect measures of administered dose in the design of radiation treatments. These measures included central-axis depth dose data, radiation-beam isodose curves, and isodose distributions for multiple-field treatments. The latter were obtained by superimposing isodose curves for individual treatment beams and determining the composite distribution of radiation dose through a manual summation process. These procedures and their experimental verification for specific treatment plans enhanced the contribution of physics to radiation therapy, because oncologists looked to physicists and their measurements and computations, rather than to skin reactions, for reassurance that treatment plans were appropriate.

In the latter 1960s, digital computers began to be used in radiation therapy to define the specific characteristics of individual radiation beams and to compile isodose distributions for treatments with multiple fields. At first, computerized treatment plans were obtained through the use of programs installed on time-sharing computers that could be accessed from distant locations.[3] In the mid-1970s, computer workstations designed specifically for treatment planning became available, and dosimetrists were trained to operate them under the parallel supervision of physicists and radiation oncologists. Today, radiation oncology facilities of even modest size employ at least one physicist and one or more dosimetrists, and they use a planning workstation for the design of radiation treatments. The computer workstation is used to select the radiation beams and treatment portals that yield dose distributions consistent with satisfactory, or in some cases optimized, therapeutic ratios for individual patients. In addition, the workstation can accept data from digital imaging units such as computed tomography (CT), magnetic resonance imagers, and PET scanners to provide an anatomic and physiologic background for superimposition of isodose distributions, as discussed earlier in this book.

In the late 1960s, a further advance in radiation therapy occurred with the development of the side-coupled linear accelerator at the Los Alamos Scientific Laboratory. This concept was rapidly incorporated into the design of compact high-energy accelerators for production of x-ray and electron beams of several MeV for use in radiation therapy. Compared with ^{60}Co, linear accelerators provided radiation beams that were more intense (higher dose rates) and sharper (well-defined edges). Over the 1970s, linear accelerators rapidly replaced ^{60}Co units as the preferred method for delivering external-beam radiation treatments to most patients. However, linear accelerators added another layer of complexity in the design and administration of external-beam therapy and required careful dosimetry and quality control by physicists. The advent of the linear accelerator is one of several steps in the transition of radiation oncology from largely an empirical and qualitative practice in its first 50 years, to a sophisticated science in the later half of the twentieth century. Advances in physics and radiation delivery systems have been accompanied by similar improvements in fundamental knowledge of cancer biology and in improved understanding of the biological effects of ionizing radiation. Considered collectively, progress in the physics and biology underlying radiation oncology was remarkable in the latter half of the twentieth century. This progress sets the stage for significant improvements in the treatment of cancer with radiation in the early part of the twenty-first century.

In the early years of radiation therapy, patients with cancers in accessible locations often were treated with radioactive sources placed in the cancers temporarily for a few days (radium sources) or permanently (radon "seeds"). These sources produced high radiation doses in their immediate vicinity and much lower doses in surrounding tissues because of the rapid falloff of dose with increasing distance. The popularity of this technique, known as brachytherapy (brachytherapy means "therapy at a short distance"), waned in the middle part of the century because (1) relatively high radiation doses were received by persons installing the sources in patients, (2) adequate radiation dose distributions were difficult to achieve in pliable tissues, and (3) external-beam radiation therapy was a reasonable replacement for radioactive implants in the treatment of cancers near the skin and in accessible organs. Only the use of radium for treatment of cervical and uterine cancer remained popular, primarily because rigid applicators could be used to retain some control over the geometry of sources inside the body.

Beginning in the 1960s, new sources of radioactivity began to be used for brachytherapy. Radium was replaced by safer ^{137}Cs sources for treatment of cancer of the cervix and uterus, and sources such as ^{125}I, ^{182}Ta, and ^{192}Ir became available for interstitial implants. In addition, computer programs were written to estimate distributions of radiation dose from sources in geometric configurations that could be determined from radiographic images. As a consequence, brachytherapy regained popularity as a method of treatment for certain cancers, including tumors of the prostate and bladder. Today, brachytherapy has experienced a substantial revival, as have the physics, dosimetry, and treatment planning aspects of this therapeutic approach.[4]

Remote afterloading equipment further improved the safety of brachytherapy procedures by providing greater protection to personnel. These devices (explained more fully in Chapters 12 and 13) allow radioactive sources to be transported through guide tubes from a shielded container into an applicator implanted within the patient. Once the sources are in place, a timer records the duration of treatment. Treatment can be interrupted by pushing a button if the patient requires medical attention. Some remote afterloading equipment is equipped with high activity (on the order of 10 Ci) sources, enabling the treatment to be delivered quickly on an outpatient basis. *High-dose-rate* (HDR) brachytherapy is now practiced in many hospitals. A similar device was made available for *pulsed-dose-rate* (PDR) brachytherapy, in which a relatively high activity (1 Ci) source is used. The source is transported into the patient for brief periods at approximately hourly intervals. In this way, the patient receives the treatment over an extended period, yet ample opportunities are provided for medical staff to attend to the patient. The biological implications and benefits of this approach to treatment are presently being investigated.

Today the practice of radiation oncology demands a solid foundation not only in medicine, but also in the physics and biology underlying medical practice with ionizing radiation. As noted by Perez,[1] "Radiation oncologists must have sound knowledge of biological concepts, and physics and dosimetry principles to enhance the appropriateness and precision with which irradiation is prescribed and delivered. Mastery of the technical aspects of treatment planning, simulation, and treatment delivery techniques with both external and internal sources is required for oncologists to supervise radiation treatments and to interact with the physics, dosimetry, and technical staff."

Over the past few decades, several experimental approaches to radiation therapy have been explored in an effort to overcome physical and biological barriers to improvements in the therapeutic ratio of cancer treatment with radiation. Some of the more promising approaches are described in the following sections.

■ ALTERED FRACTIONATION

Over the years, efforts have been directed toward achieving an inexpensive yet potentially powerful method for improving results in radiation therapy by manipulating the fractionation schedule of delivered treatments.[5] Still, the vast majority of treatment schedules vary only modestly from techniques developed in the 1920s.[6] Since that time, many biological experiments and clinical trials have been conducted to investigate the effects of changes in fractionation. It is widely believed that tissues respond to changes in fractionation according to the "four R's" of radiation therapy:

repair of sublethal damage, redistribution of cells within the cell cycle, repopulation, and reoxygenation.[7] Experiments and trials have demonstrated a number of important characteristics of tumors and normal tissues that can be summarized as follows:

- Extending the duration of a course of radiation therapy has little effect on late reactions but has a large sparing effect on early reactions.
- The severity of late effects is largely dictated by fraction size.
- Both fraction size and overall treatment time determine the response of acutely responding tissues.[8]

Clinical trials are presently being conducted using several different fractionation schemes. Most common are *hyperfractionation* and *accelerated fractionation*. The goal of hyperfractionation is to separate early and late effects on the assumption that tumor response is dictated by early effects, whereas most normal tissue complications can be characterized as late effects. The overall treatment time is maintained at conventional levels, but two treatment fractions per day (or more) are given. The dose per fraction is generally slightly more than half of conventional fraction sizes; therefore, the total dose is increased slightly over conventional fractionation schemes. Conversely, accelerated fractionation roughly involves a conventional total dose and number of fractions. However, the fractions are delivered twice or more per day, so that the overall treatment time is reduced by half or even less. The goal of accelerated fractionation is to reduce repopulation in rapidly proliferating tumors. Because the number and size of the dose fractions are unaltered, little or no change in late effects is expected. Extensive clinical trials are required to demonstrate the benefits of schemes such as these to improve clinical results by altering the fractionation schedule.

▪ BIOLOGICAL MODELING AND PLAN EVALUATION

The advent of whole-body CT in the 1970s gave radiation oncologists anatomic information that previously was unavailable. With the development of modern computer systems, CT information can be reformatted and displayed in arbitrary planes, and three-dimensional views can be created. This capability permits clear distinction between tissues involved with tumor and those that must be protected from radiation. At the same time, treatment planning software has advanced from rudimentary programs that simply superimpose measured data on anatomic information, to complicated algorithms that correct for (a) the complex shape of the patient and the tumor and (b) the presence of nonhomogeneous tissues in the vicinity of the tumor.[9–11]

The analysis of competitive treatment plans and selection of an optimal plan must consider several factors. The capabilities of the available treatment equipment must be included because certain combinations of field size, gantry angle, and couch position may not be achievable. Before implementing complex treatment configurations, one must consider the ability of the technical staff to deliver the treatment accurately on a daily basis. Also, the biological response of the tissues to the radiation must be considered. Determining the biological response requires that detailed knowledge of each tissue's response to radiation must be known as well as the changing tissue environment (considering factors such as nutrition and oxygenation). Estimates of tumor control probability (TCP) can be made from knowledge of the distribution of intratumor and intertumor radiosensitivities, initial clonogen numbers, and measured proliferation times. These models of TCP can then be applied to calculated nonuniform dose distributions. Additional models of normal tissue complication probabilities (NTCP) can be computed by similar methods. The calculated TCP and NTCP values may then be used to score competing treatment plans for an individual patient. A treatment plan selected by this method would be expected to carry the greatest likelihood for success. An example of calculated TCP and NTCP curves is

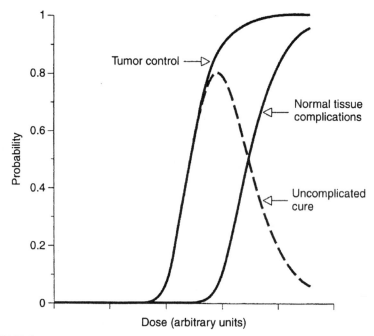

FIGURE 16-1

A representation of calculated tumor control probabilities and normal tissue complication probabilities. Also shown is a plot of the probability of uncomplicated tumor cure.

shown in Figure 16-1, together with a curve representing the likelihood of uncomplicated cure.

◼ MOLECULAR IMAGING

Molecular imaging is a rapidly emerging scientific discipline focused on the development and evaluation of new tools, procedures, and reagents to image biochemical concentrations and pathways in vivo at the cellular and molecular levels. Of particular interest are new imaging approaches for identifying key targets for diagnosis and treatment of diseases at the molecular level. The emergence of this discipline reflects the rapid growth of new knowledge stimulated by the evolution of techniques such as molecular cloning, microfabrication, chip arrays, robotics, x-ray crystallography, rapid mass spectrometry, and sophisticated and fast computer analysis.[12] These techniques provide approaches to acquiring answers to fundamental biological questions that heretofore have been unattainable. Molecular imaging is expected to impact patient care in the near future, especially through its potential to identify susceptible patients in order to prevent the occurrence of disease, and to provide earlier diagnosis and treatment in order to intercede in the progression of disease in a more effective manner. In addition, molecular imaging promises to offer more efficient approaches to monitoring the effectiveness of treatment compared with the many months, or even years, usually needed today to determine whether treatment has been effective.

To image target molecules in vivo, at least four criteria must be satisfied.[12] These criteria are the:

- Availability of high-affinity molecular probes with adequate pharmacodynamics
- Ability of molecular probes to overcome barriers (vascular, interstitial, cell membrane) to biological delivery

- Use of amplification strategies (chemical or biological) to increase signal strength
- Accessibility to sensitive, fast, high-resolution imaging techniques

These criteria are discussed below.

High-Affinity Probes

Target identification and validation with high-affinity probes is essential to interrogating target molecules in vivo. These probes can be small molecules (e.g., receptor ligands or enzyme substrates) or large molecules (e.g., monoclonal antibodies or recombinant proteins). Recent advances in the technology of drug discovery and the design of therapeutic drugs are facilitating the design of molecular probes with exquisitely high affinity for specific target molecules. To date, the development of imaging probes has lagged behind the design of therapeutic agents, primarily because of the smaller market for imaging probes. This handicap should decrease in the future as molecular imaging rises in importance as an enabling technology for molecular target identification and assessment.

Overcoming Delivery Barriers

To be effective, molecular probes must be able to reach the intended target in sufficient concentration, and remain affixed to the target for an adequate time, to produce a recognizable in vivo image. Nonspecific binding, metabolism, excretion and delivery barriers all interfere with this objective. Often delivery barriers are the most difficult obstacle to overcome. A variety of strategies are being developed to circumvent recognized barriers for in vivo imaging with molecular probes. Another problem is high background noise caused by the presence of unbound probes in the tissue. In some cases this problem may be solvable by choosing imaging times carefully; in other cases more aggressive measures may be necessary, such as the use of compounds that redirect unbound probes shortly before imaging.

Amplification Strategies

Strategies to increase the signal in order to distinguish it from noise are an essential part of the operational plan for molecular imaging. Various chemical and biological techniques for signal amplification are being developed to facilitate molecular imaging at the level of molecular proteins. They include strategies for (1) increasing probe concentration, (2) trapping probes, and (3) changing the physical behavior of probes. In addition, attention is currently focused on molecular imaging of proteins rather than on DNA and RNA, because cells contain more protein molecules compared with nucleic acids. In any future application of molecular imaging, any one or all of these approaches may be used to acquire a signal strength that is adequate for imaging.

Molecular Imaging Techniques

At this time, improvements in existing imaging techniques (e.g., MR spectroscopy and PET), along with the development of new imaging techniques (e.g., optical imaging), are the focus of research in molecular imaging. Significant improvements in speed, sensitivity, and resolution are necessary to realize the potential of medical imaging in the future.

Molecular imaging offers great promise for prevention and early intercession into disease and disability and, through this potential, for substantially improving the health and well-being of persons of all creeds, countries, and color. Realization of this promise presents a major challenge to radiation oncology and radiology, as these disciplines will need to focus increasingly on molecular biology and genetics as part of their instructional programs for physicians and scientists. Meeting this challenge is one of the great opportunities for the disciplines today.

■ PROTON THERAPY

The use of high-energy protons for radiation therapy was first proposed by Wilson in 1946[13] and was pursued in the 1950s and 1960s at five main centers: Berkeley (United States), Dubna (Russia), Uppsala (Sweden), Harvard (United States), and Moscow (Russia).[14] Progress was slow in these efforts, in part because proton dosimetry and imaging techniques for tumor localization were not well developed and in part because the accelerators used to produce the proton beams were designed as experimental facilities rather than as clinical machines. More recently, significant growth has occurred in the number of accelerators used for proton therapy, as shown in Figure 16-2. By 1997, more than 17,000 patients had been treated with protons (Table 16-1), with encouraging results reported for both malignant and nonmalignant conditions.[15–17]

Proton beams offer the potential of providing improved distributions of radiation dose compared with more traditional treatment techniques employing external beams of electrons, x rays, or even neutrons. This potential improvement is a result of the Bragg peak of the proton beam that occurs at the end of the range of protons in tissue (Figure 16-3). In the Bragg peak, the dose rises rapidly to a maximum because the protons slow down and produce more ionization along their paths. In the peak region, the dose substantially exceeds the dose at the entrance portal and at more superficial depths.

By changing the energy of the proton beam and the degree of attenuation of the beam before it enters tissue, the Bragg peak can be positioned at the center of a tumor, with greatly reduced doses to more superficial tissues. Furthermore, it can be shaped to encompass the tumor by varying the beam energy slightly so that the Bragg peak effectively scans the tumor from front to back. This approach is discussed in greater detail later in this section. Additional potential advantages of a proton beam include the rapid falloff of dose beyond the Bragg peak, minimum scattering in tissue so that the beam edge remains sharply defined at depth, and the possibility of some degree of skin sparing at the entrance surface.[14,15]

Compared in Figure 16-4 are isodose curves for a 35-MeV electron beam and a 160-MeV proton beam produced at the Harvard Cyclotron Laboratory. The large amount of scattering with the electron beam causes nonuniformity of dose over the irradiated volume of tissue and poor definition of the beam edge. Both of these features are much improved with the proton beam. Isodose distributions for parallel-opposed fields of ^{60}Co gamma rays, 20-MeV x rays, and 160-MeV protons are shown

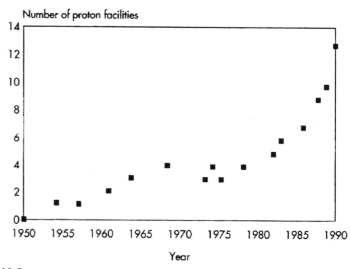

FIGURE 16-2
Number of proton facilities worldwide since 1950. (From D. E. Bonnett.[14])

TABLE 16-1   Centers Currently Operating a Proton Therapy Program

Facility	Location	Date of First Treatment	Patient Total
Berkeley	United States	1954	2084
Harvard	United States	1961	7181 (June '97)
Moscow	Russia	1969	2838 (May '96)
St. Petersburg	Russia	1975	969 (Dec. '95)
Chiba	Japan	1979	96 (Oct. 96)
Tsukuba	Japan	1983	525
PSI	Switzerland	1984	2325 (June '97)
Dubna	Russia	1967	124 (Nov. '96)
Uppsala	Sweden	1957	185 (Apr. '97)
Clattterbridge	United Kingdom	1989	764 (June '97)
Loma Linda	United States	1990	369 (Dec. '92)
Louvain-la Neuve	Belgium	1991	21 (Nov. '93
Nice	France	1991	636 (Nov. '95)
Orsay	France	1991	956 (May '97)
Faure	South Africa	1993	191 (Mar. '97)
Indiana University	United States	1993	1 (Dec. '94)
Davis CF	United States	1994	127 (Aug. '97)
TRIUMF	Canada	1995	23 (Dec. '96)
		Total	~17, 000

in Figure 16-5. Compared with the gamma rays, the x rays restrict the radiation dose more appropriately to the spherical treatment region. However, the protons are far superior to either of the other treatment techniques in this regard.

The clinical use of protons can be divided into two major applications: those using protons with energies less than 80 MeV and those employing protons with energies greater than 160 MeV. The major application of lower-energy protons is for treatment of ocular melanoma, and several centers are using low-energy accelerators, principally cyclotrons, for this application.[14] These facilities have several common

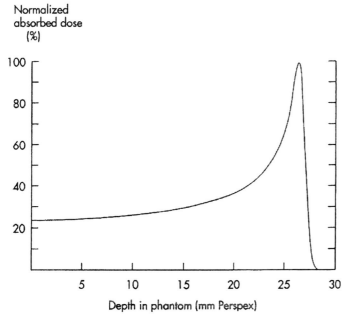

FIGURE 16-3
A proton Bragg peak (62-MeV proton beam at the Clatterbridge Center of Oncology). (Used with permission from D. E. Bonnett, et al.[18])

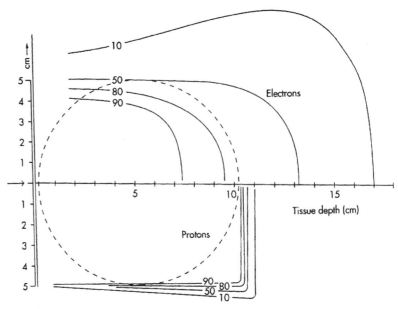

FIGURE 16-4

A comparison of isodose curves for a 35-MeV electron beam and 160-MeV proton beam. (Used with permission from A. M., Koehler, W. M., Preston.[19])

features, including a horizontal beam line with scattering foils and range modulators to shape the proton beam to the treatment region both laterally and in depth. Patients are seated in a motor-driven chair during treatment, restrained by a bit block and head restraint or face mask, and provided with a visual target such as a light-emitting diode for fixing the patient's gaze (Figure 16-6). The use of protons between 60 and 80 MeV for the treatment of ocular melanoma has experienced substantial success to date.[18]

Protons with energies of 160 MeV and above have been investigated for the treatment of a variety of deep-seated lesions.[21] The Proton Therapy Co-operative Group[22] has stated that high-energy proton therapy should be conducted with protons between 160 and 250 MeV in energy, with the beam energy variable either continuously or in steps separated by no more than a few MeV. The average beam current should be not less than 10 nA so that treatment times are reasonable. In addition, the facility should have relatively low capital and operating costs, be relatively small with minimum weight, and be reliable and easy to operate and maintain.

As described in Table 16-2, the three principal types of accelerators for high-energy proton therapy are the linear accelerator, cyclotron, and synchrotron. The cyclotron is a fixed-energy accelerator capable of beam currents much greater than those needed for proton therapy. Cyclotrons are relatively simple, reliable, and inexpensive machines that have been recommended as eminently suitable for use in clinical facilities. They tend to accumulate high internal levels of induced radioactivity, however, and may weigh as much as 150–200 tons. The synchrotron produces proton beams of variable energy and is relatively low in weight and power consumption. However, the maximum beam current is limited by the ion injector system and is on the low side even when the proton-extraction efficiency and pulse repetition rate are near maximum. The linear accelerator has adequate beam output but requires a relatively large amount of space. It can deliver beams of variable energy by extracting the beam after different stages of acceleration. Young et al.[23] have suggested that an accelerator for proton therapy should (1) furnish treatment beams by both passive scattering and beam scanning techniques, (2) be designed solely for proton therapy, and (3) furnish at least 3×10^{11} protons per second with a pulse length greater than 10 msec. These criteria would confine the choice of accelerator to either a cyclotron or a slow-cycling synchrotron.

A proton accelerator furnishes a beam with a small cross-sectional area and a sharp Bragg peak. This proton beam must be configured into one that can uniformly

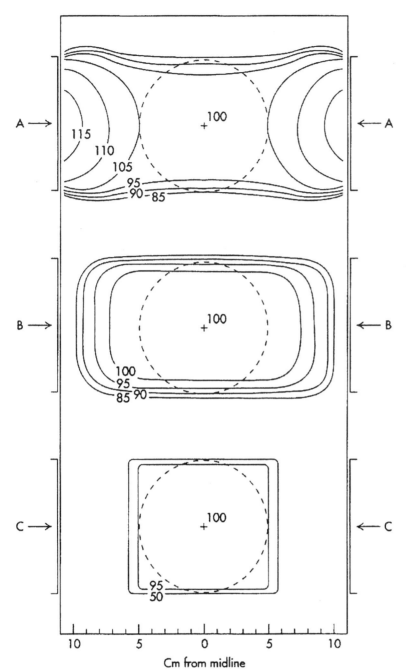

FIGURE 16-5
A comparison of iosdose contours for parallel-opposed fields for (**A**) ^{60}Co, (**B**) 20-MeV x rays, and (**C**) 160-MeV protons. (Used with permission from A. M., Koehler, and W. M., Preston. [19])

irradiate a much larger volume of tissue. That is, the proton beam must be widened in cross-sectional area, and the depth of penetration must be shaped so that a uniform distribution of absorbed dose is attained for the target volume.[14,15] The main features of various beam delivery systems to achieve uniform irradiation of tumors are depicted in Figure 16-7. The systems can be separated into two categories: those that use a fixed depth of penetration and fixed beam modulation with either passive scattering or dynamic scanning to spread the beam (*A*, *B*, and *C* in Figure 16-7) and those that irradiate the target volume with a narrow beam controlled in three dimensions (*D* in Figure 16-7), a technique referred to as three-dimensional proton conformal therapy.

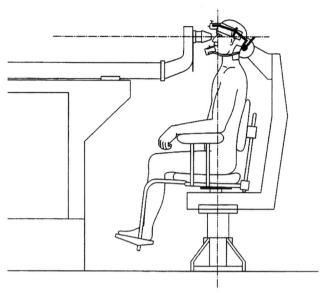

FIGURE 16-6
The patient support system for the treatment of ocular melanoma in use at the Svedberg laboratory. (Used with permission from A. Montelius, et al.[20])

As shown in Figure 16-3, the Bragg peak of a proton beam is constricted to a limited range in the absorbing medium and is too narrow in depth to provide uniform irradiation of a tumor of any significant size. Uniform irradiation can be achieved by scanning the Bragg peak across the target volume through the technique of varying (modulating) the beam energy and, therefore, the depth of penetration of the proton beam. The principle of beam modulation is shown in Figure 16-7, in which the initial Bragg peak is reduced both in energy and in relative height, and the resultant peak is added to the initial peak. This process is repeated several times until a flat dose distribution over the required range in depth is obtained. The most common method of beam modulation is use of a rotating stepped absorber (the range shifter in Figure 16-7 D) to vary the depth of the Bragg peak, together with a plastic block to limit the maximum range of the Bragg peak (the range limiter in Figure 16-7). Shaping of the field in the lateral dimension is achieved by using an irregularly shaped collimator in combination with tissue-compensating bolus individually designed for each patient. The beam is spread laterally to a clinically useful size by either passive scattering or beam scanning, as described subsequently.

Most proton treatments are conducted with a passive scattering technique to widen the lateral dimensions of the beam (Figure 16-7A,B). This technique involves the placement of high-Z foils in the beam to scatter the protons laterally. Usually, one

TABLE 16-2 Comparison of Accelerator Parameters

	Intensity (protons sec^{-1})	Energy (MeV)	Machine Power (kW)	Size (m²)	Pulse Length (msec)	Extraction Efficiency (%)	Residual Activity	Beam Emittance
Linac	5.00E + 14	250 Variable	350	150 Large	1000E + 00	100	Low	Small
Cyclotron	5.00E + 13	250 Fixed	500	25 Medium–small	CW	40	High	Large
Synchrotron	1.00E + 11 (1 Hz)	250 Variable	150	50 Medium	>50	95	Low	Medium
Synchrotron (fast cycle)	5.00E + 11 (5 Hz)	250 Variable	100–150	50 Medium	1.00E-02 1.00E-04	85–90	Low–medium	Medium–large

CW, continuous wave.

Source: P. Young et al.[23]

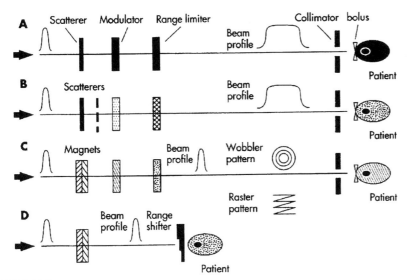

FIGURE 16-7
The main features of some of the various possible beam delivery systems for proton therapy.
A: Single scattering foil. **B:** Double scattering foil. **C:** Dynamic scatter: beam wobbler or raster
scanning. **D:** Proton three-dimensional conformal therapy. (Redrawn from Blattmann, H.,[24] as
presented in D. E. Bonnett.[14])

or two scattering foils are used in combination with the range modulator (sometimes
referred to as a range shifter) to shape the axial dimension of the Bragg peak. Several
investigators have explored the optimum design and geometry of scattering foils and
range shifters to obtain desired shapes of the high-dose region of proton beams of
different energies.[14,15,25,26]

An alternative to the passive scattering technique to expand the lateral dimensions
of a proton beam is use of an electromagnetic technique to scan the beam laterally
(Figure 16-7C). This approach is referred to as dynamic scanning, in contrast to
the technique of passive scanning described in the preceding paragraph. Several
geometries for dynamic scattering have been employed, including (a) moving a
narrow proton beam through a series of concentric circles of increasing radius (*beam
wobbling*), and (b) confining the beam to a rectangular raster scan pattern. Dynamic
scanning minimizes energy losses, preserves the maximum useful range of the
proton beam, and can be accomplished in less space than that required for passive
scattering. It requires stringent safety measures, however, to prevent overirradiation
of small volumes of tissue.[14]

Three-dimensional conformal therapy with protons (Figure 16-7D), also known
as spot or voxel scanning, involves scanning the proton beam not only laterally,
but also along the beam axis. A prototype system developed at the Paul Scherrer
Institute in Switzerland furnishes a horizontal scan by employing a sweeper magnet,
a vertical scan by moving the patient couch, and an axial scan by using a range shifter
system of individual absorption plates moved into the beam pneumatically.[27] The
relative merits of three-dimensional scanning compared with passive scattering and
two-dimensional scanning have been discussed extensively in the literature.[24,28,29]
Concerns over the effects of respiration, organ motion, and tissue heterogeneities on
the uniformity of proton dose distributions for various approaches to beam geometry
have been considered by several investigators.[30,31]

Protons have similar radiobiological properties to x or gamma rays, and the
relative biologic effectiveness (RBE) is not significantly increased in the region of the
Bragg peak, even though microdosimetric measurements have shown a slight RBE
enhancement at the end of the proton range.[32] Most proton therapy facilities use
an RBE of 1.1 relative to ^{60}Co and quote the prescribed dose in terms of the *cobalt
gray-equivalent*, which is the absorbed dose multiplied by an RBE of 1.1.[14]

Several studies have documented the superior dose distributions of protons or protons plus photons, compared with photons alone for treatment of tumors in a variety of anatomic sites, including the base of the skull and the prostate,[16] brain,[33,34] spinal cord,[35] maxillary sinus,[36] rectum,[37] tonsillar region,[38] and cervix.[39] These studies have shown that, compared with photons alone, it is possible for protons or protons plus photons to deliver a higher dose to the target volume with an equal or lower dose to critical tissues, or to give the same dose to the target volume with less dose to normal tissue. These evaluations have employed less than optimum methods for shaping the proton beam, and the potential advantages of proton therapy may be greater than those revealed by these preliminary studies.[14]

Dosimetric measurements for proton therapy can be attained with calorimeters, Faraday cups, and thimble and parallel plate ionization chambers,[40] although only calorimeters furnish absolute measurements of absorbed dose. The first protocol for proton dosimetry was produced by the AAPM in 1986, and a more recent code of practice for clinical proton dosimetry has been published by the European Clinical Heavy Particle Dosimetry Group (ECHED).[41] These publications differ in several respects, including the choice of the value of W/e for protons (AAPM value of 34.3 joule/coulomb compared with an ECHED value of 35.18 joule/coulomb). These differences are presently under review.

■ NEUTRON BRACHYTHERAPY

The element californium (Cf) was first produced in 1950 as a result of bombardment of a ^{242}Cm cyclotron target with helium ions at Berkeley. In 1952, the isotope ^{252}Cf was discovered in the debris from uranium that had been subjected to intense neutron irradiation. The finding that the isotope decays by spontaneous fission with the emission of neutrons led to speculation that compact sources of neutrons could be fabricated for various purposes, including brachytherapy.[42] ^{252}Cf decays by spontaneous fission with a half-life of 2.65 years. It emits neutrons at a rate of 2.34×10^{12} Bq g^{-1} and emits gamma rays from fission events and products at a rate of about 1.3×10^{13} Bq g^{-1}. The average neutron energy is generally taken to be 2.35 MeV.[43]

Demand for ^{252}Cf has greatly exceeded the supply, and only small quantities have been available for evaluation of its usefulness in medicine. Since 1973, the entire supply of ^{252}Cf in the Western world has been produced in the High Flux Isotope Reactor (HFIR) at Oak Ridge, Tennessee. Smaller quantities have been produced at Dimitrovgrad in Russia.[44]

The high neutron flux in the HFIR permits the production of transplutonium elements through a chain of neutron absorptions and beta decays as shown in Figure 16-8. Neutron absorption increases the mass number of the nuclide by 1, and beta decay increases the atomic number by 1. For example, curium-244 (^{244}Cm) absorbs a neutron to become ^{245}Cm, and ^{245}Cm then absorbs a neutron to become ^{246}Cm and so on up to ^{249}Cm. At this point, neutron absorption is largely replaced by beta decay because the half-life of ^{249}Cm is short enough (64.2 min) to allow many of the nuclei to decay before they can capture a neutron. The berkelium-249 (^{249}Bk) formed by beta decay captures a neutron and becomes ^{250}Bk, which, in turn, decays by beta emission to californium-250 (^{250}Cf). This isotope is altered through successive neutron absorptions to ^{252}Cf. Although ^{252}Cf decays by spontaneous fission, its 2.65-year half-life means that it can also absorb neutrons to produce heavier Cf isotopes when in the reactor. The chain reaction stops with fermium-257 (^{257}Fm) because the next isotope in the chain, ^{258}Fm, has a half-life for spontaneous fission that is so short (0.38 ms) that the nuclei disappear into fission products essentially as soon as they are formed.

Clinical brachytherapy trials with ^{252}Cf were begun in 1968 in Houston, London, and Paris. Initial results suggested that this technique yielded no clinical advantages compared with conventional radiation therapy, and the clinical trials were discontinued in the mid-1970s. At about this time, clinical trials of neutron brachytherapy

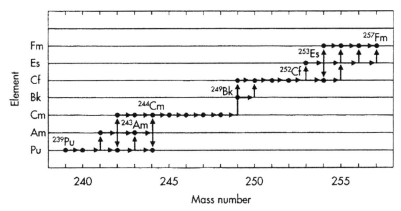

FIGURE 16-8
Nuclear reactions that produce transplutonium elements in the High Flux Isotope Reactor at the Oak Ridge National Laboratory. (From O. L., Keller.[44])

were initiated in Tokyo, but interest declined gradually until efforts were essentially discontinued in the early 1980s. Interest in ^{252}Cf for implant therapy arose in 1973 at the Academy of Medical Sciences in Obninsk but was tempered over the years by mixed results and concern of the medical staff about levels of exposure to neutrons. In 1972, studies were begun at the University of Kentucky in Lexington into the use of ^{252}Cf for intracavitary therapy. For many years, this institution was the only location in the United States that was actively pursuing neutron brachytherapy.[45] Several international conferences on neutron therapy were held in Lexington, where follow-up studies of neutron brachytherapy with ^{252}Cf sources were presented and discussed. However, neutron brachytherapy was unable to evolve beyond a highly controversial experimental technique, and with the departure of the principal investigator for ^{252}Cf brachytherapy in 1992, the program of clinical trials at Lexington was discontinued. In the later 1980s, two new investigations into ^{252}Cf were initiated, one in Vilnius, Lithuania,[46] and the other in Brno, Czech Republic.[47]

■ NEUTRON CAPTURE THERAPY

Neutron capture therapy relies on the premise that a substance can be identified that has the dual properties of (1) selective absorption in cancerous tissue and (2) release of densely ionizing, short-range radiations when the tissue is exposed to thermal (low-energy) neutrons from a nuclear reactor. The isotope of greatest promise for neutron capture therapy is ^{10}B because it releases short-range α particles by an (n, α) reaction when irradiated by thermal neutrons.

This experimental technique, known as boron neutron capture therapy (BNCT), was tried initially in the 1950s on patients with inoperable brain tumors. These experiments were unsuccessful because of (1) poor penetration of thermal neutrons through the scalp, (2) extensive damage to blood vessels in the brain owing to interactions of neutrons with boron present in the circulatory system, and (3) inadequate understanding of the biological and pharmacological properties of boron-containing compounds and their effects on radiation response. Although BNCT experiments were stopped in the United States after their initial lack of success, they have been continued in Japan for the treatment of patients with inoperable tumors of the central nervous system.[48] The 5-year survival of 20% of these patients following treatment with sodium borocaptate and neutrons is encouraging. However, the absence of a histologic breakdown of the patients makes the results difficult to interpret quantitatively.[49]

Neutron capture therapy with boron-containing compounds is a challenging endeavor. In addition to the difficulties mentioned previously, treatment beams of epithermal (1–100 keV) and thermal (0.025 eV) neutrons are poorly collimated and are contaminated with substantial numbers of gamma rays. Also, neutrons interact with other elements such as nitrogen [^{14}N (n, p)^{14}C reactions] and hydrogen [^{1}H (n, γ)^{2}H and ^{1}H (n, n)p reactions] present in significant concentrations in biological tissues. These problems require the attainment of concentration ratios of boron-containing pharmaceuticals of at least 3, and preferably 10 or more, in tumors compared with surrounding normal tissues.[49] Results with boronated lipoproteins and BOPP, a boronated prophyrin, show promise of attaining such concentration differentials in brain tumors of rodents.[50]

Interest in BNCT is experiencing somewhat of a revival, partly in response to clinical results in Japan, but also because new boron compounds show promise of providing greater concentration differentials between tumors and normal tissues. Also, sources of neutrons are being phased out of their intended purposes and are available for BNCT at locations such as the Brookhaven National Laboratory on Long Island, New York. Interest in the United States is focused principally on the use of BNCT for malignant gliomas because conventional treatment of these tumors usually fails due to lack of control of the primary tumor. BNCT promises to deliver high doses of radiation to cancer cells present in these primary tumors and to the margins of edematous tissue, while sparing surrounding normal tissue from a necrotizing dose of radiation. If this promise can be realized through development of tumor-specific boron-containing pharmaceuticals and design of appropriate neutron beams, BNCT could yet prove to be a useful technique in the treatment of certain cancers.[51]

■ NEUTRON BEAM THERAPY

The first efforts to use beams of fast neutrons to treat cancer were initiated by Stone[52] at the Lawrence Berkeley Laboratory in 1938, only 6 years after Chadwick discovered the neutron in 1932.[53] These efforts were stopped in 1942 after disastrous results with several patients caused by extensive damage of normal tissue, and because the Berkeley cyclotron was needed for the war effort. Not until 1956 was interest rekindled in neutron therapy, when a group of investigators at the Hammersmith Hospital in London developed a rationale for using high-LET radiations, including fast neutrons, in radiation therapy. The principal feature of the rationale was to take advantage of the reduction in the oxygen enhancement ratio (OER) observed for neutrons compared with photons in tissue-culture experiments. The OER is the dose required for a given biological effect when irradiation occurs under hypoxic conditions, divided by the dose needed for the same effect under oxygenated conditions. The Hammersmith rationale proceeded as follows[53]:

1. Hypoxic cells exist in most, if not all, tumors.
2. These hypoxic cells have an OER of about 3 and are relatively radioresistant to conventional forms of therapy.
3. Neutrons reduce the OER to about 1.6, yielding a therapeutic gain factor (TGF) of $3/1.6 = 1.9$.
4. The TGF of neutrons should lead to improved effectiveness of neutrons compared with photons in the treatment of most tumors.

The Hammersmith rationale is compromised by two factors: (1) Tumor heterogeneity complicates the identification of patient groups with tumors that have high levels of hypoxia, and it makes the selection of patients for neutron therapy difficult. (2) Experiments with animals have repeatedly demonstrated that reoxygenation of tumors occurs when irradiation is delivered in multiple fractions, so hypoxia may be less significant than initially assumed as a factor in the radioresistance of tumors.

Two other advantages of neutrons over photons have been proposed. The first is that repair of sublethal damage may be less efficient with neutrons compared with photons, so that cell killing with neutrons is ultimately more effective. This possibility reflects the higher LET of neutrons compared with photons. For tumors with a significant capacity for recovery from irradiation, neutrons may provide an elegant therapeutic approach because they induce more extensive irreparable damage. This increased effectiveness of neutrons is expressed as the RBE, defined as the ratio of the absorbed dose of photons required to attain a certain amount of cell killing, divided by the absorbed dose of neutrons to attain the same degree of cell death. In laboratory studies, neutrons often have an RBE of 2–3, implying that a lower absorbed dose may be required for neutrons compared with photons to achieve a desired level of cell killing in patients. The complicating factor, however, is that the RBE of neutrons may be higher for normal cells as well as for tumor cells, so the relative advantage of neutrons over photons may be less than imagined. This advantage may be particularly marginal when late effects of irradiating normal tissue are considered. Furthermore, the RBE of neutrons may differ widely for various normal tissues, and the selection of an average RBE value in the planning of neutron treatments often is a compromise between treatment effectiveness and normal tissue sparing.[54] This problem has led to difficulties in comparing the results of various clinical trials with fast neutrons.[55]

The second advantage that has been proposed for fast neutrons is the possibility that variations in radiation sensitivity of cells over different phases of the mitotic cycle may be less dramatic with neutrons compared with more conventional types of radiation.[32] For example, slowly growing, well-differentiated tumors with a large G0–G1 compartment in the cell cycle may be particularly susceptible to neutrons compared with photons.[56] This hypothesis may be the explanation for the observation that neutrons appear to be superior to photons for treatment of prostate and salivary gland cancer and soft tissue sarcoma.

As a result of radiobiological studies with neutrons at the cellular and whole-animal levels in the late 1940s and 1950s, many of the complications associated with Stone's early investigations of neutron therapy began to be better understood and appreciated. Clinical investigations of neutron therapy were started at Hammersmith Hospital in 1956, and encouraging results began to be published several years later.[57] These conclusions encouraged other institutions to initiate studies of fast neutron therapy. These studies yielded conflicting results that raised questions once again about the usefulness of fast neutron therapy.[55]

Early trials with neutrons also led to increased appreciation of the many difficulties caused by limitations in the equipment available for neutron therapy. Many of the early trials were conducted with neutrons from deuterium–tritium generators and low-energy cyclotrons. These neutrons yielded depth dose distributions more similar to orthovoltage x rays or ^{137}Cs gamma rays than to megavoltage x rays, and they produced neutron beams with diffuse edges and almost no dose buildup region at the surface. In addition, neutron therapy was conducted with horizontal or vertical fixed beams of markedly inferior geometry compared with the isocentrically mounted linear accelerators or cobalt units with which they were being compared. Also, neutron beams differed considerably among institutions, even for neutrons produced at similar energies, in contrast to highly standardized beams of photons. These differences created variations in RBE values for neutron beams that required careful radiobiological characterization of the beams before they could be employed clinically. Finally, institutions differed in the ways in which neutron dose was measured and expressed. All of these factors contributed to difficulties in evaluating the results of neutron therapy trials and comparing them among institutions and with conventional methods of radiation therapy. Some, but not all, of these problems have been addressed in the multi-institutional clinical trials of neutron beam therapy sponsored by the U.S. National Cancer Institute. Hall has summarized the desirable features of a neutron clinical facility as (1) an adequate dose rate so that treatment times do not exceed a few minutes, (2) depth doses comparable to megavoltage x rays, (3) isocentric geometry, and (4) location in or near a major medical center.[54]

Over the period 1965 through 1990, more than 12,000 patients were treated with fast neutrons, although only about 1400 were included in randomized, controlled clinical trials.[55] The trials were directed to cancers of the head and neck, brain, salivary gland, lung, cervix, rectum, bladder, prostate, and pancreas. Only two of these trials unequivocally demonstrated superior results for neutrons compared with conventional radiation therapy. Results in the other clinical trials have largely been inconclusive. The first successful study was conducted between 1980 and 1986 on the use of neutrons for treatment of inoperable tumors of the salivary gland.[58] With a follow-up period of 2 years, local tumor control was attained in 85% (11/13) of the patients treated with neutrons, compared with only 31% (4/13) in the group treated with photons. Although normal tissue complications were observed more frequently in the neutron group, their improved survival provided more time for complications to arise. The second successful clinical trial was the use of neutrons mixed with photons for treatment and follow-up of 91 patients with prostate adenocarcinoma. In a 1989 report of this trial, the 7-year disease-specific survival rates were 80% for mixed neutron–photon beams versus 55% for photons alone.[59] Although this trial has been criticized for the relatively poor results achieved with patients treated exclusively with photons, the improved survival of the neutron-treated patients is incontrovertible. In both the salivary gland and the prostate trials, relatively small numbers of patients are involved, and longer follow-up times are necessary to determine if long-term complications are greater in the neutron-treated patients.

In the United States, cooperative clinical trials of fast-neutron beams are being conducted at Fermilab outside of Chicago, the University of California at Los Angeles, MD Anderson Hospital in Houston, and the University of Washington in Seattle. Late reactions caused by the response of normal tissue to neutrons, poor treatment geometry of neutron facilities, poor dose distributions of neutron beams, and improperly designed clinical trials have compromised the demonstration of an unequivocal advantage of neutrons for radiation therapy.[60] This lack of success has undermined the enthusiasm for neutron therapy in all but a few limited applications, such as salivary gland tumors and sarcomas. Although institutions with neutron facilities will undoubtedly continue to explore these applications, it is unlikely that many new facilities for neutron therapy will be commissioned until answers about the clinical usefulness of fast neutrons become clearer.

■ HEAVY ION AND PION THERAPY

Heavy ions such as helium and neon nuclei have been used experimentally to treat selected types of cancers at physics facilities, where such ions can be accelerated to high energies. Heavy-ion beams yield Bragg peaks similar to those of protons and somewhat sharper beams because the particles are heavier and less subject to lateral scattering in tissue. A possible disadvantage of heavy ions is the production of densely ionizing fragments during interactions with tissue nuclei as the heavy ions slow down near the end of their tracks, causing irradiation of tissues beyond the Bragg peak.

Heavy-ion therapy has been underway for several years with the Bevatron accelerator at the Lawrence Berkeley Laboratory of the University of California. Although patients treated at the Berkeley facility continue to be followed, as described subsequently, the accelerator itself has been shut down. A $300 million heavy-ion medical accelerator (HIMAC) dedicated exclusively to medical applications was opened in 1994 in the town of Chiba just outside Tokyo.[61] The HIMAC accelerator has dual synchrotrons, each capable of producing high-energy ^{4}He and ^{40}Ar ion beams. A schematic of the HIMAC twin-synchrotron facility is shown in Figure 16-9. Also, a European light-ion medical accelerator (EULIMA) is being designed as a project of the Commission of the European Communities,[62] and the University Clinic of Radiology in Heidelberg and the German Cancer Research Center are planning collaborative radiotherapy research with heavy ions.[63]

At the Berkeley Bevatron, 239 patients were treated for cancers of the skin, subcutaneous tissues, paranasal sinuses, nasopharynx, salivary glands, skull base and juxtaspinal area, esophagus, pancreas, biliary tract, prostate, lung, soft tissue, and bone. These patients were treated with mixed beams that included at least 10 Gy

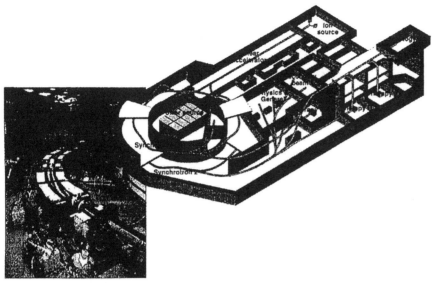

FIGURE 16-9
Twin-synchrotron HIMAC facility for heavy-ion radiotherapy at Chiba. (Used with permission from F., Myers.[61])

from neon ions. Treatments consisted of multiport irradiations, with one horizontal treatment field per day usually delivered with the patient in the sitting position. Promising preliminary results were obtained for patients with soft tissue sarcomas, prostate carcinomas, and salivary gland tumors.[64] More work, much of which will have to be conducted at the HIMAC facility in Japan, is required before the usefulness of heavy ions in radiation therapy can be thoroughly assessed.

Pions are charged particles of mass intermediate between the masses of electrons and protons that are produced in high-energy accelerators during energetic nuclear reactions. Their potential for radiation therapy was acknowledged shortly after their discovery in 1947 by Occhialini and Powell[65] and was enhanced by the description of the "star" component of the Bragg peak contributed by densely ionizing particles released as the pions caused nuclear fragmentation near the end of their tracks.[66] The pion Bragg peak with its "star" enhancement is depicted in Figure 16-10.

In 1961, Fowler and Perkins[68] proposed the development of clinical trials of pion radiotherapy, and in 1968 a clinical channel for pion radiotherapy was planned at the Los Alamos Meson Production Facility (LAMPF). The first patient was treated at LAMPF in 1974, and patient treatments were discontinued in 1981. Over this

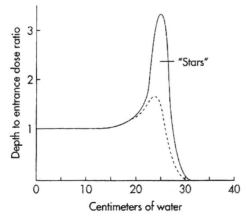

FIGURE 16-10
Pion Bragg peak with "star" enhancement contributed by nuclear fragmentation.[67]

period, 228 patients were irradiated with pions as part or all of their treatments. As concluded by von Essen and colleagues, the overall results of these treatments are not particularly impressive.[69] They range from a high rate of tumor control, but with serious complications in patients with prostate cancer, to no advantage compared with conventional treatment in patients with pancreatic cancer. Although there are individual cases with remarkable local cures in pion treatment of cancers of the prostate, head and neck, lung, bladder, and cervix, the number of patients in each category is too small to draw any conclusions. Further experiences with pion therapy at the TRIUMF accelerator in Vancouver and the S.I.N. facility in Villigen, Switzerland, have not helped resolve the uncertainty of the effectiveness of pion therapy.[51] These facilities have discontinued their clinical experiments with pion therapy and are now concentrating their efforts on proton therapy.

■ CONCLUSIONS

Radiation therapy is a dynamic discipline that is built on a solid foundation in physics. It is evolving at the leading edge of technology and computer science applied to therapeutic medicine. Persons specializing in the discipline must have a firm grasp of all of these subjects if they are to participate in state-of-the-art care of patients. This book is designed to help members of the radiation–oncology team gain an understanding of the physical foundation of the discipline and to remain alert to and knowledgeable about technical developments and experiments such as those described in this chapter. It also is intended to provide the framework necessary to remain current in a rapidly changing and technology-intensive profession.

REFERENCES

1. Perez, C. A. Quest for excellence: the ultimate goal of the radiation oncologist: ASTRO gold medal address, 1992. *Int. J. Radiat. Oncol. Biol. Phys.* 1993; **26**: 567–580.

2. Johns, H. E., and Cunningham, J. R. *The Physics of Radiology*, 3rd edition. Springfield, IL, Charles C Thomas, 1983.

3. Hendee, W. R., and Cadigan, R. A. Timesharing computers for treatment planning in radiation therapy. *Radiology* 1971; **99**:423–428.

4. Williamson, J., Thomadson, B., and Nath, R. (eds.) *Brachytherapy Physics.* Proceedings of the 1994 AAPM Summer School. Madison, WI, Medical Physics Publishing, 1995.

5. Peschel, R. E., and Fischer, J. J. A review of time-dose effects in radiation therapy. *Med. Phys.* 1980; **7**:601–608.

6. Coutard, H. Roentgen therapy of epitheliomas of the tonsillar region, hypopharynx and larynx from 1920 to 1926. *AJR* 1932; **20**:313–331.

7. Withers, H. R. The four R's of radiotherapy. In *Advances in Radiation Biology, vol. 5*, J. T. Lett, and H. Adler (eds.). New York, Academic Press, 1975.

8. Hall, E. J., and Cox J. D. *Altered Fractionation Patterns in Radiation Therapy in the 1990s: Rationale for the emerging Modalities (a categorical course in Radiation Therapy).* Oak Brook, IL, The Radiological Society of North America, 1989.

9. Lichter, A. S., and Lawrence, T. S. Recent advances in radiation oncology. *N. Engl. J. Med.* 1995; **332**:371–379.

10. Mohan, R., et al. A comprehensive three-dimensional radiation treatment planning system. *Int. J. Radiat. Oncol. Phys.* 1988; **15**:481–495.

11. Mohan, R., et al. Clinical relevant optimization of 3-D conformal treatments. *Med. Phys.* 1992; **19**:933–944.

12. Weissleder, R., and Mahmood, U. Molecular imaging. *Radiology* 2001; **219**:316–333.

13. Wilson, R. R., Radiological use of fast protons. *Radiology* 1946; **47**:487–491.

14. Bonnett, D. E., Current developments in proton therapy: A review. *Phys. Med. Biol.* 1993; **38**:1371–1392.

15. Chu, W. T. Hadron therapy. In *Biomedical Uses of Radiation Part B: Therapeutic Applications*. W. R. Hendee (ed.). New York: Wiley-VCH, 1999, pp 1057–1131.

16. Austin-Seymour, M., Urie, M., Munzenrider. J., Willett, C., Goitein, M., Verhey, L., Gentry, R., McNulty, P., Koehler, A., Suit, H., Considerations in fractionated proton radiation therapy: Clinical potential and results. *Radiother. Oncol.* 1990; **17**:29–33.

17. Munzenrider, J. E., Verhey, L. J., Gragoudas, E. S., Seddon, J. M., Urie, M., Gentry, R., Birnbaum, S., Ruotolo, D. M., Crowell, C., McManus, P., et al. Conservative treatment of uveal melanoma: Local recurrence after proton beam therapy. *Int. J. Radiat. Oncol. Biol. Phys.* 1989; **17**:493–498.

18. Bonnett, D. E., Kacperek, A. Sheen, M. A., Goodall, R. Saxton, T. E. The 62 MeV proton beam for the treatment of ocular melanoma at Clatterbridge. *Br. J. Radiol.* 1993; **66**:907–914.

19. Koehler, A. M., and Preston, W. M. Protons in radiation therapy. *Radiology* 1972; **104**:191–195.

20. Montelius, A., Blomquist, E., Naeser, P., Brahme, A., Carlsson, J., Carlsson, A. C., Graffman, S., Grusell, E., Hallen, S., Jakobsson, P. et al. The narrow proton beam therapy Unit at the Svedberg Laboratory in Uppsala. *Acta Oncol.* 1991; **30**:739–745.

21. Larsson, B. Proton therapy: Review of the clinical results. In *Proceedings of Eulima Workshop on the Potential Value of Light Ion Beam Therapy (Nice)*, P. Chauvel and A. Wambersie (eds.). Brussels, Commission of European Communities, 1989.

22. Gottschalk, B. Design of a hospital-based accelerator for proton radiation therapy: scaling rules. *Nucl. Instrum. Methods Phys. Res. (Sec. B)* 1987; **24/25**:1092–1095.

23. Young, P., Hagan, W., Morton, P., and Young, D. Comparisons of accelerator types for uses in proton therapy. Fourth workshop on Heavy Charged Particles in Biology and Medicine (GSI, Darmstradt, 1991) as referenced in Bonnett, D. E. Current developments in proton therapy. *Phys. Med. Biol.* 1993; **38**:1371–1392.

24. Blattmann, H. Beam delivery systems for charged particles. *Radiat. Environ. Biophys.* 1992; **31**:219–231.

25. Coutraken, G., et al. A prototype beam delivery system for the proton medical accelerator at Loma Linda. *Med. Phys.* 1991; **18**:1053–1099.

26. Urie, M. M., Sisterson, J. M., Koehler, A. M., Goitein, M., Zoesman, J. Proton beam penumbra: Effects of separation between patient and beam modifying devices. *Med. Phys.* 1986; **13**:734–741.

27. Bacher, R., Blattmann, H., Boehringer, T., Coray, A., Egger, E., Pedroni, E., Scheib, S., Phillips, M. Development and first results of discrete dynamic spot scanning with protons. In *Proceddings International Heavy Particle Therapy Workshop*, and H., Blattmann (ed.). Paul Scherrer Institute Report 69, Villigen PSI, 1990.

28. Goitein, M., and Chen, T. Y. Beam scanning for heavy charged particle radiotherapy. *Med. Phys.* 1983; **10**:831–840.

29. Garoley, K. U., Oeltke, U., and Lam, G. K. Range modulations in proton therapy—an optimization technique for clinical and experimental applications. *Phys. Med. Biol.* 1999; **44**:N81–N86.

30. Daftari, I., Petti, P. L., Collier, J. M., Castro, J. R., Pitluck, S. The effect of patient motion on dose uncertainty in charged particle irradiation for lesions encircling the brain stem or spinal cord. *Med. Phys.* 1991; **18**:1105–1115.

31. Phillips, M. H., Pedroni, E., Blattmann, H., Boehringer, T., Coray, A., Scheib, S. Effects of respiratory motion on dose uniformity with a charged particle scanning method. *Phys. Med. Biol.* 1992; **37**:223–234.

32. Raju, M. R. *Heavy Particle Radiotherapy*. New York, Academic Press, 1980.

33. Archambeau, J. O., Slater, J. M., Tangeman, R. Role for proton beam irradiation in treatment of pediatric CNS malignancies. *Int. J. Radiat. Oncol. Biol. Phys.* 1992; **22**:287–294.

34. Wambersie, A., Gregroire. V., and Bruckner, J. M. Potential clinical gain of proton (and heavy ion) beams for brain tumors in children. *Int. J. Radiat. Oncol. Phys.* 1992; **22**:275–286.

35. Nowakowski, V. A., Castro, J. R., Petti, P. L., Collier, J. M., Daftari, I., Ahn, D., Gauger, G., Gutin, P., Linstadt, D. E., Phillips, T. L. Charged particle radiotherapy of paraspinal tumours. *Int. J. Radiat. Oncol. Biol. Phys.* 1992; **22(2)**:295–303.

36. Miralbell, R., Crowell, C., and Suit, H. D. Potential improvement of three dimensional treatment planning and proton therapy in the outcome of maxillary sinus cancer. *Int. J. Radiat. Oncol. Biol. Phys.* 1992; **22**:305–310.

37. Tatsuzaki, H., Urie, M. M., and Willett, C. G. 3-D comparative study of proton vs x-ray radiation therapy for rectal cancer. *Int. J. Radiat. Oncol. Biol. Phys.* 1992; **22**:319–374.

38. Slater, J. M., Slater, J. D., and Archambeau, J. O. Carcinoma of the tonsillar region: Potential for use of proton beam therapy. *Int. J. Radiat. Oncol. Biol. Phys.* 1992; **22**:311–320.

39. Smit, B. Prospects for proton therapy in carcinoma of the cervix. *Int. J. Radiat. Oncol. Biol. Phys.* 1992; **22**:345–354.

40. Verhey, L. J., et al. The determination of absorbed dose in a proton beam for purpose of charged-particle radiation therapy. *Radiat. Res.* 1979; **79**:34–54.

41. Vynckier, S., Bonnett, D. E., and Jones, D. T. L. Code of practice for clinical proton dosimetry. *Radiother. Oncol.* 1991; **20**:53–63.

42. Knauer, J. B., Alexander, C. W., and Bigelow, J. E. Cf-252: Properties, production, source fabrications and procurement. *Nucl. Sci. Appl.* 1986; **2**:263–271.

43. Anderson, L. L. Cf-252 physics and dosimetry. *Nucl. Sci. Appl.* 1986; **2**:273–281.

44. Keller, O. L. Californium-252: Properties and production. *Nucl. Sci. Appl.* 1986; **2**:263–271.

45. Maruyama, Y. Preface. *Nucl. Sci. Appl.* 1986; **2**:13–18.

46. Shpikalov, V. L., Atkochyus, V. B., Valuckas, K. K. The application of Cf-252 in contact neutron therapy of malignant tumors at the Scientific Research Institute of Oncology in Vilnius, Lithuania. *Nucl. Sci. Appl.* 1991; **4**:419–424.

47. Tacev, T., Strnud, V., Vacek, A., Rasovska, O., Ptackova, B., Krystof, V. Radiotherapy of cervix uteri carcinoma with Cf-252 implant and external hypooxy radiotherapy. *Nucl. Sci. Appl.* 1991; **4**:201–212.

48. Hatanaka, H., and Nakagawa, Y. Clinical results of long-surviving brain tumor patients who underwent boron neuron capture therapy. *Int. J. Radiat. Oncol. Biol. Phys.* 1994; **28**:1061–1066.

49. Phillips, T. L. Boron neutron capture therapy: Finally come of age? *Int. J. Radiat. Oncol. Biol. Phys.* 1994; **28**:1215–1216.

50. Hill, J. S., et al. Selective tumor uptake of a boronated porphyrin in an animal model of cerebral glioma. *Proc. Natl. Acad. Sci. USA* 1992; **89**:1785–1789.

51. Raju, M. R. Hadron-therapy in a historical and international perspective. International symposium on Hadron-Therapy. Villa Olma, Como Italy, 1993.

52. Stone, R. S. Neutron therapy and specific ionization. *AJR* 1948; **59**:771–785.

53. Chadwick, J. Possible existence of a neutron. *Proc. R. Soc. Lond. A.* 1932; **136**:696.

54. Hall, E. J. *Radiobiology for the Radiologist, 3rd edition*. Philadelphia, J. B. Lippincott, 1988.

55. Duncan, W. An evaluation of the results of neutron therapy trials. *Acta Oncol.* 1994; **33**:299–306.

56. Battermann, J. J. *Clinical Application of Fast Neutrons, the Amsterdam Experience* (thesis). University of Amsterdam, Amsterdam, 1981.

57. Catterall, M., Bewley, D. K. *Fast Neutrons in the Treatment of Cancer*. London, Academic Press, 1979.

58. Griffin, T. W., Pajak, T. F., Laranire, G. E., Duncan, W., Richter, M. P., Hendrickson, F. R., Maor M. H. Neutron vs photon irradiation of inoperable salivary gland tumors: Results of an RTOG-MRC cooperative randomized study. *Int. J. Radiat. Oncol. Biol. Phys.* 1988; **15**:1085–1090.

59. Krieger, J. N., Krall, J. M., Laramore, G. E., Russel, K. J., Thomas, F. S., Maor, M. H., Hendrickson, F. R., Griffin, T. W. Fast neutron therapy for locally advanced prostate cancer: Update for post trial and future research directions. *Urology* 1989; **34**:1–9.

60. Scalliet, P. Trouble with neutrons. *Eur. J. Cancer* 1991; **27**:225–230.

61. Myers, F. A heavy ion accelerator gears up to fight cancer. *Science* 1993; **261**:1270.

62. Chauvel, P., and Wambersie, A. (eds.). Proceedings of the EULIMA Workshop on the Potential Value of Light Ion Beam Therapy, EUR 12165 EN, Brussels, Commission of the European Communities, 1989.

63. Wambersie, A., et al. The European high-LET research programs in 1991. In *Radiation Research: A Twentieth Century Perspective*, vol. II, W. C. Dewey et al (eds.). New York, Academic Press, 1991.

64. Castro, J. R. High-LET charged particle radiotherapy. In *Radiation Research: A Twentieth Century Perspective*, vol. II, W. C., Dewey et al. (eds.). New York, Academic Press, 1991.

65. Occhialini, G. P. S., and Powell, C. F. Nuclear disintegrations by slow charged particles of small mass. *Nature* 1947; **159**:186–190.

66. Perkins, D. H. Nuclear disintegration by meson capture. *Nature* 1947; **159**:126–127.

67. Curtis, S., and Raju, M. A calculation of the physical characteristics of negative pion beams—energy-loss distribution and Bragg curves. *Radiat. Res.* 1968; **34**:239.

68. Fowler, P. H., and Perkins, D. H. The possibility of therapeutic applications of beams of negative pi mesons. *Nature* 1961; **189**:524–528.

69. von Essen, C. F., Bagshaw, M. A., Bush, S. E., Smith, A. R., Kligerman, M. M. Long-term results of pion therapy at Los Alamos. *Int. J. Radiat. Oncol. Biol. Phys.* 1987 Sep; **13**:1389–1398.

ANSWERS TO SELECTED PROBLEMS

Chapter 1

1-1. $Z = 8$; $A = 17$; mass defect $= 0.141367$ amu; $E_b = 131.6$ MeV; $(E_b)_{avg/nucleon} = 7.74$ MeV

1-2. 15.999 amu

1-3. W: 58.2 keV; H 10.1 eV

1-4. e: 0.51 MeV; p: 937.7 MeV

1-5. 2.37×10^{24} fissions; 0.85 g

1-6. isotopes: $^{14}_{6}C$, $^{15}_{6}C$; $^{14}_{7}N$, $^{15}_{7}N$; $^{16}_{8}O$, $^{17}_{8}O$

   isotones: $^{14}_{6}C$, $^{15}_{7}N$, $^{16}_{8}O$; $^{15}_{6}C$, $^{16}_{7}N$, $^{17}_{8}O$

   isobars: $^{14}_{6}C$, $^{14}_{7}N$; $^{15}_{6}C$, $^{15}_{7}N$; $^{16}_{7}N$, $^{16}_{8}O$

1-7. 28.6 days; 42.9 days

1-8. 1600 years

1-9. essentially 100%

1-10. 9.5 ng; $N = 17.8 \times 10^{13}$ atoms; 49.0 ng

1-11. 37%

1-12. $\lambda = 1.24 \times 10^{-3}$ nm; $\nu = 2.4 \times 10^{20}$ s^{-1}

1-13. $^{126}_{53}I \rightarrow ^{126}_{54}Xe + ^{0}_{-1}\beta + \bar{\nu}$

   $^{126}_{53}I \rightarrow ^{126}_{52}Te + ^{0}_{+1}\beta + \nu$

   $^{126}_{53}I + ^{0}_{-1}e \rightarrow ^{126}_{52}Te + \nu$

1-14. 6.15×10^{14} atoms; 9.2×10^{-8} g

1-15. 691×10^{3} MBq

1-16. ^{131}I negatron decay; ^{125}I electron capture and possibly positron decay

1-17. 160

1-18. 0.018 MeV; 0.018 MeV

1-19. 1.98 MeV; 0.96 MeV

Chapter 2

2-1. 2.04 keV/cm

2-2. 5150 IP/cm

2-3. 1.25×10^{18}; 20 kW (20,000 J/sec)

2-4. 11.3 degrees

2-5. 250 keV; 0.023; 0.005 nm

Chapter 3

3-1. $I = (1/10)I_0 = I_0 e^{-\mu(TVL)}$
   $\ln(1/10) = 2.30 \log(1/10) = -\mu(TVL)$
   $-2.30 = -\mu(TVL)$
   $TVL = 2.30/\mu$

3-2. —

3-3. 0.59

3-4. 2.5 cm

3-5. 2 keV; 25 keV

3-6. 138 keV; 12 keV; decreased

3-7. 86.5 keV

3-8. $\Delta\lambda = 0.00243(1 - \cos \emptyset)$
   for $\emptyset \geq 60°$, $\cos \emptyset \leq 0.5$
   $\Delta\lambda \geq 0.00124$ nm
   For high-energy photons, $\lambda \ll \Delta\lambda$
   and can be ignored.
   $\lambda' = \lambda + \Delta\lambda \approx \Delta\lambda$
   $h\nu \leq 1.24/0.00124$ nm
   ≤ 1000 keV, which is below threshold for pair production

3-9. 13.2 cm

3-10. 0.9 cm^2/g

Chapter 4

4-1. 0.58 cm; 10.6 cm

4-2. a. 0.98 cm
   b. 34% smaller (0.53 cm)

4-3. 1137 Ci/g

4-4. Approximately 162 MΩ/m

4-5. 1.005; 1.15; 7.09

4-6. 7.4 cm; $14.22 - 15.78$ MeV ($\pm 5.2\%$)

Radiation Therapy Physics, Third Edition, by William R. Hendee, Geoffrey S. Ibbott, and Eric G. Hendee
ISBN 0-471-39493-9 Copyright © 2005 John Wiley & Sons, Inc.

Chapter 5

5-1. 69×10^{15} IP; 1.11×10^{-2} coulomb; 48.4×10^{-2} J/m^3; 37.4×10^{-2} J/kg; 37.4×10^{-2} Gy

5-2. 65.7 R/min

5-3. 7.8×10^{10} MeV/m^2 – sec; 15.6×10^{11} MeV/m^2

5-4. 2.28×10^{15} photons/m^2; 2.28×10^{15} MeV/m^2

5-5. 7.4

5-6. 0.28 nA

5-7. 47 pFd

5-8. 300 R or 7.7×10^{-2} coulomb/kg

5-9. 10J/kg; 8 J

5-10. 0.85

5-11. 2.5 cSv

5-12. 0.014°C

5-13. 9.6×10^{17}

5-14. 1.5 mm A1; 2.25 mm A1; 0.7

Chapter 6

6-1. 75.2 R/min; 0.95 Gy/min

6-2. 2.04; 4.37; 0.963

6-3. 0.12%

6-4. 0.996

6-5. 1.009

6-6. 80.7%; 0.972

Chapter 7

7-1. 28.2%; 129 cGy

7-2. 1.272

7-3. 353.6 cGy

7-4. 268 cGy; 102 cGy

7-5. 89% primary; 11% scatter

7-6. 10.1×10.1 cm^2; 274 cGy; 95 cGy

7-7. Increase by factor 2.12

7-8. 0.763 cGy/MU; 262 MU

7-9. 5.28 min; 0.76 rev/min

7-10. 0.54

7-11. 61.0

Chapter 8

8-1. 138 MU

8-2. 116 MU

8-3. 78.5 cGy; 102.5 cGy

8-4. 88.9 cGy

8-5. a. 0.694 cGy/mu
    b. 0.673 cGy/mu

8-6. a. 66.2%
    b. 66.7%

8-7. 5.3 cm

8-8. 1.68 cm

Chapter 9

9-1. 10:1

9-2. $X_2:X_1 = 2:1$

9-3. 1000

9-4. 0.5

9-5. 4.2 megabytes

9-6. 2.5 lp/mm

9-7. 5760

9-8. 1.8

9-9. Air − 1000; Bone + 1000

9-10. 0.23%

9-11. 160 μsec

9-12. 63.9 MHz

Chapter 10

10-1. –

10-2. Octal: 163,235; Decimal: 59037; Hexadecimal: E69D

10-3. Binary: 111 1100 1011; Octal: 3713; Hexadecimal: 7C6

10-4. –

10-5. 2000 increments are required, so a digitizer having at least 11-bits must be used (2048 values). Approximately 0.0145 V per increment.

10-6. 13.65 seconds

10-7. 3.3 seconds

10-8. 703 scans

Chapter 11

11-1. $\dfrac{(20 \times 20 \times 15)}{(10 \times 10 \times 15)} \times \dfrac{5^3}{4^3} = 4 \times 1.95 = 7.8$, or almost a factor of 8

11-2. $(15 \times 2) \times (15 \times 2) \times 9 = 8100$, or over eight thousand adjustable parameters

11-3. –

11-4. If about a third of the patients have 3 times the number of monitor units, this will effectively double the workload of the linear accelerator. A safety factor of 10 should still be able to accommodate this, but this type of analysis should be part of implementing an IMRT program in existing vaults.

Chapter 12

12-1. –

12-2. a. Once the daughters are in secular equilibrium, their activities equal that of the parent (10 mCi).

  b. 6.5×10^{-8} g (0.65 ng)

12-3. 2.6×10^{-4} cm^3. No, an inert "filler" material is mixed with the RaSO$_4$.

12-4. 1.76 mCi; 0.63 mCi

12-5. 1.27 cGy · cm^2/hr

12-6. 1.61 mCi

Chapter 13

13-1. 0.19 R/hr

13-2. a. 1.98 R/hr; 0.32 R/hr

  b. 1.85 R/hr; 0.30 R/hr

13-3. 1.08 mg; 990 hr

13-4. 2.1 cm

13-5. a. 25 mg distributed uniformly or 39 mg distributed on periphery

  b. 154 mg distributed on periphery

13-6. One solution: Single plane implant having sides 6 cm long with linear density 0.67 mg/cm and 5 internal line sources with linear density 0.5 mg/cm. Total activity is 31 mg Ra-eq. Treatment time of 86 hours.

13-7. –

13-8. One solution using the Manchester method: 30 mg on belt, 15 mg in core, 8 mg on end of cylinder 4 cm in diameter and 6.4 cm long. Treatment time of 75.1 hours.

13-9. –

13-10. One solution: two planes 1.5 cm apart, with 16 seeds on periphery and 7 seeds distributed in the central region of each plane.

13-11. –

13-12. 33,303 cGy (using the air kerma strength calculation method)

13-13. 24.4 hr; 483 cGy

13-14. 1.1 mR/hr

13-15. 5.26 cGy/hr; 197 days

Chapter 14

14-1. 5×10^{-5}; yes

14-2. 0.45 Sv (45 rem); 0.05 Sv (5 rem); 0.045 Sv (4.5 rem)

14-3. .16 mGy/hr; 2.1 cm; 1.4 cm

14-4. 165 cm concrete; 90 cm

14-5. 35 cm

14-6. 80 cm; no

Chapter 15

15-1. see page 358

15-2. 0.85 MU. Yes, end effect is less than 1 monitor unit.

15-3. a. A 4% reduction in dose.

  b. A 0.1% reduction in dose.

15-4. 146 monitor units

15-5. 739 cGy

15-6. 71 milliroentgens

15-7. ±3.3%. No, it exceeds the specification of ±3%.

15-8. –

15-9. To reduce the risk of spreading radioactive contamination

15-10. Tongue and groove effect

15-11. 0.4% or 0.8cGy; no

INDEX

AAPM-accredited dosimetry calibration laboratories (ADCLs), 91, 108–109, 361, 400–401

AAPM protocols, 115, 116, 117–126, 120, 122, 123, 159

AAPM Subcommittee on Radiation Dosimetry (SCRAD), 117

AAPM Task Groups, 117

Absolute calorimetry, 95

Absorbed dose, 92, 93, 94, 95, 106 measurement of, 99–100

Absorbing medium, 95

Absorption coefficients, values of, 112–113

Absorption edges, 41

Accelerated fractionation, 417

Accelerator gradient, 60

Accelerator guide, 4-MeV, 61

Accelerators, 422–423, 424

Accelerator waveguide, 59, 61

Achromatic magnets, 66, 67

Acoustic impedance, 204, 205

Actinium series, 17

Activity of an atom sample, 8, 9

Acute radiation syndromes, 336–337

Adaptive radiotherapy, 279

Adjacent fields, separation of, 179–180

"Afterloading" techniques, 301. See also Remote afterloading entries

Air, 85 effective atomic number of, 87–88

Air-equivalent material, 87

Air-filled cavity, ionization in, 88

Air ionization chambers, sensitivity of, 105

Air kerma, 93 calibration coefficient of, 108, 110–111 relation to exposure, 110

Air-kerma strength, 289 calculation of, 313–315

Algorithms, inaccuracies in, 393–394

Alignment lasers, 56, 57

All-digital cameras, 209

Alpha–beta ratio, 325

Alpha (α) decay, 11–12, 19

Alpha emission, 11–12

(α, n) reaction, 18

Alphanumeric data, 225

Alpha particles, 12

(α, p) reaction, 18

Alpha transition, 12

Altered fractionation, 416–417

Alternating current (AC), 28

Ambient pressure, 91

Ambient radiation, 190

American Association of Physicists in Medicine (AAPM), 108, 117. See also AAPM entries

American College of Radiology (ACR), 240

American National Standard Code for Information Interchange (ASCII), 225, 226

Americium-241, 291–292

Ampere, 33

Analog-to-digital conversion, 225–227

Analog-to-digital converters (ADCs), 242

Analytical engine, 220

Analytical method, 258

Anatomical structures, general classifications of, 270–272

Ancillary equipment, testing, 363

Anderson, C. D., 47

Andrade, Edward, 14

Anger cameras, 206

Angstrom (Å), 3, 32

Angular momentum, 212

Anisotropy factor, 314, 315

Annihilation photons, 48, 210

Annihilation radiation, 23

Anode, 28 rotating, 27

Anode x-ray tube, stationary, 26

Antineutrinos, 12, 13

Apparent activity, 289

"Apparent focal spot," 33

Applicators, for brachytherapy procedures, 399

A/P tabulation, 137

Area of uncertainty, 334

"Arithmetic processor," 232

Arpanet, 238

"Array" processor, 232

As low as reasonably achievable (ALARA) exposure, 335, 339

Assembly language, 235

Atomic attenuation, 50

Atomic attenuation coefficient, 37

Atomic mass, 3

Atomic mass unit (amu), 3

Atomic number, 2, 7

Atomic theory of matter, 2

Atoms, 3, 4

Attenuating material, electron density of, 46

Attenuation, 36–40

Attenuation coefficients, 36, 37 cross-sectional displays of, 200

Attenuation correction methods, 210

Attenuation curves, 343

Attenuation equation, differential form of, 36

Attenuation measurements, broad-beam geometry for, 36

Attenuators, HVL measurements with, 104

Auger electrons, 6–7, 41

Automatic brightness stabilization (ABS) system, 384

Automatic exposure control (AEC), 384

Autoradiograph, 293

Autowedge, 150

Average dose, 184

Average gradient, 189–190

Average life, 10

Avogadro, Amadeo, 3

Avogadro's number, 3

Azimuthal quantum number, 5

Backscatter, 134

Backscatter factor (BSF), 116 , 132–133, 140, 141, 143–144, 154

Backward-directed field, 60

Bandwidths, for closed-circuit television, 198, 199

Barn, 24

Barrier material, 346

Basal dose rate, 312

Base-2 number system, 222–223

Base-10 number system, 221–222

Base density, 190

Basic programming language, 235

Bateman equation, 15

Baud rate, 228

Beam alignment tests, 370–372, 382

Beam data entry, 247–248

Beam edge unsharpness, 55–56

Beam flatness, measurement of, 378, 379

Beam-flattening filter, 67–68

Beam modulation, 424, 425

Beam quality (Q), 114–116, 122–123

Beams, "hardened," 132. See also Megavoltage beams

Radiation Therapy Physics, Third Edition, by William R. Hendee, Geoffrey S. Ibbott, and Eric G. Hendee
ISBN 0-471-39493-9 Copyright © 2005 John Wiley & Sons, Inc.

Beam scanning systems, 363
Beam's eye view (BEV), 252–253
Beam-shaping platform, 75–76
"Beam stopper," 345
Beam surface, irregular, 168–171
Beam symmetry, measurements of, 378, 380
Beam wobbling, 425
Becquerel (Bq), 8
Becquerel, Henri, 7, 11, 19
Bending magnet, 66–67
Benzene dosimeters, 96
Berkeley, George, 2
Berkelium (Bk), 426
Beta (β) decay, 12–14
Beta-emitting sources, 352
Betatron donut, 70, 71
Betatrons, 53, 70, 71
Bethe–Block formula, 99
Bevatron, 430–431
Billiard-ball collisions, 22
Binary system, 222–223
Binding energy, 3–4, 5–6
Biochemical tracers, 206
Biological modeling, 267, 417–418
Biomedical research, 17. See also Medical
    entries
Bit (binary digit), 223, 242
Bit depth, 227, 229
Blades, collimator, 75
Bloch, Felix, 211
Blocking tray, 75–76
Bohr, Niels, 4, 7, 260
Bohr model, 4–5, 6
Bolus, 169
Bone density value, 172
Boot, H. A. H., 62
Boron (B), 352
Boron neutron capture therapy (BNCT),
    427–428
Brachytherapy, 286, 415–416. See also
    Brachytherapy treatment planning
    quality assurance procedures for,
        399–408, 409
    radioactive nuclides used in, 288
Brachytherapy sources, 289, 292–293
    inventory of, 352
    radiation dose from, 296–297
Brachytherapy treatment planning, 295–330
    air-kerma strength calculation, 313–315
    dose over treatment duration, 316
    implant design, 300–301
    interstitial implants, 302–313
    intravascular brachytherapy, 328–329
    isodose distributions, 300
    plaque therapy, 316–317
    radiographic localization of implants,
        318–322
    remote afterloading, 317–318
    therapy with radiopharmaceuticals, 327
    three-dimensional image-based implants,
        322–327
Bragg–Gray principle, 99–100, 106

Bragg–Gray relation, 118, 120
Bragg peak, 420, 421, 424, 431
Brain, radiation-induced edema in, 337
Breast brachytherapy, 327
Bremsstrahlung, 24–25
Bremsstrahlung photons, 30, 32
Bremsstrahlung spectrum, 24
Bremsstrahlung x rays, 68
Brightness gain, 197
British Journal of Radiology, 131, 135
Broad-beam geometry, 36, 104
Broad-beam transmission, 344, 348
Bucky, Gustav, 194
Bucky factor, 194
Bucky–Potter mechanism, 194
"Build-down" region, 134
Buildup cap, 88
Buildup factor, 37, 131
Buildup-up cap, 109
Buncher, 64
Bureau International des Poids et des
    Mesures (BIPM), 86, 108
Bytes, 223–224

CaF$_2$:Mn, 98
Calcium tungstate screen, 191–192. See also
    CaWO$_4$ x-ray intensifying screens
Caldwell, Eugene, 194
Calibration
    in air, 109–111, 116
    in-phantom, 116–117
    with ionization chamber in a medium, 118
    of low-energy x-ray beams, 114–117
    of megavoltage beams, 117–126
    of photon beams, 123–124
    of photon beams versus electron beams,
        117–118
    protocol for, 117
    treatment unit, 159–160
Calibration coefficient, 108, 109
Calibration conditions, versus treatment
    conditions, 159
Calibration dose rate, 159, 160
Calibration factor, 108
Calibration protocols, 159
    International Atomic Energy Agency,
        126–127
Calibration standards, 108–114
Calibration uncertainty, 109
Californium (Cf), 292, 426, 427
Calorimeter, 95
Calorimetric dosimetry, 95
Calorimetry, 95
Cameron, John R., 98, 383
Cancer, radiation-induced, 338
Carcinogenesis, 336
Cascade tube, 53
Cascading electrons, 41
Catcher cavity, 65
Cathode, 28
Cathode assembly, 27
Cathode-ray tube, 26

Cavities, 60–61
Cavity-gas calibration factor, 99, 120
Cavity-type magnetron, 62
CaWO$_4$ x-ray intensifying screens, 191.
    See also Calcium tungstate screen
CD ROMs, 234
Cellulose acetate film, 189
Centigray, 92
Central axis absorbed dose, 131
Central axis depth doses, 130, 153
Central axis percent depth dose, 135–138,
    162–163
Central processing unit (CPU), 230,
    231–232, 242
Cerebrovascular syndrome, 337
Ceric sulfate dosimeters, 96
Cerrobend blocking, 372, 373
Cervix, carcinoma of, 175
Cesium (Cs), 290
Cesium-131, 292
^{137}Cs, maximum specific activity for, 57
^{137}Cs sources, 416
^{137}Cs teletherapy units, 57, 58
Chadwick, James, 261
Chamber, sensitivity of, 89, 90
Chamber calibration factor, 91
Chamber capacitance, 88–89
"Chamber checker," 362
Chamber depth, shift in, 124
Characteristic curve, 95, 189, 190
Characteristic radiation, 41
Characteristic x rays, 6, 30, 32
"Charge-coupled" devices (CCDs), 195
Charger-reader, 90
Checksums, 393
Chemical dosimetry, 96–97
Circuitry, three-phase, 29
Circular microtron, 72, 73
Circular waveguide, 65
Circulator, 65
Clarkson scatter integration technique, 166,
    259–262
Classical scattering, 41
Clinical medicine, 17
Clinical target volumes (CTVs), 182
Closed-circuit television, 198
Cobalt (Co), 291
^{60}Co, 12, 13, 15, 18
    relative biological effectiveness of, 101
^{60}Co calibration coefficient, 121
^{60}Co gamma rays, 83–84
    isodose curves for, 152
    tissue/air ratios for, 140
Cobalt gray-equivalent, 425
^{60}Co source capsule, 55
^{60}Co sources, 81, 188
^{60}Co teletherapy units, 54, 56, 76, 414–415
Cobalt units, 54–56, 57
Coefficient of equivalent thickness (CET)
    method, 178–179
Coherent scattering, 40, 41
Cold spots, 179, 180

Collecting volume, length of, 85
Collective dose, 336
Collective model, 7
Collimator angle indicator, testing, 368
Collimator jaws, 150, 368
Collimator rotation stability, 367, 370–371
Collimators, 55, 68–69
    of a simulator, 75–76
    types of, 207–208
Collimator scatter factor, 160, 161
Collisional energy loss, 25
Collision-detection device, 75
COLOSSUS computer, 221
Committee on the Biological Effects of
    Atomic Radiation (BEAR) reports,
    337–338
Compensator material, thickness of, 170
Compiler, 235
Complementarity principle, 270
Compound contact scanning, 205
Compression cones, 169
Compton, Arthur Holly, 43
Compton electron, 43, 44–45
    ionization produced by, 87
Compton electronic attenuation coefficient,
    46
Compton interactions, 47
Compton mass attenuation coefficient, 46
Compton scattering, 40, 43, 250
    likelihood of, 48, 50
Compton shift (wavelength), 43
Computational accuracy tests, 394
Computational algorithms, 265
Computed radiography, 195, 388
Computed tomographic scanner, 201
Computed tomography (CT), 200–203
    See also CT entries; Emission
    computed tomography
Computer applications, 234
Computer-based treatment planning,
    245–282
    beam data entry, 247–248
    biological modeling, 267
    challenges of, 280
    dynamic delivery techniques, 277–278
    electron beam computational algorithms,
    265
    forward planning, 267–269
    immobilization and localization, 253–258
    intensity-modulated radiation therapy,
    270–276
    inverse planning, 270
    patient data entry, 248–251
    photon beam computational algorithms,
    258–265
    selection of ideal treatment plan, 265–267
    tomotherapy, 278–279
    virtual simulation techniques, 252–253
Computer bugs, 234
Computer hardware, 230
Computer languages, 242
Computer memory, 230–231, 242

Computers. See also Computer systems;
    Treatment planning computer
    in radiation therapy, 415
    representation of graphic data by, 227–229
    speed of, 224
Computer storage capacity, 224
Computer systems, 219–242
    architecture, 230–234
    data representation, 224–230
    history of computers, 220–221
    networking, 238–241
    programming languages, 234–237
    requirements for treatment planning,
    241
    terminology and data representation,
    221–223
Condenser chambers, 88–90
Condenser "R meter," 90
Conformal therapy, 247, 270, 280
Constancy measurements, daily, 361
Contact therapy units, 52
Continuous quality improvement (CQI),
    360–361
Contrast improvement factor, 194
Contrast resolution, 384
Conversion coefficient, 15
Conversion efficiency, 191
Convolution techniques, 202, 265
Coolidge cascade tube, 53
Coolidge hot-cathode x-ray tube, 26, 27
Copenhagen interpretation, 270
Copper absorber, 37–38
Cormack, Allen, 200
Coronary artery disease, 328
Corrected field size, 160
Correction factors, 90–91
Cost function, 274
Couch. See also Treatment couches
    positioning and calibration of, 386
    rotation stability of, 371
Coulombic interactions, 22
Cowan, Clyde L., Jr., 13
C program, 235–237
Crookes x-ray tube, 52
Cross product, 58–59
Cross section of an interaction, 24
CT images, 249–253. See also Computed
    tomography (CT)
CT information, 417
CT number, 201
CT scanners, 142
CT simulators (CT-Sim), 73, 200
    quality assurance for, 385–387, 388
CT-to-density table, 387
Cumulative dose-volume histograms, 266
Curie (Ci), 9
Curie, Irene, 13, 18
Curie, Marie, 11, 12
Curie, Pierre, 11
Curium (Cm), 426
Cutie-pie ionization-chamber survey meter,
    353

Cutoff energy, 120
Cyberknife, 399
Cyclotrons, 70–72, 422
Cylindrical chambers, 121–122

Daniels, Farrington, 98
Data blocks, 233
Data buses, 230
Data compression, 240
Data entry, inaccuracies in, 393
Data output, inaccuracies in, 393
Data transfer rate, 233
Deblurring function, 202
de Broglie, Louis, 262
Decay. See Radioactive decay
Decay constant, 8, 10, 19
Decay scheme, 11, 12. See also Decay series
Decay series, 17, 19
Decrement lines, 56, 148, 179
Deep therapy machines, 53
Dees, 71, 72
de Hevesy, Georg, 206, 260
Delayed effects, 336
Delineator wires, 75
Deliverable treatment, conversion to,
    274–275
Delivery barriers, overcoming, 419
"Density distributions," 201
Density (polarization) effect, 99
Depletion zone, 97
Depth, influence of, 131
Detail screens, 191
Detective quantum efficiency (DQE),
    388
Deuteron, 18
Device drivers, 239
Diagnostic energy range, 47
Diagnostic imaging, 187–216. See also
    Imaging
    computed tomography, 200–203
    emission computed tomography,
    209–211
    fluoroscopy, 196–199
    functional magnetic resonance imaging,
    213–214
    magnetic resonance imaging, 211–213
    nuclear medicine, 206–209
    radiography, 189–196
    treatment simulators, 199–200
    ultrasonography, 203–206
Diagnostic radiology, 31, 42
Diagnostic x-ray beam, 40
Diamagnetism, 213
Differential scatter-air ratios, 262, 263
Digital communication, options for, 240
Digital computers, 226. See also Computer
    entries
Digital detectors, 198
Digital images, 227–228, 229, 242
    spatial resolution of, 196
Digital Imaging and Communications in
    Medicine (DICOM) standard, 241

Digitally reconstructed radiographs (DRRs), 73, 253, 385
Digital radiography, 194–195
Digital-to-analog conversion, 225–227
Digital-to-analog converters (DACs), 242
Digital x-ray detectors, 195–196, 215
Digitization error, 227
Digitizers, 241
Direct accelerators, 58
Directional coupler, 65
Directly traceable instruments, 109, 114
Disintegration constant, 8
Disintegration energy, 11
Display stations, 240–241
Diverging matrix, 258–259
(d, n) reaction, 18
Dome, Steve, 95
Door shielding, 349–351
Dose buildup, 94
    region of, 131
Dose calculation
Dose computations, 142–143, 166–168
    accuracy of, 409
    algorithms for, 281
    homogeneous and heterogeneous, 250
    Sievert's method for, 297–299
Dose correction factor, 171
Dose distributions, 158
Dose equivalent, 100–102, 106
Dose estimation, from calibration in air, 109–111
Dose gradients, 148
Dose in free space, 139
Dose prescription, 246
Dose rate, 60, 134, 138
Dose-rate constant, 313
Dose rate–distance relationship, 133–134
Dose reporting, recommendations for, 183–184
Dose-shaping objectives, 273
Dose-shaping structures, 272, 275
Dose specification, 181–184, 316
Dose spread array, 263–264, 265
Dose to air, 110–111, 116, 139
Dose to medium, 111–113, 114
Dose to muscle, 111–113
Dose to tissue, 111, 116
Dose to water, 116, 117, 123, 126
    from a measurement of ionization, 118–120
    in a photon beam, 123
Dose-to-water calibration, 126
Dose-to-water calibration coefficient, 108, 120–121
Dose verification, patient-specific, 396–397
Dose-volume histograms (DVH), 265–267
Dosimeters, 94–95, 98
Dosimetric LiF, 98
Dosimetry. See also Radiation field dosimetry
    calorimetric, 95
    chemical, 96–97
    photographic, 95–96
    scintillation, 97

    semiconductor, 97
    thermoluminescence, 97–98
    validating calculations of, 136
Dosimetry indexes, 404–406, 407
Dosimetry standards, 108
Doubly achromatic magnet, 66
Drift tubes, 58–59
Dual-energy linacs, 65
Dual-field image intensifier, 197
Dual-focus x-ray tube, 27, 28
Dual-photon energy linacs, 76
Duane, William, 85, 286, 287
Dwell times, 318
Dynamic arc therapy, 277–278
Dynamic delivery techniques, 277–278
Dynamic scanning, 425

Echocardiography, 205
Edison effect, 26
"Effective area," 310
Effective atomic number, 41–42, 87, 105
Effective attenuation coefficient, 39
Effective dose equivalent, 106, 338, 339, 340, 354
Effective dose equivalent limit, 339
Effective point of measurement, 121–122, 126
Effective SSD method, 170–171
Ehrlich, Margarete, 95
Einstein, Albert, 5
Elastic electron interactions, 34
Elastic interaction, 22
Electric field
    intensity of, 65
    orientation of, 59
Electromagnetic radiation, 14–15
Electrometers, 89
    calibration of, 361–362
Electron applicator (cone), 691
Electron beam dose distribution, 15
Electron beams, 58
    calibration of, 108–127
    characterization of, 379–380
    computational algorithms for, 265
    depth dose curves for, 173
    dose calculations for, 392
    mean incident energy of, 151–152
    quality of, 123
    tissue inhomogeneities and, 172–173, 178–179
Electron binding energy, 41
Electron capture, 13–14, 18
Electron charge (e), 3
Electron cloud, 2
Electron Delay Storage Automatic Calculator (EDSAC), 221
Electron density, 46–47
Electron depth dose, isodose curves and, 151–152
Electron dose distribution, 174
Electron–electron interactions, 22–23
Electron energy, in a microtron, 72

Electron equilibrium, 85, 109
Electronic attenuation, 50
Electronic attenuation coefficient, 37, 38
Electronic collimation, 210
Electronic gain, 197
Electronic mail (e-mail), 238
Electronic Numeric Integrator and Calculator (ENIAC), 221
Electronic portal imaging detectors (EPIDs), 176
Electron linacs, 59
    medical, 60
Electron mass, 70
Electrons, 2, 4–7
    collisional and radiative energy losses of, 25
    specific ionization of, 23
Electron scattering, 172–173
    elastic, 22, 24
    by electrons, 22–23
    inelastic, 24
    by nuclei, 23–25
Electron scattering angle, 43
Electron shells, 4–5
Electron sources, x-ray tube, 27–28
Electron velocity, 72
Electron volt (eV), 3
Electrostatic force, 4
Emergency off buttons, 382
Emission computed tomography (ECT), 209–211
Emitted power, 31
End effect, 115
Energy absorption coefficient, 39
Energy conservation concept, 12
Energy-defining slit, 67
Energy-dependence curves, 98
Energy-dependent dosimetry, 96
Energy-dependent reference depth, 124
Energy-dependent scintillators, 97
Energy fluence, 81, 84
Energy flux, 81
Energy flux density, 80, 105
Energy loss, collisional versus radiative, 25
Energy of decay, 11
Energy per unit exposure, 82–84
Energy switch, 66
Energy transfer coefficient, 39
Equipment, 361. See also Ancillary equipment; Instruments; Megavoltage treatment equipment; Microwave equipment; Microwave power-handling equipment; Patient monitoring equipment; Relative dose measuring equipment; Remote afterloading equipment; RF power-handling equipment
    problems with, 360
Equivalence of mass and energy ($E = mc^2$), 4
Equivalent dose, 102, 338
Equivalent tissue/air ratio (ETAR) method, 178, 262

Erythema, 131, 414
"Erythema dose," 131
European light-ion medical accelerator
    (EULIMA), 430
Excited atoms, 22, 23
Excited energy state, 14
Exit dose, 134
Exponential attenuation, 38
Exponential equation, 38
Exposure, radiation, 82–84. See also
    Radiation protection
Exposure calibration coefficient, 108, 109
Exposure latitude, 189, 190
Exposure measurements, international
    standard for, 86
Exposure-measuring device, 89
Exposure rate, 138, 289
Exposure rate constant, 287
Exposure-to-dose conversion factor, 114
External beam therapy, dose specification
    for, 181–184
External coordinate system, 398
Extrapolation chamber, 92
Extrapolation ionization chambers, 106
Eye plaques, 292
Eye tumors, 316–317

Failla, G., 92, 130
Failla extrapolation chamber, 92
"Farmer chamber," 89
Fast film, 190
Fast neutrons, 428–430
"Fast" screen, 191
Fermi, Enrico, 12
Ferrous sulfate solution, 96
f factor, 111
F-factor, 134, 136
Fiducial localization, 398, 399
Fields, abutting, 180
Field-shaping, 160
Field size, 141, 144, 145–147, 151, 152
Field weighting, 163
Filament current, 27
Filament-emission-limited operation, 27, 34
Filaments, 27
    composition and configuration of, 28
Film
    average gradient of, 189–190
    characteristic curve for, 189, 190
    optical density of, 95
    processing of, 191
    as a "radiation sensor," 96
"Film badges," 353–354
Film fog, 190
Film gamma, 190
Film processor, 387–388
Film sensitometry, 191
Film speed (sensitivity), 190
Filtered backprojection, 203
First-generation scanner, 201, 202
First-order motion, 212
First-order reaction, 8

First-scattered radiation, 263, 264
Fission-produced nuclides, 18
Fixed-point (integer) computations, 225
^{18}F-labeled fluorodeoxyglucose (^{18}FDG),
    210
Flattening filter, 67, 147
    correction for, 262
Fletcher–Suit implant, 321–322
Floating-point operations, 225. See also
    MFLOPS (million floating-point
    operations)
Fluence maps, 274, 276–277
Fluence rate, 80
Fluorescence x rays, 6
Fluorescence yield, 7
Fluoroscope, 196
Fluoroscopic images, television display of,
    198–199
Fluoroscopic system, quality assurance for,
    384
Fluoroscopy, 196–199
Flux density, 80
Focal spot, 28, 33
    testing size of, 382–383
    Van de Graaff generator, 70
Force equation, 58
Forces in nature, 4
Forward-directed field, 59
Forward-peaked x-ray beam, 67
Forward planning, 267–269
4n + 2 series, 17
Fourth-generation scanner, 201, 203
Fractional attenuation, 37, 49
Fractional depth dose, 123, 130
Fractional transmission, 36, 176
Fractionation, altered, 416–417
Franck, James, 260
Free-air ionization chamber, 85–86
"Free" electrons, 43, 46
Frequency of precession, 212
Frequency ramp filter, 202
Fricke, Hugo, 96
Fricke dosimeter, 96–97
Full-wave rectification, 28–29
Functional magnetic resonance imaging
    (fMRI), 213–214, 215
Fusion bomb, 4

Gadolinium oxysulfide screen, 191–192
Gamma emission, 14–15
Gamma cameras, 206
Gamma knife, 399
Gamma-ray emission, 81
Gamma-ray isodose curves, measuring,
    152–153
Gamma (γ) rays, 14
    attenuation of, 36–40, 54
    detection of, 48, 208–209
    interactions of, 40–49
Gamma-ray sources, protection from,
    341–342
Gantry angle, 377, 369

Gantry isocenter, testing, 368–369
Gantry rotation, 142, 371–372
Gap width, determination of, 179
Gastrointestinal syndrome, 337
Geiger–Mueller (G–M) counters, 353
Generator, of a simulator, 75
Geometric penumbra, 55–56
Geometry function, 313, 314
Given dose, 160, 163
Glasser, Otto, 88
Gödel, Kurt, 221
Gold (Au), 291
"Good" geometry, 36, 104
Goodspeed, Alexander, 26
Gram-atomic mass, 3
Gravitational force, 4
Gray (Gy), 82, 92, 110
Gray, L. H., 82
Gray-scale display, 201
Grenz-ray units, 52
"Grid cleanup," 194
Grid cut-off, 194
Grid ratio (GR), 194
Grid strips, 194
Gross tumor volume (GTV), 182
Ground state, 12
Grubbé, Émil, 52
G value, 96
Gynecologic interstitial implant, 327

Half-life, 9–10, 19
Half-value layers (HVLs), 38, 103–105, 108
    beam quality and, 114
    measurements of, 50, 104, 383
Half-value thickness (HVT), 38
Half-wave rectification, 28, 29
Hansen, W. W., 62, 64
Hard disks, 233
"Hardened" beam, 39, 132
Hardware, 230
Heavy-ion medical accelerator (HIMAC),
    430
Heavy-ion therapy, 430–431
Heisenberg Uncertainty Principle, 255, 270
Helical tomotherapy, 278–279
Hematopoietic syndrome, 337
Hendee, Eric, xiii
Heterogeneity correction factor, 177
Heterogeneity corrections, 251, 262,
    280–281
High-affinity probes, 419
High-dose-rate (HDR) brachytherapy,
    317–318, 400. See also Prostate HDR
High-dose-rate (HDR) dosimetry check, 408
High-energy photon mantle field, 167
High-energy photons, skin-sparing effect of,
    94
High-energy proton therapy, 422
High-energy x rays, 70
    percent depth dose for, 136
High-flux isotope reactor (HFIR), 426
High-frequency x-ray generators, 30

High-level computer languages, 235
High-power klystron, 65
"High-resolution" image, 228
Hinge angle, 165
Hodgkin's disease, 167
Homogeneity coefficient (HC), 39, 103–104, 114
"Hot cathode" x-ray tube, 26
Hot spots, 164, 165, 166, 180, 182, 184
Hounsfield, G., 200
Hurter–Driffield (H–D) curves, 95, 190
Hybrid analog-digital cameras, 209
Hydrogen (H), 2, 6
    electron density of, 46–47
    magnetic moment of, 211–212
"Hydrogen" bomb, 4
Hyperfractionation, 417

Image contrast, 47, 48
Image intensification, 75, 196–198
Image-intensification fluoroscopy, 215
Image matrix, 227
Image orientation, 386
Image quality, 386–387
Image reconstruction, 202
Images, quality assurance for, 387–388
Image transmission, standards for, 242
Imaging, computer networks for, 238.
        See also Diagnostic imaging
Imaging devices, interfaces of, 239
Imaging techniques, 188–189
Immediate effects, 336
Immobilization devices, 255–258
Immobilization techniques, 281
Implants. See also Implant therapy entries
    design of, 300–301
    interstitial, 302–313
    radiographic localization of, 318–322
    sources used for, 399
    three-dimensional image-based, 322–327
Implant therapy, techniques for, 286
Implant therapy sources, 286–294
    brachytherapy sources, 289, 292–293
    implantable neutron sources, 292
    ophthalmic irradiators, 292
    radium sources, 286–288
    radium substitutes, 290–292
In-air calibrations, 116
Incident photon, Compton scattering of, 43
Indian club needles, 287
Indirectly traceable instruments, 109
Inelastic interactions, 22, 34
Infinite thickness, 143
Inflection point, 190
Inherent filtration, 30
Inhomogeneities. See Tissue inhomogeneities
Inhomogeneity effects, measurements of, 175–176
In-phantom calibrations, 116–117
Input/output (I/O) devices, 230, 232, 242
Instruments, directly and indirectly
        traceable, 109, 114. See also Equipment

Integral dose, 180–181, 247
Integrated circuits (ICs), 221
Integrated ionization chamber, 89
Intensifying screens, 191–193, 214
Intensity-modulated arc therapy (IMAT), 277–278
Intensity-modulated radiation therapy (IMRT), 68, 270–276, 281
    phantoms for, 387
    quality assurance for, 394–397, 409
Intensity-modulated treatment, 142
Interactions, cross section for, 24
Interface effects, 280
Interlocks, testing, 366–367
Internal conversion, 14–15
Internal (image-based) localization, 257–258
International Atomic Energy Agency (IAEA)
        calibration protocol, 126–127
International Commission on Radiation
        Units and Measures (ICRU), 182–183, 246
International Commission on Radiological
        Protection (ICRP), 337–338, 340
International Electrotechnical Commission
        (IEC), 150, 164
Interpreter, 235
Interstitial brachytherapy systems, 306
Interstitial implants, 286, 330. See also
        Implants
    gynecologic, 327
    uncrossed, 310
Intracavitary applicators, 300–301, 302
Intracavitary implants, 286
Intracavitary x-ray tubes, 52
Intraluminal implants, 286
Intraoperative therapy, 52
Intraophthalmic irradiator, 16
Intravascular brachytherapy, 328–329, 330
Intrinsic filtration, 30
Inverse planning, 270
Inverse-square relationship, 134
Iodine (I), 291
Ion chambers, benefits of, 92
Ionization chamber readings, 106
Ionization chambers, 85–86, 353
    absorbed dose measurements with, 99–100
    air mass inside, 108
    calibration of, 361–362
    determining characteristics of, 118
    in a medium, 118
    photon–electron interactions in, 118
    for reference dosimetry, 115
Ionization clusters, 110
Ionization measurements, 115–116. See also
        Ionizing radiation measurement
    dose to water, 118–120
Ionization ratio (IR), 123
Ionization recombination correction, 115, 116, 121
Ionized atom, 22
Ionizing radiation, xiii, 80

Ionizing radiation measurement, 79–106
    absorbed dose measurements, 99–100
    dose equivalent, 100–102
    radiation dose, 92–98
    radiation exposure, 82–92
    radiation intensity, 80–82
    radiation quality, 102–105
Ion pairs (IPs), 22, 23, 82. See also IP
        entries
Ion pairs per centimeter (IP/cm), 23
IP collection, efficiency of, 90
IP recombination, 86
Iridium (Ir), 291
Irradiated volume, 183
Irradiation, effects of, 180
Irregular beam surface, 168–171
Irregular fields
    Clarkson method for, 136–137
    dose calculations for, 166–168
Isobars, 2–3
Isocenter, 139, 140
Isocenter dose rate, 161
Isocentric beam arrangements, 163
Isocentric conditions, treatment under, 161–162
Isocentric positioning, 163
Isocentric radiation therapy, 140, 141
Isocentric techniques, 159
Isocentric treatment time, 145
Isocentric treatment units, 56, 57
Isodose charts, 170, 171
Isodose curves, 145–153, 154
    comparison of, 150–151
    electron depth dose and, 151–152
Isodose data, obtaining, 152–153
Isodose distributions, 147, 213
    for adjoining fields, 181
    corrections to, 168
    for fields at angles other than 180°, 164–166
    from individual sealed sources, 300
    for isocentric beam arrangements, 163
    for multiple fields, 162–166
    tissue inhomogeneities and, 173
Isodose plotter, 152
Isoenergy curves, 148
Isomeric transition, 12, 13, 14, 15, 17–18, 19
Isomers, 3
Isotones, 2
Isotopes, 2, 4
    produced by neutron bombardment, 17–18
Isotope teletherapy units, 54–57

Jennings, William, 26
Joliot, Frederic, 13, 18
Jukeboxes, 233

K-absorption edge, 191
K_α x rays, 6
K_β x rays, 6

K-capture, 14
K-shell electrons, 41
K-shell fluorescence yields, 7
Kell factor, 199
Kerma (kinetic energy released in matter), 92, 93, 106. *See also* Air-kerma strength
Kerma curve, 94
Kerst, D., 70
Kilocurie, 9
Kinetic energy, 3, 6–7
  in electron–electron interactions, 22
Kinetic energy equation, 58
Klystrons, 59, 64–65
kVp accuracy, 383
Laboratories, calibration, 108–114
L_α x rays, 6
Lamerton, L., 135
Larmor frequency, 212
Laser quality assurance, 385
Latent image, 189
"Lateral disequilibrium," 178, 280
Lauritsen, Charles, 53
Lawrence, Ernest O., 18, 70, 59
L_β x rays, 6
L-block, 352
L-capture, 14
LDR gynecologic interstitial implant, 327
Lead sheets, 192
Leaf transmission, 374
Leak testing, 352
Leakage radiation, 67, 347–349, 351
$Li_2B_4O_7$, 97–98
LiF, 97, 98
Lifetime risk estimation, 335–336
Light field, versus radiation field, 370, 374
Light field indicators, testing, 368
Light localizer, 53, 55
Linear accelerators (linacs), xiii, 53, 54, 57–69, 142, 398–399, 415. *See also* Electron linac
  calibrating, 126
  electric field orientation in, 59
  historical development of, 58–61
  low- and high-energy, 66
  x-ray targets of, 134
Linear accelerator waveguide, side-coupled standing-wave, 60
Linear attenuation, 37, 50
Linear density calculation, 309
Linear energy transfer (LET), 23, 34, 101
Linear hypothesis of radiation injury, 335
Linear radium sources, dose delivery by, 298–299
Linear stopping power, 23
Line focus principle, 33, 34
Line numbers, 235
"Liquid drop" model, 7
Livingston, M., 70
Load, 65
Local area networks (LANs), 195
Localization devices, 255–258
Localization (port) film, 47

Localization techniques, 281
Localizing laser alignment, testing, 370
Local standard, 361
Longitudinal relaxation time, 212, 214
Loop, 235
Los Alamos Meson Production Facility (LAMPF), 431–432
Low-dose-rate (LDR) brachytherapy, 317, 330. *See also* LDR gynecologic interstitial implant
Low-energy accelerators, 421–422
Low-energy electron beams, calibration of, 122
Low-energy photon, Compton interaction and, 45
Low-energy x-ray beams, calibration of, 114–117
Low-energy x rays, 42
Low-energy x-ray units, 52–54, 76
Low-level computer languages, 234–235
Low-N/Z nuclei, 14
Low-Z nuclides, Auger electrons in, 7
Lung tissue, 174, 175

Machine characteristics, IMRT, 395–396
Machine language (object code), 234–235
Machlett Dynamax x-ray tube, 27
Magnetic disks, 232–233
Magnetic field intensity, 65, 66
Magnetic moments, 211–212
Magnetic quantum number, 5
Magnetic resonance imaging (MRI), 211–213, 215, 251. *See also* Functional magnetic resonance imaging (fMRI)
Magnetic tape devices, 233
Magnetron microwave power tubes, 59, 62–64
Magnification correction, 319
Mainframe computers, 221
mA linearity, 383
Mammography, 32, 205
Manchester system, 305–311
Mantle field treatment, 167
Manual-method treatment planning, 158–185
  dose calculations for irregular fields, 166–168
  dose specification for external beam therapy, 181–184
  integral dose, 180–181
  multiple-field isodose distributions, 162–166
  oblique incidence and irregular beam surface, 168–171
  point dose calculations, 158–160
  separation of adjacent fields, 179–180
  tissue inhomogeneities, 172–179
  treatment at standard SSD, 160–161
  treatment under isocentric conditions, 161–162
mAs linearity, 384
Mass attenuation, 50

Mass attenuation coefficients, 37, 41, 42
  for pair production, 48
Mass data storage, 242
Mass defect, 3–4
Mass energy absorption, 50
Mass energy-absorption coefficients, 83, 111, 112–113, 117
Mass–energy equivalence formula, 4
Mass number, 2
Mass of components, 3
Mass stopping power, 23, 25, 99
Mass storage devices, 232–234
Material, tissue-equivalence of, 130
MATHCAD (Mathematics Computer-Aided Design), 235
Matrix systems, 240–241
Matrix techniques, 258–259
Matter, composition of, 2–8
Maximum contiguous dose rate, 316
Maximum cumulative dose, 338
Maximum dose, 184
Maximum energy, 12–13, 50
Maximum permissible dose (MPD), 337
Maximum photon energy, 32
Maximum significant dose rate, 316
Maximum voltage, 30
Mayneord, W. V., 54, 130, 135
Maze entrances, 349, 350, 351
Mean dose equivalent, 102
Mean life, 10
Mean path length (mean free path), 38
Measured data, inaccuracies in, 392–393
Measurement quality assurance (MQA), 108. *See also* Quality assurance (QA)
Mechanical alignment
  in megavoltage equipment, 367–370
  tests of, 380
Mechanical checks, monthly, 366
Median target dose, 184
Medical accelerators, 69–73
  major components of, 61–69
Medical electron linacs, 60, 68
Medical radiology, 188. *See also* Diagnostic imaging
Medium
  energy-absorption characteristics of, 111
  linear stopping power of, 23
  mass stopping power of, 99
Medium-dose-rate (MDR) brachytherapy, 317
Megabecquerel (Mbq), 9
Megacurie, 9
Mega ohms, 59
Megavoltage beams, calibration of, 117–126
Megavoltage CT (MVCT), 278, 279
Megavoltage radiation therapy, 76
Megavoltage treatment equipment, 132, 159, 364–380
Megavoltage x rays, flattening filters for, 147
Megavoltage x-ray machines, 53–54
Memorial system source strength recommendations, 324

Mendeleyev, Dmitri, 259
Metal-oxide-semiconductor (MOS) capacitors, 195
Metastable energy state, 14
Meter setting, 68, 159–160, 161
MFLOPS (million floating-point operations), 225, 232
Microchips, 221
Microcurie, 9
Microprocessors, 221
Microtrons, 72–73
Microwave cavity, invention of, 59
Microwave equipment, 64
Microwave frequency bands, 59
Microwave power, 59
Microwave power-handling equipment, 65–66
Microwave wavelength, 63
Millicurie, 9
Minicomputers, 221
Minification gain, 197, 198
Minimum dose, 184
Minimum wavelength photons, 32
MiniPACS (picture archiving and communications systems), 195
MLC conversion, 275
Modal dose, 184
Modem, 231, 232
Modified peripheral loading, 323
Modulation transfer function (MTF), 388
Modulator, linear accelerator, 61–62
Molecular imaging, 418–419
Molybdenum target, 32
^{99}Mo–^{99m}Tc generator, 16
Monitor chamber linearity, calibration of, 377
Monitor end effect, 377
Monitor ionization chamber, 68, 69
Monitor units, 68, 138, 246
Monoenergetic beam, HVL of, 132
Monoenergetic photons, 83
Monoenergetic x rays, 38
Monte Carlo analysis, 247, 263, 299
Moore's Law, 221
Moseley, H. G. J., 6
Multi-energy linacs, 65
Multi-leaf collimator, 372–375
Multi-MV linear accelerator, 59
Multi-MV x rays, 93
Multimodality accelerators, 65
Multiple fields, isodose distributions for, 162–166
Multiple image slices, 210
Multitasking, 232
Multitransducer arrays, 205
Multivaned collimators, 56
Muscle, dose rate in, 123
Mutagenesis, 336

Nanocurie, 9
Nanometer (nm), 3
Narrow-beam geometry, 36, 104
Nasopharyngeal applicators, 287

National Council on Radiation Protection and Measurements (NCRP), 337–338, 340, 341, 352
National Institute of Standards and Technology (NIST), 95, 108, 361
Natural radioactivity, 17
Negative beta particles (negatrons), 12, 19, 23
Negative electrode, 28
Negative ions, 2
Negligible individual dose (NID), 339
Negligible individual level (NIL), 339
Neptunium series, 17
Networking, 238–241
Networks, 239, 242
Neutrino, 12
Neutron beam therapy, 428–430
Neutron bombardment, 17–18
Neutron brachytherapy, 426–427
Neutron capture therapy, 427–428
Neutron detectors, 353
Neutron number, 2, 7
Neutron/proton (N/Z) ratio, 7
Neutrons, 2
Neutron shielding, 351–352, 354
Neutron sources, implantable, 292
(n, γ) reaction, 18
"Noisy" image, 190
Nonstochastic (deterministic) radiation effects, 336–337, 354
Normalized collimator scatter factors, 160, 167
Normalized peak scatter factor (NPSF), 143–144, 160
Normalized phantom scatter factors, 160
Normal tissue complication probability (NTCP), 267, 281, 417
Nuclear chain reaction, first man-made, 12
Nuclear diagnostic studies, 206
Nuclear fission, 4, 7, 18
Nuclear force, 4
Nuclear fusion, 4
Nuclear imaging, γ-ray energies for, 208
Nuclear medicine, 16, 206–209, 215
Nuclear medicine imaging, 207–209
Nuclear transmutation, 18
Nucleons, 2, 4
Nucleus (nuclei), 2, 7
    electron scattering by, 23–25
    stability of, 7–8
Nuclides, 3
    decay constants of, 8
    fission-produced, 18
    low-Z, 7
Number systems, 221–223, 242
Numeric data, 225
Nutation, 213
N/Z ratio, beta decay and, 12

Objective functions, 274
    dose-based or dose-volume-based, 272–273

Oblique incidence, 168–171
Occupancy factors, 343, 344
Oldendorf, William, 200
Operating system, 234
Ophthalmic irradiators, 292, 316
Opposing fields
    arrangements of, 164
    isodose distributions for, 162–163
Optical density (OD), 189, 190, 191
Optical disks, 234
Optical distance indicator, testing, 370
Organs at risk (OAR), 183, 246, 265, 272
Orthovoltage therapy units, 53
Orthovoltage x rays, 30, 152
Orthovoltage x-ray units, 54
Output monitoring system, calibration of, 375–377
Oxalic acid dosimeters, 96
Oxidation reactions, 96
Oxygen enhancement ratio (OER), 428

Packet switching, 238
Pair annihilation, 23
Pair production, 40, 47–48, 50
Palladium (Pd), 291
Parallel multihole collimator, 207–208
Parallel–opposed field, 162
Parallel-plate chambers, 121, 122, 124
Parallel-plate ionization chambers, 92, 106, 126
Parallel-processing, 232
Paramagnetism, 213
Parent atoms, number of, 9
Paris system, 311–313
Par-speed screens, 191
Particle accelerators, 18, 58
Particle bombardment, nuclear transmutation by, 18
Particle mass, 72
Particles, in a cyclotron, 71
Particle velocity, 60
Pascal's calculating device, 220
Passive scattering technique, 424–425
Past-pointed axes, 164
"Paterson–Parker" system, 305, 306
Patient contours, 248–249
Patient data entry, 248–251
Patient monitoring equipment, 367, 382
Patients, screening, 213
Patient-simulating phantom, 130
Patient-specific dose verification, IMRT, 396–397
Pauli, Wolfgang, 12
Pauli Exclusion Principle, 5
Peak scatter factor (PSF), 136, 143
Pencil beam method, 265
Penumbra correction models, 260–261
Penumbra trimmer, 55
Percent backscatter factor (%BSF), 133
Percent depth dose, 130–135, 154, 158, 171
    computing tissue/air ratio from, 140–141
    measurement of, 122–123, 378, 379

SSD and, 136
survey of, 135
tables of, 135–139
Peripheral loading, 323
Personnel
monitoring of, 353–354
quality assurance and, 360
Perturbation correction, 100, 127
PET/CT unit, 251
PET radionuclides, 210, 211
(p, γ) reaction, 18
Phantoms, 113–114, 118, 130
Phantom scatter factor, 160, 161
Pharmaceuticals, as imaging agents, 207
Phase velocity, 59
Philosophy of risk, 334
Photodisintegration, 40, 48
Photoelectric absorption, 40
Photoelectric interactions, 41–42
Photoelectric mass attenuation coefficient, 41
Photoelectrons, 41, 42
ionization produced by, 87
Photographic dosimetry, 95–96
Photographic films, 153
Photoluminescent dosimeters, 98
Photomultiplier tubes (pmts), 208
Photon beam characterization, 377–379
Photon beam computational algorithms,
258–265
Photon beam dose calculations, 392
Photon beams, 122
calibration of, 117–118, 123–124
tissue inhomogeneities and, 172, 173–178
Photon–electron conversion factor, 124, 125
Photon fluence, 80, 81
per unit exposure, 82–84
Photon flux (photon flux density), 80, 81, 85
Photon intensity, 93
Photon mass attenuation coefficients,
112–113
Photons, 36
bremsstrahlung, 24, 30, 32
Phototimer, 384
Physical half-life, 9–10
Physics instrumentation, 361–363, 409
Picocurie, 9
Piezoelectricity, 204
Pion therapy, 431–432
Plan evaluation, 417–418
Planning risk volume, 183
Planning target volume (PTV), 182
Plaques, 286, 316–317
Plastic phantoms, 114
Pneumoencephalography, 200
(p, n) reaction, 18
Point dose calculations, 158–160
"Point source" calculations, 296
Polar coordinates, 148
Polarity effect, 90–91
Polyenergetic beam, 38, 39
Polystyrene wedge, 182
"Poor" geometry, 36, 104–105

Population dose, 336
Portal imaging, 388
Port films, 47, 73, 192–193, 214, 370
Positive electrode, 28
Positive ions, 2
Positron decay, 13, 19
Positron emission tomographic unit, 72
Positron emission tomography (PET), 23,
200, 210–211, 215, 251. See also PET
entries
Positron emitters, 70
radioactive nuclides as, 13, 72
Positronium, 23
Positrons, backscattering of, 23
Positron transition, 13
Potter, Hollis, 194
Power deposition, 31
Power law tissue/air ratio method, 177–178,
262
Power splitter, 65
P_{pol}, 121
Precession, 212
Prescribed dose, 159
Pressure, standard, 23
Pressure–temperature correction factor, 91
Primary electrons, 118, 120
Primary ion pairs, 22, 82
Primary off-axis factor, 167, 260, 262
Primary radiation, 36, 133, 343–346
Primary Standard Dosimetry Laboratory
(PSDL), 108, 109, 126
Principal quantum number, 5
Programmable read-only memory chips
(PROMs), 231
Programming languages, 234–237
Prostate HDR, 325–327
Prostate seed implants, 322–325
Protection survey, 380–381
Protons, 2
Proton therapy, 420–426
Proton therapy centers, 421
(p, 2n) reaction, 18
Pulsed beams, 115
Pulsed-dose-rate (PDR) brachytherapy, 318,
400, 416
Pulse–echo sound, 204
Pulse-forming network, 61–62
Pulse-height analyzer, 208
Pulse-height distribution, 103
Pulse sequences, 213
Purcell, Edward, 211

Q (quality factor), 63, 101
Quality assurance (QA), 357–409. See also
Quality assurance procedures
brachytherapy, 399–408
components of, 359–360
CT simulator, 385–387
image, 387–388
IMRT, 394–397
megavoltage treatment equipment,
364–380

personnel, 360
physics instrumentation, 361–363
procedures, 360–361
radiation therapy simulators, 380–384
source-change, 400–401
treatment planning computer, 389–394
Quality assurance form, 403
Quality assurance procedures, 361–363
daily, 401–403
monthly, 403–407
Quality assurance program, 158
checks to include in, 406–407
Quality assurance tests, 360, 361
Quality control (QC), 358, 361
Quality conversion factor, 121, 122, 124
Quality of radiation, 102–105
Quantum computers, 225
Quantum numbers of an electron, 5
Quimby, Edith H., 130, 304
Quimby System, 303–305, 310–311

R_{50}, 123
Rabi, Isador, 211
Rad (radiation absorbed dose), 82
Radial dose function, 314, 315
Radiation barriers, 343–349
Radiation beam, cross-sectional area of, 140
Radiation detriment, 334
Radiation dose, 92–98
Radiation dosimeter, 94–95
Radiation energy/depth, influence of, 141
Radiation exposure, 7, 82–84, 105. See also
Radiation protection
control of, 340–341
limits on, 338–341
measurement of, 84–92
Radiation field dosimetry, 130–154
percent depth dose and, 130–135
Radiation fields, 73
sizes/shapes of, 131–133
Radiation hormesis, 335
Radiation intensity, 80–82
Radiation length, 67, 68
Radiation oncology, 188, 416
Radiation protection, 334–354
effects of radiation exposure, 336–337
exposure limits for, 338–341
history of standards related to, 337–338
personnel monitoring, 353–354
protective barriers, 341–352
sealed radioactive sources, 352
three options for, 341
Radiation protection surveys, 352–353,
365–366. See also Radiation safety
surveys
Radiation quality, 102–105, 106, 131
Radiation quantity, 80, 81–82, 105
Radiations, biologic effectiveness of various,
102
Radiation safety, IMRT, 394
Radiation safety surveys, 400. See also
Radiation protection surveys

Radiation sources, protective barriers for, 341–352
Radiation standards, 354
Radiation therapists, 188, 360
Radiation therapy, 10, 25, 42, 52
  advances in, 414–432
  computers and, 415
  delivery of, 73
  energy delivery during, 93–94
  evolving techniques in, xiii
  "four R's" of, 416–417
  fundamental rule of, 247
  history of, 414–416
  objective of, 414
  pair production and, 48
  stationary targets in, 32
  tissue damage and, 180
  use of energy absorption coefficient in, 39
  Van de Graaff generators in, 70
Radiation therapy calibrations, 119
Radiation therapy installation, use factors for, 343
Radiation Therapy Oncology Group (RTOG), 326, 327
Radiation therapy simulators, 73, 74
  quality assurance procedures for, 380–384
Radiation therapy unit, miscalibration of, 91
Radiation type, relative biological effectiveness of, 100
Radiation units, 52–76
  low-energy, 52–54
Radiation weighting factor, 102, 338, 339
Radiative energy loss, 25
Radioactive atoms, mean life of, 10
Radioactive decay, 7, 8–11, 19. See also Decay entries
  types of, 11–15
Radioactive equilibrium, 15–16
Radioactive implants, 286
Radioactive isotope, decay constant of, 10
Radioactive nuclei, emission of positrons from, 13
Radioactive nuclides, 72, 288. See also Radionuclides
Radioactive samples, 8
  physical half-life of, 9–10
Radioactive tracers, 18, 206, 207
Radioactivity, 7
  natural, 17
Radiofrequency (rf) range, 212. See also RF power-handling equipment
Radiographic grids, 193–194, 215
Radiographs, 75, 192–193
  diagnostic-quality, 73
  early versus modern, 189
Radiography, 189–196
  digital, 194–195
Radionuclide generator, 206
Radionuclides, 12, 17–18, 206. See also Radioactive nuclides
  dose rate constants for, 342
  PET-suitable, 210, 211

Radiopharmaceuticals, 206–207
  therapy with, 327
"Radium bombs," 54
Radium molds, 286
Radium needles, 287, 290, 307
Radium sources, 286–288, 352
Radium substitutes, 290–292
Randall, J. T., 62
Random access memory (RAM), 230, 232
Rare-earth intensifying screens, 191
Ratio of tissue/air ratios (TARs) method, 171, 176–177, 262
Raw lobe, 68
Rayleigh scattering, 41
Ray-line isodose curves, 149, 150
Read-only memory (ROM), 231
Receptor-specific radiopharmaceuticals, 207
Recoil electron, maximum energy transferred to, 45
"Recoil" nucleus, 23
Recombination errors, 86
Reconstruction algorithms, 202–203
Rectangular waveguides, 65
Rectification, 28
"Rectilinear pencil-beam scanning," 203
Reduction reactions, 96
Reference air-kerma rate (RAKR), 289
Reference depth, 124
Reference dose, 130
Reference dose rate, 312–313
Reflection target, 68
Region of dose buildup, 131
Reines, Frederick, 13
Relative biological effectiveness (RBE), 100–101, 425, 429
Relative dose measuring equipment, 363
Relative electron density, 177
Relativistic increase in mass with velocity, 72
Relaxation length, 38
Rem (roentgen equivalent man), 82
Remote afterloading, 317–318, 330, 416
Remote afterloading equipment, 399–400
Resonance frequency, 212
Resonant transformers, 53
Respiratory gating, 256, 257
Restenosis, 328–329
Restricted stopping powers, 120
Retardation, radiation-induced, 340
Retraction plane, 323
Reverse electron flow, 28
RF power-handling equipment, 65
"Rhumbatron," 63
Richards, Powell, 16
Risk, philosophy of, 334
^{222}Rn, 15, 16
Roentgen (R), 82, 110
Röntgen, Wilhelm, 25–26
Root mean square (RMS) error, 359
Rossi–Griesan equation, 67
Rotational frequency, 212
Rotational (arc) therapy, 56, 142–143

Rutherford (Rf), 8
Rutherford, Ernest, 11, 12, 14, 18, 85, 97

Safety interlocks, 381
Safety procedures
  in brachytherapy, 400
  for megavoltage treatment equipment, 365–367
  for radiation therapy simulators, 380–382
Sample of atoms, 8
  specific activity of, 9
Satellite collimators, 55, 56
Saturation voltage, 86
S-band, 63
Scanning slit radiography, 195
Scatter/air ratio (SAR), 144, 154, 167, 168
Scattered photons, 46
  limitation of, 193–194
Scattered radiation, 132–133
  secondary barriers for, 346–347
Scattering, 36
Scattering foil, 67–68
Scatter integration technique, 259–262
Scatter-maximum ratios (SMR), 144, 146
Scatter/phantom ratio (SPR), 144
Scintillation cameras, 206, 208, 209, 210
Scintillation detector, 97
Screen-film radiograph, 191
Secondary barriers, 346–349
Secondary electrons, 85, 118
Secondary ion pairs, 23, 82
Secondary radiation, 36
Secondary standard dosimetry laboratories (SSDLs), 108
Second-generation scanner, 201, 202
Second-order motion, 212
Secular equilibrium, 16, 19
Segmentation, 73
Segrè, E., 207
Self-rectification, 28
Semicircular electrodes (dees), 71
Semiconductor dosimetry, 97
Semiempirical methods, 259–263
Semilogarithmic plots, 10, 38, 39
Sensitivity centers, 189
Sensitivity of a chamber, 89
Sensitometric curves, 95, 190
Serial tomotherapy, 278, 281
"Shell model" of the nucleus, 7
Shielding barriers, 354
Shields, bladder and rectal, 303
Shifting depth ionization data, 122
Shunt impedance, 59, 60
Side-coupled linear accelerator, 76, 415
Side-coupled standing-wave accelerator, 60, 61, 76
Sievert, 82
Sievert, Rolf, 82, 299
Sievert integral, 297–299, 330
Signal amplification strategies, 419
Simple backprojection, 202
Simulated annealing method, 274

Simulators, 73–76. *See also* Treatment simulators
Single-modality accelerators, 65
Single-photon emission computed tomography (SPECT), 200, 210, 215
Skin lesions, treatment of, 52
Skin-sparing advantage, 94, 131, 132
"Skin standard dose," 131
Slice thickness, 201
"Slice therapy," 278
"Sliding window" treatment delivery approach, 277
Sloan, David, 59
Soft tissue, photon interaction in, 47
Software, 202, 230, 234
"Soft" x-ray beam, 39
Solid-state dosimeters, 98
Sorenson, R. W., 53
Sound Navigation and Ranging (SONAR), 204
Source–axis distance (SAD), 123, 140, 141
Source calibration, 400–401
Source capsule, 54
Source-change quality assurance, 400–401
Source exposure mechanism, 54–55
Source-to-calibration distance (SCD), 167
Source-to-collimator distance (SCD), 55–56
Source-to-skin distance (SSD), 55–56, 123, 140, 141, 143, 158, 159, 167, 170. *See also* Standard SSD
    effect of, 133–134
Space-charge-limited mode, 27, 34
Spatial resolution, 384
Specific activity of a sample, 9
Specific gamma-ray constant, 287
Specific ionization (SI), 23
SPECT imaging, 360°, 210
Spectral distributions, 103–105
Spencer–Attix formulation, 118
Spin density, 212
Spin–lattice relaxation time, 212, 214
Spin quantum number, 5
Spin–spin relaxation time, 212, 214
Spiral CT scanners, 201
"Split-field" test, 372
"Spoke film," 371
Sputtering, 66
Sputter-ion (Vac-Ion) pumps, 66
^{90}Sr, 16
Stability curve, 7
Standard SSD, treatment at, 160–161
Standard temperature and pressure (STP), 23, 82
Standing wave, 60
Stationary x-ray targets, 32
Station pressure, 91
Statistical decision theory, 267
Stem correction factor, 90, 91
Stem effect, 362
Stereoshift radiographs, 321
Stereotactic radiosurgery/radiotherapy, 397–399

Sterling's rule, 137, 138
Stern, Otto, 211
Stern–Gerlach experiment, 251
Stochastic (probabilistic) radiation effects, 336, 354
Stopping power ratios, 99, 126
Storage phosphor technology, 195
Structural shielding, 343
Subroutines, 234
Superficial therapy units, 52–53
Superlinearity theory of radiation damage, 335
Supervoltage therapy units, 53, 54, 70
Surface irregularities, 172
Surface lesions, treatment of, 52
Survey meters, 363
Switching tube, 62
Synchrocyclotron, 71
Synchrotron, 422
System calibration coefficient, 109
System calibration factor, 109, 111
Systeme International (SI) units, 82

Tantalum (Ta), 291
Targets, 30, 31, 67
Target thickness, 67
Target-to-axis distance (TAD), 380
Target-to-film distance (TFD), 380, 384
Target volumes, 270–272
TE_{10} mode, 65
Technetium (Tc), 207. *See also* ^{99}Mo–^{99m}Tc generator
Teleradiology links, 195
Teleradium units, 54
Teletherapy cobalt source, 56
Teletherapy units, 54–57
Television images, 198, 199
Temperature, standard, 23
10-MeV photons, 48
Tenth-value layers (TVLs), 103, 345, 346
Teratogenesis, 336
TG-21 protocol, 123, 127
TG-51 protocol, 126
Therapeutic radiology, 188
Therapeutic x-ray beam, 32, 40–41
Thermionic emission, 28
Thermistor, 95
Thermoluminescence dosimetry, 97–98
Thermoluminescent dosimeters (TLDs), 98, 354
Thermoluminescent dosimetry systems, 361
Thimble ionization chambers, 87–88, 119
Thin-wall thimble chamber, 88
Third-generation scanner, 201, 202
Thoreaus (unit), 30
Thoreaus, R., 30
Thorium series, 17
3-bit digitizer, 227
Three-dimensional image-based implants, 322–327
Three-dimensional integration methods, 263–265

Three-dimensional proton conformal therapy, 423, 425
Three-dimensional treatment planning, 247, 280, 330
Three-phase circuitry, 29
Three-phase generator, 75
Three-phase power, 29
Threshold energy, 47, 48
Threshold model of radiation injury, 334–335
Thyratron, 62
Timers, accuracy and linearity of, 383–384
Tissue/air ratio (TAR), 139–141, 154, 158, 167
Tissue-compensating filters, 169–170
Tissue depth, 134, 141
Tissue dose calorimeter, 95
Tissue equivalence, 130
Tissue-equivalent dosimeter, 95
Tissue-equivalent phantoms, 113–114, 130
Tissue inhomogeneities, 172–173
    correction for the presence of, 173–179
Tissue/maximum ratio (TMR), 144, 145–146, 154, 158, 161
Tissue penetration depth, 151
Tissue/phantom ratio (TPR), 144–145, 154
Tissues, distinguishing, 47
Toe, 189, 190
Tolerance doses, 246, 334, 337
Tomotherapy, 278–279
Tongue and groove effect, 374
Total attenuation coefficient, 50
Total biological detriment, 340
Total body irradiation (TBI), 134
Total capacitance, 89
Total mass energy absorption coefficient, 84
Total wall thickness, 115
Transducer, 204, 205
Transient equilibrium, 15–16, 19
Transistors, 221, 242
Transit dosimetry, 176
Transition energy, 11, 12, 13
Translate–rotate scanning geometry, 201, 202
Transmission media, 239–240, 242
Transmission rates, 228–229
Transmission targets, 31–32, 67
Transverse electric (TE) mode, 65
Transverse magnetic (TM) mode, 65
Transverse relaxation time, 212, 214
Transverse-section SPECT units, 210
Traveling-wave design, 60
Traveling-wave linacs, 59
Treated volume, 183
Treatment. *See also* Brachytherapy; Deliverable treatment; Isocentric entries under isocentric conditions, 161–162
    at standard SSD, 160–161
Treatment accessories, transmission factor of, 378–379
Treatment couches, 69, 369. *See also* Couch
Treatment distance, 134
Treatment fields, 161, 192, 280

Treatment planning, 188, 246–247. *See also* Brachytherapy treatment planning; Computer-based treatment planning; Manual-method treatment planning; Three-dimensional treatment planning; Treatment plans
  computed tomography and, 201
  IMRT, 395
  techniques of, 270–272
Treatment planning computer, 168, 180, 389–394
Treatment planning systems, 241
Treatment plans, analysis of, 417–418
Treatment practices, comparisons among, 181–182
Treatment simulators, 199–200, 215
Treatment time, determining, 137–139, 141
Treatment time calculations, 154, 158
Treatment unit calibration, 159–160
Treatment volumes, 182–183
Triple-field image intensifier, 197
Triple focus, 66, 67
Triplet production, 48
TRIUMF accelerator, 432
TRS-398 protocol, 126, 127
"True focal spot," 33
Tumor control probability (TCP), 267, 268, 281, 417–418
Tumor dose, increasing, 163
Tungsten (W), 6, 191
Tungsten filaments, 27
Tungsten target, 27, 31
Tungsten-target diagnostic x-ray tube, emission spectra for, 30
Turing, Alan, 221
Two-dee cyclotron, 71
"Two's complement notation," 225

Ultrasonography, 203–206, 215. *See also* Ultrasound imaging
Ultrasound imaging, 257–258
Ultrasound reflection coefficient, 204
Underlying tissue depth, effect of, 134
Unequal field weighting, 163
Uniform Distribution of Activity Test, 293
Uniform linear-density needles, 287
Universal wedge, 150
Unstable nuclei, 7
Uranium series, 17
Use factors, 343
Uterine cancer, 300–301

Vacuum pumps, 66
Van de Graaff generators, 53, 69–70
"Variable angle" method, 321
Varian, Russell, 64
Varian, Sigurd, 64
Victoreen condenser "R meter," 90
Villard, Paul, 14, 82
"Virtual needles," 327
Virtual simulation, 252–253, 281
Virtual simulator, transition to, 255
"Virtual source," 134
"Vitascope," 196
Voltage, x-ray tube, 28–30
Voltage pulses, 103
Voltage reduction, 90
Voltage waveforms, 29–30
Volume element of tissue (voxel), 201, 202
Volume rendering techniques, 252
von Laue, Max, 260
von Neumann, John, 231
Voxel scanning, 425

Waite, H. F., 26
Water, 39–40
  calibrated dose rate in, 123, 126
  as a phantom material, 114
  tissue-equivalence of, 130
Water-equivalent depth, 176
Water phantom, 116, 118, 123, 130
Waveguides, 65
Weak force, 4
Weber, 66
Wedge angle, 150
Wedge filter, 150, 151, 165, 166
Wedge filter angle, 164
Wedge isodose angle, 150, 164, 165
Wedge isodose curves, 149–150
Wedge transmission factor, 379
Whole-body dose equivalent, 101–102
Wideroe's accelerator, 58, 59
Wilkinson extended source model, 260
Word-processing program, 231
Words, 224
Work function (W-quantity), 23, 34, 82, 110
Workload, 343, 345
Workstation standards, 241
World Wide Web (WWW), 238

X-ray beam calibration, 108–127
X-ray beam data, 248

X-ray beam performance measurements, 383–384
X-ray beam qualities, 114
X-ray beams, 27
  exponential attenuation of, 38
  field size of, 145–147
  filtration of, 30
  "harder" and "softer," 30
  isodose distribution for, 162
  opposing, 164
  photodisintegration and, 48
  spectral distribution of, 103–105
  zones of, 148
X-ray CT, versus SPECT, 210
X-ray detectors, digital, 195–196
X-ray film, 189–191. *See also* Film
X-ray generators, high-frequency, 30
X-ray images, 26, 33
X-ray interactions, 36–50
X-ray isodose curves, measuring, 152–153
X-ray photons, energy distribution of, 103
X-ray plates, 189
X-ray production, efficiency of, 29, 30–31, 34
X rays, 21–34
  attenuation of, 36–40
  direct exposure to, 191
  history of, 25–26
  properties of, 26
X-ray spectra, 30–33, 34, 103
X-ray targets, 28, 67
X-ray therapy, superficial, 52
X-ray transmission computed tomography, 215
X-ray tubes, 58
  conventional, 26–30
  dual-filament, 28
  dual-focus, 28
  electron sources for, 27–28
  focal spots of, 28, 33
  modern diagnostic, 26, 27
  operation modes of, 27, 34
  of simulators, 75
  voltage of, 28–30
X-ray units, 26
  low-energy, 52–54
X-ray wavelengths, 32

^{90}Y, 16

Z, bremsstrahlung and, 24